Cancer and the Family

Second Edition

Cancer and the Family

Second Edition

Edited by

Lea Baider

Department of Radiotherapy and Clinical Oncology,
Sharett Institute of Oncology, Hadassah University Hospital,
Jerusalem, Israel

Cary L. Cooper

University of Manchester Institute of Science and Technology, UK

Atara Kaplan De-Nour

Hadassah University Hospital, Hadassah Medical
Organization, Israel

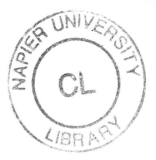

JOHN WILEY & SONS, LTD

Chichester · New York · Weinheim · Brisbane · Singapore · Toronto

Copyright © 2000 by John Wiley & Sons Ltd,
Baffins Lane, Chichester,
West Sussex PO19 1UD, England

National 01243 779777
International (+44) 1243 779777
e-mail (for orders and customer service enquiries): cs-books@wiley.co.uk
Visit our Home Page on http://www.wiley.co.uk
or http://www.wiley.com

Other Wiley Editorial Offices

John Wiley & Sons, Inc., 605 Third Avenue,
New York, NY 10158-0012, USA

WILEY-VCH Verlag GmbH, Pappelallee 3,
D-69469 Weinheim, Germany

Jacaranda Wiley Ltd, 33 Park Road, Milton,
Queensland 4064, Australia

John Wiley & Sons (Asia) Pte Ltd, 2 Clementi Loop #02-01,
Jin Xing Distripark, Singapore 129809

John Wiley & Sons (Canada) Ltd, 22 Worcester Road,
Rexdale, Ontario M9W 1L1, Canada

Library of Congress Cataloging-in-Publication Data

Cancer and the family / edited by Lea Baider, Cary Cooper, Atara Kaplan De Nour.–
2nd ed.
    p. cm.
  Includes bibliographical references and index.
  ISBN 0-471-80300-6 (alk. paper)
    1. Cancer–Social aspects. 2. Cancer–Patients–family relationships. I. Baider, Lea. II.
Cooper, Cary L. III. Kaplan De-Nour, A., 1932-
  RC262.C2695 2000
  362.1'96994–dc21
                                                                99-056524

British Library Cataloguing in Publication Data

A catalogue record for this book is available from the British Library

ISBN   0 471 80300 6

Typeset in 10/12pt Times from the authors' disks by Dobbie Typesetting Ltd, Tavistock, Devon
Printed and bound in Great Britain by Bookcraft Ltd, Midsomer Norton
This book is printed on acid-free paper responsibly manufactured from sustainable forestry,
in which at least two trees are planted for each one used for paper production.

Contents

SECTION IV   THE CHILD'S PERCEPTION OF A PARENT'S ILLNESS   199

SECTION VI   SEXUALITY: PERCEPTION OF SELF

18 Sexual self-concept for the woman with cancer
Barbara L. Andersen and Deanna M. Golden-Kreutz

19 Deciding to have children after cancer
Leslie R. Schover

SECTION VII   GENETICS: FAMILIAL RISK

20 Communication of individualized cancer risk information within the family context
Joan L. Bottorff, Pamela A. Ratner, Joy L. Johnson and Mary K. McCullum

SECTION VIII TERMINAL ILLNESS AND SYSTEMS OF BELIEF

24 The family in terminal illness

Simon Wein

25 Religion, cancer, and the family

Bernard Spilka and Scott Hartman

Contributors

Lea Baider (*Editor*) Department of Radiotherapy and Clinical Oncology, Sharett Institute of Oncology, Hadassah University Hospital, Jerusalem 91120, Israel

Cary L. Cooper (*Editor*) Manchester School of Management, University of Manchester Institute of Science and Technology, PO Box 88, Manchester M60 1QD, UK

Atara Kapan De-Nour (*Editor*) Department of Psychiatry, Hadassah University Hospital, Jerusalem 91120, Israel

Neil K. Aaronson Department of Psychosocial Research and Epidemiology, The Netherlands Cancer Institute, Plesmanlaan 121, 1066 CX Amsterdam, The Netherlands

Terrance L. Albrecht Medical Interaction Research Group, H. Lee Moffitt Cancer Center and Research Institute, Tampa, FL, USA

Barbara L. Andersen Department of Psychology, Ohio State University, 202 Townshend Hall, 1885 Neil Avenue Mall, Columbus, OH 43210–1222, USA

Kathryn H. Anderson Department of Family and Child Nursing, University of Washington School of Nursing, Seattle, WA 98195–7262, USA

Lynn C. Behar Department of Family and Child Nursing, University of Washington School of Nursing, Seattle, WA 98195–7262, USA

Christina G. Blanchard Medical Interaction Research Group, H. Lee Moffitt Cancer Center and Research Institute, Tampa, FL, USA

Eveline M. A. Bleiker Department of Psychosocial Research and Epidemiology, The Netherlands Cancer Institute, Plesmanlaan 121, 1066 CX Amsterdam, The Netherlands

Joan R. Bloom School of Public Health, University of California at Berkeley, 409 Warren Hall, Berkeley, CA 94770–7360, USA

Joan L. Bottorff School of Nursing, University of British Columbia, T201–2211 Westbrook Mall, Vancouver, BC, Canada V6T 2B5

Mary Kay Dabney Psychological Services, Beth Israel Cancer Center, 10 Union Square East—4th Floor, New York, NY 10003, USA

Emily Darby Department of Family and Child Nursing, University of Washington School of Nursing, Seattle, WA 98195–7262, USA

Maria Die-Trill Unidad de Psico-Oncologia, Departamento de Oncologia, Hospital Universitario 'Gregorio Marañón', c/Dr. Esquerdo 46, 28007 Madrid, Spain

Michael J. Dolgin Clinical and Consulting Psychology, 29 Ha'atzmaut Street, Haifa, Israel

Deanna M. Golden-Kreutz Department of Psychology, Ohio State University, 202 Townshend Hall, 1885 Neil Avenue Mall, Columbus, OH 43210–1222, USA

Carolyn Cook Gotay Prevention and Control, Cancer Research Center of Hawaii, University of Hawaii at Manoa, 1236 Lauhala Street, Honolulu, Hawaii 96813, USA

Scott Hartman Department of Psychology, University of Denver, CO 80208, USA

Josette E. H. M. Hoekstra-Weebers Department of Medical Psychology, University Hospital, PO Box 30.001, 9700 RB Groningen, The Netherlands

Jimmie C. Holland Memorial Sloan–Kettering Cancer Center, Cornell University Medical College, New York, NY, USA

Carl Christopher Hook Mayo Clinic, 200 First Street S.W., Rochester, MN, USA

Jan P. C. Jaspers Department of Medical Psychology, University Hospital, PO Box 30.001, 9700 RB Groningen, The Netherlands

Joy L. Johnson School of Nursing, University of British Columbia, T201–2211 Westbrook Mall, Vancouver, BC, Canada V6T 2B5

Marjorie Kagawa-Singer School of Public Health and Asian–American Studies, University of California at Los Angeles, PO Box 951772, Circle Drive South, Los Angeles, CA, USA

Willem A. Kamps Beatrix Children's Hospital, Division of Pediatric Oncology, University Hospital, Groningen, The Netherlands

Daniel Karus Center for the Psychosocial Study of Health and Illness, Joseph L. Mailman School of Public Health of Columbia University, 100 Haven Avenue (Suite 6A), New York, NY 10032, USA

Kathryn M. Kash Psychological Services, Beth Israel Cancer Center, 10 Union Square East—4th Floor, New York, NY 10003, USA

S. Bryant Kendrick Primary Care Residency Program, Wake Forest University School of Medicine, Winston-Salem, NC, USA

David W. Kissane Centre for Palliative Care, St. Vincent's Hospital, 104 Studley Park Road, Kew, Victoria 3101, Australia

Ed C. Klip Department of Medical Psychology, University Hospital, PO Box 30.001, 9700 RB Groningen, The Netherlands

Harold G. Koenig Center for the Study of Religion/Spirituality and Health, Duke University Medical Center, GRECC, VA Medical Center, Durham, NC 27710, USA

Nangel Lindberg Department of Psychiatry and Biobehavioral Science, School of Medicine, University of California at Los Angeles, CA 90024–1759, USA

Peter Maguire CRC Psychological Medicine Group, Stanley House, Christie Hospital NHS Trust, University of Manchester, Wilmslow Road, Manchester M20 4BX, UK

Tomoyuki Mantani Department of Psychiatry and Neurosciences, Hiroshima University School of Medicine, 1–2–3 Ksumi, Minami-Ku, Hiroshima 734, Japan

Frances Marcus Lewis Department of Family and Child Nursing, University of Washington School of Nursing, Seattle, WA 98195–7262, USA

Mary K. McCullum Hereditary Cancer Program, British Columbia Cancer Agency, Vancouver, BC, Canada

Daniel G. Miller Strang Cancer Prevention Center, New York, USA

Tu-Uven Nguyen School of Public Health and Asian–American Studies, University of California at Los Angeles, PO Box 951772, Circle Drive South, Los Angeles, CA, USA

Michael P. Osbourne Strang Cancer Prevention Center, New York, USA

Jamie Ostroff Department of Psychiatry, Memorial Sloan–Kettering Cancer Center, 1275 York Avenue, New York, NY 10021, USA

Andrea Farkas Patenaude Psycho-oncology Research in Pediatric Oncology, Dana-Farber Cancer Institute, 44 Binney Street, Boston, MA 02115, USA

Sean Phipps St. Jude Children's Research Hospital, Memphis, TN, USA

Carolyn Pitceathly CRC Psychological Medicine Group, Stanley House, Christie Hospital NHS Trust, University of Manchester, Wilmslow Road, Manchester M20 4BX, UK

Renée Proulx Intensive Ambulatory and Palliative Care Services, Montreal Children's Hospital, McGill University, 2300 Tupper Street–A201, Montreal, Quebec, Canada H3H 1P3

Pamela A. Ratner School of Nursing, University of British Columbia, T201–2211 Westbrook Mall, Vancouver, BC, Canada V6T 2B5

Victoria H. Raveis Center for the Psychosocial Study of Health and Illness, Joseph L. Mailman School of Public Health of Columbia University, 100 Haven Avenue (Suite 6A), New York, NY 10032, USA

David Reiss Department of Psychiatry and Behavioral Sciences, George Washington University Medical Center, Ross Hall, Room 612B, 2300 Eye Street N.W., Washington, DC 20037, USA

Stephanie Ross Department of Psychiatry, Memorial Sloan–Kettering Cancer Center, 1275 York Avenue, New York, NY 10021, USA

John C. Ruckdeschel Medical Interaction Research Group, H. Lee Moffitt Cancer Center and Research Institute, Tampa, FL, USA

Toshinari Saeki Department of Psychiatry and Neurosciences, Hiroshima University School of Medicine, 1–2–3 Ksumi, Minami-Ku, Hiroshima 734, Japan

Leslie R. Schover University of Texas, M.D. Anderson Cancer Center, TX, USA

Mary Ellen Shands Department of Family and Child Nursing, University of Washington School of Nursing, Seattle, WA 98195–7262, USA

Karolynn Siegel Center for the Psychosocial Study of Health and Illness, Joseph L. Mailman School of Public Health of Columbia University, 100 Haven Avenue (Suite 6A), New York, NY 10032, USA

Janet A. Sinsheimer Department of Family and Child Nursing, University of Washington School of Nursing, Seattle, WA 98195–7262, USA

Barbara M. Sourkes Intensive Ambulatory and Palliative Care Services, Montreal Children's Hospital, McGill University, 2300 Tupper Street–A201, Montreal, Quebec, Canada H3H 1P3

Bernard Spilka Department of Psychology, University of Denver, CO 80208, USA

Peter Steinglass Ackerman Institute for the Family, 146 East 78th Street, New York, NY 10021, USA

Antonella Surbone Memorial Sloan–Kettering Cancer Center, Cornell University Medical College, New York, NY, USA

Karen Weihs Department of Psychiatry and Behavioral Sciences, George Washington University Medical Center, Ross Hall, Room 612B, 2300 Eye Street N.W., Washington, DC 20037, USA

Simon Wein Department of Oncology, Shaarei Zedek Medical Center, PO Box 3235, Jerusalem, Israel

David K. Wellisch Department of Psychiatry and Biobehavioral Science, School of Medicine, University of California at Los Angeles, CA 90024–1759, USA

Yosuki Uchitomi Psycho-oncology Division, National Cancer Center Research Institute East, Kashiwa, Japan

Shigeto Yamawaki Department of Psychiatry and Neurosciences, Hiroshima University School of Medicine, 1–2–3 Ksumi, Minami-Ku, Hiroshima 734, Japan

Ellen H. Zahlis Department of Family and Child Nursing, University of Washington School of Nursing, Seattle, WA 98195–7262, USA

Foreword

I am privileged to present the Foreword to this second edition. The first one filled a much needed niche in the literature on cancer and the family. The authors of the chapters have updated their information, giving us an idea of the new research that has been done. Once again, we see the present state of our knowledge about the impact of cancer on the family brought together. As one would expect from the editors, they have paid attention to cross-cultural issues. The authors represent a range of countries and cultures which gives attention to the societal impact upon families and their beliefs about cancer.

Proper attention is also given to the impact of cancer at different stages of the life cycle. Families too are going through their own life cycle so that cancer impacts differently, depending on its developmental phase: the young couple with cancer in a child: the older couple with cancer in a spouse; the young adult who faces cancer in the context of attempts at intimacy and career; the child who faces death of a parent. Each situation involves family issues which are universal but also different. The editors have used good judgment in the choice of authors to address the range of family issues. One can be confident that this updated volume gives us an important look at the field, the literature and its interpretation.

This book attests to the fact that psychosocial oncology, or psycho-oncology, is coming of age and that the family is assuming its proper role as a basic topic in the field. *Cancer and the Family* provides a clinician or investigator, anywhere in the world, with a background from which to study a difficult case, or to access information needed to design a study. I strongly hope that the book stimulates a vigorous research effort in families coping with cancer. The need is great and the effort small at present. We are indeed indebted to the editors and to the authors for giving us a refreshing and thorough view of the family, and its members, as it is affected by cancer today around the world. The fields of psycho-oncology and oncology in general are the beneficiaries, as well as patients and their families who should experience better care.

Professor Jimmie C. Holland
Chair, Department of Psychiatry & Behavioral Sciences
Wayne E. Chapman Chair in Psychiatric Oncology
Memorial Sloan–Kettering Cancer Center
New York, USA

Introduction

Cancer remains one of the most common diseases in both men and women of all age groups, affecting one third of families in the Western world. Improved methods of prevention, detection and treatment have, however, created a seismic shift in emphasis in coping with cancer, from how to die with the disease, to how to live a full life with it. What has become clear with time is that, far from being an isolated experience for the patient, coping with cancer affects every individual within the family as well as the family system itself.

Despite widespread evidence of the profound impact of serious medical illness on family life, as well as equally compelling data concerning the role of family behavior in shaping both detection and the clinical course of medical illness, families are still often ignored or, at best, tolerated in many health-care settings.

In our years of clinical and research experience, we have learned the vital importance of the family as an intricate system of both potential distress and effective support when confronted with the reality of cancer. This is repeatedly borne out by the extensive knowledge accumulated on family communication, modes of interaction, quality of life, and in other instances, its impact on the patient and their family members—across a wide cultural and social spectrum. Some families will react to cancer as a frightening crisis best met with a conspiracy of silence; in others, families consciously make themselves extended agents of the patient and medical care system; and there are all shades in between.

Our belief that such knowledge should be shared and exchanged led to the publication of the first edition of this book in 1996. The field, however, is developing rapidly. In the four years since *Cancer and the Family* was published, thinking on the subject has broadened substantially, new applications and conceptualizations have been developed, and an extensive new understanding of the role of the family has been acquired through both research and clinical trials.

This second edition has been extensively updated for all those involved in the field of chronic illness in the family. Some chapters from the first edition have been omitted, all those that remain have been updated, and numerous new topics have been added—among them, the role played by culture and by belief systems in coping with cancer, the efficacy of specific family interventions, and the impact of genetics on the response of patients and their families to cancer.

The book is divided into nine sections, each comprising several chapters.

- The first section is mainly theoretical: it conceptualizes the behavior and dynamics of the family when one of its members is chronically ill; it highlights methodological problems in family research; and it describes, in particular, family functioning when coping with chronic disease.

- The second section focuses on cultural differences relating to the causes of cancer and its prognosis, and how such differences impact on both social support for patients and their families, and their ability to cope with the disease within different cultures and different belief systems within society.
- Psychological intervention to help patients and their families with cancer is an area that has undergone marked development since the earlier edition of our book, and it now constitutes a section in its own right. It looks at the effectiveness of different interventions in preventive care, coping and grief therapy in the process of terminal illness.
- The fourth section describes the reactions of children and adolescents to cancer in a parent, and the impact of the disease on the stability of the family as a whole. It eloquently depicts the perception of the child to the behavior of the parent, and how this boomerangs back on the sick parent.
- Section five looks at what happens to families in which it is the child who has cancer. These chapters suggest how parents can be helped to make the psychological adjustment and how they can effectively help their children in problem-solving, expression of fears and uncertainties, and the overt need for control and protection.
- Because cancer is a family affair, the sexuality of patients and their partners is explored as a basic family issue. The sixth section presents studies of sexual self-image in the woman with cancer, and examines decision-making about pregnancy after cancer, and other self-concepts of sexual identity.
- Part seven deals with another area that has developed exponentially since the book was first published: genetics and familial risk. Psychosocial and ethical aspects are both considered, including communication of individualized cancer-risk information among family members, genetic counseling for cancer, and clinical and therapeutic approaches to patients.
- Another area whose importance for patients and their families has only been recently recognized, is the belief system or religious practices embraced by the patient and his family members. Three chapters examine the role of religious or other systems of belief as a resource for patients and families coping with cancer and terminal illness—a resource that can be a tool for enhancing quality of life and well-being and an instrument of family integration.
- The final section deals with another important but insufficiently studied topic: health-care communication with the patient and within the patient's family. This section looks at why there are problems in communication, how much to tell, to whom it should be told and who should tell it. It touches on ethical concepts of paternalism versus individual autonomy, integrating the family's ethic of care with that of the patient, patient–family communications with physicians, and the medical oncologist's ethical dilemmas.

While the second edition has been updated and expanded, the nine sections into which it is divided are not, of course, comprehensive, nor is the coverage within each of them exhaustive. Limitations of space compel us to be selective, excluding highly relevant topics within family and chronic illness. Despite all that has been learned, further psycho-oncological research and clinical understanding about cancer within the family spectrum is still needed. We hope that this second edition of our book will, like the first, stimulate and encourage future professional collaboration on the central role of the family as a conceptual system in cancer.

L. Baider
A. Kaplan De-Nour

Section I
FAMILIES: THEORETICAL AND METHODOLOGICAL ISSUES

1

Family Processes and Chronic Illness*

PETER STEINGLASS
Executive Director, Ackerman Institute for the Family,
and Cornell University Medical College, New York, USA

In 1962, two American pediatricians, Meyer and Haggerty, published a paper reporting findings from a study examining the relationship between family stress and susceptibility to streptococcal infection (Meyer and Haggerty, 1962). Their at the time rather provocative findings indicated that the incidence of clinical streptococcal infections in mothers and their children could not be predicted from positive throat cultures, neither could it be predicted from such host-related variables as family history of repeated infections, personal allergy history, family size or the like. Instead, the incidence of clinical infections was most strongly associated with a very different type of 'challenge'—an episode of acute family stress, as measured by interview and diary data about the occurrence of life events that had disrupted family life. An acute family crisis was four times more likely to have occurred during the pre-illness period than the two weeks post-illness.

Although viewed with considerable skepticism because its findings seemed so counter-intuitive (the prevailing belief system of most medical researchers in 1962 was that all disease would ultimately be totally explainable at a molecular level), the family stress study, as it was called, was in retrospect actually alerting us to a new and intriguing possibility—that the quality of a person's primary social environment might be a determinant of the clinical incidence of disease. Further, it also presaged such current interests as the inter-relationships between stress, social support, and immunological competency (i.e., psycho-immunology).

Now let us move ahead 25 years and look at another study, this one was carried out by David Reiss and his colleagues at George Washington University's Center for Family Research (Reiss et al., 1986). In this particular study, one of a series of studies looking at the relationships between family factors and medical illness, the subjects were patients on chronic hemodialysis and their families. The findings,

*A version of this chapter was presented at the 4th International Congress of Psycho-oncology, Hamburg, Germany, September 3–6 1998

focusing on the association between three types of family factors—the family's problem-solving style; the strength of the family's extended family network; and the family's level of accomplishment (measured via income and educational levels)—and early death of patients, turned out to be quite startling.

I say 'startling' because: (a) these three family-level factors were able to predict early death of patients with 100% accuracy; (b) patient medical status variables had 0% predictive accuracy; and (c) in all three cases the direction of the association between the family variables and clinical course was counter-intuitive. For example, it turned out that meaningful contact of family members across three generations (the family network variable) predicted *early death*. In like fashion, the more highly coordinated the family was in its problem-solving style (usually considered a positive trait), the greater the likelihood the patient would be dead at the time the research team did their 2-year follow-up. And it was also the case that level of accomplishment was *negatively* correlated with clinical course. That is, the higher the family's level of accomplishment, the more likely the patient would have died by follow-up. And at the same time, physician ratings of the patient's disease severity proved useless as predictors of illness course (whether the patient was alive or dead 3 years after initially being recruited into the study).

Because the Reiss et al. study was of a relatively small sample of families, its dramatic findings would need to be replicated before one would consider them as having been firmly established. However, at least two tentative conclusions seemed warranted, even given the pilot nature of these findings: first, family factors are critically important in influencing the course of end-stage renal disease (ESRD); and second, prior ideas about what types of family behaviors are most adaptive in dealing with medical illness might not be applicable in severe chronic illnesses like ESRD.

If we now move to the present, one might reasonably think, given examples such as the Meyer and Haggerty study, and the Reiss et al. study cited above, that interest in family behavior as it relates to medical illness should be very high. But such is still not yet the case. Instead, it is more accurate to say that despite the growing evidence of the profound impact of serious medical illness on family, and the equally compelling evidence of the role of family behavior in shaping the clinical course of medical illness, when compared to the attention given to the person with the illness (or at least to his/her body) (Campbell, 1986; Fisher et al., 1992; Litman, 1974; Patterson and Garwick, 1994), families are often either ignored or at best tolerated in many medical settings. In the USA there are probably many reasons for this, including: the lack of training health care professionals receive in how to relate to families; the logistical difficulties in interfacing the complex schedules of medical personnel and family members; and the widely held view that families should take a back seat to patient needs at times of medical illness.

And in addition to these prejudices and training deficiencies, it is also the case that very few programs are currently available that have been specifically designed to help families wend their ways through the complexities of dealing with serious medical illness. Although many clinical and hospital settings have improved the types of educational programs and support groups they have available for families, these programs typically *exclude* patient family members and are only rarely administered by professionals with training in family systems treatment approaches.

Hence, given the subject for this book—an examination of the evidence linking family psychosocial factors and cancer diagnosis, clinical course, and treatment—it behooves us to place the cancer story in the more general context of chronic medical illness. To do so, I will take on two tasks: first, to provide a brief overview of the research and clinical literature on this subject; and second, to give some views about how one might go about designing and implementing generic psychosocial programs for chronic medical illness families.

A BRIEF OVERVIEW OF THE FAMILY AND ILLNESS CLINICAL LITERATURE

What can we glean from the literature to date addressing issues relating families and medical illness? This literature has pointed to four ways in which family factors affect the onset and course of chronic medical illnesses: (a) family pathology/dysfunction as a contributing factor in the development of chronic illness; (b) the family as a resource for the individual coping with medical illness; (c) family factors as determinants of differential clinical course of specific chronic illnesses; and (d) family characteristics as they influence relationships with health care delivery systems. I would propose that the above four areas also reflect four different *perspectives* on family factors and chronic medical illness, which we could call, respectively: the 'deficit' perspective; the 'resource' perspective; the 'clinical course' perspective; and the 'impact' perspective.

THE 'DEFICIT' PERSPECTIVE

This approach has focused on family pathology. The basic idea is that the family is a potentially negative force in medical illness situations, in that dysfunctional family behavior psychologically and physically debilitates its members, thereby increasing the risk for physical illness.

Perhaps the best known of these 'deficit' models is the 'psychosomatic family' model of Minuchin et al. (1978). It has provided the underpinnings for much of the family and illness research carried out in the 1970s and 1980s. The basic conceptual approach in all of these investigations is the same—because families in which there is a chronically ill member seem to share certain structural properties and characteristic response styles, it is hypothesized that these factors are critical in rendering an individual family member susceptible to disease.

As characterized by Minuchin and his colleagues, four family characteristics were crucial: (a) enmeshment and over-involvement of family members; (b) over-protection; (c) rigid transactional patterns aimed at maintaining the status quo; and (d) denial or avoiding of conflict. The overall result is a family that presents itself as a conflict-free unit whose only concern is the presence of a chronic illness in one of its members. Although others have suggested modifications of this model, for our purposes we can think of all this work as hypothesizing an *etiological* role for the family, both in the onset of illness and in the exacerbation of chronic episodic medical conditions like labile diabetes, auto-immune diseases, and chronic pain syndromes.

The psychosomatic family model outlined above has come under considerable criticism for three main reasons: (a) the lack of clear operational definitions of its core dimensions (e.g., enmeshment); (b) its tendency to pathologize families; and (c) its failure to appreciate how stressful chronic illness can be for families (Coyne and Anderson, 1988; Kog et al., 1985; Wood, 1993). Thus, it is probably of primary interest to us at this point because of its historical significance and its influence on the family therapy field. While it held sway, clinical efforts were directed at identifying problematic families (e.g., enmeshed or over-rigid families) and offering them family therapy. That is, the working assumption seemed to be that families who were having problems coping with medical illness were by definition dysfunctional.

Although this view is now balanced by others to be described below, efforts to identify aversive family characteristics associated with poor illness outcomes has continued apace. Current candidates, each supported by empirical research evidence, include such family environmental properties as interpersonal criticism and hostility (Fiscella et al, 1997; Gowers et al., 1995; Gustafsson et al., 1994; Hermanns et al., 1989) and such behavioral properties as recurrent family conflict, withdrawal and isolation (Wamboldt and Wamboldt, 1995). A popular current explanation for why such negative family emotional and behavioral characteristics might influence illness course is the purported relationships between affect regulation and autonomic physiological reactivity, and immunological competence (Burman and Margolin, 1992; Levenson and Gottman, 1983; Kiecolt-Glaser et al., 1994). Presumably, family emotional climate is a key factor in determining whether affect (especially negative affect) is adequately regulated or spirals into dangerous extremes.

THE FAMILY AS RESOURCE

More recently, a very different perspective has emerged in examining the relationships between families and medical illness, this time focused on the family as a potential resource for coping with chronic illness (Walsh and Anderson, 1988; Wood, 1993). In a number of respects, this second perspective is merely the opposite side of the one we have already discussed. This time, for example, it is the ability of the family to create a positive emotional climate that in turn is purported to help individual family members successfully regulate emotional, physiological, and immunological functioning (which in turn helps attenuate disease impact). But also of central importance here is the compelling evidence about the powerful role played by *social support* in influencing overall disease morbidity and mortality, as well as the course of most chronic illnesses (Uchino et al., 1996). And if one then acknowledges that the importance of the family as a resource is its role as the primary source of social support for family members coping with illness, the family then sits at the center of health issues.

Many readers may be familiar with the House et al. (1988) review of these data, published in *Science*, that concluded with the following dramatic statement:

> The evidence regarding social relations and health increasingly approximates the evidence in the 1964 Surgeon General's report that established cigarette smoking as a cause or risk factor or morbidity and mortality from a range of diseases. The age-adjusted risk ratios are stronger than the relative risks for all causes of mortality reported for cigarette smoking (p. 543).

The basic argument is that the family serves either a protective or preventive role in strengthening individual resistance to illness, and a determinant role in successful adherence to treatment regimens once illness is present. In both of these roles it is the family that to a large extent teaches and reinforces health behaviors related to diet, tobacco and alcohol use, and exercise, plus collaborates with health care professionals in shaping and adhering to medical treatment regimens.

THE CLINICAL COURSE PERSPECTIVE

This third perspective looks at how the family influences the differential course of chronic illness, and argues that because different illness characteristics and phases place different demands on the family, the manner in which the family responds to these challenges may therefore have a profound impact on the individual's adjustment to the illness.

The research and clinical work stimulated by this perspective looks at the interface between family behavior and illness characteristics, and asks questions about how family and illness variables mutually reinforce one another as the illness moves into its chronic phase (Steinglass et al., 1987; Wynne et al., 1992). Often the question being asked is what aspects of family behavior serve to *maintain* the chronicity of medical illnesses, and vice versa. I will return to this issue when I move on to talk about intervention.

Briefly, it is proposed that as an illness moves into its chronic phase, families gradually (some would also say insidiously) come to reorganize their daily lives around illness demands (Reiss et al., 1993). For example, daily routines are reorganized to accommodate illness demands (sleep–wake cycles, mealtime schedules, etc.). Space within the home is reorganized to accommodate treatment needs (wheelchair accessibility, bedroom reassignments to minimize physical exertion of patients, etc.). Socializing changes are based on the energy level of the patient. Emotional expression often becomes restricted out of a concern that too much anger or excitement might re-exacerbate a flare-up of an episodic illness like labile diabetes or asthma. As this process takes hold, the family more and more becomes focused on illness issues as a central theme in its life. It has been pointed out that once this process takes hold, it actually becomes difficult for families to find the right balance between illness and non-illness issues in their lives (Gonzalez et al., 1989). It is in this sense that one can then think about the family as actually *maintaining* a chronic illness course, even when changes in the medical condition might have allowed the family to diminish the amount of time and attention being paid to illness demands.

THE IMPACT PERSPECTIVE

This fourth perspective focuses not so much on the way family factors influence the onset or course of chronic medical conditions, but rather on the impact of the illness on the family. Suffice it to say that a large body of data now exists attesting to the profound impact of chronic illness on family life (Patterson and Garwick, 1994). In fact, in some instances it may well be that the impact of medical illness on the family as a group is equal to or even more devastating than it is for the patient alone.

Certainly this has been the case in cancer, where psychological distress levels among family caregivers are typically comparable to or higher than those levels reported by cancer patients (Harrison et al., 1995; Kazak et al., 1992; Nijboer et al., 1998; Northouse et al., 1998), and where estimates are that 20–30% of family caregivers report clinically significant levels of mood disturbance (Blanchard et al., 1997; Siegel, et al., 1996).

There are a number of ways of characterizing this literature. The one I want to emphasize is the growing trend away from studies organized around specific diseases (e.g., the impact of diabetes on the family; the impact of cardiac disease on the family; the impact of cancer on the family), toward a focus instead on generic approaches to chronic illness impact. The argument is that a preferable approach to the 'impact' issue is to develop typologies of medical illnesses based on the types of *psychosocial* challenges presented by the illness (Rolland, 1984; 1987). Within this perspective, for example, it would be proposed that whether an illness has a predictable, unremitting course vs. an unpredictable, episodic one might be a powerful determinant of what types of challenges the illness presents for the family. In like fashion, whether the illness has an acute or insidious onset, whether its clinical course is one of gradual deterioration or potential improvement in functioning would also mean more to the family than the specific disease itself (say, diabetes vs. asthma).

The implication here is not only that the degree and type of impact would be based on psychosocial illness dimensions, but also that clinical interventions for families should focus more on these types of issues than on the specific illness diagnosis the family faces. Yet this is clearly not the case. In most medical settings, clinics are organized around type of disease (the arthritis clinic; the cardiac rehabilitation service, etc.). Although this approach allows for the availability of specialized services appropriate to specific diseases (e.g., physical therapy for joint disease; diet management for diabetes), at the same time it precludes easy access to a focus on psychosocial issues generic to chronic medical illness. Nor does it lend itself toward a family-level conceptualization of treatment plans. A simple example here might be the tendency to discuss alteration of diet with the patient alone, rather than with the whole family, even though in most families shopping and meal preparation is rarely the sole responsibility of the patient (Cousins et al., 1992).

Further, this disease-specific approach also reinforces the focus on the index patient (and his/her needs), with the rest of the family increasingly being treated as adjunctive paraprofessionals (e.g., the assumption that families should be 'required' to redesign their living spaces to accommodate complicated rehabilitation or life support equipment, or the trend toward encouraging family members to become quasi-nurses, administering intravenous medications or managing high-tech equipment like dialysis machines).

INTERVENTIONS FOR FAMILIES—
THE MULTIPLE FAMILY DISCUSSION GROUP MODEL

So with this overview in mind, let us now move on to focus on clinical interventions for chronic medical illness families. Family-oriented clinicians have pointed to four different ways in which such interventions might be beneficial: first, in helping the family mobilize its shared resources toward the goal of chronic disease management;

second, to help prevent isolation of the patient and family from its natural social supports; third, to reduce the negative impact of chronic illness on family life; and fourth, to create a better understanding between the family and health care professionals about the goals for treatment (especially the establishment of shared goals that make sense to patient, family members, and professionals).

As has already been mentioned, intervention programs for medical illness families are not yet routinely incorporated as standard components of treatment protocols in chronic illness clinical settings. This seems to be particularly true when the index patient is an adult member of the family, and is assumed to be 'in charge' of his/her disease management issues and decision-making. That is, if and when family-focused treatment services become available, it is usually because the patient is a child or elderly family member and the medical team expects that it will be calling on the family to carry out long-term disease management. But even in these cases, if a family-focused intervention is present, it is most likely to be organized as a 'support group' for non-ill family members, and is rarely based on a carefully thought-out family systems model of illness and the family.

An encouraging exception to this picture is the growing interest in the use of what has been called psycho-educational multiple-family groups (MFGs) (Gonzalez and Steinglass, in press). These groups draw on two of the traditions (perspectives) about families I have just reviewed—the family-as-resource perspective and the clinical course perspective. For those readers unfamiliar with MFGs, the basic idea is to bring together a number of families, dealing with either comparable illness conditions or similar clinical course issues, and encourage them to share experiences and ideas about coping with illness. The notion is that although the group leaders will be providing some educational material about illness issues, it is the families themselves who will provide most of the 'data' about the impact of illness on family life, what issues have been most problematic, and how to best cope with them. In this type of setting, families are able to make powerful connections with one another, and the stigmatizing aspects of medical illness are diminished. Further, by learning that families share common experiences, they are able to appreciate that much of the 'problem' lies with the illness and not with their inability to cope with it.

Multiple-family groups have a long history in psychiatric settings, dating back to the 1960s and 1970s when they were being experimented with in conjunction with long-term treatment for chronic schizophrenia (O'Shea and Phelps, 1985). Although many versions of MFGs have been proposed, the most promising seem to be those that have been labeled 'psychoeducational,' which in controlled clinical trials have been found to have powerful effects in both reducing relapse rates and improving patient social functioning (Goldstein and Miklowitz, 1995; McFarlane et al., 1995). Particularly important in accounting for the power of these groups appears to be the *inclusion* of the patient in the group (many family support groups typically exclude patient family members), a clearly delineated protocol for the structure and content of group sessions, trained group facilitators with family therapy as well as medical experience, and an emphasis on family interaction to facilitate sharing of experiences and knowledge (utilizing actual or potential alliances among members of different families based on similarities of age, sex, focal problem or family role).

The use of such psychoeducational MFGs in medical settings is more recent, but early indications are that they may be ideally suited to helping families deal with the isolation they often experience in coping with medical illnesses (especially chronic illnesses), in reducing stress-related anxiety and depression in non-patient family members, and in facilitating a collaborative stance between family and health care professionals (Biegel et al., 1991; Gonzalez et al., 1989). Thus these groups seem effective in addressing at least three of the four stated objectives listed above for family-oriented interventions in medical settings.

Most versions of MFGs used in medical settings draw on two main perspectives in their design and clinical goals—(a) a family systems perspective, and (b) a cognitive–social learning perspective. The family systems perspective is utilized both to determine how the MFG is structured and to identify those aspects of family behavior to target in developing the overall MFG protocol. The cognitive–social learning perspective is reflected in the content areas to be included in the MFG, the focus on a strengthening of cognitive and interpersonal communication skills, and the incorporation of behavioral tasks to reinforce content taught within the group sessions.

Thus far, these groups have been used with families coping with diabetes (Satin et al., 1989; Steinglass, 1998), asthma (Wambolt and Levin, 1995), end-stage renal disease (Steinglass et al., 1982), HIV/AIDS (Pomeroy et al., 1995; 1996), inflammatory bowel disease (Takacs and Kollman, 1994) and, of course, cancer (Ostroff and Steinglass, 1996; Stuber et al., 1995; Wellisch et al., 1978). Clearly if the early encouraging reports about the effectiveness of MFGs in helping families better cope with the challenges presented by chronic medical illnesses hold up to further scrutiny, it would obviously be a highly welcome antidote to the way families are currently dealt with in medical settings.

My own work with multiple-family discussion groups encompasses a decade of research, first at the Center for Family Research (CFR) of the George Washington University Medical Center (GWU) in Washington, DC, and then at the Ackerman Institute for the Family in New York City, and in Ackerman's collaboration with the Sloan–Kettering Cancer Center. Because the development of our version of an MFDG for medical illness families was carried out within the context of an ongoing research program, the concepts underlying the group design were heavily influenced by findings emerging from CFR studies of chronic psychiatric and medical illness and the family (Reiss, 1981; Reiss et al., 1986; Steinglass et al., 1987).

The chronic illness family model that emerged from this work hypothesized that families living with chronic illness often react by trying to accommodate family life to the challenges and demands of the illness. Over time, this process of accommodation leads to major changes in such aspects of family life as daily routines, family rituals, and styles of problem solving. As the stimulus for these changes is the desire to neutralize and minimize the impact of the illness on family life, the family tends to become overly focused on the here and now—a focus on the present at the expense of long-term growth. We called this process a 'reorganization of the family around the illness,' the result being that the family drifted away from other priorities that had previously been important parts of their lives.

So a model that calls our attention to: (a) an elevation of illness issues to a pre-eminent position in the family's hierarchy of priorities; (b) a restructuring of family regulatory behaviors to accommodate illness demands; and (c) a consequent alteration in family growth patterns as the family allows itself to be dictated to by the ebbs and flows of the illness' clinical course, would help direct our attention to the issues that should be addressed in a multiple-family discussion group for families trying to cope with a chronic medical illness. For example, it is easy to see how family attempts to accommodate to an illness, once in place, can easily take on a life of their own.

Particularly important here is an understanding of the developmental processes at work within the family. An ability to see how a family's initial efforts to reorganize its daily routines around illness-related needs (diet; maintaining stable routines; modification of physical activities; hyper-alertful behavior) can easily, over time, become a semi-permanent way of life, *even though the acute crisis has long since passed and these behaviors are no longer medically necessary*, also suggests a possible agenda for a MFDG—to somehow reverse this process and help the family restore a better balance to their lives.

Put another way, we can assume that one of the consequences of *all* medical illnesses for families is a need to bring increased order and regularity to daily life. However, for most illnesses this over-regulation of family life in the service of illness management is a temporary need. Once the illness has stabilized, a more balanced pattern of illness/non-illness activities can be restored. If that re-balancing process does not occur, we can conclude that the family has become 'stuck' around illness issues. Getting the family 'unstuck' then becomes the primary goal for the MFDG.

After a decade of work with multiple-family discussion groups, we are now able to report that a very substantial series of experiences with our MFDG model suggests that the version of the group we have developed seems to be applicable not only to very different types of illness experiences, but also to circumstances in which the index patients occupy different generation roles within the family. In each of the situations for which we have used our MFDG model—these have included heterogeneous chronic illness groups (Gonzalez et al., 1989), cancer groups (Ostroff and Steinglass, 1996), and diabetes groups (Steinglass, 1998)—families have reported that they have found the experience very useful, and have urged that these groups be made available to all families trying to cope with the long-range issues associated with serious medical illness.

Although we have not yet been able to design and implement a research protocol to systematically examine how and why, and to what degree, the MFDG is having its impact on families, we can easily speculate about the sources of its potential power. Particularly salient seem to be the following:

1. *The establishment of a **community of families** with shared experiences.*   Families in the MFDG not only wind up feeling less isolated, they also come to realize that their reactions, feelings, and struggles are normal. The group experience therefore leads to a sense of positive affirmation for families, rather than the sense of guilt and powerlessness that often dominated family life before their participation in the MFDG.
2. *The underlying **conceptual model** for the groups.*   Our model of how families come to reorganize their lives around a chronic illness, and the need to re-examine illness vs. non-illness priorities in family life makes sense to the families with which we have worked. Both the non-pathologizing nature of the conceptual model, and the ease with which the model's key constructs can be translated into an accessible, metaphoric language, helps create a relaxed

atmosphere within the group. Within this atmosphere, it becomes feasible to address issues that might otherwise be seen as forbidden territory (e.g., apprehensions about a possible re-exacerbation of the illness).

3. *The structural richness of the MFDG allows **multiple perspectives** on illness issues and management to be generated.* Members of MFDGs are simultaneously individuals with their own experiences of illness, people influenced by their family's unique culture, people tied to certain illness roles (patient, non-patient, caregiver, and so forth), and individuals identified by the family role they occupy (parent, child, spouse). Thus, MFDGs are replete with possible combinations of illness and family roles, each of which carries with it different perspectives on the illness experience. Leaders of our MFDGs repeatedly comment about how powerful an experience it is for families to participate in collaborative problem-solving efforts, not only within their own family, but also across families, and between families and the group leaders.

4. *The ability to take an **observational stance**.* In most interactions that occur in clinical settings, individuals are expected to be 'present' participants in the interaction. If a physician asks a question, patients are expected to provide an answer. If a family is being given instructions about a treatment regimen, they are expected to absorb the information and then follow the instructions. Even in most group therapy settings, people are often challenged by others in the group, and feel a need to defend themselves. In our MFDG model, by way of contrast, this more typical experience is balanced by a series of experiences in which both individuals and families are also encouraged to take an observational stance. For example, during the group-within-a-group exercises, each member of the MFDG is at one point invited to become a member of an 'observing team,' and to then comment on what they feel they have seen. In like fashion, in the session in which families create their before-illness and after-illness montages, they are each invited in turn to join with the rest of the group in commenting about these visual representations (metaphors) of their family and its experiences.

Our strong sense from watching families go through this 'observational' process, is that it facilitates an opening up of the family to new perspectives that simply would not be possible if they were feeling a need to defend their behavior and life choices to others. We would speculate, therefore, that it is this ability to 'step back' from oneself, especially within a group atmosphere emphasizing collaborative problem-solving, that creates the opportunity for families to consider a new and better balance between illness vs. non-illness needs and priorities in their lives.

CONCLUDING COMMENTS

This brief walk through the research and clinical literature on families and medical illness suggests: (a) that the evidence for the reciprocal impact of illness on families and families on important clinical course issues is compelling; (b) that it is not an exaggeration to propose that, for chronic medical illness situations, it is the family rather than the individual alone who should be seen as the unit of care; and (c) that the experience with using MFGs for medical illness families indicates this family-as-the-unit-of-care model can be translated into meaningful intervention programs.

But in addition to these conclusions, it might be useful to close by reminding ourselves of a number of trends that are currently unfolding that will in all likelihood only magnify the importance of the family in the medical treatment environment of the next decade. These include:

- Aging population—prolonged old age and attendant medical illness.
- Conditions that used to be acute and possibly terminal are now increasingly becoming chronic, e.g., ESRD, HIV, cancer.
- Impact of high-technology treatments on the family, including increasing use of the family as an extension of the health care team (for home treatment).
- Growing appreciation of the importance of health behaviors in the prevention of illness.
- Death and dying decision-making.
- Genetic predisposition to illness, and the implications of genetic testing for the family.

REFERENCES

Biegel, D.E., Sales, E. and Schulz, R. (1991). *Family Caregiving in Chronic Illness: Alzheimer's Disease, Cancer, Heart Disease, Mental Illness and Stroke*. Newbury Park, CA: Sage.

Blanchard, C.G., Albrecht, T.L. and Ruckdeschel, J.C. (1997). The crisis of cancer: psychological impact on family caregivers. *Oncology* 11: 189–94.

Burman, B. and Margolin, G. (1992). Analysis of the association between marital relationships and health problems: An interactional perspective. *Psychological Bulletin* 112: 39–63.

Campbell, T.L. (1986). Family impact on health: a critical review. *Family Systems Medicine* 4: 135–200.

Cousins, J., Rubovits, D. et al. (1992). Family versus individually oriented intervention for weight loss in Mexican–American women. *Public Health Reports* 107: 549–555.

Coyne, J.C. and Anderson, B.J. (1988). The 'psychosomatic family' reconsidered: diabetes in context. *Journal of Marital and Family Therapy* 14: 113–123.

Fiscella, K., Franks, P. and Shields, C.G. (1997). Perceived family criticism and primary care utilization: psychosocial and biomedical pathways. *Family Process* 36: 25–41.

Fisher, L., Ransom, D.C., Terry, H.E., Lipkin, M Jr. and Weiss, R. (1992). The California Family Health Project: I. Introduction and a description of adult health. *Family Process* 31: 231–250.

Goldstein, M.J. and Miklowitz, D.J. (1995). The effectiveness of psycho-educational family therapy in the treatment of schizophrenic disorders. *Journal of Marital and Family Therapy* 21: 361–376.

Gonzalez, S. and Steinglass, P. (in press). Application of multifamily groups in chronic medical disorders. In: W.R. McFarlane (Ed.), *The Multifamily Group*. New York: Oxford University Press.

Gonzalez, S., Steinglass P. and Reiss, D. (1989). Putting the illness in its place: discussion groups for families with chronic medical illnesses. *Family Process* 28: 68–87.

Gowers, S., Jones, J. et al. (1995). Family functioning: a correlate of diabetic control. *Journal of Child Psychology and Psychiatry* 36: 993–1001.

Gustafsson, P.A., Bjorksten, B. et al. (1994). Family dysfunction in asthma: a prospective study of illness development. *Journal of Pediatrics* 125: 493–498.

Harrison. J., Haddad, P. and Maguire, P. (1995).   The impact of cancer on key relatives: a comparison of relative and patient concerns. *European Journal of Cancer*, **31A**(11): 1736–1740.

Hermanns, J., Florin, I. et al. (1989).   Maternal criticism, mother–child interaction, and bronchial asthma. *Journal of Psychosomatic Research* **33**: 469–476.

House, J.S., Landis, K.R. and Umberson, D. (1988).   Social relationships and health. *Science* **241**: 540–545.

Kazak, A.E., Stuber, M., Torchinsky, M., Houskamp, B., Christakis, D. and Kasiraj, J. (1992).   Post-traumatic stress in childhood cancer survivors and their parents. Annual Meeting of the American Psychological Association. Washington, DC: American Psychological Association.

Kiecolt-Glaser, J.K., Malarkey, W.B. et al. (1994).   Stressful personal relationships: Immune and endocrine function. In: R. Glaser and J.K. Kiecolt-Glaser (Eds.), *Human Stress and Immunity*. San Diego, CA: Academic Press.

Kog, E., Vandereycken, W. and Vertommen, H. (1985).   The psychosomatic family model: a critical analysis of family interaction concepts. *Journal of Family Therapy* **7**: 31–44.

Levenson, R.W. and Gottman, J.M. (1983).   Marital interaction: physiological linkage and affective exchange. *Journal of Personality and Social Psychology* **45**: 587–597.

Litman, T.J. (1974). The family as a basic unit in health and medical care: a sociobehavioral overview. *Social Science and Medicine* **8**: 495–519.

McFarlane, W.R., Link, B. Dushay, R., Marchal, J. and Crilly, J. (1995).   Psychoeducational multiple family groups: four-year relapse outcome in schizophrenia. *Family Process* **34**: 127–144.

Meyer, R.J. and Haggerty, R.J. (1962).   Streptococcal infections in families. Factors altering individual susceptibility. *Pediatrics* **29**: 539–549.

Minuchin, S., Rosman, B.L. and Baker, L. (1978).   *Psychosomatic Families*. Cambridge, MA: Harvard University Press.

Nijboer, C., Tempelaar, R., Sanderman, R., Triemstra, M., Spruijt, R.J. and van den Bos, G.A.M. (1998).   Cancer and caregiving: the impact on the caregivers's health. *Psycho-Oncology* **7**: 3–13.

Northouse, L.L., Templin, T., Mood D. and Oberst, M. (1998).   Couples' adjustment to breast cancer and benign breast disease: a longitudinal analysis. *Psycho-Oncology* **7**: 37–48.

O'Shea, M.D. and Phelps, R. (1985).   Multiple family therapy: current status and critical appraisal. *Family Process* **24**: 555–582.

Ostroff, J. and Steinglass, P. (1996).   Psychosocial adaptation following treatment: a family systems perspective on childhood cancer survivorship. In L. Baider, C.L. Cooper and De-Nour, A.K. (Eds.), *Cancer and the Family*. New York: Wiley.

Patterson, J.M. and Garwick, A.W. (1994).   The impact of chronic illness on families: A family systems perspective. *Annals of Behavioral Medicine* **16**: 131–142.

Pomeroy, E.C., Rubin, A. and Walker, R.J. (1995).   The effectiveness of a psychoeducational task-centered group intervention for family members of persons with AIDS: an evaluation. *Journal of Social Work Research* **19**: 142–152.

Pomeroy, E.C., Rubin, A. and Walker, R.J. (1996).   A psychoeducational task-centered group intervention for family members of persons with HIV/AIDS: strategies for intervention. *Family Process* **35**: 299–312.

Reiss, D. (1981).   *The Family's Construction of Reality*. Cambridge, MA: Harvard University Press.

Reiss, D., Gonzalez, S. and Kramer, N. (1986).   Family process, chronic illness and death. *Archives of General Psychiatry* **43**: 795–807.

Reiss, D., Steinglass, P. and Howe, G. (1993).   The family's organization around the illness. In R.E. Cole, D. Reiss (Eds), *How Do Families Cope with Chronic Illness?* (pp. 173–213). Hillsdale, NJ: Erlbaum.

Rolland, J.S. (1984).   Toward a psychosocial typology of chronic and life-threatening illness. *Family Systems Medicine* **2**: 245–263.

Rolland, J.S. (1987).   Chronic illness and the life cycle: A conceptual framework. *Family Process* **26**: 203–221.

Rolland, J. (1994). *Families, Illness, and Disability: An Integrated Treatment Model*. New York: Basic Books.

Satin, W., LaGreca, A.M., Zigo, M.A. and Skyler, J.S. (1989). Diabetes in adolescence: effects of multifamily group intervention and parent simulation of diabetes. *Journal of Pediatric Psychology* **14**: 259–275.

Siegel, K., Karus, D.G., Raveis, V.H., Christ, G.H. and Mesagno, F.P. (1996). Depression distress among the spouses of terminally ill cancer patients. *Cancer Practice* **4**: 25–30.

Steinglass, P. (1998). Multiple family discussion groups for patients with chronic medical illness. *Families, Systems & Health* **16**: 55–70.

Steinglass, P., Bennett, L.A., Wolin, S.J. and Reiss, D. (1987). *The Alcoholic Family*. New York: Basic Books.

Steinglass, P., Gonzalez, S., Dosovitz, I., & Reiss, D. (1982). Discussion groups for chronic hemodialysis patients and their families. *General Hospital Psychiatry* **4**: 7–14.

Stuber, M.L., Gonzalez, S., Benjamin, H. and Golant, M. (1995). Fighting for recovery: Group interventions for adolescents with cancer and their parents. *Journal of Psychotherapy Practice and Research* **4**: 286–296.

Takacs, L.F. and Kollman, C.E. (1994). An inflammatory bowel support group for teens and their parents. *Gastroenterology Nursing* **17**: 11–13.

Uchino, B., Cacioppo, J. et al. (1996). The relationship between social support and psychological processes: a review with emphasis on underlying mechanisms and implications for health. *Psychological Bulletin* **119**: 488–531.

Walsh, F. and Anderson, C. (1988). Chronic disorders and families: An overview. In F. Walsh, C. Anderson (Eds), *Chronic Disorders and the Family* (pp. 1–23). New York: Haworth.

Wamboldt, M.Z. and Levin, L. (1995). Utility of multifamily psychoeducational groups for medically ill children and adolescents. *Family Systems Medicine* **13**: 151–161.

Wamboldt, F. and Wamboldt, M.Z. (1995). Parental criticism and treatment outcome in adolescents hospitalized for severe, chronic asthma. *Journal of Psychosomatic Research* **39**: 995–1005.

Wellisch, D., Mosher, M. and Scoy, C. (1978). Management of family emotional stress: Family group therapy in a private oncology practice. *International Journal of Group Psychotherapy* **28**: 225–231.

Wood B. (1993). Beyond the psychosomatic family: a biobehavioral family model of pediatric illness. *Family Process* **32**: 261–278.

Wynne, L.M., Shields, C.G. and Sirkin, M. (1992). Illness, family theory, and family therapy: I. Conceptual issues. *Family Process* **31**: 3–18.

2

Family Reorganization in Response to Cancer: A Developmental Perspective

KAREN WEIHS and DAVID REISS

George Washington University Medical Center, Washington, DC, USA

Cancer brings some families together. Others are torn apart, and none escape the changes resulting from the intrusion of this life-threatening illness. Each family is a unique relational system, and the outcomes of multiple family members are interlocked during cancer care. These outcomes include mental health and role function which are sustained by family relationships (Baider and Kaplan De-Nour, 1984; Gotay, 1984; Given et al., 1993).

The majority of families mount a resilient response, despite the suffering which is universal for those living with cancer (Arpin et al., 1990). They report feeling closer to one another after marshaling resources to fight the disease (Taylor and Brown, 1988; Zemore and Shepel 1989; Lewis et al., 1989). Cancer-induced emotional, behavioral and physical health problems have been found to cluster in a minority of families (Baider and Kaplan De-Nour, 1984; Cassileth et al., 1985). Multiple investigators have reported that one-third of adult cancer patients, their spouses and their children have clinically significant distress and psychosocial dysfunction (Maguire, 1981; Northouse and Swain, 1987; Omne-Ponten et al., 1993).

The quality of the family environment affects the outcome of its members. Family environments experienced as cohesive and low in conflict include family members who are less distressed and have better coping than patients, partners and children whose families are detached and/or high in conflict (Bloom et al., 1984; Lieber et al., 1976; Lichtman et al., 1984; Neuling and Winefield, 1988; Friedman et al., 1988; Arpin et al., 1990; Lewis et al., 1989; Fritz et al., 1988). These family characteristics have also been linked to behavioral disorders in children whose parents have cancer (Lewis et al., 1989). When the child is a cancer survivor, clear and direct communication within the family about the illness seems to prevent depression in the child (Spinetta and Maloney, 1978; Koocher and O'Malley, 1981). The importance of family function for the psychological adjustment of its members becomes evident when it is assessed along with physical disability in the same patient population. Family function has a much greater effect than physical disability on the patient's mental health (Ell and Nishimoto, 1989; Vinokur et al., 1989).

Cancer and the Family, 2nd Edn. Edited by L. Baider, C. L. Cooper and A. Kaplan De-Nour
© 2000 John Wiley & Sons, Ltd

Compromised mental health continues for at least 3 years after diagnosis and during remission of the disease for many cancer patients and their spouses. These mental health problems are associated with decreased closeness in family relationships (Ell et al., 1989). A study of patients with metastatic breast cancer is consistent with this finding. Patients with declining mood, over the course of a year, were those with higher conflict and lower expressiveness in their family environment (Spiegel et al. 1983).

Another intriguing body of knowledge involves the prediction of higher rates of disease progression and death for cancer patients based on poorer social and family relationships (Funch and Marshall, 1983). The Almeda county study of social connections and cancer incidence, mortality and prognosis followed 6848 adults for 17 years. Women who had smaller networks and who felt isolated were at significantly increased risk of dying from cancer of all types. Social connections were not prospectively associated with cancer incidence or mortality among men, but men with few social connections showed significantly poorer cancer survival rates (Reynolds and Kaplan, 1990).

Marriage also has an effect on cancer outcomes. Studies including men and women have shown a survival advantage to being married (Goodwin et al., 1987), whereas studies of women with breast cancer show no effect, or negative effects of marriage on length of life (Forsen, 1991). Marriage may be more burdensome and stressful than supportive for women, with the opposite more generally the case for men. Only when widows represented the comparison group to married female cancer patients has marriage shown a survival advantage for breast cancer patients (Neale et al., 1986). Two separate investigators report an *advantage* in survival time for *unmarried* women with breast cancer compared to those who are married (Waxler-Morrison et al., 1991; Ell et al., 1992). More research is needed to differentiate between genders in the study of relationship effects on cancer outcomes. These discrepancies may be better explained if the *quality* of marital relationships, rather than their existence, is made the predictive variable in future studies.

The literature summarized above makes it clear that cancer affects the mental health and perhaps the physical health, of spouses and children as well as patients. It also tells us that families whose members have the best mental health are likely to perceive their family environments to be cohesive and expressive, without the burden of excessive conflict. Correlations of depression and anxiety among family members suggest that something shared by members of the same family influences the mental health of its members. Some attributes of the family may also influence the course of the biologic disease process. It is not yet clear whether the latter attributes are the same as those which correlate with psychological adjustment.

We have focused on psychological adjustment related to family function in this phase of our work. Our second phase ties these adjustment processes to influences of the family on the course of the disease. We see psychological adjustment of family members as an indicator of emotional resilience in the family. It can be understood as a manifestation of personal and family development over the course of the illness.

In this chapter, we will present our current views on cancer-related changes in families. They have arisen from our attempt to specify more clearly the qualities of family relationships that differentiate vulnerable families from those who are emotionally resilient in response to cancer. These qualities are likely to be related to family characteristics that existed prior to the onset of illness. We have also begun to explore how these family qualities, and their changes across time, might influence the clinical course of the patient, along with the mental health of everyone in the family.

The essence of our current hypothesis is as follows: cancer poses the risk of separations and losses which can best be contained in relationships which are secure. Psychological adjustment depends on adaptation of family relational processes in response to these threatened separations and losses that are related to cancer. The specific nature of the cancer threat, because of its potential for loss and separation, can set in motion either constructive or destructive transformations of family relationships. These transformations occur through the activation of attachment and caregiving relationships which give rise to new forms of communication, joint problem solving, mutuality and, at times, intimacy.

CANCER AS A THREAT TO THE LIFE COURSE OF THE FAMILY

The trajectory of chronic illness assimilates to a life course, contributing so intimately to the development of a particular life that illness becomes inseparable from life history
(Arthur Kleinman, 1988).

Cancer threatens the family with separations and losses. Such threats can seriously divert the life course of the family. Secure family relational processes steady the life course through containment of distress generated by threats. Relational processes within the family are internalized as working models of attachment relationships in the minds of individual family members. These mutually reinforcing attachment processes within the family and within the individual bind family members together and stabilize the composition of the family (Figure 2.1). The *life course of the family* is manifest in its continuity over time. The life course of each family arises from its particular history and it is guided toward the future by shared values and goals. These include the maintenance of health, personal development, productivity in education and in work, recreation, community involvement and preservation of family integrity.

Our concept of *threat* is informed by the work of Brown and Harris (Brown, 1989) who designate the magnitude of *threat* on the basis of the *meaning* of life events and difficulties in the context of close relationships, personal history and social circumstances. How can we make a judgment about threat based on meaning? Weber dealt with this issue in terms of 'explanatory understanding' (*erklarendes verstehen*: Weber, 1964). Explanatory understanding relates the particular situation to its meaning based on the values, plans and goals of the family. A critical feature of explanatory understanding is the self-evident character of its assessment of meaning.

The self-evident nature of meaning is clarified by Alfred Schutz (1971), who described it as the result of being brought up in a particular world. He emphasizes the public quality of understanding in which everyone participates on the basis of being human, part of a family and part of society. The validity of this approach is supported by Reiss' report of congruence in judgments about the severity of stressful life events and the level of personal responsibility for these events among members of a suburban community in the USA (Reiss and Oliveri, 1983, 1991). The assessment

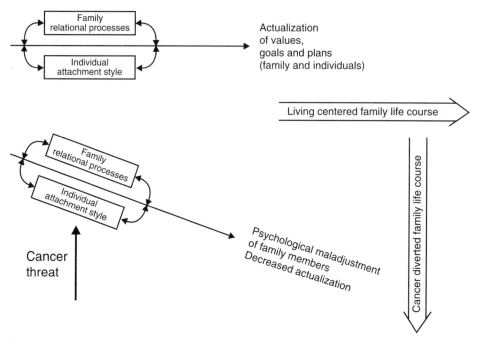

Figure 2.1   Life course of the family

of *threat* in psycho-oncology is, therefore, likely to be a useful way to bring together the tangible facts about the cancer experience and their human context, in order to study their effects on the family over time.

The threat of cancer to the family can best be estimated by understanding the personal and social contexts in which it arises. Threats to the life course of the family occur within *cancer-related systems* (Figure 2.2). The cancer-related system has several levels of organization within a hierarchically arranged continuum. It includes: the cancer, the patient's overall health, the person with cancer, the patient's family, and the community. Each level is regarded as an organized whole, with distinctive properties that are altered by interchange with other levels, but with no level reducible to simpler levels. Cyclical and repetitive patterns of interaction promote homeostasis within each level and between levels as well (von Bertalanffy, 1968). The *cancer-related system* emerges as the individual, the family and the community come together to respond to the effects of malignant cells in the body of the cancer patient. Influences from all levels combine to produce the cancer-induced threat.

Characteristics at each level of the system which increase the threat of loss and separation during cancer are included in Figure 2.3. We will describe each level, beginning at the bottom of the hierarchy of natural systems.

Threat from the level of *organs, tissues and cells* influences the family when the biologic meaning of the cancer becomes known. The type and location of the tumor, the stage of cancer spread throughout the body, and the availability of treatments for the disease form the basis for therapeutic recommendations, rehabilitation potential and prognosis. The patient and the family become joined to the medical team as the

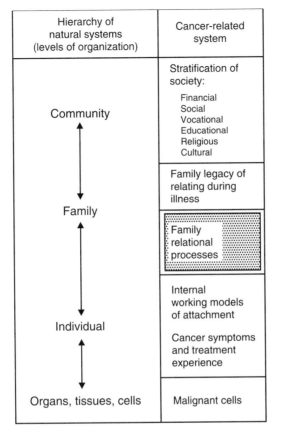

Hierarchy of natural systems (levels of organization)	Cancer-related system
Community ↑↓	Stratification of society: Financial Social Vocational Educational Religious Cultural
Family ↑↓	Family legacy of relating during illness
	Family relational processes
Individual ↑↓	Internal working models of attachment Cancer symptoms and treatment experience
Organs, tissues, cells	Malignant cells

Figure 2.2   The cancer-related system

nature of the disease is determined and the plan for treatment is developed. The biologic realities contribute heavily to the range of possibilities for the family life course once cancer is diagnosed.

The *unpredictable nature of the cancer experience* is a threat to family function. Cancer unfolds with a rhythm of its own, to which families must adjust their steps. Most cancer patients have periods of crisis separated by quiescent times. These crises occur in unexpected episodes to which families must react quickly. Intense involvement with doctors and 'high-tech' treatments continue for months, followed by periods of waiting to see if survivorship or recurrence will define their futures. Death and a premature resolution of their life story is the final phase of the cancer experience for many patients and their families. Ambiguity has been shown to be the most stressful aspect of situations in which families must adapt to loss of a member (Boss and Greenberg, 1984; Boss, 1987). Thus, the unpredictability of the illness challenges the ongoing security of the family to defend its vital functions against the cancer intruder.

The *individual* person with cancer is threatened by the intrusion of cancer into his/her body. The magnitude of physical intrusion depends on the biologic properties of the tumor, the side effects of treatment and the person's overall health. The extensive

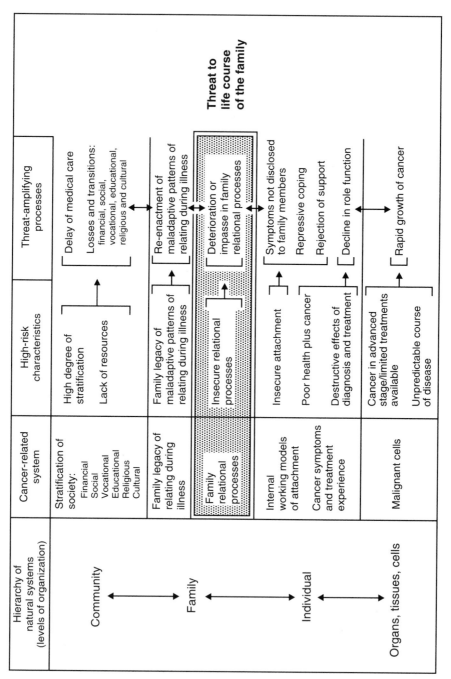

Figure 2.3   The cancer-related system: sources of threat to the life course of the family

literature on individual patient coping, adjustment and experiences of social support which shape his/her psychological reaction to cancer cannot be reviewed here. We will address only a few characteristics of the individual responses to cancer which have particular relevance to family process.

Working models of relationships in the minds of individuals have been described as attachment schemas. Those with insecure working models of attachment are most at risk for prolonged distress from cancer that is not assuaged by social support. The uniqueness of the cancer experience leaves most patients feeling as if no other person could understand his/her terror and alienation (Bahnson, 1975). A person with insecure working models of attachment relationships would expect misunderstanding, criticism, rejection and/or burdensome care seeking from others in response to his/her disclosure of distress (Bretherton, 1988; Levitt et al., 1994). He/she would, therefore, limit self-disclosure and requests for support (Mikulincer and Nachshon, 1991; Simpson et al., 1992). Such behavior may take the form of repressive coping which is thought to be a risk factor for more rapid disease progression by some investigators (Weinberger, 1990; Jensen, 1987). Alternatively, it may be expressed as depressed mood, irritability, and decreased social functioning.

The patient is challenged to 'put the cancer in its place' by separating a healthy self from the body which seems to have betrayed him/her (Nerenz and Leventhal, 1983). Family members who relate to the patient, separate from the disease, help him/her to firmly plant him/herself against the cancer 'enemy' (Gonzalez et al., 1989). This process is crucial in reducing the threat of patient isolation and depression.

Moving to the level of the family, it is important to acknowledge that the threat to the life course of the family varies with the *phase of cancer treatment*. The family must move between 'living-centered' and 'cancer-centered' life courses with the course of the disease. An example of changes in the family life course when an adult family member has cancer is illustrated in Figure 2.4. When the demands of the disease are high and the family becomes 'cancer-centered' the risk of poor psychological adjustment increases. Personal and financial resources are devoted to fighting the cancer, leaving other goals of the family unaddressed. The life course of the family shown in Figure 2.4 is as follows:

The whole family is drawn abruptly into a close connection with the medical team, becoming cancer-centered during the acute phase of cancer care. As the treatment phase emerges, the patient stays more connected than the rest of the family to the medical team. The family as a whole returns to a more living-centered course, but not to its course prior to the diagnosis. The patient enters remission and a living-centered course is resumed, but it is more influenced by cancer than before the illness. A recurrence of disease pulls the whole family back to the cancer-centered course for a short period of time followed by a balance of both cancer- and life-centered orientation. The terminal phase involves another move toward a cancer-centered life course, along with distancing of the patient from the rest of the family and from the medical team. Grieving keeps the family on a cancer-centered life course for a period of time after the death of the patient and is followed by a return to a living-centered course. The family must reorganize in order to pursue its goals and to express its values through activities that no longer include the patient.

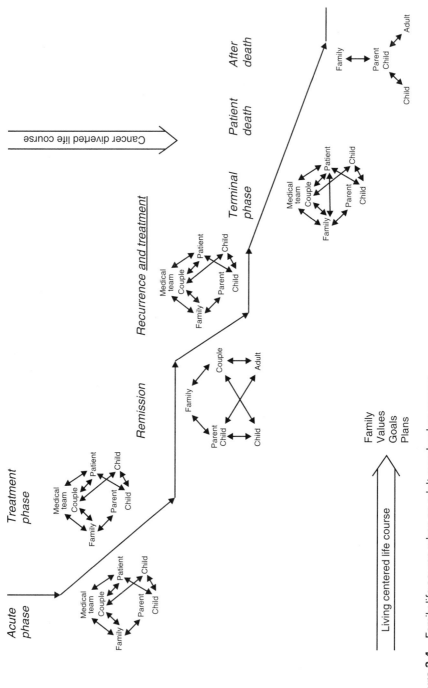

Figure 2.4   Family life course when an adult member has cancer

FAMILY LEGACY OF RELATING DURING ILLNESS

The threat of cancer depends on the meaning of the *particular* cancer to the *particular* family. Kleinman (1988) describes illness as a 'transactional communicative experience. Illness meanings are shared and negotiated. They are an integral part of lives lived together.' These socially constructed meanings of illness include understandings of how family members are expected to relate to one another when someone is ill. They invoke a family legacy which is passed down from one generation to the next (Bowen, 1978; Mullins and Christie-Seely, 1984; Rolland, 1994).

Unfavorable cancer meanings contribute much more strongly than socio-economic status or disease severity to patient distress and poor adjustment to illness (Arpin et al., 1990). Nevertheless, over half of cancer patients reported substantial *improvement* in their lives since the illness. Improvement was related to the belief that the illness is a challenge which can yield personal growth.

A 'cancer legacy' from the past may introduce distortions in otherwise secure family relationships. Cancer-related losses of relationships, or painful, maladaptive interchanges during the illness of loved ones in the past may increase the sense of danger from cancer to the family. Patients who fear that they will be a burden to their family may avoid disclosure of distress and thereby foreclose opportunities for comforting responses. Such withholding can signal family members to separate themselves from the patient, creating an avoidant pattern of relating, with decreased communication about the cancer and decreased availability of joint problem solving for addressing the treatment needs of the patient.

Alternatively, *increased* security in a family with such 'cancer legacies' may came about with a new episode of cancer, if sensitive supportive responding is used to calm the distress of members threatened with separation or loss. In this way, the cancer experience is an opportunity to *revise* the 'cancer legacy'.

Penn (1983) has described relationship patterns which appear during illness which are mirror images of patterns in previous generations of the family. This observation is consistent with Steinglass et al.'s (1987) notions of multigenerational transmissions of relationship patterns which are affected by illness. They studied adult offspring of alcoholic parents. Some of these adults formed their marital families with *distinctive* ways of relating which were separate from the alcohol-induced patterns of the previous generation. Other families developed relationship patterns which were *subsumed* by alcoholic behaviors or by zealous efforts to ward off alcoholism.

Families in which the threat of cancer is associated with emotionally charged patterns of relating from previous generations may be more likely to have their current ways of relating *subsumed* by the disease-related patterns. The healthy development of individuals and relationships in a family subsumed by cancer is likely to be compromised. Wellisch documented the long-term, negative influence of maternal death from breast cancer on the later relationships of daughters. Decreased sexual satisfaction in the daughters' adult marital relationships was among the more common problems in these women compared to those who had not experienced a mother's cancer. This impact is stronger if the daughter is a teenager, rather than an adult, at the time of the mother's illness and death, and if her feelings of emotional distress remain unresolved as she enters adulthood (Wellisch et al., 1991, 1992).

Finally, we must address the societal level of the cancer-related system. The threat of cancer to the life course of the family depends on the degree of *stratification in the society and its overall resources*. For example, low-income young families in the USA are at especially high risk for loss of the family's savings during cancer treatment. This heavy impact of illness in families was documented in a study of 2661 chronically ill adults (Covinsky et al., 1994). Twenty percent of families reported a family member who quit work to provide care for the patient. One-third had a loss of most or all of the family savings and/or loss of the major source of income. One-third of cancer patient families, especially those who are younger and have lower income, face a substantial threat to their financial security from cancer in the USA. Stratification by race, ethnicity and geographic location also contributes to differences in threat from cancer to families (Ell et al., 1992; Cella et al., 1991).

The threat of cancer to the family is the composite of stresses and losses from all levels of the larger cancer-related system as it moves through each phase of the illness experience.

FAMILY RELATIONAL PROCESSES BASED ON ATTACHMENT

We use the word 'family' to designate a group of individuals with close personal relationships whose identities develop in conjunction with one another over time. The family affects the lives of its members through the patterning and quality of relatedness, more than through the number of members or its formal designations (marriage, family, intimate partnership, etc.). This definition allows us to use a common approach to 'families' across different cultural and ethnic groups.

Cancer threatens to separate the patient from his/her family members, both emotionally and physically. Family relational processes modulate the impact of the cancer-related threat on the life course of the family (see Figure 2.1). Serious deflection of the family's life course is likely to include distress and dysfunction for family members, and perhaps compromised medical outcome for the patient.

Secure family relationships protect the family from the destructive impact of threats on the psychological adjustment of family members and on the family life course. Conger et al. (1994, 1995) studied 225 Iowa families and showed that economic threat increases marital conflict and parental depression. The same families were visited one year after establishing this association. Increased marital conflict, documented in the previous year, predicted hostility in the parent–child relationship, along with depression and antisocial behavior in adolescents at 1 year follow-up. A direct effect of economic stress on the outcomes of the the children was not detected, supporting the notion that changes in the security of marital and parent–child relationships are the mediators of the destructive effects of economic threat on adolescent psychological adjustment (Whitbeck et al., 1991).

Relationships which are *insecure* may be especially vulnerable to the destructive effects of threats.

In order to understand the family's response to the cancer threat, we looked to studies of human development which explain individual differences in responding to distress and separation between family members. Bowlby described such a behavioral, motivational system, which he called the 'attachment system'. Attachment processes were found to guide infant behavior during times of danger or threatened separation from the primary care provider. Expressing distress and seeking closeness to a significant other triggered the complementary 'caregiving response' in the person with whom an attachment relationship had been previously established. Attachment and caregiving are mutually reinforced reciprocal patterns in an attachment relationship (Hinde, 1982) which has enduring and irreplaceable bonds (Bowlby, 1969, 1988).

Bowlby proposed an orderly developmental sequence in which human beings acquire the emotional and behavioral capacities for relatedness. For example, children develop internalized mental schemas of the attachment relationship, which allow them to remember their care providers when they are separated. This internal model is used as a substitute for the actual attachment and caregiving exchange as a method of calming distress. This capacity for self-calming frees the child for further development through exploratory behavior (Ainsworth et al., 1974).

Attachment style has been described as a person's stable way of relating to an attachment figure who provides the 'subjective potential for physical and/or psychological safety and security' Berman and Sperling, 1994). Attachment style is thought to be guided by an individual's internal working models of attachment.

Differences in style of attachment for individuals develop out of attachment experience in each person's life. They form the basis for the epigenetic unfolding of family relational processes, which we believe to be highly relevant to psychological adjustment in the cancer setting. We will briefly describe the four styles of attachment in order to assist the reader to consider our hypotheses most fully.

Ainsworth et al. (1978) developed an experimental procedure called the Strange Situation, which enabled her to document that children have consistent differences in the use of their parents for calming and resumption of exploratory behavior. Observations of reunion behavior after an experimental separation were used to classify differences in both the infant and the parental behavior.

Secure attachment style was designated in children who were found to greet the returning parent with open arms. The parents of these secure children noticed their infants' signals, interpreted them accurately (by taking the infants' perspective), and then responded reasonably, promptly and appropriately. The infant was easily calmed and able to return to exploration.

Three patterns of *insecure* attachment were also identified through the use of the Strange Situation. Children who turned their backs or avoided their mothers at the reunion were designated an *avoidant* style of attachment. Their mothers provided less affectionate holding and rejected their bids for close bodily contact. These mothers also mentioned their dislike of close contact with their babies in conversations with the observer. Mothers of *ambivalent* babies, by contrast, were inconsistently sensitive, and frequently ignored their babies' signals. They did not, however, reject close bodily contact. Their infants were clingy and remained distressed for long periods of time after reunion (Ainsworth and Bell, 1969; Ainsworth et al., 1974, 1971; Blehar et al., 1977). Main and Hesse (1990) later identified a fourth group of infants termed *insecure-disorganized*, who displayed strongly avoidant *and* resistant reunion behavior, along with a variety of disorganized behaviors.

Studies with preschoolers, kindergartners and adults support these categorizations of four styles of attachment behavior and support Wynne's developmental model of relational processes. *Secure* children, parents and young adults are able to communicate coherently without necessarily insisting that they or their attachment figures are absolutely perfect. By contrast, children and adults with *insecure-avoidant/dismissing* attachment styles tend to defend themselves against closeness by processes that restrict the flow of ideas about attachment relationships interpersonally. They tend to give an aloof and non-empathic impression. At the same time, they have a strong tendency to idealize parents or themselves when giving general statements without being able to illustrate these global judgments with autobiographical memories (the memories may be absent or contradict the generalizations). The third attachment style, *ambivalent/preoccupied*, is characterized by preoccupation with conflictual attachment. In a fourth style, *disorganized*, the underlying problem in the adults has been described as unresolved mourning for a childhood attachment figure. At 6 years of age, the children who are classified as disorganized in attachment style are overly controlling of relationships—using either a care-giving or a punitive mode of interaction with the parent in the separation–reunion procedure (Main and Cassidy, 1988).

Lyman Wynne (1988) applied the findings of attachment researchers in his epigenetic model of enduring *family* relational systems. This model informs our understanding of the dynamic unfolding of family relationships during the cancer experience. He expanded on Bowlby's observations of a developmental hierarchy of capacities within the individual to describe development within *relationships*. He describes change in family systems as *epigenetic*. Epigenesis refers to . . .

> 'events of *becoming* (*genesis*) that build *upon* (*epi*) the immediately preceding events. Constitutional and experimental influences recombine in each phase to create new potentialities. This determines the next phase. If the transactions at any given phase are distorted or omitted, all the subsequent phases will be altered because they build upon a different substrate' (Wynne, 1965).

The threat of separation and loss from cancer can be understood as an activator of attachment and caregiving responses in the family. Relationship experiences from the past which involved cancer or serious illness are remembered through situation-specific internal working models which combine with existing patterns at the time of the cancer.

We would then predict that activation of attachment relational processes in response to the cancer threat would set in motion an epigenetic sequence of development in relational capacities in the family. If secure attachments are activated and reinforced through the sensitive responsiveness of family members to the distress generated by the cancer, then revisions of other relational capacities are likely to occur without distortion or impasse. Expressions of distress and caregiving responses in insecure attachment relationships would appear as one of three types: (a) ambivalent—emotionally over-involved (b) avoidant—'flat' detached; or (c) disorganized—critical and hostile.

Secure attachment	Insecure attachment		
Individual attachment style – analogous to relational process	• Ambivalent/ preoccupied	• Avoidant/ dismissing	• Disorganized
Attachment/ caregiving	• Emotional over-involvement	• 'Flat' detachment	• Criticism/hostility
Communication	• Amorphous communication deviance	• Constricted guarded communication	• Fragmented communication deviance
Joint problem-solving	• Cyclic 'solutions' and ruptures	• Evasion of problem-solving	• Disruptive disagreement
Mutuality	• Unstable pseudomutuality	• Rigid syntonic pseudomutuality	• Pseudohostility
(Intimacy)	• (Romanticized relatedness)	• ('Ho-hum' relatedness)	• (Coercive/submissive relatedness)

Figure 2.5   Family relational processes—an epigenetic model. Reprinted by permission from Falicov, C. J. (Ed.), *Family Transitions: Continuity and Change over the Life Cycle* (pp 81–106) New York: The Guildford Press

Attachment relational processes, in Wynne's epigenetic model, are the substrate from which other family processes are developed (Wynne, 1988). Four capacities for relating within the family that arise in the epigenesis of enduring relational systems are shown in Figure 2.5. They are: attachment/caregiving, communication, joint problem-solving, and mutuality. Each process can be thought of as the positive side of a domain which also includes its converse. For example, separation is the converse of attachment and optimal relationship function includes fluctuations between separation and attachment behaviors. Each attachment relationship has a range of closeness and separation which is altered over time and changes in social circumstances. Through recursive, 'circular' processes, each level of relational process influences adjacent levels. For example, the quality of communicating shapes the security of attachment within relationships.

Communication is characterized as optimal when there is shared focusing of attention and a belief in a shared social reality. If this communicative sharing is not accomplished, then the security of attachment will not be reinforced, and eventually it will deteriorate to some derivative of insecurity or the relationship will be abolished.

Joint problem-solving involves shared engagement in tasks that create the potential for relational growth (Wynne, 1970). Over time, roles develop as a result of the repetition of task-related transactions to accomplish tasks. Joint problem-solving has been described as the bridge between relational processes and family structures, such as roles.

Mutuality is the 'flexible, adaptive pattern of relational continuity that incorporates change' Wynne and Wynne, 1986). Mutuality incorporates both distancing or disengagement and constructive re-engagement as new circumstances make old ways of communicating and solving problems ineffective. A family which is able to relate with mutuality maintains its composition of membership but changes the form or content of relationships in response to a new situation.

Cancer requires the family to revise its ways of relating and, therefore, mutuality is a crucial determinant of the threat to the family life course from cancer. Problems related to cancer care require family members to move into roles which must be mutually determined by the people involved. If common ground is not created, the relationship is at risk for rupture or for the development of pseudomutuality.

Pseudomutuality occurs when family composition is maintained but a secure and responsive base for relating has been lost. An example comes from the common experience reported in a study by Wilson (1991) of men whose wives develop breast cancer. Many men reported great feelings of alienation from their wives, finding their attempts at empathy to often miss the mark, leaving them feeling bewildered, helpless and guilty. Despite these highly uncomfortable emotions, many men did not share their feelings with their wives, who they viewed to be already emotionally overtaxed with the illness.

Some husbands committed themselves to enduring the illness, not so much out of love for their wives as out of obligation. These men were likely to move into the helper role, feeling distant emotionally but tuning in to concrete demands of the situation in order to fulfill personal expectations for decent behavior in the illness situation. This pseudomutual solution to the challenge of cancer results in insecurity of the attachment relationship, which is likely to leave both partners feeling detached or misunderstood. The threat to the life course of their family is increased as they face new problems without the resources of a secure and resourceful relationship.

Our observations of differences in family patterns of engagement, when cancer threatens to separate them from the patient, are consistent with the differences in attachment-based family relational processes described above. Each phase of illness presents the possibility of revision in attachment styles within the family, and thereby the substrate for resilience or vulnerability to destructive changes in life course in response to cancer.

CANCER-RELATED TRANSFORMATIONS OF ATTACHMENT RELATIONSHIPS

Attachment relationships within the family are either reinforced or revised in response to cancer when attachment and caregiving systems are activated by the threat of cancer (Figure 2.5). Change in attachment styles occurs as the product of both developmental history and current circumstances (Sroufe et al., 1990).

There are three distinguishing features of the attachment system that are helpful in understanding its operation in the cancer setting. First, the attachment behavioral system may or may not be active at any given time. Second, attachment is manifested in, but not defined by, a limited set of characteristics that arise when distance from or accessibility of the attachment figure exceeds some individually defined limit. These characteristics include overt behaviors, emotional reactions, and cognitive activity. Finally, internal working models of relationships are based on prior history of attachment relationships, in some cases situation-specific, as with cancer, plus current interactions between the self and the attachment figure when the attachment behavioral system is activated (Berman and Sperling, 1994).

Families in which insecure attachment patterns predominate would be expected to exhibit distortions such as over-involvement, avoidance or criticism in response to expressions of distress about cancer symptoms or diagnosis. Wynne's model suggests that subsequent dysfunctions of communication, problem-solving and mutuality would also occur in these families.

Insecure relational processes fail to provide a 'holding environment' in which the distress associated with cancer can be shared and relieved, for some or all family members. The distressed person does not receive a comforting and accepting response. Others might become distressed and focused on their own strong feelings (emotional over-involvement), they might be withdrawn from the distressed person ('flat' detachment), or they may become controlling or hostile to the person expressing distress. These responses do not promote security in the relationship. Whether they transform the nature of the previous relationship depends on the meaning of the exchange to the family members involved.

The following vignette from our current study of families of breast cancer patients includes avoidant insecure relational processes and demonstrates the cumulative destructive effect of inadequate attachment and caregiving exchanges. Patients who appear to function well under day-to-day circumstances may feel out of control and unable to respond to their own emotions and those of family members when they are asked about their cancer. This can leave others in the family feeling shut out and worried. Mrs L and her daughter found themselves in this situation 2 years after Mrs L was diagnosed with breast cancer. Her daughter told us, 'On the surface, mom has faith, but underneath she's worried and concerned. She doesn't talk about it, maybe so it won't come back.'

This daughter's ongoing distress about the relationship with her mother 2 years after the cancer diagnosis can be understood from her account of the early phase of the illness. 'Mom did not accept the diagnosis. She didn't even tell me when she found out. My brother did. She was overloaded with caring for my father, who had a stroke, so she didn't "have time" to talk about herself. I'm glad she at least got the full treatment recommended.' Insecurity in this mother–daughter pair is generated by their lack of acknowledgment of a serious threat to the mother's health and, thereby, the threat to the continuation of the mother–daughter relationship.

The daughter's need for caring and reassurance in the face of her mother's illness arises from her fears about her own health. 'I am fearful I could get breast cancer, too. I see what she has gone through, and I don't really understand it. I would like to talk about what her doctors are saying. I only know bits and pieces.' The threat of losing her own health, along with the loss of security in the relationship with her mother, remains high.

This mother–daughter relationship exemplifies an insecure avoidant attachment relationship. Constricted communication about cancer prevents the reciprocal exchange of distress and caregiving. The lack of openness about the cancer increases insecurity in the mother–daughter attachment and perpetuates anxiety for the daughter. Continued development in the mother–daughter relationship awaits the calming of fears which arose 2 years earlier, at the time of the diagnosis.

In another case, an insecure, detached relationship style deteriorates to hostility and criticism with the threats of death engendered by cancer. The Miller family demonstrates relational processes which are based on hostile and critical caregiving responses to expressions of distress. Mrs Miller is a 48 year old African–American woman who was seen with her husband of 16 years. They are a middle class family without other major stressors at the time of the cancer diagnoses. Their 15 year-old daughter was also present for the family discussion of the stresses in the family related to the breast cancer.

Patient: My stress is directly related to the results of my surgery, and from finding out that it was a malignant biopsy. So my stress was, sort of like, I used the word 'depression', which you (husband) never wanted me to use, but I used it because that's how I felt. Because for a while I thought I would die.
Spouse: Which was normal. It's normal for you to think like that.
Patient: First reaction when you hear the word 'cancer'.
Spouse: Yeah.
Patient: So, I had to, my stresses and adjustments were mostly getting myself out of the doldrums so I wouldn't have everybody else feeling bad.
Spouse: Well, most of mine were the fact that you had cancer, you know, and not knowing what the results were going to be, whether you could be cured or not and what the effect of the treatment would be on you, and the impact on the kids. Because I knew that they were taking it very hard and it was very stressful to me just knowing that you had it and then going for the operation, and on with the treatment. It was just a time for me I just didn't know what was going to happen—a new experience, something that I had never gone through before. So,...I think in my mind, I had set up some criterion for how I was going to handle myself and how I was going to handle the situation no matter what happened. The stress was really there until you completed the treatment.
Daughter: Well, when you first told me I felt sad but I can't say that I really felt really sad, I guess because of the way you handled it. You didn't handle it like you was going to die. In front of me you didn't give me the impression, like you was like, 'Oh baby girl, I'm gonna die, what you gonna do? Let me start making out my will..." you know and stuff like that. Crying in front of me and stuff like that. Unless you was just worried about me...and I wasn't sad because I didn't think like that.

First of all, I don't know much about cancer. I know what it is for a person to die but I just couldn't...picture my momma dying? I just didn't, that's why I didn't let it hurt me that much, I just knew, for some reason, I just knew that you weren't leaving (Mother and daughter pause with warm and direct eye contact here).
Spouse: See, most of the time mine would come out like when I would be at work or when I would be alone. I wouldn't do it around you all or around anybody, you know.
Spouse: I had it in my mind that as long as you looked healthy, and you were healthy, I was not going to let you get into a state where you started feeling sorry for yourself...You still have to function and you have to do and rely on yourself. And I think that is one of the best things that I could do, is to force you to continue to do the things that you've always done.

I feel that was healthy for you. I do. And you got mad at me a lot and fussed with me and stuff about it. I was glad to see that, because, at work, several people who had cancer actually died, and I could see them just wither away . . . You have said to me many times that you knew you were going to die, or you thought you were going to die, that I knew you were going to die, which wasn't true. Why would you make a statement like that? What prompted you to make a statement like that? I mean why did you feel . . . .

Patient: I said that I was going to die?

Spouse: You would make statements that I was just waiting for you to die, or that I knew you were going to die because you had cancer. Did you really feel that or did you just say that out of anger? Or were you being despondent, or being doubtful, or . . .

Patient: The way your self-therapy that you were giving me, the way you were treating me, that you said you thought was helping me. I didn't think it was helping me.

Spouse: I know you didn't, I know you didn't.

Patient: With you not supporting me the way I wanted you to, you made me feel, it felt like you were preparing yourself to live without me. And you were. And I guess that's a normal reaction too.

Spouse: You have to. I thought, 'What if it came out that you *did* die?' I thought about the kids. Now I had the responsibility of raising the kids myself. Was I capable of doing that?

This couple was *not* successful in responding to one another's distress. Their differences left the patient feeling depressed, angry and burdened with the need to 'get herself out of the doldrums so that everybody else wouldn't be feeling bad'. The husband's controlling behavior leaves both him and the patient alone with unmodulated distress. Their daughter, also, has not discussed her fears about cancer, leaving her in a more infantile stance of 'pretending' that her mother 'wouldn't leave her', when she knows this could happen and would benefit from a clearer discussion of her feelings which *could* be worked through in a secure, empathic family environment.

This interview reveals the increasing insecurity in the couple's relationship, which the wife expresses as her sense that her husband had separated from her and was preparing to live without her. This resulted in her expressing her distress and worry more strongly. She seems to have been saying, 'I want you to comfort me', but her husband heard her continued fears for death as evidence of her weakness, irrationality and need for further 'forcing' away from depression. The widening gulf resulting from a cycle of husband's control and wife's smothered cries of distress exemplifies the deterioration of already insecure attachment between this husband and wife. Neither parent is able to calm down and feel secure, and it is not likely that their daughter will move beyond detachment to share her distress regarding the threatened loss of her mother. This may retard her normal adolescent development. Unmodulated fears are likely to prevent her from establishing the secure base from which to undertake the adolescent developmental tasks of independence and autonomy. The quality of relating for this family could be classified in the *insecure* section, based on criticism and hostility.

Another course is possible for families with insecure attachment styles who face cancer. The uniqueness of needs which arise because of a malignant disease may elicit new and more productive caregiving responses within the family. A more fruitful pattern of communicating with shared attention and meaning could then arise, feeding back to reinforce a more secure attachment. It is likely that this would occur in situations where cancer is a novel threat, which can be responded to outside the family's usual patterns of behavior. Families in which a cancer issue has shaped their understanding of themselves would be expected, on the other hand, to have amplified fears and are more likely to develop insecure attachment patterns as a result of the cancer diagnosis.

Silberfarb et al. (1980) report the phase of disease recurrence to be the most distressing for patients and families. Security in family relationships is crucial at later stages of disease when the family may already be severely taxed by the illness experience. If security in the family is low during remission of the cancer, the family could face recurrent disease without the ability to function together. Preservation and restoration of family function during each phase of illness is needed to prevent the progressive deterioration of relationships as the disease marches forward with the family struggling to maintain its integrity along the way.

When disease severity is high, secure relationships may be insufficient to contain the distress. The transformation of relationships over the course of cancer is illustrated in the following family, whose secure attachments were challenged by the severity of the patient's illness. The patient, her husband Al and their 14 year-old daughter, Jessica, were included in the research interviews. Laura, the patient, began by saying she was grateful to be alive and with her family. 'It's destructive to react with self-pity. I don't want to do it, but I have to fight it. The first time I was diagnosed I *needed* Al to be sticky and emotional and he wanted to get on with life. I thought he should supply me with support, and I couldn't see what he needed. I was very angry and depended on him to take care of everything. Eventually I realized that I didn't feel good about myself when that was happening. Now I'm more accepting and we share more.'

'You learn things from going through these terrible times . . . like tenderness, care, grief. My kids were *furious* with me for being sick, and I had to find a way to comfort them. Jessica fell apart the first time. She tells me now that she felt left out and misunderstood—like we hadn't talked in a year. But when I'd try to talk to her, we'd just get into a fight. She's much stronger now, I think just from growing up.'

The patient's daughter told us:

> 'It changed my world view. I have to be more serious. It deepened me. I feel different from my friends who haven't gone through this. But I can't say it's hard for me, it's hard for *her*. I used to cry a lot when I was talking to mom. So now we only mention the cancer briefly and in passing. I'm less dependent now. My folks don't need to focus on me anymore, because I am more independent than before. I remember wanting to be told more about the cancer when it came back the first time. This time I really don't want to know any more. The things I saw, I did not want to know about.'

This patient's spouse and daughter distanced themselves from her at the time of her initial recurrence, because her self-absorption, anger and demands for emotional involvement were beyond their abilities to respond. The remission of illness demands, the secure foundation of relationships, and the maturing of an adolescent allowed this family to accommodate after the first recurrence, thereby establishing new relationships which functioned to address all family members' needs without further insecurity at the time of the second recurrence. The daughter's "independence" and change in desire for information about the cancer can be seen as healthy self-protection in the face of a painful situation. The mutuality of family processes allowed her to change the form of her relationships in a way that was understandable to everyone.

CONCLUSION

We have described a model of relational development in families when a member has cancer. It is founded on the notion that the threat of cancer has a particular effect on the security of attachment, such that attachment and care-giving systems are activated in most patients and their family members at times when cancer-related risks of separation and loss become apparent. The magnitude of threat experienced by each patient and family is the product of high-risk characteristics at several levels in the hierarchy of natural systems. That cancer-related system is specific to each patient and varies greatly from patient to patient and family to family. Threats from many levels interact and balance within a living, natural system. It is within this social system that the threat of cancer arises for a particular patient.

Threatened loss and separation are prevented from taking the family off course when family relational processes stabilize the family and calm the distress of individual family members. Wynne's epigenetic model of relational processes is proposed as a template for distinguishing the stage of development and the type of distortions which might be found in a population of cancer patients.

Our theory is aimed at improving the care of cancer patients through identification of families with the greatest threat of cancer-induced separations and losses. Highly threatened families, with insecure relational processes, are at greatest risk for being diverted from their life course by the cancer experience and are at risk for psychological maladjustment (Sheldon et al., 1970).

Family therapists suggest that intervention which addresses the specific level of distortion or impasse in family development will free the natural developmental processes in relationships to flourish. The Fundamental Interpersonal Relations Orientation (FIRO) is one such relational–developmental method which has been used effectively with families who have destructive transformations or impasses in relationships (Doherty et al., 1991). Further application of an epigenetic model of family relational processes is likely to be fruitful for understanding and promoting resilience in the cancer patient and his/her family.

REFERENCES

Ainsworth, M.D.S. and Bell, S.M. (1969). Some contemporary patterns in the feeding situation. In A. Ambrose (Ed.), *Stimulation in Early Infancy* (pp. 133–170). London: Academic Press.

Ainsworth, M.D.S., Bell, S.M., Blehar, M.C. and Main, M. (1971). Physical contact: a study of infant responsiveness and its relation to maternal handling. Presented at *The Biennial Meeting of the Society for Research in Child Development*, Minneapolis, MN.

Ainsworth, M.D.S., Bell, S.M. and Stayton, D. (1974). Infant–mother attachment and social development. In M.P. Richards (Ed.), *The Introduction of the Child into a Social World* (pp. 99–135). London: Cambridge University Press.

Ainsworth, M.D.S., Blehar, M.C., Waters, E. and Wall, S. (1978). *Patterns of Attachment: A Psychological Study of the Strange Situation*. Hillsdale, NJ: Erlbaum.

Arpin, K., Fitch, M., Browne, G.B. and Corey, P. (1990). Prevalence and correlates of family dysfunction and poor adjustment to chronic illness in specialty clinics. *Journal of Clinical Epidemiology* **43**(4): 373–383.

Bahnson, C.B. (1975). Psychologic and emotional issues in cancer: the psychotherapeutic care of the cancer patient. *Seminars in Oncology* **2**(4): 293–309.

Baider, L. and Kaplan De-Nour, A. (1984). Couples' reactions and adjustment to mastectomy: a preliminary report. *International Journal of Medicine and Psychiatry* **14**(3): 265–276.

Berman, W.H. and Sperling, M.B. (1994). The structure and function of adult attachment. In M. B. Sperling and W. H. Berman (Eds), *Attachment in Adults* (pp. 1–30). New York: Guilford.

Blehar, M.C., Lieberman, A.F. and Ainsworth, M.D.S. (1977). Early face-to-face interaction and its relation to later infant–mother attachment. *Child Development* **48**: 182–194.

Bloom, J.R., Pendergrass, S.M. and Burnell, G.M. (1984). Social functioning of women with breast cancer: validation of a clinical scale. *Journal of Psychosocial Oncology* **2**(1): 93–101.

Boss, P. (1987). Family stress. In M. Sussman and S. Steinmetx (Eds), *Handbook of Marriage and the Family* (pp. 695–723). New York: Plenum.

Boss, P. and Greenberg, J. (1984). Family boundary ambiguity: a new variable in family stress theory. *Family Process* **23**: 535–546.

Bowen, M. (1978). *Family Therapy in Clinical Practice*. New York: Jason Aronson.

Bowlby, J. (1969). *Attachment and Loss, Vol. 1: Attachment* (2nd Edn). New York: Basic Books.

Bowlby, J. (1988). *A Secure Base*. New York: Basic Books.

Bretherton, I. (1988). Open communication and internal working models: their role in the development of attachment relationships. In R. Thompson (Ed.), *Nebraska Symposium on Motivation: Socio-emotional Development*. Lincoln NE: Lincoln, NE: University of Nebraska Press.

Brown, G., Harris, T. (1978). *Social Origins of Depression: A Study of Psychiatric Disorder in Women*. New York: Free Press.

Brown, G.W. (1989). Life events and measurement. In G.W. Brown and T.O Harris (Eds), *Life Events and Illness* (pp. 3–48). New York: Guilford.

Cassileth, B.R. et al. (1985). Psychosocial status of cancer patients and next of kin: normative data from the profile of mood states. *Journal of Psychosocial Oncology* **3**(3): 99–105.

Cella, D.F. et al. (1991). Socioeconomic status and cancer survival. *Journal of Clinical Oncology* **9**(8): 1500–1509.

Conger, R., Ge, X., Elder, G., Lorenz, F. and Simons, R. (1994). Economic stress, coercive family process and developmental problems of adolescents. *Child Development* **65**(3): 541–561.

Conger, R., Patterson, G. and Ge, X. (1995). Parental stress and child adjustment: an across-site replication. *Child Development* **66**(1): 80–97.

Covinsky, K.E., Goldman, L., Cook, E.F., Oye, R., Desbiens, N., Reding, D., Fulkerson, W., Connors, A.F.J., Lynn, J. and Phillips, R.S. (1994). The impact of serious illness on patients' families. *JAMA* **272**(23): 1839–1844.

Doherty, W., Colangelo, N. and Hovander, D. (1991). Priority setting in family change and clinical practice: the family FIRO model. *Family Process* **30**: 227–240.

Ell, K., Nishimoto, R., Mediansky, L., Mantell, J. and Hamovitch, M. (1992). Social relations, social support and survival among patients with cancer. *Journal of Psychosomatic Research* **36**(6): 531–41.

Ell, K., Nishimoto, R., Morvay, T., Mantell, J. and Hamovitch, M. 1989a. A longitudinal analysis of psychological adaptation among survivors of cancer. *Cancer* **63**: 406–413.

Ell, K.O. and Nishimoto, R.H. (1989b). Coping resources in adaptation to cancer: Socioeconomic and racial differences. *Social Services Review* **63**: 433–446.

Forsen, A. (1991). Psychosocial stress as a risk factor for breast cancer. *Psychotherapy and Psychosomatics* **55**: 176–85.

Friedman, L., Baer, P., Nelson, D., Montague, L., Smith, F. and Dworkin, J. (1988). Women with breast cancer: perception of family functioning and adjustment to illness. *Psychosomatic Medicine* **50**: 520–528.

Fritz, G., William, J. and Amylan, M. (1988). After treatment ends: psychosocial sequelae in pediatric cancer survivors. *American Journal of Orthopsychiatry* **58**: 552.

Funch, D.P. and Marshall, J. (1983). The role of stress, social support and age in survival from breast cancer. *Journal of Psychosomatic Research* **27**(1): 77–83.

Given, C.W., Stommel, M., Given, B., Osuch, J., Kurtz, M.E. and Kurtz, J.C. (1993). The influence of cancer patients' symptoms and functional states on patients' depression and family caregivers' reaction and depression. *Health Psychology* **12**(4): 277–285.

Gonzalez, S., Steinglass, P. and Reiss, D. (1989). Putting the illness in its place: discussion groups for families with chronic medical illness. *Family Process* **28**: 69–87.

Goodwin, J.S., Hunt, W.C., Key, C.R. and Samet, J.M. (1987). The effect of marital status on stage, treatment, and survival of cancer patients. *JAMA* **258**(21): 3125–3130.

Gotay, C.C. (1984). The experience of cancer during early and advanced stages: the views of patients and their mates. *Social Science in Medicine* **18**(7): 605–613.

Hinde, R.A. (1982). Attachment: Some conceptual and biological issues. In C.M. Parks and J. Stevenson-Hinde (Eds.), *The Place of Attachment in Human Behavior* (pp. 31–35). New York: Basic Books.

Jensen, M.R. (1987). Psychobiologucal factors predicting the course of breast cancer. *Journal of Personality* **55**(2): 317–342.

Kleinman, A. (1988). *The Illness Narratives*. New York: Basic Books.

Kobak, R., Cole, H., Ferenz-Gillies, R. and Fleming, W. (1993). Attachment and emotion regulation during mother-teen problem solving: a control theory analysis. *Child Development* **64**(1): 231–245.

Koocher, G. and O'Malley, J. (1981). *The Damocles Syndrome*. New York: McGraw-Hill.

Leiber, L., Plumb, M., Gerstenzang, M. and Holland, J. (1976). The communication of affection between cancer patients and their spouses. *Psychosomatic Medicine* **38**(6): 379–389.

Levitt, M., Coffman, S., Guacci-Franco, N. and Loveless, S. (1994). Attachment relationships and life transitions: an expectancy model. In M.B. Sperling and W.H Berman (Eds.), *Attachment in Adults* (pp. 232–255). New York: Guilford.

Lewis, F. and Bloom, J. (1978–79). Psychosocial adjustment to breast cancer: a review of selected literature. *International Journal of Psychiatry in Medicine* **9**(1): 1–17.

Lewis, F.M., Woods, N.F., Hough, E.E. and Bensley, L.S. (1989). The family's functioning with chronic illness in the mother: the spouse's perspective. *Social Science and Medicine* **29**(11): 1261–1269.

Lichtman, R., Taylor, S., Wood, J., Bluming, A., Dosik, G. and Leibowitz, R. (1984). Relations with children after breast cancer: the mother–daughter relationship at risk. *Journal of Psychosocial Oncology* **2**(3/4): 1–19.

Maguire, P. (1981). The repercussions of mastectomy on the family. *International Journal of Family Psychiatry* **1**: 485–503.

Main, M. and Cassidy, J. (1988). Categories of responses to reunion with the parent at age 6: predictable from infancy and stable over a one-month period. *Development Psychology* **24**: 415–426.

Main, M. and Hesse, E. (1990). Parents' unresolved traumatic experiences are related to infant disorganized attachment status: is frightened and/or frightening parental behavior the linking mechanism? In M. Greenberg, D. Cicchetti and E. Cummings (Eds), *Attachment in the Preschool Years* (pp. 161–185). Chicago, IL: University of Chicago Press.

Mikulincer, M. and Nachshon, O. (1991). Attachment styles and patterns of self-disclosure. *Journal of Personality and Social Psychology* **61**(2): 321–331.

Mullins, H.C. and Christie-Seely, J. (1984). Collecting and recording family data: the genogram. In J. Christie-Seely (Ed.) *Working With the Family in Primary Care: A Systems Approach to Health and Illness* (pp. 179–191). New York: Praeger Publishers.

Neale, A.V., Tilley, B.C. and Vernon, S.W. (1986). Marital status, delay in seeking treatment and survival from breast cancer. *Social Science and Medicine* 23(3): 305–312.

Nerenz, D.R. and Leventhal, H. (1983). Self-regulation theory in chronic illness. In T.G. Burish and L.A. Bradley (Eds.), *Coping with Chronic Disease* (pp. 13–37). New York: Academic Press.

Neuling, S.J. and Winefield, H.R. (1988). Social support and recovery after surgery for breast cancer: frequency and correlates of supportive behaviors by family, friends and surgeon. *Social Science and Medicine* 27(4): 385–92.

Northouse, L. and Swain, A. (1987). Adjustment of patients and husbands to the initial impact of breast cancer. *Nursing Research* 36(4): 221–227.

Omne-Ponten, M., Holmberg, L., Bergstrom, R., Sjoden, P. and Burns, T. (1993). Psychosocial adjustment among husbands of women treated for breast cancer: mastectomy versus breast conserving surgery. *British Journal of Cancer* 29A(10): 1393–197.

Penn, P. (1983). Coalitions and binding interactions in families with chronic illness. *Family Systems Medicine* 1(2): 16–25.

Reiss, D. and Oliveri, M.E. (1983). Family stress as community frame. In H.I. McCubbin, M.B. Sussman and J.M. Patterson (Eds), *Social Stress and the Family* (pp. 61–83). New York: Haworth Press.

Reiss, D., Oliveri, M.E. (1991). The family's conception of accountability and competence: a new approach to the conceptualization and assessment of family stress. *Family Process* 30: 193–214.

Reynolds, P. and Kaplan, G. (1990). Social connections and risk for cancer: prospective evidence from the Alameda County Study. *Behavioral Medicine* (Fall): 101–110.

Rolland, J.S. (1994). *Families, Illness, and Disability: An Integrative Treatment Model*. New York: Basic Books.

Schutz, A. (1971). Concept and theory formation in the social sciences. In A. Schutz (Ed.), *Collected Papers* (pp. 48–98). The Hague: Nijhoff.

Sheldon, A., Rysier, C. and Krant, M. (1970). An integrated family oriented cancer care program: the report of a pilot project in the socio-emotional management of chronic disease. *Journal of Chronic Disease* 22: 743–755.

Silberfarb, P.M., Maurer, L.H. and Crouthamel, C.S. (1980). Psychosocial aspects of neoplastic disease: I. Functional status of breast cancer patients during different treatment regimens. *American Journal of Psychiatry* 137(4): 450–455.

Simpson, J., Rholes, W. and Nelligan, J. (1992). Support seeking and support giving within couples in an anxiety-provoking situation: the role of attachment styles. *Journal of Personality and Social Psychology* 62(3): 434–446.

Spiegel, D., Bloom, J. and Gottheil, E. (1983). Family environment as a predictor of adjustment to metastatic breast carcinoma. *Journal of Psychosocial Oncology* 1(1): 33–44.

Spinetta, J. and Maloney, L. (1978). The child with cancer: patterns of communication and denial. *Journal of Consulting and Clinical Psychology* 46: 1540.

Sroufe, L.A., Egeland, B. and Kreutzer, T. (1990). The fate of early experience following developmental change: longitudinal approaches to individual adaptation in childhood. *Child Development* 6: 1363–1373.

Steinglass, P., Bennett, L.A., Wolin, S.J. and Reiss D. (1987). *The Alcoholic Family*. New York: Basic Books.

Taylor, S. and Brown, J. (1988). Illusion and well-being: a social perspective on mental health. *Psychological Bulletin* 103(2): 193–210.

Vinokur, A.D., Threatt, B.A., Caplan, R.D. and Zimmerman, B.L. (1989). Physical and psychosocial functioning and adjustment to breast cancer. *Cancer* 63: 394–405.

von Bertalanffy, L. (1968). *General Systems Theory*. New York: Braziller.

Waxler-Morrison, N., Hislop, G.T., Mears, B. and Kan, L. (1991). Effects of social relationships on survival for women with breast cancer: a prospective study. *Social Science and Medicine* 33(2): 177–183.

Weber, M. (1964). In T. Parsons (Ed.), *The Theory of Social and Economic Organization*, London: Collier, Macmillan.

Weinberger, D.A. (1990). The construct validity of the repressive coping style. In J.L. Singer (Ed.), *Repression and Dissociation Implication for Personality Theory* (pp. 337–386). Chicago, IL: University of Chicago Press.

Wellisch, D.K., Gritz, E.R., Schain, W., Wang, H.-J. and Siau, J. (1991). Psychological functioning of daughters of breast cancer patients. Part I: Daughters and comparison subjects. *Psychosomatics* **32**(3): 324–336.

Wellisch, D.K., Gritz, E.R., Schain, W., Wang, H.-J. and Siau, J. (1992). Psychological functioning of daughters of breast cancer patients. Part II: Characterizing the distressed daughter of the breast cancer patient. *Psychosomatics* **33**(2): 171–179.

Whitbeck, L., Simons, R., Conger, R., Lorenz, F., Huck, S. and Elder, G. (1991). Family economic hardship, parental support and adolescent self-esteem. *Social Psychology Quarterly* **54**(4): 353–363.

Wilson, S. (1991). The unrelenting nightmare: husbands' experience during their wives' chemotherapy. In J.M. Morse, J.L. Johnson (Eds), *The Illness Experience: Dimensions of Suffering* (pp. 237–313). Newbury Park, CA: Sage.

Wynne, L.C. (1965). Some indications and contra-indications for exploratory family therapy. In I. Boszormenyi-Nagy and J. Framo (Eds), *Intensive Family Therapy: Theoretical and Practical Aspects, with Special References to Schizophrenia* (pp. 289–322). New York: Harper and Row.

Wynne, L.C. (1970). Communication disorders and the quest for relatedness in families of schizophrenics. *American Journal of Psychoanalysis* **30**: 100–114.

Wynne, L.C. (1988). An epigenetic model of family processes. In C.J. Falicov (Ed.), *Family Transitions: Continuity and Change Over the Life Cycle* (pp. 81–106). New York: Guilford.

Wynne, L.C. and Wynne, A.R. (1986). The quest for intimacy. *Journal of Marital and Family Therapy* **12**: 383–394.

Zemore, R. and Shepel, L. (1989). Effects of breast cancer and mastectomy on emotional support and adjustment. *Social Science and Medicine* **28**(1): 19–27.

3

Cancer and Couples—Its Impact on the Healthy Partner: Methodological Considerations

LEA BAIDER

Professor, Director, Psycho-Oncology, Sharett Institute of Clinical Oncology and Radiotherapy, Hadassah University Hospital, Jerusalem, 91120 Israel

ATARA KAPLAN DE-NOUR

Professor, Department of Psychiatry, Hadassah University Hospital, Jerusalem, 91120 Israel

Our first study on couples' reaction to cancer was published 15 years ago and included a small group of 20 post-mastectomy women and their husbands (Baider et al., 1984). Surprisingly, we found that the psychological distress of the husbands, as measured by the Brief Symptom Inventory (BSI) (Derogatis and Spencer, 1982), was as high as that of the patients. However, husbands revealed as many adjustment problems, along the Psychological Adjustment to Illness Scale (PAIS) (Derogatis and Lopez, 1983), as the women patients. At that time, it was easy to review the relevant literature, since not many papers had yet been published on this subject.

A decade later, we reviewed published reports on the impact of cancer on couples (Baider et al., 1993). At that time, approximately 20 studies were available, of which about half referred to breast cancer patients and their husbands. Furthermore, the studies were of small samples, none of which included as many as 100 couples.

Five years later there was some limited improvement with the appearance of more wide ranging studies, but still with the main concentration on breast cancer (Manne, 1998). The lack of sufficient information was further highlighted by the recent review by Nijboer et al. (1998) on Cancer and Caregiving. Only about one-third of the reviewed papers actually covered the caregivers of cancer patients.

It is, therefore, considered appropriate to try once more to address these issues, concentrating on two main subjects: (a) methodological problems that could explain the lack of sufficient information, possibly resulting in contradictory results; (b)

Cancer and the Family, 2nd Edn. Edited by L. Baider, C. L. Cooper and A. Kaplan De-Nour
© 2000 John Wiley & Sons, Ltd

psychological reactions of couples to cancer and the factors that influence or modify these reactions.

METHODOLOGICAL PROBLEMS

The methodological problems will be presented in three sections: sampling, instruments and design.

SAMPLING PROBLEMS

The magnitude of the sample is still a major problem. Presently, there are some reports that include 100 patients or more (Ell et al., 1988; Pistrang and Barker, 1995; Hoskins 1995; Baider and Kaplan De-Nour, 1988a; Baider et al., 1995a, 1998a), but in some others there are less spouses than there are patients. The fact that spousal refusal is higher than that of the patients has received only scant attention. In our first report of couples, 12 out of 32 husbands (nearly 40%) refused to participate. We found no basic difference between the women whose husbands did participate and those who did not.

At a later stage, in a report of melanoma patients, 28 out of 78 spouses (36%) refused to participate (Baider et al., 1995a). Again, it was difficult to determine the reason for the high spouse refusal, other than the fact that more husbands than wives refused to participate. A recent study revealed that only 30 out of 163 spouses (approximately 18%) refused to participate, and again there were significantly more husbands than wives in that group (Baider et al., 1998a). It is highly recommended that the problem of the refusals be borne in mind. There is always the possibility of some patients' refusal to participate in psychological studies, and in addition, there is often a higher spousal refusal. Therefore, all our studies on couples deal with a self-selected group. The possibility does exist that some of the contradictions in findings could be the result of different levels of 'self-election' of couples.

Diagnosis of the sample is another major problem. Many studies are of breast cancer patients and their husbands (including a few of the recent ones: Hoskins 1995; Baider and Kaplan De-Nour, 1988b; Northouse et al., 1998) which, of course, yield valuable information on this specific and large group of couples. Whether the findings of these studies can be applied to other patient populations seems doubtful, although efforts have been made to assemble a group of spouses of women with breast cancer and compare them with wives of men with prostate cancer (Ptacek et al., 1997).

Another method of gathering information about couples with cancer has been to examine groups of 'mixed' cancer diagnoses, but is this analysis valid? Can a patient/spouse with colon cancer be compared to a patient/spouse with melanoma or lymphoma? It is suggested that some of the contradictions might be due to these differences in 'mixing' patients.

To highlight this problem, we summarized the results of some of our studies of couples with cancer about whom we had information concerning psychological distress as assessed by the Brief Symptom Inventory (BSI). The first two studies are of small samples of male and female patients and their spouses within one cancer diagnosis. The results seem quite clear, i.e., female patients report higher psychological distress than male patients, while husbands report higher psychological distress than wives. Actually, the husbands report higher psychological distress than the male patients. The next two studies are of larger samples of mixed cancer diagnoses, including cancers of both genders (e.g., gastrointestinal, lymphomas, melanoma). The findings of the first two studies are not replicated. There is no difference in the psychological distress of male and female patients: in one study, the husbands are somewhat more distressed than any other group; and in the second study, the wives' group reports the greatest distress. The reason for this confusion may be the different composition of the groups in the different studies.

We would suggest that in order to achieve a better understanding of patients' and spouses' reactions representing both genders, there should be large-scale studies of male and female cancer patients within a specific diagnosis and stage of cancer.

The medical condition of the patients is another major problem. Studies that concentrate on one diagnosis often provide information regarding the relationship between the specificity of the diagnosis and the psychological state of the patient. On the other hand, those that report about 'mixed' cancers do not use the illness variable as a possible causal factor in the patient's adaptive behavior to a new situation. Few studies provide information about the functional status of the patient, such as Karnofsky scores, and nothing could be found in the literature about co-morbidity. Studies usually provide information about the date of the diagnosis of the cancer and less frequently about the current treatment the patients receive, its duration, frequency and/or additional simultaneous treatments.

One could, therefore, conclude that we are dealing with investigations of the psychological reactions of couples to a severe, and often life-threatening, disease, which include paradoxically little information about that disease and its treatment regimens.

ASSESSMENT INSTRUMENTS

Very many instruments have been used to assess the psychological reactions and the adjustment of couples. Due to the extreme heterogeneity of measures, including those developed for a specific study, we will review only the more commonly used self-report instruments for assessment of mood and psychological distress, psychosocial functioning, coping, and assessment of family support systems.

Mood and/or psychological distress have been assessed by self-reports in nearly all the literature. Earlier studies often used the Spielberger State/Trait Inventory (STAI) to assess anxiety, and the Beck Depression Inventory (BDI) (Beck et al., 1974) to assess depression (Christensen 1983; Cassileth et al., 1985; Oberst and Scott, 1988). We, too, were inclined to use these measures in some of our earlier work, and found that breast cancer patients were significantly more depressed than their husbands but not more anxious (Baider et al., 1988). We cannot but wonder to what extent these findings are due to the many 'physical' items in the BDI. Some studies used the Profile of Mood Status (POMS) (Cassileth et al., 1985; Dar et al., 1992; Pistrang and Barker, 1995). It seems, however, that the focus has shifted from the examination of depression and anxiety to a broader concept of psychological distress.

One finds, therefore, increasing use of the Symptom CheckList (SCL-90) (Heinrich and Schag, 1985; Keitel et al., 1990; Hannum et al., 1991; Carter and Carter, 1993) and even more of the shorter version—the Brief Symptom Inventory (BSI). We believe that this shift—from assessing symptoms of psychopathology to assessing psychological distress—is not merely technical, but represents a shift in our concept that psychological problems of cancer couples are more ones of adjustment and adaptation and less of psychopathology.

Converting the SCL-90 or BSI raw scores to standardized T scores enables comparison of male and female subjects. The psychometrics of the measures is beyond the scope of the present report. We would like to note our findings, however, that the internal reliability of the BSI is extremely high in very different populations; and we look forward to the time when there will be enough studies using the BSI for meta-analysis.

Assessment of psychosocial adjustment is more difficult than assessment of mood and psychological distress. The most commonly used self-report has been the Psychosocial Adjustment to Physical Illness Scale (PAIS) (Northouse et al., 1988; Kaye and Gracely, 1993; Hoskins, 1995). We, too, have been using the PAIS repeatedly (Baider et al., 1984, 1988a, 1988b, 1989). It is a fairly long measure that requires good literacy. On the other hand, we cannot recommend any other instrument for assessing psychosocial adjustment. In the last few years, we have concentrated on assessing and reporting that psychosocial adjustment is directly linked to the emotional and medical physical conditions.

It would seem that anyone interested in stress would also be concerned with coping with stress. However, perhaps because of the complexity of studying couples with cancer, few studies have tried to assess coping mechanisms in couples. Oberst and James (1985) tried to assess coping by interviews, Christensen (1983) administered self-reports for locus of control and Northouse et al. (1998) measured hopelessness by the Beck Hopelessness Scale (Beck et al., 1974).

We have attempted, although without much success, to assess coping in a number of ways. In an earlier study of breast cancer patients and spouses (Baider et al., 1986), we administered the semi-structured Sentence Completion Test to measure categories of coping as well as the investment of energy. It yielded interesting results, for example husbands were found to be more defensive but coping more efficiently, especially in active coping. While the investment of energy into interpersonal activities and instrumental activities of the patients and husbands was about the same, patients showed high investment of energy in themselves.

However, the test seems to have created more resistance than other self-reports, with only 43 of the 62 couples participating. Furthermore, no relationship was found between coping as assessed by the test and depression and anxiety of patients or spouses. Only in the spouses' group was a significant relationship found between this measure and psychosocial adjustment as assessed by the PAIS. In addition, highly skilled and expensive scorers are required, therefore this measure was not used again.

In a study of melanoma couples (Baider et al., 1995a), we applied the Dealing with Illness Coping Inventory (Fawzy et al., 1990) and found that wives reported higher cognitive coping than their ill partners. For many years, we have administered the Impact of Events Scale (IES) (Horowitz et al., 1979) and regard it as a coping measure. There is no doubt that the IES provides meaningful information and that it is very strongly correlated with psychological distress (BSI). The question is whether the Intrusion and Avoidance of this scale are indeed coping mechanisms or rather symptoms or syndromes of distress. In recent times, we have been inclined to regard the IES—and especially the Intrusion sub-scale—as a measure of distress and not coping, and as a measure that may be more sensitive to the patients' psychological condition than the BSI.

Our last station in the search for coping measures was the Mental Attitude to Cancer Scale (MAC) (Greer et al., 1989) which provides information about four attitudes: Fighting Spirit, Anxious Preoccupation, Hopelessness/Helplessness and Fatalistic (Stoic) Acceptance. Up to the present time, we have administered it only to patients, and not to their spouses, with some apparently meaningful results (Baider et al., 1998b).

Thus far, we have elaborated on the problems of assessing coping. We believe that if we want to go beyond descriptive studies and gain some understanding about 'why' and the 'how', suitable coping measures must be found.

Family support is considered to be most effective in the adjustment of patients, and it has been suggested that it may also be very helpful for the spouses; although it is acknowledged that measuring family support is not a simple task. Several studies have used the Dyadic Adjustment Scale (DAS) (Spanier, 1976) which measures relationship satisfaction but not support.

Over the years, a number of measures have been tried, and the fact that some of these measures have been changed is a reflection of the problem. We started with the Family Environment Scale (FES) (Moos and Moos, 1981). It was considered unsuitable, because it is long and gives information along 10 separate subscales. Recently, Kissane et al. (1998) proposed using four items from only three subscales (cohesion, expressiveness and conflict) as a measure, called the Family Relationship Index (FRI), for screening families.

We moved from the FES to Olson's Family Adaptability and Cohesion Scale (FACES III) (Olson et al., 1985). There is no doubt that this measure gives much information. However, in a clinical study of cancer couples, does one use the raw scores or the discrepancies between the Real and the Ideal, or the discrepancies between the partners' perception of the real or wishes for the ideal? With these questions in mind, we finally moved on to a less ambitious scale—Perceived Family Support (PFS) (Procidano and Heller, 1983; Baider et al., 1995a, 1995b, 1998b). The main drawback of changing the measures is that we are unable to compare our own past studies.

The dissatisfaction with measures of family support led researchers to develop their own measures: Hoskins (1995) designed the Partner Relationship Inventory that has Emotional Needs and Interactional Needs subscales. Manne et al. (1997) adapted and developed a scale for Perceived Supportive Spouse Behaviors and another for Perceived Negative Spouse Behaviors. Ptacek et al. (1997) also used some scales, such as the Social Provision Scale (Cutrona and Russell, 1990) and a questionnaire designed for use in this study.

There seems to be difficulty in finding two studies that use the same measure to assess family support. We would suggest that there is little chance of improving the understanding of the relevance of family support as long as there is no agreement on a basic measure of support that could be included as part of a core assessment of cancer couples.

DESIGN OF STUDIES

In this section, we will address two issues: (a) administration of self-reports, and (b) cross-sectional vs. longitudinal studies.

Not all studies report clearly how the self-reports were administered—by personal interview, mail or telephone. There is no doubt that interviews are expensive and require skilled manpower. While the use of mailed self-reports can be described as cost effective, we believe that if we want to learn about the partners' individual reactions, having them complete the questionnaires by themselves might provide slanted information.

Concerning cross-sectional vs. longitudinal studies, the overwhelming majority of studies are cross-sectional. We believe that there is no need to elaborate on the importance of longitudinal studies if we want to progress beyond descriptive studies. Most of the longitudinal studies cover only short periods. A few reports (Hoskins 1995; Northouse et al., 1998) followed up the couples for at least a year. We started with 133 couples, and after two years had only 67 couples not only because patients' mortality but also due to patient's refusal (15) and spouses' refusal (20) (Baider et al., 1998a). In all longitudinal studies, participants drop out due to change of abode, death, or simply refusal to continue with the project. Dealing with couples increases the problem almost two-fold. Nevertheless, we believe that longitudinal studies are absolutely crucial.

THE PSYCHOLOGICAL REACTIONS OF COUPLES AND THE FACTORS THAT MODIFY THESE REACTIONS

At this stage, it is generally accepted that spouses experience at least as much psychological distress as patients. Most studies report a similarity or relationship between the distress of patients and spouses. On the other hand, Hannum et al. (1991) found a negative correlation between the distress of patients and spouses (using the SCL-90), and Dar et al. (1992) reported lack of correlation between the distress of patients and spouses (using the POMS). Although the findings on the relationship between partners' distress are not always consistent, we agree with the majority. In a group of breast cancer patients and their husbands, we found moderate but significant correlations both on depression and state of anxiety (Baider et al., 1988b). The same was true (using BSI) for small groups of male and female colon cancer patients and their spouses (Baider et al., 1989). In melanoma patients, however, the correlation was significant only for the male patients and their wives, but not for the female patients and their husbands (Baider et al., 1995a). In a study of 'mixed' cancer (Baider et al., 1995b), significant correlations were found between partners; but when studied by multiple regression, wives' General Symptom Index (GSI) failed to influence the male patients' distress. This finding is somewhat contradictory to the above in the melanoma group. Even more confusing is that in a recent study (Baider et al., 1998a) no correlations were found between the distress (using BSI) of patients and spouses. Recently, we analyzed data for fairly large groups of patients with 'mixed' cancer and found a significant correlation on the BSI of 0.48 for 118 male patients and their wives, and 0.44 for 169 female patients and their husbands.

The question of whether there is a relationship between the levels of distress within couples is extremely important because of the possible significant implications for any planned intervention. Even if there is a relationship between the levels of distress of couples, the moderate correlations suggest that in some couples there is no relationship at all, or even a negative one. Northouse et al. (1998) raised this question when she presented data for only part of her original sample in which it was revealed that, in 11 out of 29 couples, only one of the partners was in deep distress.

These results, which are both interesting and important, pose the question of whether there is really a transmission of distress and/or well-being in couples. If there is, what is its direction? Furthermore, how does one identify whether it is the patient or the spouse who is in distress?

Most studies suggest that the level of distress (measured by BSI or POMS) is moderate. One wonders whether that is so or whether the results are slanted by self-selection of the patients and the spouses who agree to participate in psychological studies. We do know that certain populations, such as Holocaust survivor and Russian cancer patients, are in very deep distress. This assertion appears to suggest that the question of whether a group of cancer patients (or spouses) is in deep distress is not as relevant as which of the patients/spouses are in deep distress or at risk of falling into the category. In other words, the crucial problem seems to be the identification of vulnerability (Baider et al., 1992, 1993, 1996a, 1996b; Peretz et al., 1994).

The situation becomes even more complex when trying to identify the factors that might affect the psychological distress of patients and spouses. There seems to be unanimity that age and education have little, if any, effect on their psychological distress. For some unknown reason, the possible effects of gender have received no attention. As mentioned earlier, in our studies of couples within one cancer diagnosis, we found (using the BSI) clear gender effects, with female patients doing significantly less well than male patients and husbands doing significantly less well than wives. Completely different results on the same measure were found in a group of 'mixed' cancer patients and their spouses, with no gender differences in the patients' group but significant differences in the spouses' group, with the wives doing less well. There appears to be no explanation for this discrepancy.

Medical factors received insufficient attention. There seems to be unanimous agreement that the time factor with regard to the diagnosis of cancer to the psychological assessment is not highly relevant. The few longitudinal studies present contradictory results, with some reporting increase in distress over time (Ell et al., 1988), increase in distress only in patient (Kaye and Gracely, 1993), and decrease in distress of both patients and spouses (Hoskins, 1995). For example, Northouse et al. (1998) found no significant change in psychological distress over time.

It is difficult to reconcile such contradictory results. A possible explanation is that the populations studied are different and, therefore, time means different things to each of them (e.g., one can expect increased distress in patients with advanced disease or undergoing aggressive treatments, and decreased distress in patients who are in follow-up with no evidence of disease).

Some studies did not report the patient's functional state nor provide the Karnofsky scores. When the Karnofsky score was included, results were not identical. In two research reports (Baider et al., 1998a, 1998b), the Karnofsky score had no effect on either patients' or spouses' distress. In another, the score caused distress only to the male patients, and in our latest study (Baider et al., 1999) it caused distress to both male and female patients but not to spouses. We are inclined to suggest that the effects of the functional state on psychological distress depend on the level of the functional state, i.e., when it is very good, it has no effect on either patients or spouses; when it is somewhat compromised, but still with Karnofsky score of 80 +, it has some effect on patients' psychological distress, but not on that of spouses. Spouses' distress would be affected only when the functional state is poor (below 80). However, this suggestion still has to be tested.

We would like to address briefly the question of coping and psychological distress. Not much has been written on this subject, probably because of the previously mentioned difficulties in measuring coping. In an earlier cross-sectional study of breast cancer, patients' and their husbands' coping was measured by The Sentence Completion Test. In both groups, no relationship was found between depression and anxiety, and coping (although a relationship was found between coping and psychosocial adjustment, as assessed by the PAIS). In another cross-sectional study, the MAC was used to assess the coping of patients only. Anxious Preoccupation contributed significantly to distress in both genders, while Fighting Spirit had protective effects only in the female patients (Baider et al., 1998a). However, one has to be very careful with correlations between distress and coping in cross-sectional studies. We do not yet have longitudinal studies that include coping mechanisms other than the IES. It is true that, on the IES, Intrusion, and to some extent also Avoidance, predicts psychological distress. However, as stated earlier, we are inclined to regard Intrusion and Avoidance as symptom clusters (of distress) and not as coping mechanisms (Baider and Kaplan De-Nour, 1997).

The last question concerns the effects of family support and psychological distress on patients and spouses. Is there enough hard evidence to confirm the often repeated statement that support—especially from the family—is very important for the emotional welfare of the cancer patient? What about the spouse and the effects of family support on his/her distress?

In cross-sectional studies, we found that Perceived Family Support had a protective effect, i.e., lower psychological distress, for spouses but not for patients. However, it could be that spouses who are more distressed perceive themselves as less supported. What became very clear in our studies is that partners' distress contribute massively to each other, i.e., spouses' distress to patients' distress, and patients' distress to spouses' distress. This finding of partners' reciprocal contribution to distress was found also in a prospective study at Time 1 but disappeared at the two-year follow-up, nor did partners' distress at Time 1 contribute to distress at follow-up.

Notwithstanding our hesitancy about cross-sectional studies, we would like to mention two of them. Ptacek et al. (1997) examined only spouses of cancer patients using the Dyadic Adjustment Scale (DAS) and the Mental Health Inventory (MHI). Support received was assessed as well as satisfaction with the received support. Very strong gender differences were found. The wives' MHI was influenced by support from others, which did not affect their DAS. Neither DAS nor MHI were affected by support from their sick partners. On the other hand, the husbands' DAS and MHI were strongly affected by the support of their sick partners. Does this really mean that wives of sick male patients can enjoy support from other sources while husbands continue to need the support of their sick female patients? Manne et al. (1997) assessed the association between positive and negative aspects of spouse response and psychological adjustment among 158 individuals with cancer. The results of this cross-sectional study suggest very strongly that positive support has practically no effect on psychological distress or on psychological well-being. On the other hand, the negative responses seem to have a very strong influence both on psychological distress and psychological well-being.

Thus, there does seem to be some strong preliminary evidence that family support may have an influence on the adjustment of patients and spouses. However, large-scale, prospective and methodologically sound studies are badly needed.

The research and methodological limitations of the work presented in this paper could lead to reformulating ideas for future development in the field of psychological research of patients and families confronted by the stress of cancer. We suggest the following parameters for research: (a) selection of specific measurements; (b) prospective longitudinal studies; (c) criteria for sample selection, diagnosis and stages; (d) causality and contagious effect of psychological distress; (e) dysfunctional coping in one or both spouses; (f) gender differentiation with similar diagnosed illness; and (g) emphasis on psychological, high-risk groups (e.g., minorities, Holocaust and other victimized populations).

The challenge to gain more knowledge and better understanding of how to provide the most appropriate care may lie in the implementation of some or all of the above research ideas.

REFERENCES

Baider, L. and Kaplan De-Nour, A. (1984). Couples' reactions and adjustment to mastectomy. *International Journal of Psychiatry in Medicine* **14**(3): 265–276.

Baider, L. and Kaplan De-Nour, A. (1986). Family perception and adjustment in post-mastectomy women. *International Journal of Family Psychiatry* **7**: 439–447.

Baider, L. and Kaplan De-Nour, A. (1988a). Adjustment to cancer: who is the patient, the husband or the wife? *Israel Journal of Medical Sciences* **24**(9–10): 631–636.

Baider, L. and Kaplan De-Nour, A. (1988b). Breast cancer: a family affair. In C.L. Cooper (Ed), *Stress and Breast Cancer* Chichester: Wiley.

Baider, L., Peretz, T. and Kaplan De-Nour, A. (1989). Gender and adjustment to chronic disease: a study of couples with colon cancer. *General Hospital Psychiatry* **10**(5): 1–8.

Baider, L., Peretz, T. and Kaplan De-Nour, A. (1992). Effect of the Holocaust on coping with cancer. *Social Science and Medicine* **34**(1): 11–15.

Baider, L. and Kaplan De-Nour, A. (1993). Impact of cancer on couples (invited paper). *Cancer Investigation* **11**(6): 706–713.

Baider, L., Peretz, T. and Kaplan De-Nour, A. (1993). Holocaust cancer patients: a comparative study. *Psychiatry—Interpersonal and Biological Processes* **56**(4): 349–355.

Baider, L., Perry, S., Holland, J., Sison, A. and Kaplan De-Nour, A. (1995a). Couples and gender relationship: a sample of melanoma patients and their spouses. *Family Systems Medicine* **13**(1): 1–9.

Baider, L., Manor, O., Ever-Hadani, P., Kaufman, B., Peretz, T. and Kaplan De-Nour, A. (1995b). Mutuality of fate: adaptation and psychological distress in cancer patients and their partners. In L. Baider, C.L. Cooper and A. Kaplan De-Nour (Eds), *Cancer and the Family*, Chichester: Wiley.

Baider, L., Kaufman, B., Ever-Hadani, P. and Kaplan De-Nour, A. (1996a).   Coping with additional stresses: comparative study of Israeli and new immigrant cancer patients. *Social Science and Medicine* **42**(7): 1077–1084.

Baider, L., Ever-Hadani, P. and Kaplan De-Nour, A. (1996b).   Crossing new bridges: the process of adaptation and psychological distress of Russian immigrants in Israel. *Psychiatry* **59**: 175–183.

Baider, L. and Kaplan De-Nour, A. (1997).   Psychological distress and intrusive thoughts in cancer patients. *The Journal of Nervous and Mental Disease* **185**: 346–348.

Baider, L., Koch, U., Esaacson, R. and Kaplan De-Nour, A. (1998a).   Prospective study of cancer patients and their spouses: the weakness of marital strength. Invited paper. *Psycho-Oncology* **7**: 49–56.

Baider, L., Walach, N., Perry, S. and Kaplan De-Nour, A. (1998b).   Cancer in married couples: higher or lesser distress? *Journal of Psychosomatic Research* **45**(1): 1–11.

Beck, A.T., Weissman, A., Lester, D. and Trexler, L. (1974).   The measurement of pessimism: the hopelessness scale. *Journal of Consulting and Clinical Psychology* **42**: 861–865.

Carter, R.E. and Carter, C.A. (1993).   Individual and marital adjustment in spouse pairs subsequent to mastectomy. *American Journal of Family Therapy* **21**: 291–300.

Cassileth, B.R., Lusk, E.J., Brown, L.L. and Cross, P.A. (1985).   Psychosocial status of cancer patients and next of kin. *Journal of Psychosocial Oncology* **3**: 99–105.

Christensen, D. (1983).   Post-mastectomy counseling: an outcome study of structured treatment protocol. *Journal of Sex and Marital Therapy* **9**: 266–275.

Cutrona, C.E. and Russell, D.W. (1990).   Type of social support and specific stress: toward a theory of optimal matching. In B.R. Sarason, I.G. Sarason and G.R. Pierce (Eds), *Social Support: An Interactional View*, New York: Wiley.

Dar, R., Beach, C., Barden, P. and Cleeland, C. (1992).   Cancer pain in the marital system: a study of patients and their spouses. *Journal of Pain Symptom Management* **7**: 87–93.

Derogatis, L.R. and Spencer, P.M. *The Brief Symptom Inventory (BSI): Administration, Scoring and Procedures Manual*. Johns Hopkins University: Baltimore, 1982.

Derogatis, L.R. and Lopez, M.C. *Psychological Adjustment to Illness Scale (PAIS): Administration, Scoring and Procedures Manual*. Clinical Psychometric Research, Johns Hopkins University, Baltimore, 1983.

Ell, K.O., Nishimoto, R.H., Mantell, J.E. and Hamovitch, M.B. (1988).   Psychological adaptation to cancer: a comparison among patients, spouses and nonspouses. *Family Systems Medicine* **6**: 335–348.

Fawzy, I.F., Cousins, N., Fawzy, N.W., Kemeny, M.E., Elashoff, R. and Morton, D.A. (1990).   A structured psychiatric intervention for cancer patients. *Archives of General Psychiatry* **47**: 720–730.

Greer, S., Moorey, S. and Watson, M. (1989).   Patients' adjustment to cancer: the Mental Adjustment to Cancer Scale (MAC). *Journal of Psychosomatic Research* **33**: 373–377.

Hannum, J.W., Giese-David, J., Harding, K. and Hatfield, A.K. (1991).   Effects of individual and marital variables on coping with cancer. *Journal of Psychosocial Oncology* **9**: 1–20.

Heinrich, R.L. and Schag, C.C. (1985).   Stress activity management: group treatment for cancer patients and spouses. *Journal of Consulting and Clinical Psychology* **53**: 439–446.

Horowitz, M., Wilner, N. and Alvarez, W. (1979).   Impact of Events Scale (IES): A measure of subjective stress. *Psychosomatic Medicine* **41**(3): 209–218.

Hoskins, C.N. (1995).   Adjustment to breast cancer in couples. *Psychological Reports* **77**: 435–454.

Kaye, J. and Gracely, E. (1993).   Psychological distress in cancer patients and their spouses. *Journal of Cancer Education* **8**: 47–52.

Keitel, M., Zevon, M., Rounds, J., Petielli, N. and Kousis, C. (1990).   Spouse adjustment to cancer surgery: stress and coping responses. *Journal of Surgical Oncology* **43**: 148–153.

Kissane, D.W., Bloch, S., McKenzie, M., McDowall, A.C. and Nitzan, R. (1998).   Family grief therapy: a preliminary account of a new model to promote healthy family functioning during palliative care and bereavement. *Psycho-Oncology* **7**: 14–25.

Manne, S.L. (1998).   Cancer in the marital context: a review of the literature. *Cancer Investigation*, **16**: 188–202.

Manne, S.L., Taylor, K.L., Dougherty, J. and Kemeny, N. (1997). Supportive and negative responses in the partner relationship: their association with psychological adjustment among individuals with cancer. *Journal of Behavioral Medicine* **20**(2): 101–125.

Moos, R.H. and Moos, B.S. *Family Environment Scale*, Consulting Psychologists Press, Palo Alto, California, 1981.

Nijboer, R., Tempelaar, R., Sanderman, R., Triemstra, M., Spruijt, R.J. and Van Den Bos, G.A.M. (1998). Cancer and caregiving: the impact on the caregiver's health. *Psycho-Oncology* **7**: 3–13.

Northouse, L.L., Templin, T., Mood, D. and Oberst, M. (1998). Couple's adjustment to breast cancer and benign breast disease: a longitudinal analysis. *Psycho-Oncology* **7**: 37–48.

Oberst, M. and James, R. (1985). Going home: patient and spouse adjustment following cancer surgery. *Topics in Clinical Nursing* **7**: 46–57.

Oberst, M.T. and Scott, D.W. (1988). Post-discharge distress in surgically treated cancer patients and their spouses. *Research in Nursing Health* **11**: 223–233.

Olson, D., Portner, J. and Lavee, Y. *FACES III*, Family Social Science, University of Minnesota, St. Paul, Minnesota, 1985.

Peretz, T., Baider, L., Ever-Hadani, P. and Kaplan De-Nour, A. (1994). Psychological distress in female cancer patients with Holocaust experience. *General Hospital Psychiatry* **16**: 413–418.

Pistrang, N. and Barker, C. (1995). The partner relationship in psychological response to breast cancer. *Social Science Medicine* **40**: 789–797.

Procidano, M. and Heller, K. (1983). Measures of perceived social support from friends and from family: three validation studies (PFS). *American Journal of Community Psychology* **11**: 1–24.

Ptacek, J.T., Pierce, G.P., Dodge, K.L. and Ptacek, J.J. (1997). Social support in spouses of cancer patients: what do they get and to what end? *Personal Relationships* **4**: 431–449.

Spanier, G.B. (1976). Measuring dyadic adjustment: new scales for assessing the quality of marriage. *Journal of Marriage and the Family* **38**: 15–28.

Section II
SOCIAL SUPPORT AND CULTURAL PERSPECTIVE

4

The Role of Family Support in Cancer Control

JOAN R. BLOOM

School of Public Health, University of California, Berkeley,
Berkeley, California 94720-7360, USA

The family plays a critical role for individuals both in the early detection of cancer, and its treatment. Social support provided by family members is a resource for the individual and, in the best circumstances, reinforces individuals in their efforts to stay healthy. Social support provided by family members differs from support provided by friends or similar others (individuals who are in a similar situation, e.g., have the same type of cancer). The family member may be closer (or more distant) psychologically to the individual, and thus can be the individual's confidant, becoming aware of the individual's innermost thoughts and feelings. Thus, the family member is in a position to provide comfort and a sense of security to the individual. At the same time, family members also have their own fears and concerns, which may reduce their effectiveness in assisting the individual to cope with the stresses involved in the detection, diagnosis and treatment of cancer.

The trauma of cancer is experienced not only by the individual, but also to varying degrees by other family members. In fact, it is estimated that three out of every four families will one day be touched by cancer. Virtually everyone can expect to be involved in at least one close relationship with someone who has the disease (Lichtman and Taylor, 1986). The individual has almost always been studied in isolation, separate from the family and other elements of his/her social context. However, a life-threatening illness such as a cancer diagnosis is an event that forces the cancer patient to rely more on family resources, and therefore affects the family as well as the patient. The reactions of these family members to the cancer experience and their interactions with the patient affect the psychosocial adjustment of the individual with cancer (Spiegel et al., 1983). Thus, the nature of the individual's social network and the resources the individual is able to draw from it constitute the context necessary to the cancer experience from the time of detection forward (Brown and Gary, 1987).

Cancer and the Family, 2nd Edn. Edited by L. Baider, C. L. Cooper and A. Kaplan De-Nour
© 2000 John Wiley & Sons, Ltd

In the past few years it has become increasingly clear that other factors either facilitate or hinder the process of adjustment and the ultimate quality of life of the individual with cancer. These factors may be either internal to the individual or external. Examples of internal factors include the individual's coping style (Lazarus, 1982), perceived control (Wallston et al., 1976), sense of efficacy (Bandura, 1977), and sense of coherence (Antonofsky, 1993). The most obvious external factors are the resources the individual has, including material/fiscal resources such as educational attainment, income and health insurance and social resources such as loving and supportive relationships with family and friends to whom the individual can turn in times of need for information, emotional support, and assistance, and, for those who are employed, a warm and supportive work environment (House and Kahn, 1985).

The structure of the family environment is important because it can facilitate or hinder the provision of supportive interactions. Some families exhibit openness between family members, increasing the ability to express one's feelings and resulting in a sense of cohesiveness (Holahan and Moos, 1981; Moos, 1976). Other families do not exhibit such an open environment, making it difficult for the individual to ask for or receive supportive exchange. For example, in a study of the psychological adjustment of women with metastatic breast cancer, better adjustment was found to be predicted by more expressiveness, less conflict and moral–religious orientation in the family (Spiegel et al., 1983). These findings are consistent with those for Hodgkin's disease survivors, where greater psychological well-being 1 year following diagnosis was associated with high family cohesion and low family conflict at the time of diagnosis (Fobair et al., 1986). Both cultural factors and family composition may affect the families' ability to provide support (Wellisch et al., 1999; Bloom et al., 1999b). A new study by Wellisch and his colleagues provides intriguing data indicating that there are cultural differences in how a patient is included in the family's social network. This affects the individual's ability to draw on social resources both inside and outside the family circle. In a current study, we find that younger women with a diagnosis of breast cancer experience one child as 'supportive,' while more than one child increases family conflict. Thus, to understand the individual's path from detection onward, both the composition of the family and its cultural context must be known.

The purpose of this chapter is to assess the role of social support, especially support derived from the family system, on the well-being and, ultimately, the quality of life of the individual as he/she progresses along the path from detection through rehabilitation and long-term survival or continuing care. Two roles of the family as a provider of social support provide the focus. The first role is as an initiator or reinforcer of the individual's attempts to keep healthy. The second role is as a provider of emotional support, information and assistance following the diagnosis of cancer.

The chapter is divided into three sections. The first section is a general discussion of the important conceptual and methodological issues relevant to social support as a construct. The second section focuses on the importance of the family in cancer detection. In the third section, the family's role during diagnosis, treatment, rehabilitation and, in the case of recurrence, continuing care provides the focus of research and discussion.

SOCIAL SUPPORT AS A RESOURCE

DEFINITION OF SOCIAL SUPPORT

Definitions of social support vary in both their precision and generality. Social support is commonly defined as information that leads individuals to believe that they are cared for and loved, are esteemed and valued, and belong to a network of communication and mutual obligation (Cobb, 1976). This definition is very specific as it is limited to perceived support, but it incorporates the notion that there are multiple types of support. A more general definition had been proposed by Kaplan et al. (1977). They define social support as the degree to which an individual's needs for affection, approval, belonging, and security are met by significant others. Both definitions define social support as the *perception* of support by the individual rather than whether or not support attempts are made by members of the individual's network of family and friends.

TYPES OF SUPPORT

Researchers have shifted from considering social support as a unitary concept to the conclusion that there are different types of support. Today, the view is that that social support is multi-dimensional (Bloom, 1982, 1986; House, 1981; Wortman, 1984; Cutrona and Russell, 1990). Schaefer et al. (1981) suggested that there are three types of support—informational, tangible, and emotional. *Informational support* refers to the provision of knowledge relevant to the situation the individual is experiencing such as whether and where to go for cancer screening or what the side effects of various treatment options are (Bloom, 1986; Cutrona and Russell, 1990). Information may alter a harmful or threatening evaluation of a difficult situation to a more benign one. For example, a woman facing a mastectomy may see the surgery as a threat to her body image until her spouse or partner points out that she may be a candidate for a lumpectomy or, if she does have a mastectomy, that reconstructive surgery is available which will restore her breast. Thus, a threatening appraisal is lessened. Tangible or *instrumental support* refers to specific assistance that others may provide for the individual which are considered to be helpful, such as transportation to a medical appointment, child care, financial assistance or a temporary loan. Thus, support provides coping assistance (Thoits, 1995). *Emotional support* is the perceived availability of thoughtful, caring individuals to whom one can share one's innermost thoughts and feelings. Listening, caring, and reassuring a loved one that he/she is worthy and loved can directly bolster self-esteem and thereby influence well-being (Pearlin and Johnson, 1977). House (1981) includes *appraisal support*, a fourth type of information providing affirmation and feedback. Wortman (1984) includes the encouragement of open expression, a type of support closely related to appraisal support. Cutrona and Russell (1990) call this type of support *esteem support* or the bolstering of a person's sense of competence by other people.

Today, the preceding types of support are considered functional support and are differentiated from *social affiliation or network support* (Thoits, 1995). While these types of *functional support* are conceptually distinct, attempts to empirically distinguish between them have been only partially successful. Thus, Schaefer and her colleagues (1981) found that informational support was both conceptually and empirically distinct from four other measures that their research team used. Recently, Bloom and her colleagues (1999b) found that when principal components analysis was conducted on their measure of emotional support, which seemed to have elements of information provision as well as instrumental support, all items loaded on a single factor.

As indicated above, functional support is distinguished from the network of relationships that exist between people. This aspect of the support system is referred to as *structural support*. Structural support is defined as being part of a system of mutual obligations and reciprocal help with other individuals and groups who have common interests and concerns (Bloom, 1986; Cutrona and Russell, 1990; Thoits, 1995). Early sociologists such as Emile Durkheim (Durkheim and Simpson, 1951), first noted that interpersonal relations between individuals had critical consequences for people's health and survival. Individuals who were marginal to their community were more likely to commit suicide than individuals who were well integrated into the community. This observation has been confirmed by others considering other outcomes as diverse as rates of miscarriage, deaths following bereavement, and all-cause mortality (Nuckolls et al., 1972; Berkman and Syme, 1979, House, 1981).

Structural support has been measured by the number of relationships or social roles that an individual has as well as the frequency and intensity with which the individual interacts with network members. Network measures capture the individual's degree of social isolation or social embeddedness. From her review of the literature, Thoit (1995) concludes that 'measures of social integration directly and positively relate to mental and physical health, including lower mortality'. She also notes that social integration does not buffer the physical or emotional impacts of major stressful life events or chronic difficulties in people's lives. In other words, the size and degree of integration within one's social network is a necessary condition, but not a sufficient condition, for gaining resources such as instrumental, informational and emotional support to buffer the stressful live events one encounters in everyday life.

Less studied is how the structural and functional aspects of social support are related to one another. That is, how the size of the network and the types of relationships within the network influence the type and amount of support that the network can potentially provide. For example, two studies of chronically ill individuals provide evidence that the increasing isolation due to illness can reduce the amount of perceived support provided (Bloom and Spiegel, 1986; Wiley and Sillman, 1990; Bloom and Kessler, 1994). The obverse is also true, that is, persons with larger social networks perceive greater mounts of various types of social support (Berrera, 1986; Wellman and Wortley, 1990; Lin and Westcott, 1991). In other words, the structure of an individual's network of social ties provides the potential for an individual to obtain functional support, but how this happens is unclear. The empirical studies suggest that the amount of perceived support is due to the size of the network. Direct confirmation of this relationship between the size and integration of the social network and the amount of instrumental and emotional support an individual can draw from the network has been reported in two studies (Bloom et al., 1991, 1998). In the first study, the size of the social networks of patients following the diagnosis and treatment of Hodgkin's disease predicted the amount of emotional support and instrumental support they perceived. In the second study, a similar finding was reported for women newly diagnosed with breast cancer, even though the measure of network size was different. Thus, the structure of one's network has two different effects: direct, affecting the individual's mental and physical health (Thoits, 1995) and indirectly, affecting the amount of functional support received, which provides additional social resources during life crises.

NEGATIVE EFFECTS OF SOCIAL SUPPORT

There is not a one-to-one correspondence between the purported provision of supportive behaviors such as information, assistance, and emotional affirmation and their perception as being supportive. In addition, the manner in which family members and friends respond to the individual with cancer may be intentionally unsupportive. The spouse or other family members may criticize the individual's attempts at coping with the diagnosis and treatment of the disease. Second, genuine attempts at being helpful are sometimes perceived as unhelpful. Support attempts most commonly identified as unhelpful were giving advice, encouragement of recovery, minimization/forced cheerfulness, and identification with feelings. On the other hand, opportunities for the open expression of feelings and contact with others experiencing a similar life crisis were perceived as helpful (Wortman and Lehman, 1985). Finally, family members may respond insensitively to the individual, albeit the response was not meant to upset or hurt the individual, for example exaggerating threatening aspects of the situation or conveying discomfort during attempts on the part of the individual to talk about the cancer experience (Dakof & Taylor, 1990; Manne et al., 1997; de Ruiter et al., 1993).

Only a few researchers have studied the effects of negative support on the cancer patient and others coping with other stressful life events such as serious illness. Negative support, especially from the spouse, have been associated with decreased well-being (de Ruiter et al., 1993; Manne et al., 1997). In one study, unsupportive interactions have been found to have a greater impact on cancer patients' well-being than supportive interactions (Manne et al., 1997). Inept supportive behavior may result in poorer well-being via the same mechanisms as positive social support. Thus, in one study avoidant coping was found to mediate the relation between spouse criticism and avoidance and psychological distress among women with arthritis (Manne and Zautra, 1989). A second possible mechanism is that the negative responses by one's partner and family reduce the opportunities to talk about feelings and concerns. Without outlets for expressing or sharing thoughts and feelings, individuals are more likely to engage in avoidance rather than directly working on solving their problems (Clark, 1993; Horowitz, 1986).

SOCIAL SUPPORT AND EARLY CANCER DETECTION

An important role of the family is supporting the individual's attempts at keeping healthy. One way of keeping healthy is through seeking medical care when it is warranted. Routine screening is important in the earlier detection of cancer when outcomes are better and more treatment options exist. There are at least two ways that the family and its members support the health-seeking behavior of its members—as a resource in the help-seeking process and as a cultural symbol of the reason to stay healthy.

Many Americans with non-European backgrounds have been described as placing higher value on interdependence and strong family ties than do middle-class, non-Hispanic Euro-Americans. For these groups and especially for new immigrants, one's family network is believed to be an important resource for individuals seeking medical care (Meyerowitz et al., 1998). In fact several studies have documented the importance of a family recommendation to seek screening mammography (Zapka et al., 1991; Lerman et al., 1990).

Jackson and his colleagues (Kang and Bloom, 1993) argue that the care-seeking process contains two steps. First, the individual goes to family and friends to seek advice. Family members and friends assist the individual in determining whether the signs and symptoms are of sufficient concern to require follow-up. Family members may provide information as to where the necessary care can be found or may accompany the individual seeking care. Only when family members reinforce or encourage the care-seeking decision is care sought from the medical care system.

The importance of one's social network in receiving preventive health care has been documented in two studies of mammography for African–American women. In the first study, almost 30% of women with the largest social networks had a routine mammogram compared with less than 11% of women with smaller networks (Kang and Bloom, 1993). This relationship does not hold for routine Papanicolau screening (Pap smear) or breast self-examination (BSE), neither are functional measures of the social support network (instrumental support and emotional support) related to utilization of screening tests. In the second study, the same relationship was found when mammography and fecal occult blood tests (FOBT) were compared to other screening tests (Kang et al., 1994). With the exception of a study by Norman and Tudiver (1986), this finding did not hold up for other screening tests such as Pap smears, clinical breast examinations, and BSE where less complex behaviors are required. For the latter three tests, a decision to seek medical care is required since the screening test is generally received at the same visit, using the same physician, and in the same geographic location. For mammography, FOBT and, possibly, screening sigmoidoscopy, more complex decisions and sequential decisions need to made as the screening test is done at a different time and generally in a different location (Kang and Bloom, 1993; Kang et al., 1994). For some screening tests, such as a clinical breast examination or a Pap smear, the major issue is the individual's decision to seek care. Once at the physician's office, the major barrier is eliminated. For other tests, such as mammography and flexible sygmoidoscopy, a second appointment is required which, according to Jackson and colleagues, would require the individual to gain support of the family to follow through on the screening recommendation.

Our current research indicates that one's social network is more important in getting women to enter the medical care system to seek the initial mammogram than in rescreening. Presumably, one's network of immediate and more distant kin provides information, encouragement and, perhaps, the importance of screening to stay healthy for the 'family's sake.' Other factors, including one's initial experience in getting the mammogram and family obligations, come into play in seeking repeat screening (Bloom, et al., 1999b). Thus, for example, Moritz and Satariano (1993) found that elderly women who were their husband's caregivers, were either slower in seeking care or less likely to seek care even when they had breast symptoms. Consequently, their breast cancer was detected at a later stage. In our current research, obligations to other members of the family may also act as distractors from following preventive medical practices. Thus, we found that having more than one child prevented the low-income women in a current study from getting a screening mammogram (Bloom, et al., 1999b).

The family can play a symbolic role in facilitating early detection of cancer through screening. In many non-European cultures, the concept of 'familialism' is very important. Familialism refers to intra-family relationships, emphasizing the obligations of the individual to the family unit (Napoles-Springer, 1998). In her review of the literature, Napoles-Springer reported on findings from Hope and Heller's (1975) study of 197 Mexican–American women from San Antonio, Texas, The association between familialism and utilization was dependent on the type of care being sought. In the case of prenatal care, both social class and familialism were positively associated with earlier timing of prenatal care. However, individuals who were higher on the familialism scale were less likely to seek care for episodes of illness. Instead, advice was sought from relatives prior to seeking health care. In another study, Napoles-Springer reports that compared to African–Americans and non-Latino whites, Latinos reported a higher regard for the overriding interests of the family over individuals. Latino families also had the highest levels of geographically local extended family with whom they interacted frequently. Finally, a study by Suarez and Pulley (1995) found that a woman's adherence to a traditional family structure became independently and positively associated with recency of mammography screening, after controlling for the effects of socio-economic and language factors. The measure of family attitudes included four items that assess immediate family and extended family ties and three items about gender roles. More traditional family attitudes may be indicative of increased social support, which, in turn, may facilitate cancer screening.

In families that are very interdependent, members will do things for the good of the family rather than for themselves. Appealing to family membership then becomes an important way to encourage both men and women to get screened. This is especially important for screening tests that are uncomfortable and unappealing to carry out (Napoles-Springer, 1998; Perez-Stable et al., 1994).

In a sample of 106 low-income Mexican–American women attending a health clinic, Kang and Bloom (1993) found no association between the perceived quality of social support and the frequency of BSE. By contrast, Norman and Tudiver (1986) developed a measure of social support specific to BSE (e.g. the proportion of female family members and friends who practice BSE, husband/partner's attitude toward BSE, and physician's attitude) which was highly correlated with the frequency of the procedure. Napoles-Springer reported on the health screening behavior of 977 Latino women ages 40 to 74 who were interviewed by phone through random digit dialing in the San Francisco Bay area of northern California. Structural measures, such as the number of friends and relatives one sees, were not predictive of screening. However, elements of the family structure, such as being single or having fewer children, were related to not getting a Pap smear. Being single was also significantly associated with not having had a mammogram in the past 2 years (Napoles-Springer,

1998). Thus, it appears that, for Hispanic populations in California, the association is between the structural elements of the social network and screening rather than the functional aspects of social support.

SOCIAL SUPPORT AND CANCER TREATMENT

The roles that family members play following a cancer diagnosis may vary depending on the time post-diagnosis. Time following the cancer diagnosis can be conceptually divided into three conceptually distinct stages. In the current analysis, these stages—acute, extended, and permanent survival—will be used to better understand the role of family support. The possibility of recurrence cannot be overlooked. The role of family support following recurrence of the cancer will also be assessed. Finally, the use of interventions to increase well-being are becoming more common. The evidence that such interventions provide social support will be examined.

The acute stage of survival extends from the time of diagnosis through the first year. During this time the disease is diagnosed, the course of treatment is selected, and the treatment plan is implemented. Extended survival begins at the end of the first year and continues through the third year. For many types of cancer, this is the time when recurrences are detected. Permanent survival begins when concerns regarding recurrence diminish. This stage of survival extends into the future. Recurrence and the need for continuing care can occur at any time on the disease trajectory. Group interventions, or support groups, are also offered at any time.

ACUTE STAGE OF SURVIVAL

The time period during which cancer is being diagnosed, treatment is being proposed, and the selected treatment is in progress is a time of acute distress for both the newly diagnosed individual and the family. How the individual responds to the treatment and its side-effects is partially dependent on his/her normal way of coping with stressful life events. However, recent research also implicates the individual's relationship and interactions with key elements of his/her social network. In one study, for example, Neuling and Winefield (1988) determined that the spouse/partner was nominated by over 90% of married subjects as the most supportive family member. In this study, the type and amount of support was assessed in the hospital, 1 month and 3 months following surgery. The frequency of all sources of support dropped off over time. However, the patterns and types of support are of interest. Empathetic support was desired most from family members. Informational support was desired from the surgeon rather than the family. Satisfaction with support was related to reductions in anxiety and depression. In the hospital, satisfaction was based on the amount of perceived support of family members. At 1 month, satisfaction with support was based on the amount of informational support received from the surgeon. At 3 months, satisfaction with support was based on the patient's perception of the amount of support received not only from the family, but also from the the surgeon.

Analyses from the PABC (Psychological Aspects of Breast Cancer Study, 1987), also provide evidence of the importance of family support during the acute stage of survival. According to the statistical technique of a path model, family support explained most of the variance in social health (26%). While having a problem-oriented coping style was the strongest predictor of psychological well-being, family support was the second second strongest predictor, explaining 22% of the variance. Consistent with other research, the relationship between social support and psychological well-being was mostly indirect through its relationship to coping style (Bloom, 1982, 1993).

The quality of the woman's relationship with her family has powerful and direct effects on psychological well-being. The importance of the relationships to one's family was not predicted in this study (Bloom, 1993). Interactions with family members improve when the woman perceives herself to be emotionally supported. Older women reported better family relationships than younger women. Compared to divorced women, married, widowed and single women also reported better family relationships, whereas women who were more externally oriented and more anxious in their approach to problems described poorer relationships with family members. These findings suggest that the family is a primary source of support for the cancer patient throughout the first year following diagnosis.

EXTENDED STAGE OF SURVIVAL

Once active treatment ends, a major source of support for the cancer survivors also goes away. The supportive interactions with members of the medical team, including oncologists, nurses, and social workers, that occurred during treatment decrease. Visits to the oncologist for follow-up actually become sources of anxiety and distress as each test can potentially reveal disease recurrence. Family and friends become the major source of support for the recovering cancer patient.

However, from the family member's perspective, the end of treatment signals that the individual has recovered. The side effects of treatment have dissipated, energy has returned, emotions have stabilized, and the family is ready to move on. Family members may also expect the cancer survivor to move on and ruminate less about the cancer experience. Unfortunately, the patient may not be on the same wavelength. And, rightly or wrongly, the cancer patient may actually perceive that the amount of support he/she is receiving has diminished.

For example, in another analysis of the PABC data, Penman et al. (1986) found that women who received adjuvant therapy reported the highest levels of social support during treatment. Their analyses suggest that it is this additional support that seems to fall off, albeit to levels consistent with women who received surgical treatment for gall bladder disease and benign breast disease during the year after the diagnosis and treatment of their condition (Bloom and Kessler, 1994). In other words, compared to the amount of emotional support received during treatment, there is a decrease in the amount of support a woman with breast cancer receives following the end of treatment. However, the amount of support received compares favorably to women who have had surgery for a non-cancerous condition. The perceived (and actual) reduction in support may be compounded by an additional factor—reductions in social activity due to the consequences of treatment. Until the individual's energy levels return, she may only have resources to maintain obligatory activities such as work and may not be able to resume social activities (Bloom et al., 1991). Improvements in role functioning in daily activities and decreases in social isolation due to role constrictions are also related to increases in perceived emotional support (Bloom and Kessler, 1994).

In a recent pilot study of social support comparing Asian and Anglo women up to 3 years post-treatment, Anglo women reported having larger networks of family and friends than either Chinese or Japanese women. Japanese women had the smallest network outside of the family. Further, Anglo women reported needing social support more than Asian women for private feelings, advice (Anglos more than Chinese women), physical assistance, and positive feedback (Anglos more than Japanese women). Chinese and Japanese women did seek support from female relatives more than Anglo women, although this was not a statistically significant difference. One Japanese–American spouse wrote to the investigators explaining that information about one's illness is kept within the immediate family because advising family and friends of one's illness is interpreted as an 'imposition' on others, as well as an obligation to visit and bring a 'get-well' gift. The investigators interpret these findings as due to the belief that help-seeking behavior outside the family, let alone in the family, is seen as an act of embarrassment to the individual and to the family (Wellisch et al., 1999).

PERMANENT SURVIVAL

As time from treatment increases and the possibility of recurrence decreases, the expectation of family and friends is that the individual will resume his/her former roles. For some, this is possible. For others, physical changes wrought by cancer and its treatment are permanent. Energy level never completely returns to the pre-morbid state, the late effects of treatment are chronic and may progress becoming life-threatening over time (such as in cardiac disease), or, as in second cancers may be life threatening from the time of diagnosis (such as lung cancer, leukemia, or breast cancer which are late effects of Hodgkin's disease).

Since there is less research on long-term survivors, it is not surprising that even less is known about the support needs of this group (Bloom et al., 1999a). Some information is available from a large clinical series of Hodgkin's disease patients at Stanford University Medical Center, where seminal treatment advances took place. Hodgkin's disease is a form of lymphatic cancer. Once incurable and inevitably fatal, treatment advances have resulted in a current survival rate of over 80%. Thus, this clinical series provides a large number of cancer survivors in which the effects of social support can be examined.

The first study is a cross-sectional survey of 403 survivors who were assessed an average of 7.22 years after treatment (Bloom et al., 1991). About one-third of these survivors have been reassessed 12 years later, providing information on their change in support networks (Bloom et al., 1999a). Six different measures of social support were investigated and predicted to have different effects on social and psychological well-being. Findings indicated that the size of the network, as well as how integrated an individual is within the network provide a mechanism through which the survivor gains helpful advice and information, instrumental support, and emotional support. Network size and integration were found to have both direct and indirect effects on well-being. Size of the network had indirect effects on social functioning, while the integration into the network (Berkman and Symes, 1979) measure of social ties directly affected social functioning. Consistent with the work of others, emotional support and family support reduced depression and global mood distress (Schaefer et al., 1981; Bloom, 1982; Bloom and Spiegel, 1984).

Inconsistent with the work of Seeman and Syme (1987) and Finlayson (1976), greater use of instrumental support was related to poorer rather than better social functioning. Individuals who were further from treatment and women were more likely to report the greater use of instrumental supports suggesting that what was being measured was dependency rather than potential network support (Bloom et al., 1991).

Follow-up of 141 long-term survivors, now an average of 12 years post-treatment, indicates that significant reductions have occurred in the size of their social network. This reduction was found for both number of friends one sees and to whom one feels close and the number of relatives one sees and to whom one feels close. Since there was an increase of more than 10% in the number of survivors who got married and less than 3% who were divorced during this period, it is difficult to attribute the reduction in network size to family changes that are attributable to growing older (the median age of the sample was 33 years) (Bloom et al., 1999a). However, it is also unclear what this apparent social constriction means and what, in any, consequences it will have.

CONTINUING CARE

When cancer has recurred, the need for social support from family and friends may become even more important. As the individuals experience disease-induced reductions in social activities, their opportunities to interact with others are also reduced. Thus, as was discussed above, the amount of social support they receive will also be reduced. Therefore, it is important not to discourage individuals to continue with their social and work activities as long as possible. To offset the negative consequences of increased disability due to cancer, providing additional support through home visitation becomes very important.

Data from a study of 86 women with metastatic cancer of the breast provides some empirical verification (Bloom and Spiegel, 1984). Emotional support provided by the family was significantly related to outlook on life (this measure was negatively correlated with depression). Social activity, such as visiting and being visited by friends, going marketing and shopping, was also related to one's outlook on life. Individuals receive support from their social involvements within the family as well as outside the home. Both affect one's satisfactions with life and sense of fulfilment. One's outlook on life as well as one's opportunities to engage in social exchanges outside the home affect one's sense of how one is functioning.

Provocative findings have recently been published using SEER (surveillance, epidemiology, and end results) tumor registry data, which indicate that married individuals diagnosed with late stage cancer live longer than individuals who are single, divorced, or widowed (Lai et al., 1999). This finding is stable across cancer sites. The beneficial effect of marriage is stronger for men than for women. Marital status accounted for up to 19% of mortality differences among men and up to 9% among women; 16% of the difference is attributable to marriage for men and 8% for women. The most dramatic difference is for cancer of the urinary bladder, where median survival for married persons was 6 months whereas it was 2 months for single persons. We can only guess at the mechanisms that underlie this finding. The effects of social support, having a confidant, and the lack of social isolation may account for the favorable effect of being warned (Berkman and Syme, 1979). The effect may also be due to better eating habits or greater adherence to the medical regimen due to having a partner reinforcing the physician's recommendations.

SUPPORT INTERVENTIONS

Two different approaches to providing informational and emotional support for people undergoing stressful life experiences are described in the literature—individual counseling and support groups. Support groups provide opportunities for individuals to interact with 'similar others,' people who have gone through, or are going through, a similar experience and can relate to the cancer patient in a way that family and friends cannot.

Results of several studies indicate that these interventions are perceived as enjoyable, increase knowledge about cancer and its treatment, reduce the severity of cancer symptoms such as pain, reduce dysphoria, improve self-esteem and sense of efficacy, and may even lengthen survival in cancer patients (Jacobs et al., 1983; Spiegel et al., 1981, 1989; Spiegel and Bloom, 1983; Ferlic et al., 1979; Heinrich and Schag, 1985; Telch and Telch, 1986; Fawzy et al., 1993; Richardson et al., 1990). None of these studies explains the mechanism by which these beneficial effects occur, neither do they provide evidence that positive outcomes accrue for all participants, nor whether changes in the support system have occurred. It is also unclear whether interventions are more effective with individuals who are socially isolated than with individuals who perceive that they are receiving less support than they desire. Results from a survey of individuals attending support groups indicates that cancer patients turn to support groups because they perceive that their needs are being inadequately met by their support system, rather than because they are isolated (Falk and Taylor, 1983).

To date, most intervention studies have either not been concerned about the support system *per se* or have assumed, but not measured, deficiencies in the support system as an indication of the need for intervention. A study of recent widows by Raphael (1977) is an notable exception. Most respondents (86%) who perceived their support systems to be inadequate reported their health to be poor, while only 22% of respondents who perceived their support systems to be adequate reported poor health. When supportive counseling was provided to those with inadequate support systems, the percentage reporting poor health decreased significantly. Unfortunately, in this study the widows did not report whether their support system improved as a function of the intervention. Two recent studies of support group interventions provide further insights into the effects of support group interventions for cancer patients. The first is a carefully designed study which focused on the effects of information, peer support, and information plus peer support for women following a breast cancer diagnosis. Consistent with the findings of Jacobs and her colleagues (1983), Helgeson (1999) found that the information intervention was most effective, while the peer support group was the least effective, and the combination of education and peer support was intermediate. However, she also found that individuals with low emotional support benefited from the peer support intervention. In other words, the group with the lowest emotional support benefited the most. Preliminary evidence from a current study (Bloom et al., 1999b) which provided education plus coping skills is consistent with this. Women diagnosed with breast cancer when they were 50 or younger and who reported low emotional support benefited the most from the intervention. Anecdotal evidence suggests that the members of the support groups provided both emotional support and tangible support, such as rides to medical appointments and child care.

DISCUSSION AND CONCLUSIONS

These data provide preliminary evidence of the importance of social support in the recovery process. Individuals who belong to a network of relationships and receive emotional and instrumental resources from their family and friends have better social functioning, regardless of the time since diagnosis, the stage at which their cancer was diagnosed, or the type of treatment needed to control the disease. In addition, these data provide information of theoretical interest, referred to earlier, suggesting how the support system operates. Structural measures of social support, such as the size of one's social network and one's integration within the network, provide survivors with opportunities to receive functional support. Functional support can be in the form of information regarding the availability and location of resources, as well as how to interpret information, such as symptoms which might require further follow-up. It can also be in the form of emotional support, such as information that one is cared for and valued. And the resources one draws from the network can be in the form of instrumental support—the availability of personal sources of assistance, such as someone who can run an errand, or provide transportation, provide assistance with child care. These sources of functional support affect outcomes such as emotional and physical well-being. This model seems as true for individuals during the acute stage of survival as it is for individuals in the permanent stage of survival, as well as for individuals needing continuing care.

From a theoretical perspective, three issues stand out. First, epidemiological data provide compelling evidence for the importance of family support in cancer survival. For all cancer sites, married individuals with late-stage cancer live longer than do those who are single, widowed, or divorced. The marital advantage is greater for men than for women. What these data do not indicate is the mechanism by which marital status confers this advantage. Is having an intimate confidant who can provide emotional support the key? Alternatively, marital status may be a proxy for having someone available to provide needed resources, including nutrition and taking medications when appropriate. Nevertheless, these data are provocative and suggest directions for future research and the provision of services for those who are not married.

Second, the data reviewed suggest that the size of one's social network has both direct and indirect consequences. People in larger networks report better physical and social functioning. Larger social networks provide more opportunities for support provision. Individuals who have social constrictions in their networks which are either illness-imposed or culturally-imposed may be at greater risk for low social support and its consequences on coping and mental and physical well-being. Further research is needed to understand better how (a) culture defines one's illness experience and (b) differences in culture may affect one's ability to utilize social support resources provided outside the family circle.

Finally, recent randomized trials on the impact of support groups suggests that they do play an important role for individuals who are at high risk for physical and mental dysphoria, those with low social support. The outcomes for individuals who report low emotional support were significantly better than for comparable individuals who did not participate in the groups. Further, research is needed to develop methods to screen individuals for low social support that can be used in clinical settings.

REFERENCES

Antonofsky, A. (1993).   The structure and properties of the Sense of Coherence Scale. *Social Science and Medicine* **36**(6): 725–733.

Bandura, A. (1977).   Self-efficacy: toward a unifying theory of behavior change. *Psychology Reviews* **84**: 191–215.

Berkman L. and Syme S.L. (1979).   Social networks, host resistence and mortality: a nine-year follow-up study of Alameda County residents. *American Journal of Epidemiology* **109**: 186–204.

Berrera, M. Jr, (1986).   Distinctions between social support concepts, measures, and models. *American Journal of Community Psychology* **14**(4): 413–445.

Bloom, J.R. (1982).   Social support, accommodation to stress and adjustment to breast cancer. *Social Science and Medicine* **16**: 1329–1338.

Bloom, J.R. (1986).   Social support and adjustment to breast cancer. In B.L. Andersen (Ed.), *Women with Cancer: Psychological Perspectives*. pp. 204–229. New York: Springer-Verlag.

Bloom, J.R. (1993).   Social support of the cancer patient: the role of the family. In L. Baider, C.A. Cooper and A.K. De-Nour (Eds), *Cancer and the Family*. Chichester: Wiley.

Bloom, J.R. and Spiegel, D. (1984).   The effect of two dimensions of social support on the psychological well-being and social functioning of women with advanced breast cancer. *Social Science and Medicine* **19**(8): 831–837.

Bloom, J.R., Fobair, P., Spiegel, D., Cox, R.S., Varghese, A. and Hoppe, R. (1991).   Social supports and the social well-being of cancer survivors. *Advances in Medical Sociology*, **2**: 95–114.

Bloom, J.R. and Kessler, L. (1994).   Emotional support following breast cancer: a test of the stigma and social activity hypotheses. *Journal of Health and Social Behavior* **35**: 118–133.

Bloom, J.R., Stewart, S.L., Johnson, M. and Banks, P.J. (1998).   The intrusiveness of illness and quality of life of young women with breast cancer. *Psycho-Oncology* **7**(2): 89–110.

Bloom, J.R., Fobair, P., Hancock, S., Stewart, S.L. and Varghese, A. (1999a).   Psychosocial and physical well-being of long-term survivors from Hodgkin's disease. Conference on Long-Term Cancer Survivors, National Cancer Institute, National Institutes of Health, Bethesda, MD.

Bloom, J.R., Stewart, S, Banks, P.J., Johnston, M. and Peterson, I. (1999b).   Design and impact of a psycho-educational group intervention on the quality of life of young women with breast cancer. American Psychological Association Annual Meeting, Boston, MA.

Brown, D.R. and Gary, L.E. (1987).   Stressful life events, social support networks and the physical and mental health of urban black adults. *Journal of Human Stress* **13**(4): 165–174.

Clark, L. (1993).   Social cognition and health psychology. In R.S. Wyer and T.K. Stull (Eds), *Handbook of Social Cognition*, 2nd edn (pp. 239–288). Hillsdale, NJ: Erlbaum.

Cobb, S. (1976).   Social support as a moderator of life stress. *Psychosomatic Medicine* **38**(5): 300–314.

Cutrona, C. and Russell, D. (1990). Type of social support and specific stress: toward a theory of optimal matching. In B.R. Sarason, I. G. Sarason and G.R. Pierce (Eds), *Social Support: An Interactional View* (pp. 319–366). New York: Wiley.

Dakof, G.A. and Taylor, S.E. (1990). Victims' perceptions of social support: what is effective to whom? *Journal of Personality and Social Psychology* **58**: 80–89.

de Ruiter, J., deHaes, J. and Tempelaar, R. (1993). Cancer patients and their network: the meaning of the social network and social interactions for quality of life. *Supportive Care in Cancer* **1**: 152–155.

Durkheim, E. and Simpson, G. (Eds) (1951). *Suicide: A Study in Sociology*. Glencoe: Free Press.

Falk, R.L and Taylor, S.E. (1983). Support groups for cancer patients. *UCLA Cancer Bulletin* **10**: 13–15.

Fawzy, F.I., Fawzy, N.W., Hyum, C.S., Elashoff, R., Guthrie, D., Fahey, D.L. and Morton, D.L. (1993). Malignant melanoma. Effects of an early structured psychiatric intervention, coping and affective state on recurrence and survival 6 years later. *Archives of General Psychiatry* **50**: 681–689.

Ferlic, M., Goldman, A. and Kennedy, J.J. (1979). Group counseling in adult patients. *Cancer* **43**: 760–766.

Finlayson, A. (1976). Social networks as coping resources. *Social Science and Medicine* **10**: 97–104.

Fobair, P., Hoppe, R.T., Bloom, J.R., Cox, R., Varghese, A., Spiegel, D. (1986). Psychosocial problems among survivors of Hodgkin's disease. *Journal of Clinical Oncology* **4**(5): 805–814.

Heinrich, R.L. and Schag, C.C. (1985). Stress and activity management: group treatment for cancer patients and spouses. *Journal of Consulting Clinical Psychology* **53**: 439–446.

Helgeson, V.S., Cohen, S., Schultz, R. and Yasko, J. (in press). Effects of education and peer discussion group interventions on 6-month adjustment to breast cancer. *Archives of Psychiatry*.

Holahan, C.J. and Moos, R. (1981). Social support and psychological distress: longitudinal analysis. *Journal of Abnormal Psychology* **90**: 365–370.

Hope, S.K. and Heller, P.L. (1975). Alienation, familism, and the utilization of health services by Mexican Americans. *Journal of Health and Social Behavior* **16**: 304–314.

Horowitz, M.J. (1986). *Stress Response Syndromes* (2nd edn). Northvale, NJ: Jason Aronson.

House, J.S. (1981). *Work, Stress, and Social Support*. Reading, PA: Addison Wesley.

House, J.S. and Kahn, R.L. (1985). Measures and concepts of social support. In S. Cohen and S.L. Syme (Eds), *Social Support and Health* (pp. 83–108), New York: Academic Press.

Jacobs, C., Ross, R.D., Walker, I.M. and Stockdale, F.E. (1983). Behavior of cancer patients: a randomized study of the effects of education and peer support groups. *Journal of Clinical Oncology* **6**: 347–350.

Kang, S.H. and Bloom, J.,R. 1993). Social support and cancer screening in older African Americans. *Journal of the National Cancer Institute* **85**(9): 737–742.

Kang, S.H., Bloom, J.R. and Romano, P.S. (1994). Cancer screening among African American women: their use of tests and social support. *American Journal of Public Health* **84**(1): 104–106.

Kaplan, B.H., Cassel, J.C. and Gore, S. (1977). Social support and health. *Medical Care* **15**(5), (Suppl.): 47–57.

Lai, H., Lai, S., Krongrad, A., Trapido, E., Page, J.B. and McCoy, C.B. (1999). The effect of marital status on survival in late stage cancer patients: an analysis based on surveillance, epidemiology, and end results (SEER) data, in the United States. *International Journal of Behavioral Medicine* **6**: 150–177.

Lazarus, R. (1982). Stress and coping as factors in health and illness. In J. Cohen, J. Cullen, and R.M. Martin (Eds), *Psychosocial Aspects of Cancer* (pp. 163–190), New York: Raven.

Lerman, C., Rimer, B., Trock, B., Balshem, A., Engstrom, P.F. (1990). Factors associated with repeat adherence to breast cancer screening. *Preventive Medicine* **19**: 1–12.

Lichtman, R.R. and Taylor, S.E. (1986) Close relationships and the female patient. In B.L. Andersen (Ed.), *Women with Cancer: Psychological Perspectives*, New York: Springer-Verlag.

Lin, N. and Westcott, J. (1991). Marital engagement/disengagement, social networks, and mental health. In J. Eckenrode and S. Gore (Eds), *The Social Context of Coping* (pp. 213–237). Plenum: New York.

Manne, S.L., Taylor, K.L., Dougherty, J. and Kemeny, N. (1997). Supportive and negative responses in the partner relationship: their association with psychological adjustment among individuals with cancer. *Journal of Behavioral Medicine* **20**(2): 101–125.

Manne, S.L. and Zautra, A.J. (1989). Spouse criticism and support: their association with coping and psychological adjustment among women with rheumatoid arthritis. *Journal of Personality and Social Psychology* **56**: 608–617.

Meyerowitz, B.E., Richarson, J., Hudson, S., Leedham, B. (1998). Ethnicity and cancer outcomes: behavioral and psychosocial considerations. *Psychological Bulletin* **123**: 47–70.

Moos, R. (1976). *The Family Environment Scale*. Palo Alto, CA: Consulting Psychologists' Press.

Moritz, D.J. and Satariano, W.A. (1993). Factors predicting stage of breast cancer at diagnosis in middle-aged and elderly women: the role of living arrangements. *Journal of Clinical Epidemiology* **46**: 443–453.

Napoles-Springer, A. (1998). The effects of cultural factors on the health screening behaviors of Latino women. Unpublished doctoral dissertation, University of California, Berkeley, CA.

Neuling, S. and Winefield, H. (1988). Social support and recovery after surgery for breast cancer: frequency and correlates of supportive behaviors by family, friends, and surgerons. *Social Science Medicine* **27**: 385–392.

Norman, R.M.G. and Tudiver, F. (1986) Predictors of breast self-examination among family practice patients. *Journal of Family Practice* **22**(2): 149–153.

Nucholls, K.B., Cassel, J. and Kaplan, B. (1972). Psychosocial assets, life crises, and the prognosis of pregnancy. *American Journal of Epidemiology* **95**: 431–441.

Pearlin, L.I. and Johnson, J.S. (1977). Marital status, life-strains and depression. *American Sociological Review* **42***: 704–715*.

Penman, D., Bloom, J.R., Fotopolis, S., Cook, M., Murowski, B., Gates, C., Holland, J., Ross, R. and Flamer, D.P. (1986). The impact of mastectomy on self-concept and social function: a combined cross-sectional and longitudinal study with comparison groups. *Women and Health* **2**: 3–4.

Perez-Stable, E.J, Otero-Sabogal, R., Sabogal, F., McPhee, S.J. and Hiatt, R.A. (1994). Self-reported use of cancer screening tests among Latinos and Anglos in a prepaid health plan. *Archives of Internal Medicine* **154**: 1073–1081.

Psychological Aspects of Breast Cancer Group (1987). Psychological response to mastectomy. *Cancer* **59**(l): 189–196.

Raphael, B. (1977). Preventive intervention with the recently bereaved. *Archives of General Psychiatry* **34**: 1450–1454.

Richardson, J.L., Shelton, D.R., Krailo, M. and Levine, A.M. (1990). The effects of compliance with treatment on survival among patients with hematologic malignancies. *Journal of Clinical Oncology* **8**(2): 356–364.

Schaefer, C., Coyne J. and Lazarus, R. (1981). The health-related functions of social support. *Journal of Behavioral Medicine* **4**: 381–406.

Seeman, T.E. and Syme, S.L. (1987). Social networks and coronary artery disease: a comparison of the structure and function of social relations as predictors of disease. *Psychosomatic Medicine* **49**: 341–354.

Spiegel, D., Bloom, J.R. and Gottheil, E. (1983). Family environment as a predictor of adjustment to metastatic breast carcinoma. *Journal of Psychosocial Oncology* **1**(1): 33–44.

Spiegel, D., Bloom, J.R. and Yalom, I. (1981). Group support for patients with metastatic cancer. *Archives of General Psychiatry* **38**: 527–533.

Spiegel, D., Bloom, J.R., Kraemer, H.C. and Gottheil, E. (1989). Effect of psychosocial treatment on survival of patients with metastatic breast cancer. *Lancet* **2**: 888–891.

Suarez, L. and Pulley, L. (1995). Comparing acculturation scales and their relationship to cancer screening among older Mexican–American women. *Journal of National Cancer Institute Monographs* **18**: 41–47.

Telch, C.F. and Telch, M.J. (1986). Group coping skills instruction and supportive group therapy for cancer patients: a comparison of strategies. *Journal of Consulting and Clinical Psychology* **54**(6): 802–808.

Thoits, P. (1995). Stress, coping and social support processes: where are we? What next? *Journal of Health and Social Behavior* **Special Issue**: 53–79.

Wallston, B.S., Wallston, K.A., Kaplan, G.D. and Maides, S.A. (1976). Development and validation of the Health Locus of Control (HLC) Scale. *Journal of Consulting Clinical Psychology* **44**(4): 580–585.

Wellman, B. and Wortley, S. (1990). Different strokes for different folks: community ties and social support. *American Journal of Sociology* **96**(3): 558–588.

Wellisch, D., Kagawa-Singer, M., Reid, S.L., Lin, Y., Nishikawa-Lee, S. and Wellisch, M. (1999). An exploratory study of social support: a cross-cultural comparison of Chinese, Japanese, and Anglo-American breast cancer patients. *Psycho-Oncology* **8**: 207–219.

Wiley, C. and Sillman, R. (1990). The impact of disease on the social support experiences of cancer patients. *Psycho-Oncology* **8**(1): 79–96.

Wortman, C.B. (1984). Social support and the cancer patient: conceptual and methodological issues. *Cancer* **53**(Suppl.): 2339–2360.

Wortman, C.B. and Lehman, D.R. (1985). Reactions to victims of life crises: support attempts that fail. In I.B. Sarason & B.R. Sarason (Eds), *Social Support: Theory, Research and Application* (pp. 463–489). The Hague: Martinus Nijhof.

Zapka, J.G., Stoddard, A., Maul, L. and Costanza, M.E. (1991). Interval adherence to mammography screening guidelines. *Medical Care* **29**(8): 697–707.

5

A Cross-cultural Comparison of Social Support Among Asian–American and Euro–American Women Following Breast Cancer

MARJORIE KAGAWA-SINGER and TU-UYEN NGUYEN

School of Public Health and Asian–American Studies,
University of California, Los Angeles, USA

Several reviews exist on family dynamics and coping with cancer in Western cultures (Lewis, 1986; Germino, 1993; Kristjansen and Aschroft, 1994, Baider, 1994), and social support for Anglo–American women with breast cancer has been extensively studied and demonstrated to be a positive factor in health outcomes (Chipp and Green, 1980; Rosaldo and Lamphere, 1974). For example, the positive effects of social support in breast cancer have been noted with regard to emotional well-being as well as with regard to length of survival following diagnosis (Spiegel, 1990). Lack of social support for recently diagnosed breast cancer patients was predictive of high distress upon follow-up 2 years later. Although the construct of social support has been demonstrated to be beneficial, its effect appears to occur at multiple levels in multiple forms and the pathway between social involvement (social ties) and social functioning appears direct, and others indicate that the pathway between social support and psychological well-being appears to be mediated by coping (Lichtman and Taylor, 1986, Bloom, 1986). Thus, social support is multidimensional, and involves tangible, emotional, informational, and physical assistance. Moreover, social support is commonly recognized to be provided by a network of individuals who play a significant role in the recipient's life (Marshall and Funch, 1983). Common to all forms of social support is the family.

Researchers and practitioners recognize, that the function of social support may be universal, but the form it takes differs among cultural groups: who constitutes the social support network, what is considered to be appropriate social support and help, how this need for social support is communicated, and how the needs are met appear to differ. In this chapter, we will address these differences by comparing Asian and Western cultures.

Cancer and the Family, 2nd Edn. Edited by L. Baider, C. L. Cooper and A. Kaplan De-Nour
© 2000 John Wiley & Sons, Ltd

Except for Gotay's chapter in the first edition of Baider's books, however, reviews in the literature provide limited information specifically on families from non-Western cultures, and even fewer studies have explored the construct and effect of social support on adjustment to breast cancer in Asian–American (AA) families (Long and Long, 1982; Ohnuki-Tierney, 1984; Kleinman, 1980; Kalish and Reynolds 1976; Shon and Ja, 1982). Interventions designed by mainstream US practitioners and researchers seem ineffective for AAs as a group and individually as well (Alagaratnam and Kung, 1986; Kagawa-Singer, 1988; Lin, 1990). For example, Solis et al. (1989) reported difficulties in attempting to start an 'I Can Cope' program in an Asian community. The intent of this chapter is to broaden the research and practice paradigms for family support during the cancer experience for AA breast cancer patients.

AAs are the fastest growing ethnic populations in the USA, and are quite diverse. The AA category is an aggregated political construct comprising over 50 distinct cultural groups. Our initial discussion focuses on some of the commonalties among the major AA cultures to highlight significant differences between Asian and Western constructs of both the individual self and the family.

We begin with a brief overview and comparison of Asian cultures with Western traditions, define family and social support from an anthropological perspective, and then provide a case example of a comparison of social support among Chinese–American, Japanese–American and Euro–American women following breast cancer treatment to emphasize the need to differentiate among the subgroups of AAs to avoid stereotypical responses. Following this discussion, we outline some implications for practice with different populations of AA breast cancer patients. Attention to these differences will promote culturally informed, and potentially more accurate, patient and family assessments. We close the chapter with a discussion of recommendations for future research in family therapy with AA cancer patients.

DEFINITIONS OF SOCIAL SUPPORT

We will first provide a brief overview of social support, and then describe how varying structures and communication patterns in families in various cultures frame the source, form and process of providing social support.

Social support has emerged as a significant and positive moderator of illness, including breast cancer (Berkman, 1982; DiMatteo and Hays, 1981). Cobb (1976) found that social support mediated the effects of stress on health. Bloom (1982) found that social support directly affected coping and indirectly affected psychological adjustment in breast cancer patients, and others have shown that support networks that provide emotional and/or tangible support create a stress-buffering effect (Dunkel-Schetter, 1984; Hirsch, 1981; Wethington and Kessler, 1986).

Family, friends, and health professionals have been identified as the most important sources of support for patients with serious illnesses (DiMatteo and Hays, 1981; Wortman and Conway, 1985). Among these three sources of support, families are perceived as most helpful in most cultures (Tebbi et al., 1985; Dunkel-Schetter, 1984; Nueling and Winefield, 1988; Rose, 1990).

Definitions of social support have ranged from the specific (information that one is cared for; Cobb, 1976) to the general (any input which moves an individual towards a desired goal; Tolsdorf, 1976). For the purpose of the present review, the types of functions comprising social support were identified as: emotional, material aide, advice and information, positive feedback, physical assistance, and social participation (Barrera et al., 1981), and the support network includes all individuals who constantly provide support among an individual's social contacts (Ell, 1984). Because of the limited understanding of the nature of social support in Asian–American populations, this more general and comprehensive definition will be used (Ell et al., 1988; Lauver and Ho, 1993), especially since 'family' constructs are quite varied among cultures and the patterns of communicating care differ considerably as well.

In order to study social support in AA cultures, two assumptions must be questioned. The first is the assumption that the dependent variable measured, usually individual well-being, is the same in all cultures, and the second is the assumption that social support is free.

Social support is assumed to promote emotional, physical and social well-being equally in all cultures, but a Western construct of individual well-being has been used to operationalize this construct. In this chapter, we provide an alternative construct of personhood based in an anthropological or psychocultural framework which is described in greater detail below.

The second assumption is that social support is provided altruistically and can be accepted without a cost. Implicit in the construct of social support is an exchange, be it material, informational, physical assistance or emotional support. The exchange of the support implies a cost that is often overlooked. When considering cultures that are sociocentric or network-focused compared to those that are individualistic, the exchange is central to the bonds among its members and should be made explicit to also understand the patient's ability or desire to receive or accept the support offered, as well as its perceived effectiveness.

Four types of exchange theory have been described for social support (Shibusawa and Kagawa-Singer, 1999):

- *Symmetrical exchange.* The recipient reciprocates by providing the giver with the equivalent amount which he/she received in the form of materials goods or emotional or instrumental support. This is seen in contractual relationships, and is the type of relationship most often assumed to be the dominant form in Western, Euro–American relationships. Both individuals enter into the exchange freely and with the expectation that the recipient will reciprocate in kind.
- *Asymmetrical exchange based on intimacy or 'amae'* (Doi, 1971). The recipient receives help while acknowledging that he/she is presuming on the caregiver's kindness and generosity. There is an implicit understanding that the recipient does not have to reciprocate. The caregiver gains satisfaction from the sense of connectedness and intimacy that results from this exchange. The reciprocation, however, takes the form of indebtedness or obligation. The recipient must be genuine in receiving the support provided. Overt acts of reciprocation would be perceived as denying the 'intimacy' that is presumed to exist between them.
- *Asymmetrical exchange based in indebtedness.* The recipient becomes indebted to the caregiver because he/she cannot reciprocate for the support provided. This leads to passive dependency in which recipients do not feel that they have the right to assert themselves or complain since they are indebted to the provider. When they cannot reciprocate the care they receive, the feeling may well be one of shame.

- *Asymmetrical exchange based on non-reciprocated receiving or 'banking'.* The recipient does not reciprocate because he/she gave in the past, and feels that he/she is collecting on the 'banked' support and services provided in the past. This is often seen in parental response to the care and support provided by grown and independent children. The recipient does not feel obligated or ashamed.

These four types of exchange are obviously ideals. The sense of 'balance' in reciprocation, either in kind or timing, is rarely so neatly perceived. Nonetheless, the differentiation allows for further discussion of variations between Asian and dominant Euro–American styles (Williams, 1997). All forms, however, emphasize the relationship inherent in any provision of social support. What must be kept in mind is that the cost of the exchange on the relationship depends upon the congruence of expectations between the recipient and the provider, and how these expectations are communicated.

CROSS-CULTURAL DEFINITIONS OF FAMILY

The primary source of social support provided to individuals experiencing distress in all cultures is from the family, but 'family' constructs are quite varied among cultures and the patterns of communicating care differ considerably as well. Anthropologically, the family is the unit of care that ensures the survival and well-being of its descendents. From this ecologic perspective, 'family' can mean a group of individuals who work together for sustenance and survival as well as a community to which the family and its individuals belong for security and well-being.

From a psychodynamic perspective, 'family' can be broadly defined as 'two or more people in a committed relationship from which they define a sense of identity' (Chilman et al., 1988). This distinction is important to recognize because the structure, purpose, and dynamics of families differ from culture to culture. Therefore, an understanding of the cultural milieu of behavior is fundamental to the provision of social support in times of crisis, for appropriate, adaptive and culturally congruent means to provide social support within the family are defined within this social framework.

Families differ significantly among cultures along several dimensions that affect how social support is provided. For example, difference can occur along the dimensions of structure, life cycle stage, roles, and communication norms. American culture places value on youth; consequently, the elderly are often devalued (Gotay, 1996). In most other cultures of the world, however, the elderly are respected and accorded a coveted status which comes with their age and experience. As Sue and Sue (1987) point out, Confucian philosophy helps to structure family roles and authority and power relationships by providing a set of rules aimed at promoting loyalty, respect, and harmony among family members. In Chinese and Japanese cultures, particularly, familial obligations are of utmost importance, including the filial duty to care for parents in their old age. As a result, social support structures in Asian cultures are built-in through cultural norms and rules.

Families have been studied structurally (who makes up a family) as well as interactionally (how these individuals relate with one another) (see Acock and Demo, 1994; Chilman et al., 1988; Rolland, 1994; Tseng and Hsu, 1991), but few psycho-oncology studies have placed the function of the family within a cultural context. To begin, we provide a definition of culture that will form the framework within which social support is discussed in this chapter.

CULTURE

Culture can be described as comprising seven nested layers that form an ecologic context for its members: Environment, Economy, Technology, Religion/World View, Language, Social Structure, and Beliefs and Values (Hammond, 1978). Evaluation of each layer provides sets of variables that can be measured, and the observed individual or family behavior should be interpreted within the cultural context using an analysis of the interaction among the variables. Thus, the cultural context is dynamic and defines reality for its members to assure their survival. Within this reality or world view, the individual's purpose in life is defined, and proper, sanctioned behavior is prescribed. These beliefs, values, and behaviors of a culture provide its members with some degree of personal and social meaning for human existence, learned through tradition and transmitted from generation to generation through sanctioned modes of communication that are learned from people whom the culture has deemed essential for desired 'personhood' (Kagawa-Singer and Chung, 1994).

Culture, then, serves two functions: (a) it provides the integrative beliefs and values that provide an individual a sense of identity, and (b) it provides the rules for behavior, the functional aspects, that enable the group to survive physically, provide for its welfare, and provide the means for the individual to gain a sense of self-worth, belonging, and continuity. Incorporation or enculturation facilitates social integration and communication among its members.

An ethnic group is a self-perceived cultural group that resides within another society and permits appropriate interactive behavior among its members with a sense of belonging, meaning in life, and ultimate loyalty (Berreman, 1982; DeVos and Romanucci-Ross, 1995). This concept of ethnicity, or subcultural identity, is much more fundamental to a person's identity than the more superficial glossing of the practice of identifiable cultural traditions (e.g., Zane and Sue, 1991) or the erroneous interchangeable use of ethnicity, culture, and race (Gregory and Sanjek, 1996). Ishi, the last Yaqui Indian of his tribe in California, stated the fundamental nature of cultural identity to personhood when he commented on the death of his culture:

> [Ethnic] identity is found in the 'cup of custom' passed on by one's parents from which one drinks the meaning of existence. Once the cup is broken, one can no longer taste life (DeVos and Romanucci-Ross, 1982, p. 388).

Individual identity, according to this interpretation, is dependent upon a construct of self that is defined and nurtured within a cultural milieu. Culture, as noted, is designed to ensure the survival and well-being, emotionally and physically, of its members. As such, cultures are designed to provide for three basic human needs: a sense of safety, a sense of integrity, and a sense of belonging (Kagawa-Singer, 1993), and most behavior among its members is directed to maintain these three essentials of life (DeVos and Romanucci-Ross, 1982; Durkheim, 1947, Goldschmidt, 1959; Maslow, 1973). Safety is defined as a sense of physical security and well-being. A sense of integrity is achieved by being a productive and integral member of one's social group, and a sense of belonging is to be a desired and nurtured member of a group with which one wishes to identify. Culture provides the definitions and means to fulfill these three basic needs, and as such, both the specific objectives for emotional well-being and the appropriate means to achieve those ends will vary according to the pattern of each group's world view.

Clinically and theoretically, practitioners and researchers must understand that cultures are not monolithic, static, or homogeneous, and neither do the individuals within any cultural group hold the beliefs and value system to the same degree that is characterized by the group as a whole.

The validity of an analysis of behavior taken out of context is questionable, even within one culture. When cross-cultural assessments are made without understanding the modifications that occur within a context, the validity of the analysis is significantly threatened. Moreover, the changes that occur during acculturation in any individual who lives in a multicultural society are not unidirectional, i.e., acculturation only in the direction of that of the dominant culture. In actuality, cultures blend at the 'edges' of interaction (Hallowell, 1955) and are continually transformed through interactions with each other unless there is conscious effort to be insulated and exclusive. Most immigrants and refugees in the USA have become at least bicultural—even generations later. That is, they have learned the dominant set of beliefs, values and behaviors well enough to function in mainstream society, but they have maintained their traditional beliefs and values as well. They become adept at switching from one set of values and behaviors to another, according to the demands of the social situation. An individual's identity may well be a synthesis of two or more cultures. Difficulties and miscommunication arise, however, when cues of communication are misread or misinterpreted by using the wrong template of interpretation, or individuals are not aware of competing sets of cultural edicts that they hold for identity and behavior.

VARIATIONS IN FAMILY STRUCTURE

Modal family structure differs considerably in different cultures. Traditionally, the most prominent family unit in North America is the nuclear family, consisting of parents and their immediate children. In contrast, the concept of 'family' in other cultures of the world carries a broader definition, which may include grandparents, aunts and uncles, cousins, and (in many Asian cultures) ancestors. The dominant American definition focuses on the intact nuclear family. Black families tend to focus on a wide network of kin and community. For Italians, the 'nuclear' family has little meaning; to them, 'family' means a strong, tightly knit, three- or four-generational family which also includes godparents and old friends (McGoldrick et al., 1982).

It is important to note, however, that each group's way of relating to a crisis situation and help-seeking will reflect its differing attitudes toward family, group identity, and outsiders, even though certain family characteristics, such as male dominance and role complementarity, are somewhat similar.

The Chinese include in their definition of 'family' all their ancestors and all their descendants. Their conception of time is very different and death does not create the same distinction it does for Westerners (Shon and Ja, 1982, Chapter 10).

The Japanese construct of the family is similar to the Chinese. One 'household' includes the extended lineage. Marriages are patrilineal, and a woman's role is to uphold the honor of the family. Japanese and Chinese cultures are traditionally similar in the role of the women, and the implications for meeting dependency needs in the cancer situation should include knowledge of gender role requirements.

Another important component of family structure is who holds the power in family decision-making. For instance, gender may dictate inheritance and kinship patterns, while dynamics between husband–wife, parent–child and brother–sister bonds may dictate roles of social support and decision-making (Tseng and Hsu, 1991). In addition, age is a critical component in the power equation within family interactions.

COMMUNICATION AND HELP SEEKING

Family relationships are built through culturally prescribed communication patterns for affection (including both verbal and non-verbal expressions), rituals, and roles among different family members. Adaptability and cohesiveness are significant aspects of how well a family can adjust to stress. Therefore, serious illness in a family member is a stressor that will most likely disrupt normal family interaction patterns and role relationships. Nevertheless, the ways families in different cultures adjust their interaction patterns and role relationships in response to cancer in AA families has not been well-studied. Nilchikovit et al. (1993) compared 'sick role behavior' in Anglo and Asian cultures. They stated that in Asian cultures, a person who is sick is given much more permission for regression than is granted or tolerated in American culture. In fact, the way that the family takes care of the patient in Asian cultures may seem 'infantilizing' to the American observer (p. 47). As a result, family functioning can change either for the better or for the worse when family attention is focused on a serious disease like cancer. That is, in dealing with cancer, a family can become closer and develop more appreciation and understanding of the family unit and each other or it is possible that under the same stressful conditions, a family may assume traditional practices of their culture, even if they adhere to 'modern' values under normal circumstances, and this dissonance can create division and increased distress. Conflicts in objectives among the family and health practitioners compounds the difficulty.

To understand how social support is provided among members of a cultural group, the rules of communication within the social network provide therapists and researchers with windows into the structure of personhood, self-worth and sense of integrity for each culture. One model that facilitates understanding of different cultural nuances and the purposes of particular styles is Doi's (1985) construct of the self, which is divided into the public self (tatemae) and the inner or true self (honne). Cultures vary in the degree to which one aspect supersedes the other in social interactions. Using this model, the Euro–American is expected to present his/her true inner self in most encounters and not use a public presentation of self. The use of the public self is considered deceptive or insincere. In contrast, the Asian individual would be expected to conceal his/her true self out of respect for the 'other'. Open communication of the 'true self' only occurs once the 'other' has become part of the inner circle, and then only on rare occasions. In an Asian culture, one uses the public presentation of self even with family, in order to maintain the 'face' or social integrity of the 'other', and nurtures the ability to communicate non-verbally to discern the true essence of the communication behind the words. Such differences in modes and expectations of communication create significant barriers to the provision of social support by families with therapists from cultures different than their own, or among family members with varying expectations of communicating caring. When other essential modifying factors in cross-cultural encounters are added into the family construct, such as varying levels of acculturation to mainstream US norms of communication that exist among parents and children or siblings, language use, degree of traditionalism held among family members, gender, and age, effective communication and the provision of perceived support becomes even more challenging.

Family cohesiveness and conformity are fundamental Asian values and practices, and the style of indirect or public presentation of self is highly valued. Direct communication of emotional feelings is discouraged. The preferred modes of emotional communication are through non-verbal indirect behaviors, rather than direct verbalization (Johnson et al., 1974; Morris, 1990; Uba, 1994). In social interactions, Asians try to anticipate the needs of others so that people do not have to directly verbalize their needs and thereby appear demanding, and impose their needs onto others. Ho (1990) discusses how Eastern beliefs see meeting adversity without complaint as a sign of dignity, while the converse is seen as weakness. Thus, these cultural proscriptions and values underlying behavior may stifle one's ability to seek support, not only from friends and professionals, but from family members as well. Expressing such needs might be interpreted as a lack of character.

The literature indicates that Anglo–American breast cancer patients utilize formal support groups as well as talking with friends and health care professionals as effective and modal responses to the emotional and social upheaval created by the cancer experience (Ell, 1984; Taylor et al., 1986). Clinical studies of mental health, however, indicate that Asian communities under-utilize available mental health services, according to their representation in the general population (Leong, 1986; Durvasula and Sue, 1992, Okazaki, 1994; Sue, 1977; Sue and Sue, 1974).

These variations in communication style arise from the hierarchical social rules of communication in Asian cultures and are most clearly seen in the traditional family—the microcosm of the greater social structure. The person in authority is expected to anticipate the needs of the dependent individual (Doi, 1971; Kim et al., 1992). Thus, if the patient overtly requests help, such a request would indicate that the provider was unable to successfully anticipate the needs of the sick individual. Such requests must either be made discreetly or indirectly or not made at all.

FAMILY INTERACTION

A very important consideration in understanding family functioning in all cultures is the developmental stage of the family life cycle. This life cycle is commonly divided into six stages, with corresponding major tasks: young single adults, new marriage, family with young children, family with adolescents, launching the children, moving on, and later life (cf. Danielson et al., 1993; Rolland, 1994). Of course, while these stages provide useful ways to view challenges faced by families dealing with cancer, Tseng and Hsu (1991) point out that life cycles vary considerably across cultures. While different milestones may be meaningful cross-culturally, 'transition between stages may be clear-cut or blurred, and each stage may be short, long, or even absent' (p. 46). For example, in the Hmong culture, youth traditionally married at 13–15 years of age, and had children soon after (Donnely, 1994). In contrast, the average age of marriage in Japan is 28 for women and 30 for men, and in the USA the average age at marriage occurs at a similar time. The age at first pregnancy for professional women in the USA is rising, and women are often in their mid-30s when their first child is born. Traditional Hmong women might theoretically be grandmothers at this same age. The dissonance in implicit expectations between the Western-trained practitioner of proactive, assertive expression of need by patients, and the Asian–American woman who expects her needs to be anticipated by the person in authority, can adversely affect the accuracy of assessments of need, the design of appropriate interventions, and the quality of the care provided (Lai and Yu, 1990).

EFFECTS OF FAMILY STRUCTURE ON SOCIAL SUPPORT WHEN CONFRONTING CANCER

The psychosocial cancer literature in the USA stresses the centrality of family to support, but also recognizes professional and lay support mechanisms as essential to a breast cancer patient's support network. Several assumptions are implicit in this model, however, that may not translate as effectively for AA women, because AA families are central to a woman's identity in a manner that is foreign to Western constructs of the self in relation to the family, roles of women and communication styles (Kagawa-Singer, 1988; Chung and Kagawa-Singer, 1994). The form of social support, who provides it, and how it is provided may differ considerably among Judeo–Christian Euro–American women and AA women.

First, for AA families from cultures influenced by Confucianism and Buddhism, family includes ancestors and descendents. The burden of behavior and character reflects on the honor of ancestors and on the continuity of the family line. Second, women have a subordinate role in these cultures that place additional constraints on behavior and communication.

In contrast, differing outlooks on life or cultural world views create varying lenses on the sanctioned way members of that cultural group perceive life and, as noted in the definition earlier, the ways of coping with adversity that support the cultural construction of individual integrity, proper role fulfillment, and rules of belonging (Kluckhohn and Strodbeck, 196?). Psychosocial assessment in oncology would be strengthened by placing emotional responses within an accurate cultural context. For example, McGoldrick (1982) describes different cultural outlooks on life by various subcultural or ethnic groups within the 'white' category. WASP (white Anglo-Saxon Protestant) optimism leads to confidence and flexibility in taking initiative, but such cheerfulness also leads to the inability to cope with tragedy or to engage in mourning (McGill and Pearce, 1982; Chapter 21, this volume). Optimism becomes a vulnerability when they must contend with tragedy. Their world view provides few philosophical or expressive ways to deal with situations in which optimism, rationality, and belief in the efficacy of individuality are insufficient. In some situations independence and individual initiative work well, but in situations in which dependence on the group is the only way to ensure survival, members of the WASP culture may feel lost and inadequate.

Feelings of dependency or emotionality create a sense of being 'out of control' for WASPs, whereas the Irish may be more concerned about 'making a scene', and Italians may feel guilty about sharing emotions with 'outsiders' that may indicate disloyalty to the family, because they feel they should only use outsiders as a last resort. Greeks, in a similar fashion, may feel that divulging personal emotional needs to outsiders would result in an insult to their pride or *filotimo*, for the message would be that their families were not strong enough to meet their needs. We use these examples to stress that the dominant US culture is not homogenous either, and comparative studies of white and AA cultures need to be more specific as well to account for subcultural differences in the US white population.

The Chinese may somatize when they are under stress and may seek medical care rather than mental health services. Somatization, however, does not mean that they are not aware of their psychological distress, but rather that they see the physical body to be the appropriate vehicle through which to address their psychological distress. This is somatopsychic, rather than psychosomatic, distress (Kawanishi, 1992). The distinction is critical, because too often, the connotation of psychosomatic disorders is that the individuals are not aware of the 'true' psychological basis of their distress. Somatopsychic distress, on the other hand, acknowledges that the individuals recognize their psychological pain, but they may see their physical body as the appropriate medium to both express and heal this inter-related distress. Notably, in a study by Kagawa-Singer et al. (1996), no differences were noted among Chinese–American, Japanese–American and Anglo–American women following breast cancer treatment in the report of symptoms, but the Asian–American women did not seek assistance for their somatic problems, whereas the Anglo–American did. Perhaps the difference is more in the assumptions or stereotypes of the practitioners than in the actual reporting of the women.

COMPARISONS OF SOCIAL SUPPORT FOR ANGLO- AND ASIAN–AMERICAN WOMEN

Thus far we have created the context within which social support in AA families is provided. Each cultural world view prescribes the structure of the family, the roles of its members, and the norms of the provision of both the form and mode of social support. In this section, we present the findings of one study that demonstrated the culturally framed provision of social support for AA women.

Very little work has been published in the Western literature to describe the form or manner in which social support is obtained for AA women in general (Uba, 1994). The few studies that have examined the impact of cancer in different cultural and ethnic groups emphasize that caution must be exercised when using Western conceptual categories and instruments for measurement with groups for which they have not been validated (Lee et al., 1989; Kesserling et al., 1986; Dodd et al., 1985; Cohen et al., 1988). Only two studies have examined the impact of cancer on AAs (Japanese–Americans and Chinese–Americans) (Kagawa-Singer, 1988; Kagawa-Singer et al., 1996). These studies indicated that the social support system for AAs with cancer differed from that of the Anglo–American, mainstream culture in the USA upon which most studies of social support were based. Japanese–American and Chinese–American cancer patients reported the same degree of side effects and disruption from treatment as the Anglo–American patients, but requested much less assistance. Their networks were significantly smaller, and the members of the network consisted of primarily immediate female family members.

The symbolic meaning of cancer also affects how patients and their families react to the cancer experience. In Asian cultures, cancer is viewed as a disease brought on by character weaknesses, genetic predisposition, and perhaps by personal lifestyle choices such as diet and employment. In the Western ethos, health is considered a natural part of life while illness is not, and interventions are focused more upon the pathology of organs or organ systems than the individual (Murphy, 1990). Anglo–Americans, then, tend to view cancer in a mechanistic fashion. Cancer is caused by external factors outside one's personal control that must be cured with proper Western medical treatments and cures (Sontag, 1977; Kagawa-Singer, 1988). The Asian perspective of a personal, intrinsic, moral causation of cancer would discourage seeking medical advice and social support outside one's immediate circle because of the social stigma attached to the disease.

In contrast, the more external, mechanistic perspective held by younger, more educated Anglo–Americans, permits a plea for assistance to be made to a broader network because there is less personal responsibility attached to the causation (Gordon, 1990). As AAs acculturate, they may hold views more closely resembling that of the dominant cultural perspective. Importantly, Western modes of dealing with breast cancer also encourage interpersonal interaction in the family through discussing and sharing aspects of the breast cancer experience (Northouse, 1994), whereas, as noted earlier, AA families tend not to practice or value highly, an open style of communication.

Although language and financial barriers do exist, cultural barriers also seem to be a major factor that militates against the use of mental health services. For example, Asians are taught to be self-sufficient and to seek help only from within the family if they cannot cope with the situation on their own (Uba, 1994). Seeking help outside of the family indicates weakness in character and would be perceived as shameful and disgraceful to the family (Lee, 1982; Araneta, 1982; Tung, 1985).

Each ethnic group's culture provides sanctioned modes of coping with the cancer experience (Kagawa-Singer, 1995). AAs, however, have an added burden of conflicting styles of coping between Western and Eastern cultures, as described earlier (e.g., assertiveness vs. humility; expressiveness vs. discreteness) that may add to the stress experienced from the disease. Kagawa-Singer (1988) found that Japanese–American and Anglo–American cancer patients perceived their cancer differently and used culturally identifiable means of adapting to the illness experience. Neither style of coping would have been appropriate for the other: coping modes that were effective for the Anglo–American cancer patients would not have been as effective for the Japanese–American patients and vice versa. These cultural differences in communication and coping styles can create conflicts not only between practitioners but among patients and their family members as well, depending upon their varying levels of acculturation and assimilation (Lavizzo-Mourey and Mackenzie, 1996).

Given the lack of data on AA social support factors in breast cancer and the differences in cultural styles of patterns between Asian and Anglo–Americans, the first author and colleagues conducted a pilot study investigating the differential impacts of breast cancer among Asian–American and Anglo–American women and their families (Wellisch et al., 1999).

Forty-six Anglo– and Asian–American women (13 Anglo–American, 18 Chinese–American, and 15 Japanese–American women) were assessed 6 months to 3 years post-treatment. Assessments consisted of a semi-structured interview plus standardized psychological tests that measured social support networks and interactions. The results showed: (a) Anglo–American women indicated greater need for social support than either of the two Asian–American groups in 66% of the categories; (b) no differences were found between the three ethnic groups in receipt of emotional or tangible social support; and (c) the network size and composition differed significantly in 83% of the categories between the Anglo group and at least one of the Asian groups. Significantly, differences were also found between the Chinese–American and Anglo–American groups as well.

Differences among all three groups in social support were in size and make-up of the networks, mode or types of social support provided, and perceived adequacy of social support.

RESULTS

The three groups were similar in terms of marital status, educational level, and degree of acculturation (Suinn et al., 1987), but differed significantly by age, with Japanese women being significantly older than both Anglo and Chinese women. Further investigation of educational levels revealed no noteworthy difference between our sample and US Bureau of Census records on Asian and Pacific Islander women. We found that 25% of our AA sample were high school graduates vs. 26.7% of the census data sample. We also found that 49% of our Asian–American sample were college graduates vs. 37.2% of the census data sample. Thus, the sample appeared to closely parallel that of the US Bureau of Census records on Asian–American women's educational levels (US Bureau of the Census, 1994).

The data in Table 5.1 indicate that AA women to have greater difficulty in requesting help than Anglo–American women following breast cancer. Of the six categories of types of social support, none of the six showed a significant difference among the three study groups on the 'wanting' ('Would you have liked?') support dimension; however, of the six categories of social support, four of six showed a significant difference between Anglos and one or both Asian study groups on the 'needing' ('Do you think you needed?') support dimension. In each of these four categories, the Anglo group was significantly greater in indicating 'needing' social support.

Contrary to our expectation that the appropriate form of social support after breast cancer would be different for Anglo–American women and AA women, and specifically that AA women would receive greater tangible support than

Table 5.1 Differences in reports of want and needing social support between Asian and Anglo groups

Categories of support	Anglo (A) (%) (n = 13)	Chinese (C) (%) (n = 18)	Japanese (J) (%) (n = 15)	C vs. J	Exact p value C vs. A	J vs. A
Private feelings						
Would have more	23.1	22.2	15.4	1.00	1.00	1.00
Needed more	100.0	72.2	53.8	0.449	0.058	0.015
Material aid						
Would have liked more	0	0	0	+ +	+ +	+ +
Needed more	23.1	14.3	38.5	0.209	0.648	0.673
Advice						
Would have liked more	38.5	11.8	16.7	1.00	0.190	0.378
Needed more	91.7	52.9	69.2	0.465	0.043	0.322
Physical assistance						
Would have liked more	38.5	31.3	23.1	0.697	0.714	0.673
Needed more	100.0	56.3	61.5	1.00	0.008	0.039
Social participation						
Would have liked more	25.0	41.2	30.8	0.708	0.449	1.00
Needed more	100.0	76.5	92.3	0.355	0.113	1.00
Positive feedback						
Would have liked more	41.7	17.6	16.7	1.00	0.218	0.371
Needed more	100.0	76.5	53.8	0.255	0.113	0.015

*p Values for differences between Chinese and Anglos and for differences between Japanese and Anglos using Fisher's exact test (two-tailed significance); no significant differences between Chinese and Japanese were found.
+ + No statistics are computed because all subjects reported their level of material aid in terms of what they wanted as 'just about right.'
'want' = how much would you have liked?: 'need' = how much do you think you needed?

Anglo–American women, who would receive greater emotional support, we found that the data did not support these assumptions. No significant differences in any of the five types of social support were found among the three study groups. The data in Tables 5.2 and 5.3 reflect types of social support (emotional vs. tangible), the categories of providers, and total support scores. No significant differences were found.

The data in Table 5.4 show the composition of the social support of the AA groups compared to Anglo–American women following breast cancer. The tables show that the mean size (overall) of the Anglo–American social network was significantly larger than either of the AA study groups, and in three of the network categories (friend/co-worker, professionals, and extended family) Anglo–Americans had significantly larger networks than at least one of the AA study groups. The Anglo–American study group was significantly different on five of six categories of network composition beyond the immediate family. Data in Tables 5.2, 5.3, 5.4, and 5.5 show the significance of the physician as a source of social support. Table 5.2 shows that Anglo women perceived significantly higher support from their physicians than the Chinese women, and a trend towards higher support than the Japanese women. However, when the percentage of tangible support is considered

Table 5.2　Mean frequency of emotional support by providers

	n	Hus-band	SE	Doctor	SE	p^*	Family	SE	Friends	SE	p	Co-workers	SE	Total support	SE
Chinese	18	1.94	0.31	1.61	0.23	0.005	2.11	0.23	1.72	0.23	0.000	0.88	0.22	1.66	0.26
Japanese	15	1.50	0.36	1.87	0.31	0.11	2.00	0.34	2.00	0.35	0.016	0.92	0.37	1.68	0.34
Anglo	13	1.38	0.37	2.62	0.24		2.31	0.33	2.92	0.08		1.67	0.38	2.19	0.33

$^*p$ Value shows significant difference compared to Anglos.

Table 5.3　Mean frequency of tangible support by providers

	n	Hus-band	SE	Doctor	SE	p^*	Family	SE	Friends	SE	p	Co-workers	SE	Total support	SE
Chinese	18	1.76	0.33	0.33	0.18	0.004*	1.61	0.29	1.28	0.27	0.017	0.47	0.21	1.09	0.29
Japanese	15	1.79	0.38	1.67	0.39	0.036	1.73	0.38	1.60	0.38		0.77	0.32	1.53	0.37
Anglo	13	1.62	0.38	0.58	0.30		1.85	0.37	2.31	0.31		1.25	0.36	1.54	0.37

p Value shows significant difference compared to Anglos.
$^*p$ Value indicates difference between Chinese and Japanese.
Rating scale of social support: 0 = none, 1 = little, 2 = moderate, 3 = a lot.

Table 5.4　Mean network size

	Chinese ($n = 18$)	SE	Range	p Value C vs. A*	Japanese ($n = 15$)	SE	Range	p Value J vs. C*	Anglo ($n = 13$)	SE	Range	p Value A vs. J*
Mean net-work size	6.61	0.43	3–9	0.000	3.92	1.22	0–15	0.046	14.92	1.50	7–29	0.000
Spouse	10.1%	0.11	0–1		7.3%	0.13	0–1		4.1%	0.14	0–1	
Family (nuclear)	36.1%	0.46	0–6		25.7%	0.55	0–8		16.5%	0.46	0–5	
Friend/co-worker	37.0%	0.44	0–6	0.004	61.5%	1.23	0–14		55.2%	1.77	1–26	
Professionals	3.4%	0.10	0–1	0.055	1.8%	0.09	0–1		7.2%	0.42	0–5	0.035
Extended family	13.4%	0.28	0–4	0.026	3.7%	0.12	0–1	0.048	17.0%	0.65	0–6	0.002

*C = Chinese, A = Anglo, J = Japanese.

Table 5.5　Percentage who received support from each category in network

	Chinese (%) ($n = 18$)	p^*	Japanese (%) ($n = 15$)	p^*	Anglo (%) ($n = 13$)
Spouse	66.7		53.3		61.5
Nuclear family	77.8		66.7		84.6
Friend/co-worker	77.8	0.07	73.3	0.044	100.0
Professionals	22.2	0.07	13.3	0.002	53.8
Extended family	50.0		26.7	0.025	69.2

$^*p$ Value shows significant difference compared to Anglo.

(see Table 5.3), Japanese rated their experiences with doctors as significantly higher than Anglos ($p = 0.03$). The data in these tables seems to indicate that physicians were a greater source of social support for the Anglo women than for the Asian women, but, overall, physicians provided very little support to any of the groups.

DISCUSSION

The general findings of this study represent an initial attempt to understand better the breast cancer experience in AA populations. Asian–Americans appeared to have greater difficulty requesting or accepting help from others than Anglo–American women following breast cancer. No interethnic differences are present in terms of wanting more opportunities for social support, but in almost every category of social support Anglos indicated a greater *expressed* need. Advice and feedback are two of the modes of social support that were statistically greater for the Anglo–American women than the Asian–American (AA) women. These two strategies are primary examples of effective social support used in Western psychotherapy and support groups. These two strategies, however, are more compatible with the Western value placed on talking as a way of solving problems and obtaining self-affirmation for social support (Thoits, 1995). Talking, as noted, is not as much a part of traditional AA styles of giving or receiving support and may partially explain the statistical difference. Another explanation for the difference between the AA and Anglo–American groups may involve Asian cultural norms of hierarchical role expectations, interpersonal etiquette, and family obligation.

The Chinese–Americans may have wanted more support, but their support network consisted primarily of nuclear family members. The Japanese–American women utilized family (nuclear and extended) the least of the three groups. The response of the two Asian groups would be consistent with other studies indicating a fundamental value of self-sufficiency for AA women in their role as 'nurturer', not receiver of care (Kagawa-Singer, 1988; Ito et al., 1997). These women may have hesitated to impose additional requests because they felt such requests would be more of a burden. The dichotomization of the results with regards to the Anglo–Americans saying they 'needed' significantly more support may stem from the Western ethos of assertiveness of one's individual need compared to the Eastern ethos of maintaining harmony, allowing others to anticipate one's needs, and abstaining from demanding behaviors in interpersonal relationships (Doi, 1971; Ho, 1990).

Additionally, the variation in size and make-up of the support networks may illuminate the lower utilization of social support outside of the spouse and family network and was consistent with the literature on AA cultures. Anglo–Americans had the largest support networks ($M = 14.92$), Chinese–Americans had smaller networks ($M = 6.61$) and Japanese–Americans had the smallest support networks ($M = 3.9$). As described earlier, these two AA groups may share the belief that help-seeking behavior outside the family, let alone in the family, is seen as an act of embarrassment to the individual and family members (Araneta, 1982; Lee, 1982; Chung and Kagawa-Singer, 1994). A striking example of this is a letter sent to one of the investigators from the husband of one Japanese–American woman who took the time to write a three-page letter to the authors to explain why his wife's social network was so small and provided so little support:

If the person being interviewed did not inform her friends about her situation before or after her surgery, then, all the questions about moral or physical or monetary or material support would be irrelevant. Take my wife's case. She did not tell anyone prior to surgery about her condition except her husband and two children. She did not tell anyone about her surgery until about a year later. Why? [Because] the code of conduct in her parents' family was not to inconvenience others for personal reasons; not to burden others if avoidable; etc. (I could go on and on) . . .

If [my wife] had told her friends about her malignancy, the people who were informed . . . would have been obliged . . . to visit her in the hospital or home to show their support and wishes for a swift recovery. [They] would take the time off to visit the friend with a get-well gift. The result is an imposition on your friend's goodwill.

The behaviors described in this excerpt illustrate two of the major AA cultural values of: (a) recognizing the cost of social obligation and indebtedness; and (b) not going outside the family for assistance with dependency needs. In fact, these AA women did have significantly lower rates of requests for help for problems encountered in the breast cancer experience. Both AA and Anglo–American women reported similar problems created by the cancer experience, but the AA women requested assistance at a much lower rate (Kagawa-Singer et al., 1996).

It should be noted, however, that there is a statistically significant difference between the Chinese–American and Japanese–American groups in number of single women [$n = 1$ (6%) and $n = 4$ (26.7%)] in the groups. Since the sample sizes are small, this difference may be one explanation for the smaller social support network size for Japanese–American women. Although these single women were living in close proximity to family, and participating in all family functions, the cultural prescriptions for self-sufficiency may limit the ability of these women to impose upon their families for assistance. Further clarification of the social support network size would require a larger sample size.

The apparent connotations of the two words ('want' and 'need') on the Arizona Social Support Interview Schedule (ASSIS) (Table 5.1) (Barrera, 1986) appear to have been sensitive enough to detect these potentially culturally based interpretations, but differences in response cannot be assessed from the results of the questionnaires. We did not test the instruments for conceptual equivalency. Construct equivalency should be assessed in subsequent studies.

No statistically significant differences were found to support the notion that Anglo–American women would perceive more emotional support from their network compared to the AA groups, but trends were found to indicate that different sources and levels of support existed for AA women compared to Anglo–American women. Notably, the two AA groups were in opposition to each other in every category, with the Anglo–American women between the two AA groups. The sole exception to this pattern was in perceived support for emotional distress, for which the Anglo women ranked highest.

The presence of an active network, however, was not equivalent to perceived support. From the patient's responses, it appears that efforts to provide social support were not expressed in a manner that was as helpful as desired. The discrepancy between what is provided compared to what is desired may indicate, for example, that a Chinese–American woman could not utilize or modify a particular support offered. Such requests on her part might offend her family members or cause

Table 5.6   Amount of negative interactions from social support network

	n	Yes	No	p^*
Chinese	18**	1	15	0.000
Japanese	15	1	14	0.000
Anglo	13	10	3	
Total	28	12	32	

$\chi^2 = 24.29$, $p < 0.0001$, d.f. = 2.
*p Value shows significant difference compared to Anglo.
**Only 16 of 18 responded to this question.

them to lose face, as their efforts would be seen as inadequate. Therefore, the frequency of support may be high, but the perceived quality of support received may not be commensurate.

Although there were no statistical differences in the perceived amount of social support received, it appears from the results in Table 5.6 that social support is obtained at a higher emotional cost in terms of negative interactions for the Anglo–American women than the AA women. According to the exchange concept described earlier, negative aspects of social support can have more impact than positive aspects (Williams, 1995, Chung and Kagawa-Singer, 1994). DiMatteo and Hays (1981) reported that social conflict may sometimes be a better predictor of adjustment than social support.

Asian cultures formally recognize the 'cost' of accepting assistance in the form of indebtedness or obligation. The smaller social support networks of the Asian women compared to the Anglo women may reflect the conscious choice to avoid the added burden (Nemoto, 1989). The intricate interrelationships of obligation, dependency, and hierarchical interpersonal etiquette may be demonstrated in the make-up of the social support network between nuclear and extended family, as presented in Table 5.4. There were no differences in the ratio of nuclear and extended family networks for Anglo–American women (16.5% vs. 17%), a moderate difference for Chinese–American women (36.1% vs. 13.4%), and a large difference for Japanese–American women (25.7% vs. 3.7%).

IMPLICATIONS FOR PRACTICE AND RESEARCH

From the information presented in this chapter, three factors emerged as salient to increase the ability of clinicians to facilitate culturally informed decisions. One is that the form of social support is likely to vary by ethnic group. For example, the data showed Japanese women to need less positive feedback, and Chinese women to need less advice. A second is that the source and size of the social support network is likely to vary by ethnic group. For example, Japanese women are likely to obtain social support from friends/co-workers and less so from immediate or external family. They are also likely to have the smallest social support network. Anglos, by contrast, have a larger network and utilize more varied sources of support. A third is that while most Anglo women expect and perceive support from professionals, most Asian women in the study did not. This implies that the notion of 'plugging in' an

Anglo woman to a professionally-led support group may be acceptable and even expected. For the majority of Asian women in this study, such a mode of support may not be familiar, acceptable or appropriate. It is noteworthy that no ethnic group perceived professionals as intrinsic members of their social support matrix, but that Anglo women were significantly more likely to perceive support coming from professionals.

A more culturally-tailored approach to social support is interrelated with issues of culturally-based communication skills. However, caution must be taken because such interventions may be hampered on two levels: (a) Asian idioms of distress and discomfort—both physical and emotional—may not be understood by Western-trained providers; and (b) the cultural modes of obtaining support and counsel for AA women militate *against* seeking help from outside their immediate social nexus, including physicians. With these cultural differences in mind, we recommend the following interrelated modifications in current practice:

1. Forms of assistance must be designed to be culturally congruent to be effective. Treatment decisions and follow-up care require that a more individually tailored and culturally contextualized approach be taken. This involves the clinician appropriately facilitating the patient's support network. As the data in this study showed, for Chinese–American women this will primarily be the family, for Japanese–American women it will primarily be friends and co-workers, and for Anglo–American women this may include elements of both.
2. Culturally-specific idioms of communication of distress must be learned and the strategies in counseling need refocusing. This requires specifically knowing proper cultural idioms of distress. It also may require shifting the focus of counseling for Asian women from a focus on individual wishes and needs to a focus on how her illness may impact on her social network. One might also facilitate group decision-making rather than the autonomy model that could be both intimidating and alienating to Asian–American women (Lavizzo-Moury and Mackenzie, 1996).
3. Assessment techniques must be modified to use more neutral modes of communication to elicit culturally expressed distress. Providers are advised to actively ask patients about their needs and give patients permission to tell their stories. This may present more time pressure for the clinician because of copious material, but will be more likely to facilitate trust and more accurate information. Standardized interviewing styles taught in the West will elicit indirect 'middle of the road' responses rather than more valid disclosure in many Asian women.
4. Social support interventions must be culturally congruent to be appropriate, acceptable, and useful. If strategies based in Western concepts of individualism are used to support the sense of integrity and well-being of individuals who hold traditional Asian beliefs and values, most AA individuals will leave therapy. Support of AA families requires interventions consonant with their expectations of communication etiquette, as well as initial objectives.

Finally, the differences noted in this study between the Japanese–Americans and Chinese–Americans caution against the tendency to combine these two groups of AA women into one without first assessing the intragroup differences. Significant within-group variation must be recognized and assessed. For example, individuals from any one culture will vary in their cultural identity according to variations in levels of acculturation and assimilation, country of origin, and individual personality. For example, the Chinese diaspora indicates that Chinese in the USA may originate from the USA (e.g., sixth generation Chinese–Americans), Africa, Panama, the UK or almost anywhere else in the world and the large populations of South American Japanese who have immigrated to the USA constitute a very different Japanese–American population than the USA-born Japanese–Americans. Intra- and inter-group variations among AAs require conscious attention to these differences in both practice and research.

Cross-cultural research in AA families is needed, but researchers must be aware of the different basis upon which positive coping and adaptation is based. We have presented a definition of culture that provides direction for comparative studies and a model for assessing these differences. The statistical techniques of multilevel analysis provide a means to begin testing this theoretical framework to enable researchers and practitioners to better meet the needs of their Asian–American breast cancer patients and their families.

REFERENCES

Acock, A.C. and Demo, D.H. (1994). *Family Diversity and Well-being*. Thousand Oaks, CA: Sage Publications.

Alagaratnam, T.T. and Kung, N.Y.T. (1986). Psychosocial effects of mastectomy: is it due to mastectomy or to the diagnosis of malignancy? *British Journal of Psychiatry* **149**, 296–299.

Araneta, E. Jr (1982). Filipino American. In Albert Gaw (Ed.), *Cross-Cultural Psychiatry* (pp. 55–68). Boston, MA: John Wright.

Baider, L., Cooper, C. L. et al. (1996). Cancer and the family. Chichester: New York, Wiley.

Barrera, M. (1986). Distinctions between social support concepts, mesures and models. *American Journal of Community Psychology* **14**(4): 413-445.

Barrera, M. Jr, Sandler, I.N. and Ramsay, T.B. (1981). Preliminary development of a scale of social support: studies on college students. *American Journal of Community Psychology* **9**: 435–447.

Berkman, L.F. (1982). Social network analysis and coronary heart disease. *Advanced Cardiology* **29**, 37–49.

Berreman, G. (1982). Bazar Behavior: Social identity and social interaction in urban India. G. Devos & L. Romanucci-Ross (Eds.) Chicago: University of Chicago Press, 71-105.

Bloom, J.R. (1982). Social support, accommodation to stress and adjustment to breast cancer. *Social Science and Medicine* **16**: 1329–1338.

Chilman, C.S., Nunnally, E.W. and Cox, F.M. (1988). *Chronic Illness and Disability*. Newbury Park, CA: Sage.

Chung, R. and Kagawa-Singer, M. (1995). Gender differences in the predictors of psychological distress among South-east Asian Refugees. *Journal of Nervous and Mental Disease* **183**: 639–648.

Bloom, J. R. (1982). Social support, accommodation to stress and adjustment to breast cancer. *Social Science & Medicine* **16**(14): 1329–1338.

Chung, R.C., Bemak, F., Kagawa-Singer, M. (1998). Gender differences in psychological distress among Southeast Asian refugees. *Journal of Nervous and Mental Disease* **186**(2): 112–119.

Cobb, S. (1976). Social support as a moderator of life stress. *Psychosomatic Medicine* **38**(5), 300–314.

Danielson, C.B., Hamel-Bissell, B. and Winstead-Fry, P. (1993). *Families, Health, and Illness: Perspectives on Coping and Intervention*. St. Louis, MO: Mosby.

DeVos, George A. (1982).   Adaptive strategies in U.S. Minorities. Minority Mental Health. E. Jones and S. J. Korchin (Eds.) Praeger: 74-117.

DeVos, G. and Rommanucci-Ross, L. (1982).   Ethnic Identity. Chicago, University of Chicago Press.

DiMatteo, M.R. & Hays, R. (1981).   Social support and serious illness. In B. H. Gottlieb (Ed.), *Social Networks and Social Support* (pp. 117–148). Beverly Hills, CA: Sage.

Dodd, M.J. (1985).   Attitudes of patients living in Taiwan about cancer and its treatment. *Cancer Nursing* **8**(4): 214–220.

Doi, T. (1971).   *The Anatomy of Dependence.* Tokyo: Kodansha Press.

Donnelly, N.D. (1994).   Changing Lives of Refugee Among Women. Seattle: Washington University Press.

Dunkel-Schetter, C. (1984).   Social support and cancer: Selected findings and recommendations on three key issues. *Journal of Social Issues* **40**: 29–35.

Durvasula, R.S. and Sue, S. (1992).   Severity of psychiatric disorder among white and Asian outpatients. Paper presented at American Psychological Association Annual Convention, August.

Ell, K. (1984).   Social networks, social support, and health status: a review. *Social Service Review* **March**, 133–149.

Ell, K.O., Mantell, J.E. and Hamovitch, M.B. (1988).   Socioculturally sensitive intervention for patients with cancer. *Journal of Psychosocial Oncology* **6**(3–4), 141–155.

Germino, B.B. (1993).   Quality of life for families with cancer: Research issues. *Quality of Life: A Nursing Challenge* **2**(2), 39–45.

Gordon, D.R. (1990).   Embodying illness, embodying cancer. *Culture, Medicine and Psychiatry* **14**(2): 275–297.

Gotay, C.C. (1996).   Cultural variation in family adjustment to cancer. In L. Baider, C.L. Cooper and A. Kaplan De-Nour (Eds), *Cancer and the Family*, 1st edition (pp. 31–52). Chichester: Wiley.

Gregory, S., Sanjek, R. (1996).   Race. New Brunswick: Rutgers University Press.

Hallowell, A.I. (1955)   *Culture and Experience.* Pittsburgh: University of Pennsylvania Press

Hammond, P.B. (1978).   An introduction to cultural and social anthropology. New York: McMillan Co. vol. XIV; 2nd. Ed.

Ho, M.K. (1976).   Social work with Asian Americans. *Social Casework* **57**(3): 195–200.

Ho, M.K. (1989).   Applying family therapy theories to Asian/Pacific Americans. Annual Program meeting of the council on social work education.

Ito, K., Kagawa-Singer, M. and Chung, R. (1997).   Asian/Pacific American Group. In *Women's Health: Dynamics of Diversity*, S. Ruzek, V. Olesen and A. Clarke (Eds), Philadelphia, PA: Temple University Press.

Johnson, F.A., Marsella, A.J. and Johnson, C.L. (1974).   Social and psychological aspects of verbal behavior in Japanese–Americans. *American Journal of Psychiatry* **131**, 580–583.

Kagawa-Singer, M. (1988).   Bamboo and oak: differences in the adaptation to cancer between Japanese–American and Anglo–American patients. Unpublished dissertation, University of California at Los Angeles.

Kagawa-Singer, M. (1993).   Redefining health: living with cancer [see comments]. *Soc Sci Med* **37**(3): 295–304.

Kagawa-Singer, M. (1995).   Socioeconomic and cultural influences on cancer care of women. *Seminars Oncological Nursing?* **11**(2): 109–119.

Kagawa-Singer, M., Chung, R. (1994).   A Paradigm for Culturally Based Care for Minority Populations. *Journal of Community Psychology* April **22**(2): 192–208.

Kagawa-Singer, M. Wellisch, D.K. et al. (1997).   Impact of breast cancer on Asian–American and Anglo–American women. *Culture, Medicine and Psychiatry* **21**(4): 449–480.

Kalish, R.A., Reynolds, D.K. (1976).   Death & Ethnicity: A Psychocultural Stud, Ethel Percy Andres Gerontology Center, Univ So Calf.

Kawanishi, Y. (1992).   Somatization of Asians: An artifact of Western medicalization? *Transcultural Psychiatric Research Review* **29**: 5–36.

Kesserling, A., Dodd, M. et al. (1986).   Attitudes of patients living in Switzerland about cancer and its treatment. *Cancer Nursing* **9**(2): 77–85.

Kim, S., McLeod, J.H. and Shantzis, C. (1992). Cultural competence for evaluators working with Asian-American communities: some practical considerations. In M.A. Orlandi, R. Weston and L.G. Epstein (Eds), *Cultural Competence for Evaluators: A Guide for Alcohol and Other Drug Abuse Prevention Practitioners Working with Ethnic/Racial Communities* (pp. 261–292). Rockville, MD: US Department of Health and Human Services.

Kleinman, A. (1980). *Patients and Healers in the Context of Culture* (pp. 104–118). Berkeley, CA: University of California Press.

Kluckhohn, F., Strodtbeck, F. (1961). Variations in value orientations. Evanston, Ill., Row, Peterson.

Kristjansen, L.J. and Ashcroft, T. (1994). The family's cancer journey: a literature review. *Cancer Nursing* **17**: 1–17.

Lai, M.C. and Yue, K.K. (1990). The Chinese. In N. Waxler-Morrison, J. Anderson and E. Richardson (Eds), *Cross-cultural Caring: A Handbook for Health Professionals in Western Canada* (pp. 68–90). Vancouver, BC: University of British Columbia Press.

Lauver, D. and Ho, C.H. (1993). Explaining delay in care seeking for breast cancer symptoms. *Journal of Applied Social Psychology* **23**(21): 1806–1825.

Lavizzo-Mourey, R. and Mackenzie, E.R. (1996). Cultural competence: essential measurements of quality for managed care organizations. *Annals of Internal Medicine* **124**(10): 919–921.

Lee, E. (1982). A social system approach to assessment and treatment of Chinese American families. In M. McGoldrick, J. Pearce and J. Giordano (Eds), *Ethnicity and family therapy* (pp. 527–551). New York: Guilford.

Leong, F. (1986). Counseling and psychotherapy with Asian–Americans: review of the literature. *Journal of Counseling Psychology* **33**, 196–206.

Lewis, F.M. (1986). The impact of cancer on the family: a critical analysis of the research literature. *Patient Education and Counseling* 269–289.

Lewis, F.M. (1996). The impact of breast cancer on the family: Lessons learned from the children and adolescents. Cancer and the family. E. Lea Baider, E. Cary L. Cooper and et al., Chichester, England UK: 271–287.

Lin, K.M. (1990). Assessment and diagnostic issues in the psychiatric care of refugee patients. In W. Holtzman and T. Bornemann (Eds), *Mental Health Immigrants and Refugees* (pp. 198–206). Austin, TX: Hogg Foundation for Mental Health.

Long, S., Long, B.D. (1982). Curable cancer and fatal ulcers: attitudes toward cancer in Japan. *Social Science and Medicine* **16**: 2101–2108.

McGill, D.P., JK (1982). British Families. Ethnicity and Family Therapy. J.P.J.G. McGoldrick M. New York, The Guilford Press: 457–482.

McGoldrick, M., Pearce, J.K. and Giordano, J. (Eds). (1982) *Ethnicity and Family Therapy* (pp. 3–30). New York: Guilford.

Marshall, J.R., Funch, D.P. (1983). Social environment and breast cancer. A cohort analysis of patient survival. *Cancer* **52**(8): 1546–1550.

Maslow, A. H. (1954). Motivation and personality (2nd ed.). New York, Harper and Row.

Morris, T. (1990). Culturally sensitive family assessment. *Family Process* **29**(1), 105–116.

Murphy, R.F. (1990). *The Silent Body*. New York: W.W. Norton.

Nemoto, T. (1989). Social support and norms toward mobilizing social support among Japanese American elderly. Doctoral dissertation, New York University.

Neuling, S.J., Winefield, H.R. (1988). Social support and recovery after surgery for breast cancer: frequency and correlates of supportive behaviours by family, friends and surgeon. *Social Science and Medicine* **27**(4): 385–392.

Nilchaikovit, T., Hill, J.M. and Holland, J.C. (1993). The effects of culture on illness behavior and medical care: Asian and American differences. *General Hospital Psychiatry* **15**: 41–50.

Northhouse, L. (1994). The family impact of cancer in women. Paper presented at the Third National Conference on Cancer Nursing Research. Newport Beach, CA, January 27–29.

Ohnuki-Tierney, E. (1984). Illness and Culture in Contemporary Japan: An Anthropological View. London, Cambridge University Press.

Okazaki, S. (1994).   Cultural considerations in treating Asian Americans. Paper presented at the Second Annual Conference on Psychopathology, Psychopharmacology, Substance Abuse and Culture, Los Angeles, October.

Rolland, J.S. (1994).   *Families, Illness, and Disability*. New York: Basic Books.

Romanucci-Ross, L., Devos, G. (1995).   Ethnic Identity. Walnut Creek, Altamira Press, A division of Sage Publications, Inc.

Shibusawa, T., Kagawa-Singer, M.   Social support for disabled elderly Japanese-Americans. Gerontology and Geriatrics Education (in revision).

Shon, S.P. and Ja, D.Y. (1982).   Asian Families. In M. McGoldrick, J.K. Pearce and J. Giordano (Eds). (1982)   *Ethnicity and Family Therapy* (pp. 208–228). New York: Guilford.

Sontag, S. (1978).   *Illness as Metaphor*. New York: Farrar, Straus and Giroux.

Sontag, S. (1978).   *Illness as Metaphor*. New York, Farrar, Straus and Giroux.

Spiegel, D. (1990).   Can psychotherapy prolong cancer survival? [editorial] [see comments].⁻ *Psychosomatics* **31**(4).

Sue, S. (1977).   Community mental health services to minority groups: some optimism, some pessimism. *American Psychologist* **32**: 616–624.

Sue, S. & Sue, D.W. (1974).   MMPI comparisons between Asian American and non-Asian students utilizing a student health psychiatric clinic. *Journal of Counseling Psychology* **21**: 423–427.

Sue, D. and Sue, S. (1987).   Cultural factors in the clinical assessment of Asian Americans. *Journal of Consulting and Clinical Psychology* **55**: 479–487.

Sue, S., Zane, N. (1991).   The role of culture and cultural techniques in psychotherapy. *American Psychologist* **42**(1): 37–45.

Suinn, R.M., Rickard-Figueroa, Lew, S. and Vigil, P. (1987).   The Suinn–Lew Asian Self Identity Acculturation Scale: an initial report. *Educational and Psychological Measurement* **47**(2): 410–407.

Taylor, S. E., Falke, R. L. et al. (1986).   Social support, support groups, and the cancer patient. *Journal of Consulting and Clinical Psychology* **54**(5): 608–615.

Taylor, S.E., Shoptaw, S.J. and Lichtman, R.R. (1986).   Breast cancer patients' participation in cancer support groups. Unpublished raw data.

Tebbi, C.K. et al. (1985).   The role of social support systems in adolescent cancer amputees. *Cancer* **56**(4): 965–971.

Thoits, P.A. (1995).   Stress, coping, and social support processes: where are we? What next? *Journal of Health and Social Behavior* (Special Issue): 53–79.

Tolsdorf, C.C. (1976).   Social networks, social support, and coping: an exploratory study. *Family Process* **15**: 407–417.

Tseng, W.S. and Hsu, J. (1991).   *Culture and Family: Problems and Therapy*. New York: The Haworth Press.

Tung, T.M. (1985).   Psychiatric care for South-east Asians: how different is different? In T. Owan (Ed.), *South-east Asian Mental Health: Treatment, Prevention, Services, Training, and Research* (pp. 5–40). Washington, DC: US Department of Health and Human Services.

Uba, L.(1994).   *Asian Americans: Personality Patterns, Identity, and Mental Health* (pp. 196–213). New York: Guilford.

US Bureau of the Census (March, 1994).   *Educational Attainment of Persons 25 Years Old and Over, by Sex, Religion, and Race*.

Wellisch, D.K, Kagawa-Singer, M., Reid, S. et al. (1999).   An Exploratory study of social support: A crpss-cultural comparison of Chinese-, Japanese-, and Anglo-American breast cancer patients. *Psycho-Oncology* **18**(3): in press.

Wethington, E. and Kessler, R.C. (1986).   Perceived support, received support, and adjustment to stressful life events. *Journal of Health and Social Behavior* **27**(March): 78–89.

Williams, H.A. (1995).   There are no free gifts! Social support and the need for reciprocity. *Human Organization* **54**(4): 401–416.

6

Culture, Cancer, and the Family

CAROLYN COOK GOTAY

Cancer Research Center, University of Hawaii,
Honolulu, Hawaii, USA

Across the globe, the experience of cancer is a family affair. Not only patients, but also their loved ones, are affected by cancer, as they attempt to deal with the potential loss of a family member and the day-to-day stresses of cancer treatment and care. Very little research has focused on how cancer affects families in non-Western cultures, and even literature on Western families has devoted scant attention to cultural issues. As the world becomes increasingly multicultural, due to factors such as widespread mass communication and immigration, understanding more about cultural variation in family adjustment to cancer becomes more important for researchers and clinicians alike.

This chapter provides an overview of cultural variation in family adjustment to cancer and draws on literature from anthropology, epidemiology, health services research, cross-cultural psychology, and psychosocial oncology, including a few overviews (Die Trill and Holland, 1993; Die-Trill, 1998; Kleinman, 1986). Illustrative material is drawn from sources worldwide to demonstrate the powerful interaction between cancer, family, and culture. Suggestions for areas that warrant increased emphasis by both researchers and clinicians will be proposed.

WHAT IS CULTURE, AND HOW DOES IT DIFFER FROM ETHNICITY AND ETHNIC IDENTIFICATION?

Although there is no 'gold standard' definition of culture, most theorists agree on what makes it up. Culture includes both subjective elements (e.g., values, attitudes, norms, roles, and beliefs) and objective elements (e.g., buildings, roads) (Triandis, 1994). These elements are transmitted from generation to generation symbolically, through language, and through social institutions, particularly the family.

Many countries include one or more subcultures. In the USA, 'Anglo' culture, based in Western European roots, has been predominant historically. However, within the USA there are many other groups with different traditions, including African–Americans and rapidly growing numbers of individuals of Hispanic and

Cancer and the Family, 2nd Edn. Edited by L. Baider, C. L. Cooper and A. Kaplan De-Nour
© 2000 John Wiley & Sons, Ltd

Asian origins who have often retained elements of their original culture while at the same time adapting to the dominant Anglo culture.

Much of the research investigating attitudes, behaviors, and health outcomes among different subgroups has relied on ethnicity to define group membership. Ethnicity is most frequently defined by blood quantum: that is, the ethnicity of parents, grandparents and previous generations. However, individuals, especially those of mixed ethnic background, may identify with their ancestry to varying degrees. 'Ethnic identification,' or the ethnic, racial, or cultural label an individual chooses for him/herself, may be a better indicator of cultural values and associated outcomes. Even in uniracial regions or countries (e.g., Japan), where virtually all residents report the same ethnic identification, it is likely that differences in religious affiliation, personal preferences, and other factors give rise to variations in individual and family 'cultures.' Understanding the inter-relationships between race, ethnicity, self-identity, and associated behaviors and outcomes is an active area of research (Leong, 1998).

WHAT ARE CULTURALLY LINKED PREDICTORS OF A FAMILY'S EXPERIENCE WITH CANCER?

INTERNATIONAL VARIATION IN CANCER INCIDENCE RATES

Although cancer is found in virtually every area of the world, there is marked geographic variation in incidence rates. For example, cancer tends to be more common in developed countries than developing countries; average age-standardized incidence rates per 100 000 population are 299.6 in developed countries and 151.9 in developing countries, and rates range from a low of 105.6 in Northern Africa to 369.9 in North America. With respect to specific cancers, considerable variation is evident across the world; for example, while Japan reports low rates for many cancers, Japanese men and women have the highest stomach cancer rates in the world. Breast cancer is common in North America and Europe, but infrequent in Asia. Liver cancer is prevalent in China and parts of Africa, but rare in Northern Europe and North America (all statistics are from Parkin et al., 1999).

Regionally-linked cancer incidence rates can sometimes be explained by, for example, low life expectancy (meaning that people die prior to age 65, when the majority of cancers are diagnosed), genetics (e.g., Ashkenazi Jews have a higher likelihood of having one of the genes linked with breast cancer), or behaviors (e.g., diet, tobacco use). In addition, screening recommendations vary greatly from one country to the next, and screening tests common in one country [such as prostate-specific antigen (PSA) screening for prostate cancer in the USA] may be virtually unknown elsewhere. In many countries, there are few resources devoted to early cancer detection, and as a consequence cancers are diagnosed late. According to Stjernsward and Teoh (1993): 'For a long time to come, as many as 80–90% of cancer patients in the developing countries will probably continue to be diagnosed with far-advanced, incurable cancer, if they are diagnosed at all' (p. 340).

INTERNATIONAL VARIATION IN CANCER MORTALITY RATES

Similar variation is found regarding cancer mortality and survival. Because cancer is more common in developed regions, the mortality rate tends to be higher; for example, cancer mortality is 116.7 (per 100 000 population) in developing countries and 182.8 in developed countries. However, average 5-year survival rates tend to be much higher in developed countries. For example, 84% of women diagnosed with breast cancer in the USA live 5 years or longer after diagnosis, compared to 49% in India. Whereas 44% of Australians diagnosed with leukemia live 5 years or more, only 10% of Chinese survive that long (all statistics are from Parkin et al., 1999).

Mortality rates are affected both by stage at diagnosis and availability of treatment. The sophisticated and expensive cancer treatments widely available in developed countries are simply not an option for many individuals in developing countries [even in developed countries, lack of health insurance may present an insurmountable barrier to receiving available treatments (Meyerowitz et al., 1998)]. For example, Eisenbruch and Handelman (1990) report that there is no Cambodian term for 'radiation therapy.' Resources for cancer control also need to be considered in the context of other national priorities: defense and food availability may take precedence over health, and health concerns about infant mortality and infectious diseases may have priority over cancer care. Stjernsward and Teoh (1993) have pointed out that:

> '...in the year 2015, it is predicted that two-thirds of all cancers...will occur in the developing countries. Although more than half of the world's cancer patients presently live in developing countries, less than 5% of the resources committed to cancer control are available to them' (p. 340).

Whether cancer is common or rare in a given culture, and whether cancer survival is a recognized possibility or is unheard of, may affect how the family and patient can explain and cope with the disease, as well as what resources are available. In countries where cancer is inevitably linked with pain and death [especially considering that pain is inadequately managed in most parts of the world, (Stjernsward and Teoh, 1993)], patient and family anxiety and expectations will suffer accordingly.

INTERNATIONAL VARIATION IN FAMILY ROLES IN HEALTH CARE

The expectations for family participation in cancer care are also culturally-conditioned. Ali et al. (1993) report that Egyptian families have a social obligation to provide hospital care, including food and hygiene, as well as emotional and spiritual support. As they remark, 'Cancer is a chronic disease that causes greater disruption to the family than to the patient' (p. 195). In contrast to the situation in Egypt, US hospital rules frequently limit the time and hours that patients can spend with others, and visitors are often not allowed to bring food to inpatients. Strains may be experienced both by families who are prohibited from providing care and by those where provision of such care is obligatory.

Traditional medicine is often an important component of cancer care, with implications for the family as well as for the patient. Published reports of complementary and alternative medicine use (including traditional remedies and other approaches) in US cancer patients vary; a recent review of 26 studies reported use rates ranging from 7% to 64%, with an average of 30% across studies (Ernst and Cassileth, 1998). Rates in excess of 50% have been reported in other developed countries, including France (Schraub and Helary, 1991) and Germany (Morant et al., 1991). It is likely that in cultures which have a strong tradition of indigenous medicine, there is considerable use of approaches such as acupuncture, herbs, and native plants. For cultures where the predominant belief is that cancer (and other illness) results from imbalance among demands (including the physical and spiritual environment), such as Native Hawaiians and Ojibways (Day, 1992), appropriate remedies include interpersonal approaches to restoring spiritual harmony within the family. For example, *ho'oponopono* is a traditional technique used by Native Hawaiians, alone or in conjunction with other remedies, to restore harmony and health. Under the direction of a leader, all family members are involved in identifying problems, seeking solutions, making restitution, and asking forgiveness, all within a spiritual context (Shook, 1985). In an approach like this, the family assumes quite a different role in patient treatment, compared to when the cancer is treated by therapies directed exclusively at the patient, delivered by medical experts.

MIGRATION, ACCULTURATION, AND GENERATIONAL STATUS

Studies examining cancer incidence and mortality rates among individuals who migrate from one region to another help to elucidate interactions between lifestyle, environment (including health care) and genetic/constitutional factors as they affect cancer rates. In general, rates of cancers that occur infrequently in countries of origin tend to be higher in migrants, and rates of relatively common cancers in countries of origin appear to be lower among migrants. In addition, rates among migrants tend to approach those found in the general population with each succeeding generation (Thomas and Karagas, 1996).

Acculturation is one factor that contributes to the closer correspondence in cancer rates between immigrant groups and the general population over time. 'Acculturation' refers to the process whereby an individual becomes fluent in the beliefs, behaviors, and values of the host culture. Individuals may become acculturated to different degrees; for example, an immigrant may assimilate (native culture is replaced by culture and customs of the mainstream society), separate (when individuals choose to segregate themselves from the mainstream society), become marginalized (when individuals are unable to fit in with either the native or mainstream society) or reflect integration/biculturalism (aspects of native culture are maintained while at the same time values and behaviors of the mainstream culture are adopted) (Berry et al., 1986). Measures of acculturation typically include the degree to which an individual uses his/her native language, number of years spent in the new country, ethnicity of close friends, and level of pride in one's heritage (e.g., Cuellar et al., 1980).

Much of the available research investigating acculturation has been based in the USA. In most studies, increased acculturation has been shown to increase cancer knowledge and decrease negative attitudes (e.g., Hubbell et al., 1996), increase cancer screening rates (e.g., Yi, 1995) and result in cancer risk factor rates (such as diet and tobacco use) that increasingly resemble those in the dominant culture (Otero-Sabogal et al., 1995). There is virtually no information about how acculturation affects family relationships and a family's adjustment to cancer. However, values and practices governing family relationships may be among the most persistent aspects of culture retained over generations.

HISTORICAL FACTORS

Different cultural groups have distinct histories, and it is important to consider political and historical contexts in understanding reactions to cancer. For example, it is standard in many medical settings to ask a cancer patient to identify his/her family members. However, this may be threatening for someone who has fled an oppressive political regime where naming one's family led to their imprisonment. Baider and her colleagues have investigated how a major twentieth century event, the Holocaust, has affected Holocaust survivors' coping with cancer. Their results indicate that Holocaust survivors who are subsequently diagnosed with cancer experience much higher levels of stress, compared to cancer patients who have not been through the Holocaust and healthy Holocaust survivors (Peretz et al., 1994). A tailored psychological intervention was unable to confer long-lasting reductions in patient distress, supporting the pervasive traumatic effect of the Holocaust on these patients (Baider et al., 1997). Mark and Roberts (1994) discuss how shaved heads and loss of hair during cancer treatment, coupled with hospital identification bracelets and gowns, may trigger flashbacks to Holocaust experiences. Although effects on the family were not discussed in these papers, it is reasonable to expect that any family member's having experienced the Holocaust may affect distress in families and patients alike when cancer is diagnosed.

WHAT ARE CULTURALLY LINKED MEDIATORS OF A FAMILY'S EXPERIENCE WITH CANCER?

There are many dimensions that vary cross-culturally and have relevance for how families cope with cancer. We will discuss several especially important considerations: attitudes toward autonomy, desired medical communication, explanatory models of illness, and family structure and roles.

ATTITUDES TOWARD AUTONOMY

One of the most striking and broad contrasts between Anglo and Asian values can be seen in the value of autonomy and the emphasis on the individual. In Anglo cultures, the rights of the individual and the emphasis on individual independence are of major importance, whereas in Asian cultures and many others, the interdependence—or 'connectedness' (Tamura and Lau, 1992)—among individuals is much more important. Whereas Anglos place emphasis on individual achievement, Asians and others are much more likely to value group achievement. In fact, doing something that will make one 'stand out' from others is actively avoided by some groups, such as Japanese and Native Hawaiians (McDermott et al., 1980).

Cancer may have its greatest impact on an Anglo by threatening his/her independence and autonomy. It is not coincidental that the largest number of items on many questionnaires used to assess quality of life in cancer patients relate to physical functioning, and a patient's ability to act independently (Donovan et al., 1989), since the majority of these scales were developed by researchers in North America. In contrast, Chaturvedi (1991), in a sample of Indian patients, family members, and caregivers, found that individual functioning was rated as the least important among 10 aspects of quality of life: 58% said that level of individual functioning was 'not important,' whereas 60% or more rated 'peace of mind,' 'spiritual satisfaction,' 'satisfaction with religious acts' and 'happiness with family' as 'very important.' While it may be argued (in all likelihood correctly) that spiritual and family concerns have been under-emphasized in North American research, it is still likely that independence is more highly valued by patients in this milieu than in many other places in the world.

DESIRED MEDICAL COMMUNICATION

In terms of the information they wish to have about their diagnosis and prognosis, Anglo patients and families present a striking and well-documented contrast to other cultural groups. In general in the USA, a value is placed on openness and full disclosure of information about the fact that the diagnosis is cancer. Patients are also seen as active participants in treatment decisions, which is clearly illustrated by legal mandates; for example, 18 US states have passed legislation that requires physician disclosure of treatment options to breast cancer patients prior to receiving therapy (Nayfield et al., 1994). While family members are generally included in discussions about cancer, the patient's right to know receives primary emphasis.

However, the assumption that 'truth-telling' is or should be a universal practice, either nationally or globally, has been contested. Mitchell's (1998) review demonstrates widely differing patterns of disclosure of information about cancer between countries, as well as cultural differences within the USA. This review distinguished between 'disclosure-dominant cultures,' including Australia and Northern Europe, in which most practitioners and patients valued open communication about a cancer diagnosis, and 'non-disclosure-dominant cultures,' in which disclosure was not the rule, such as Japan and a number of Southern and Eastern European countries. For example, a 1994 study of 792 Estonian physicians found that 42% 'almost never' tell patients they have cancer, while only 10% 'always' inform the patient (Barr, 1996). Physicians in such cultures are likely to believe that non-disclosure upholds Hippocratic principles of non-maleficence (by not depressing the patient) and beneficence (by maintaining hope). Mitchell categorized the USA somewhere in between the two groups of cultures; despite the widespread practice of fully informing patients, some population subgroups (e.g., Anglos and African–Americans) are more likely to report that they want full information than others, e.g., Asian–Americans, Hispanics (Blackhall et al., 1995) and Native Americans (Kaur, 1996).

Mitchell (1998) also points out that a number of elements of disclosure may vary cross-culturally, including what is disclosed (i.e., a diagnosis of cancer vs. a terminal prognosis), the accuracy and level of detail of the information, and with whom details are shared. Cultural expectations, such as the right of the family to protect the patient, are prevalent in many Asian and Hispanic cultures, implying that the family member, not the patient, should be informed. In addition, sociodemographic characteristics of the patients were found to be a consistent influence across cultures; for example, older and less educated patients were less likely to be informed of their diagnosis.

EXPLANATORY MODELS FOR CANCER

Theories of cancer etiology are linked to general cultural explanations for health and illness. In this century, a rational scientific model has prevailed in the Anglo culture, which holds that disease results from a specific cause which can be identified and explained through scientific theories and addressed through scientifically-based medical technologies and treatments. Cancer research seeks causes, such as faulty genes and environmental carcinogens, and solutions, such as surgery, chemotherapy, and radiation. This 'medical model' has proved valuable worldwide for many diseases. However, the search for cause-and-effect relationships for etiology and/or treatment has not yielded clear and positive results for most cancers to date. This may be one reason why record numbers of Americans are seeking alternative approaches, many of which are based in theories of illness etiology from other cultures.

Asian cultures traditionally place more emphasis on the interaction between mind, body, and environment, with illness a result of disharmony among elements. Treatment emphasizes restoration of balance, through therapies which affect the body and mind as a whole (e.g., meditation, acupuncture, herbs combined with prayer, Indian Ayurvedic medicine, yoga) (Marsella and Higginbotham, 1984). Other cultures view cancer as bad karma: punishment for transgressions in a previous life. Still other cultures attribute disease to magical causes, such as sorcery and witchcraft. Such beliefs are still prevalent in some regions, such as New Guinea (Feinberg, 1990; Lepowsky, 1990).

In order to understand family coping strategies, it is critical to understand patients' and families' theories of cancer causation. Families who believe that the cancer occurred because of something they or the patient did (e.g., an Anglo family in which a smoker is diagnosed with lung cancer) will in all likelihood experience different degrees of stress and enact different coping strategies than a family who believes that the cancer arose from bad karma due to failures in a previous life.

FAMILY STRUCTURE AND ROLES

Cross-cultural studies of family structure have shown that in much of North America, the most important family unit has traditionally consisted of the nuclear family of parents and children. The American family has become increasingly diverse in recent years, due to the frequency of single parenthood, divorce, remarriage, and 'blended' families, adoptions by gay and lesbian couples, and other social phenomena. As a consequence, the definition of 'American family' has become much more heterogeneous and flexible, but a two-generation model remains pre-eminent. In most other cultures of the world, consideration of 'family' has traditionally been much broader, including grandparents, aunts and uncles, cousins, and in many Asian cultures, ancestors. While linkages by blood generally are sufficient to define family, some cultures consider the broader community as part of the family constellation, such as Native Hawaiians (McDermott et al., 1980) and Israel's kibbutzim communities (Tseng and Hsu, 1991). Another important aspect of family structure is who holds the power in family decision making. Gender may dictate inheritance and kinship patterns (e.g., patriarchal or matriarchal societies). The most critical family axis also differs, with the husband–wife, parent–child, and brother–sister bonds being most important for Anglos, Asians, and Micronesians, respectively (Tseng and Hsu, 1991).

Shankar (1997) has examined the role of different family members in providing support to cancer patients in different cultural groups in a fascinating pilot study. She asked breast cancer patients from Japan ($n=30$), India ($n=9$), and the USA ($n=10$) to indicate who provided them with support in coping with different aspects of their diagnosis and treatment experience. The patients were asked about five different aspects of support and four different sources of support (husband, children, relatives, and friends). Results indicated both similarities and differences in patterns of support in the three groups of women. All three groups indicated that their husbands, by far, provided the most personal, emotional, and social support. The Japanese women were most likely to cite their husbands as providing support in all areas. However, Indian women were far more likely to say that their relatives helped them to maintain fulfilling relationships and self-esteem and discuss surgery, whereas American women were more likely to mention their friends, especially regarding discussion of surgery. More than 85% of Japanese and American women said their husbands were most helpful in developing a positive attitude for the future, whereas Indian women overwhelmingly endorsed their children. While this study does not provide definitive answers to the question of how families provide social support for cancer patients in different cultures, it implies that there is considerable variation across groups.

CASE STUDIES OF FAMILIES IN DIFFERENT CULTURES COPING WITH CANCER

Often, cultural values remain unexamined when they are widely shared. In fact, differing cultural practices may become most evident when cultural systems confront one another. The following case studies are based on the experience of cancer patients and their families whose traditional cultures come into conflict with the Western biomedical health care system. The experiences of these families illustrate a number of points discussed above.

CASE 1

Muller and Desmond (1992) report on the case of Mrs Lee (a pseudonym), a 49 year-old woman who had emigrated from the People's Republic of China to San Francisco 8 years previously. Mrs Lee was diagnosed with metastatic lung cancer, and a number of issues emerged during her diagnosis and treatment, particularly related to communications with her family. Both she and her husband spoke only Cantonese, and her 22 year-old son Arnold (the youngest child, who lived with his parents and was the family member most conversant in English) was the primary communicator and decision maker. He was adamant that Mrs Lee should not be informed of her diagnosis or be allowed to make treatment decisions, which was a continuing source of discomfort for the physicians, who believed the patient had the right to make choices on her own behalf. There was considerable dissent between Arnold and the health care team over the 6.5-month period between the time Mrs Lee was diagnosed and when she died. Arnold consistently insisted on the most aggressive care possible; he refused the physicians' recommendations for hospice care and a 'do not resuscitate' order (which the physicians imposed anyway) and during the final phases of treatment demanded the use of a ventilator and other heroic measures to prolong his mother's life.

This case was examined in detail by the treating team and the hospital. It illustrated several concerns relative to cancer, culture and the family. Communication was a key issue; whereas the Western health care providers believed the patient had the right to know her diagnosis, the patient's family did not agree (and evidently, a Cantonese-speaking interpreter was never introduced to ask Mrs Lee's opinion). Consistent with mores about 'truth telling' in other parts of the world, the Lees believed patients should be protected from being told they had cancer. Another issue relates to family roles. In this family, the son took over the primary management of his mother's care for the family. As discussed earlier, in some cultures, a son is the recognized 'head of the family' and may assume this authority in spite of relative youth. A final interesting facet of this case is the family's demand for aggressive treatment. As the authors remark, this behavior seems inconsistent with a more typical Chinese response of accepting death. However, Braun and Nichols (1996) point out that Chinese Buddhism considers premature death bad luck, and Mrs Lee was only 49 years old. Thus, Arnold may have been attempting to do everything possible to avoid such an outcome and assure his mother reincarnation at a higher level in her next life.

CASE 2

Eisenbruch and Handelman (1990) present a case study of a Cambodian adolescent with advanced brain cancer. The 'Oeur' family (a pseudonym) had lived in Australia for several years after fleeing from the Pol Pot revolution and spending several years in border camps. Their 16 year-old son, Bunn, was treated with surgery, radiation, and medication and had a year's remission before suffering a relapse and passing away. A psychiatrist and anthropologist (both of whom were fluent in Khmer, the Cambodian language), and members of the south-east Asian community provided a 'cultural consultation service' during Bunn's care to address a number of culturally-linked concerns faced by the family. For example, Bunn's surgery required that half of his head be shaved, and he was concerned that he would be thought to be *chkouet*, (crazy), since only prisoners and the mentally ill would have heads partially shaven in Cambodia. This potential barrier was addressed by encouraging him to shave his entire head, since that is considered reverent and will enhance future incarnations.

The family sought an explanation for Bunn's illness, which was one of several negative events (including another child being hit by a car and the father having an automobile accident) that had occurred since the family moved to a new house. They relied on a combination of explanations, including the Buddhist tenet of karma (demerits inherited from a previous life) and folk beliefs in house spirits and the spirit of Bunn's grandfather (which had occurred to Bunn in a dream). The Oeurs invited two monks to conduct a ceremony to sanctify their home and vanquish evil spirits, and they continued prayers and rituals afterwards. Interestingly, the physicians attributed Bunn's remission to the biomedical care they had provided, Mrs Oeur to the religious ceremonies she had sponsored, and Bunn to a macrobiotic diet he had adopted based on the recommendation of an Australian friend!

In this case, the participation of knowledgeable health care providers who could speak the language and were aware of the family's beliefs and value system undoubtedly contributed to as positive an experience as possible, although the outcome was unfortunately not cure. As the authors point out, they were able to support the family's use of both traditional and Western systems of care.

CASE 3

Pelusi (1994) presents a case study and commentary regarding RB, a 23 year-old Native American (Hopi) woman who had been diagnosed with cervical cancer. She had received surgical treatment (radical hysterectomy) and radiation therapy. RB, who spoke little English, lived with her family on a reservation 250 miles away from the treatment center and stayed alone in a hotel for the several months needed to complete therapy. RB suffered from severe diarrhea during her treatment. She refused to use prescribed medications for diarrhea control, but herbal teas supplied by her family controlled her symptoms. RB became very depressed during treatment because she was now 'unmarriageable,' and in fact told the staff that 'she had decided not to return to the reservation because she would be a disgrace to her family' (p. 10). Further, RB said that the health care providers did not understand how important it was that she remained fertile, and that they had not adequately prepared her for the outcome of her treatment.

This case illustrates how cancer can threaten important family roles that provide self-worth and status in a culture. In Hopi culture, being a wife and mother are the most highly valued roles for women. The patient's surgery rendered her infertile and closed the possibility that RB could assume this role. A commentary about this case points out the importance of the patient's being able to identify other culturally accepted ways to contribute to her community (Soldavini et al., 1994). If the health care providers had better understood the significance of fertility for the patient and her family, perhaps they could have addressed the issue from the outset and included cultural liaisons (or, at a minimum, people who could speak Hopi) in the treatment team. This case also illustrates how family members can participate in care and provide alternative, indigenous interventions (herbal tea that appeared to work in this situation). It should be noted that RB was isolated from this potential support throughout most of her treatment.

IMPLICATIONS FOR RESEARCH AND CLINICAL PRACTICE

We will focus on three areas where additional emphasis by both researchers and clinicians could provide important contributions to this field.

NEED FOR ADDITIONAL ATTENTION TO FAMILY ISSUES

How do families from different cultures cope with cancer? Empirical literature to answer this question is sorely lacking at the present time. There is limited information about cultural variation, even within North American families, where the majority of family-level research has been reported. In other parts of the world, data are absent altogether. Research that focuses on the family unit can be challenging to conduct. Such studies require active involvement of multiple individuals and pose logistical and methodological challenges. For example, questionnaires and interviews must be appropriate to family members' developmental stage, language, and understanding. In order to have available measurement tools appropriate to all individuals within a family (as well as to make cross-cultural comparisons), translation may be necessary in order to achieve equivalence. Several types of equivalence are desirable (Guillemin et al., 1993): semantic equivalence (do the words and phrases have similar meaning?); idiomatic equivalence (do any idioms or colloquialisms have the same meaning?); experiential equivalence (are illustrative situations comparable, such as asking if family members can drive as an indication of access to transportation may not be meaningful in a culture where personal automobiles are rarely used); and conceptual equivalence (is the concept being measured equally meaningful in both cultures?). Given the current state of the field, research using a variety of study designs could make a significant contribution. Descriptive studies that include cultural variables, such as the meaning of cancer to the family, and impact of cancer on family functioning, are sorely needed for most cultures. Qualitative methods may be particularly appropriate in hypothesis generation in order to capture more fully the perspectives of the individuals themselves.

Clinicians also need to consider carefully cultural variations in family involvement in cancer care. The case studies varied in how well culturally-based family considerations were integrated into communication of the diagnosis, treatment decision making and supportive care. At a minimum, the availability of someone who can speak the language (or languages) of patients and family members seems critical to provide the family and patient with an understanding of the biomedical aspects of the disease and treatment. If such a person is not on staff at a treatment facility, bringing in a consultant or even a telephone or electronic mail contact would seem to be a standard of care. Recognition and acknowledgement of important cultural values in cancer care is also critical. This kind of 'cultural competence' can be incorporated within the training of health care providers. For example, Carrillo et al. (1999) describe a curriculum they developed for 'cross-cultural primary care.' This curriculum includes five thematic modules including the basic concepts of culture, core cultural issues (e.g., authority, physical contact, communication styles, gender, sexuality, family), understanding the meaning of illness, social contacts, and techniques for negotiating across cultures. While this curriculum was designed for medical students, residents, and practicing physicians, it seems like a useful model for training the wide range of health professionals who are involved in providing cancer care.

RECOGNITION THAT CULTURAL CONSIDERATIONS ARE IMPORTANT FOR ALL PATIENTS AND FAMILIES

It is important to recognize that *every* patient and family has a culture, not only individuals who belong to minority groups, people who live in other countries, or those who are immigrants. Cultural aspects of values and appropriate behaviors are often invisible to members of 'majority' groups, or when all individuals share the same values; however, through comparison with other groups, implicit cultural assumptions become apparent. These cultural factors are key variables, along with life experiences, socio-economic status, and personality differences, that affect the meaning of cancer for individuals and families, as well as how they cope with the disease. As Burkett (1991) points out, 'culture . . . is not an optional factor that only sometimes influences health and illness; it is a prerequisite for all meaningful human experiences, including being ill . . . among all people, not just members of "exotic" cultures' (p. 287).

For researchers, the challenge is to understand how culture is linked to particular perspectives and behaviors. For example, socio-economic factors comprise a set of critical variables which need to be carefully considered in understanding the relationships between culture and family coping. Freeman's (1989) review of the marked racial differences in cancer incidence and survival in the USA concluded that low socio-economic status, rather than minority culture membership *per se*, was the primary reason for unfavorable cancer rates. Even though groups like African–Americans and Native Hawaiians reported much higher cancer rates, 'within one race, economic status is the major determinant of cancer outcome. Therefore, the target for correction is poverty, regardless of race' (p. 284). Investigators need to exercise great caution in drawing conclusions that observed differences between cultural groups are a function of cultural differences, since culture may co-vary with many other variables. Direct measurement of the values, attitudes, and behaviors for which 'culture' serves as a shorthand will enable identification of the most crucial differences between groups and individuals for which appropriate interventions can be developed. Measurement of such constructs will also facilitate theory development and testing, an area where little attention has been directed (Betancourt and Lopez, 1993).

For clinicians, there is need to ask patients and family members questions to provide an understanding of their unique family culture. For example, it is important to ask questions such as 'have you tried to understand why you got cancer? What ideas do you have about this?' and 'are there other members of your family who should be here when we talk about your treatment choices?' or, simply, 'what concerns does your mother (father/spouse/son/daughter/etc.) have about your illness?' Families within a culture are as variable as families between cultures, and family individuality must not be overlooked in an attempt to understand cultural patterns. Personality traits, economic factors (including education, occupation, and income), individual and family experiences, past interactions with the health care system, length of current residence (e.g., recent immigration), and subgroup membership within a larger culture (e.g., indigenous status) are among the factors which may affect a family's reaction to cancer.

NEED TO DEVELOP CULTURALLY APPROPRIATE SUPPORTIVE INTERVENTIONS FOR CANCER PATIENTS AND THEIR FAMILIES

The benefits psychosocial interventions provide for cancer patients have been amply documented (Andersen, 1992). Such interventions include behavioral approaches, non-behavioral counseling and therapy, informational and educational methods, and organized peer support (Meyer and Mark, 1995). However, few non-white patients have participated in such studies (Meyer and Mark, 1995), few interventions have been directed at the patient–family unit, and very few interventions have been reported outside North America and Europe. As a result, information is not available about which approaches are more effective in different cultures, what additional strategies may be warranted, and how existing models could be modified to make them more appropriate across populations. The challenge to researchers is clear.

For clinicians, the need to provide support to patients and families that is comfortable, accepted, and therapeutic to the patient and family is also clear. In addition to obvious concerns, such as making interventions available in the patient's preferred language, other cultural factors may affect whether an intervention is effective in a particular cultural group. For example, the direct and open communication that often characterizes support groups in the USA may not be as comfortable or supportive for Asian–American or Native American patients (or in people from non-disclosing cultural heritages). Different approaches to providing support may be needed. A possible model may be found in interventions to increase participation in breast and cervical cancer screening in USA minority populations. A number of such programs in the USA have been built around social support within ethnic communities, including African–Americans, Hispanics, Native Americans, and Asian and Pacific Islanders. Strategies such as using pre-existing social networks, natural strengths of community leaders, and cultural traditions have been shown to be effective in improving cancer-related outcomes in these populations (Gotay and Wilson, 1998). Similarly, when it comes to coping with cancer, interventions that build on the ties between individuals, the importance of the family, and traditional cultural values may improve well-being in both patients and family members.

CONCLUSION

In this chapter, we have described the enormous cross-cultural variation in cancer incidence and mortality, approaches to cancer treatment, attitudes toward autonomy, desired medical communication, explanatory models for cancer, and family structure and roles. We have also discussed some factors that influence responses to cancer, such as acculturation and historical events. The case studies provided poignant examples of how cultural conflicts may emerge when cultures with very different expectations related to cancer and the family come head-to-head.

At the same time, the case studies provide clues about how to build in cultural concerns to cancer care. With the increasing multiculturalism throughout the world, understanding how to provide culturally competent models of family-centered cancer care has become an urgent issue. Both researchers and clinicians have important contributions to make in this area.

ACKNOWLEDGEMENTS

The preparation of this paper was partially supported by an award from the National Institute on Aging (AG 16601). The assistance of Joan Holup, Miles Muraoka, Sarah Bruner, and Alison Dame is gratefully acknowledged.

REFERENCES

Ali, N.S., Khalil, H.Z. and Yousef, W. (1993). A comparison of American and Egyptian cancer patients' attitudes and unmet needs. *Cancer Nursing* 16: 193–203.

Andersen, B.L. (1992). Psychological interventions for cancer patients to enhance the quality of life. *Journal of Consulting and Clinical Psychology* 60: 552–568.

Baider, L., Peretz, T. and Kaplan De-Nour, A. (1997). The effect of behavioral intervention on the psychological distress of Holocaust survivors with cancer. *Psychotherapy and Psychosomatics* 66: 44–49.

Barr, D.A. (1996). The ethnics of Soviet medical practice: behaviors and attitudes of physicians in Soviet Estonia. *Journal of Medical Ethics* 22: 33–40.

Berry, J., Trimble, J. and Olmedo, E. (1986). Assessment of acculturation. In W. Lonner and J. Berry (Eds), *Field Methods in Cross-Cultural Research*, Newbury Park, CA: Sage.

Betancourt, H. and Lopez, S.R. (1993). The study of culture, ethnicity, and race in American psychology. *American Psychologist* 48: 629–637.

Blackhall, L.J., Murphy, S.T., Frank, G., Michel, V. and Azen, S. (1995). Ethnicity and attitudes toward patient autonomy. *Journal of the American Medical Association* 274: 820–825.

Braun, K.L. and Nichols, R. (1996). Cultural issues in death and dying. *Hawaii Medical Journal* 55: 260–264.

Burkett, G.L. (1991). Culture, illness, and the biopsychosocial model. *Family Medicine* 23: 2867–2891.

Carrillo, J.E., Green, A.R. and Betancourt, J.R. (1999). Cross-cultural primary care: a patient-based approach. *Annals of Internal Medicine* 130: 829–834.

Chaturvedi, S.K. (1991). What's important for quality of life to Indians—in relation to cancer. *Social Science and Medicine* 33: 91–94.

Cuellar, I., Harris, L.C. and Jasso, R. (1980). An acculturation scale for Mexican–American normal and clinical populations. *Hispanic Journal of Behavioral Sciences* 2: 199–217.

Day, T.W. (1992). Cross-cultural medicine at home. *Minnesota Medicine* 75: 15–17.

Die Trill, M.D. and Holland, J. (1993). Cross-cultural differences in the care of patients with cancer. A review. *General Hospital Psychiatry* 15: 21–30.

Die-Trill, M. (1998.) The patient from a different culture. In J.C. Holland (Ed). *Psycho-Oncology*, New York: Oxford University Press.

Donovan, K., Sanson-Fisher, R.W. and Redman, S. (1989). Measuring quality of life in cancer patients. *Journal of Clinical Oncology* 7: 959–968.

Eisenbruch, M. and Handelman, L. (1990). Cultural consultation for cancer: astrocytoma in a Cambodian adolescent. *Social Science and Medicine* 31: 1295–1299.

Ernst, E. and Cassileth, B.R. (1998). The prevalence of complementary/alternative medicine in cancer. *Cancer* 83: 777–782.

Feinberg, R. (1990). Spiritual and natural etiologies on a Polynesian outlier in Papua New Guinea. *Social Science and Medicine* 30: 311–323.

Freeman, H.P. (1989). Cancer in the socioeconomically disadvantaged. *CA—A Cancer Journal for Clinicians* **39**: 266–288.

Gotay, C.C. and Wilson, M.E. (1998). Social support and cancer screening in African–American, Hispanic, and Native American women. *Cancer Practice* **6**: 31–37.

Guillemin, F., Bombardier, C. and Beaton, D. (1993). Cross-cultural adaptation of health-related quality of life measures: literature review and proposed guidelines. *Journal of Clinical Epidemiology* **46**: 1417–1432.

Hubbell, F.A., Chavez, L.R., Mishra, S.I. and Valdez, R.B. (1996). Beliefs about sexual behavior and other predictors of Papanicolaou smear screening among Latinas and Anglo women. *Archives of Internal Medicine* **156**: 2353–2358.

Kaur, J.S. (1996). The potential impact of cancer survivors on Native American cancer prevention and treatment. *Cancer* **78**: 1578–1581.

Kleinman, A. (1986). Culture, the quality of life and cancer pain: anthropological and cross-cultural perspectives. In V. Ventafrida, F.S.A.M. Van Dam, R. Yancik and M. Tamburini (Eds), *Assessment of Quality of Life and Cancer Treatment*. Amsterdam: Elsevier Science Publisher B.V.

Leong, F. (1998). Special issue on acculturation and ethnic identity among Asian–Americans. *Asian American and Pacific Islander Journal of Health* **6**: 3–4.

Lepowsky, M. (1990). Sorcery and penicillin: treating illness on a Papua New Guinea island. *Social Science and Medicine* **30**: 1049–1063.

Mark, N. and Roberts, L. (1994). Ethnosensitive techniques in the treatment of the Hasidic patient with cancer. *Cancer Practice* **2**: 202–208.

Marsella, A.J. and Higginbotham, H.N. (1984). Traditional Asian medicine: application to psychiatric services in developing nations. In P. Pedersen, N. Sartorius and A. Marsella (Eds), *Mental Health Services: The Cross-cultural Context*. London: Sage.

McDermott, J.F., Tseng, W. and Maretzki, T.W. 1980. *People and cultures of Hawai'i: A Psychocultural Profile*. Honolulu:University of Hawaii Press.

Meyer, T.J. and Mark, M.M. (1995). Effects of psychosocial interventions with adult cancer patients: a meta-analysis of randomized experiments. *Health Psychology* **14**: 101–108.

Meyerowitz, B.E., Richardson, J., Hudson, S. and Leedham, B. (1998). Ethnicity and cancer outcomes: behavioral and psychosocial considerations. *Psychological Bulletin* **123**: 47–70.

Mitchell, J.L. (1998). Cross-cultural issues in the disclosure of cancer. *Cancer Practice* **6**: 153–160.

Morant, R., Jungi, W.F., Koehli, C. and Senn, H.J. (1991). [Why do cancer patients use alternative medicine? (in German)]. *Schweizerische Medizinische Wochenschrift* **121**: 1029–1034.

Muller, J.H. and Desmond, B. (1992). Ethical dilemmas in a cross-cultural context. A Chinese example. *Western Journal of Medicine* **157**: 323–327.

Nayfield, S.G., Bongiovanni, G.C., Alciati, M.H., Fischer, R.A. and Bergner, L. (1994). Statutory requirements for disclosure of breast cancer treatment alternatives. *Journal of the National Cancer Institute* **86**: 1202–1208.

Otero-Sabogal, R., Sabogal, F., Perez-Stable, E.J. and Hiatt, R.A. 1995. Dietary practices, alcohol consumption, and smoking behavior: ethnic, sex, and acculturation differences. *Journal of the National Cancer Insitute Monographs* **18**: 73–82.

Parkin, D.M., Pisani, P. and Ferlay, J. (1999). Global Cancer Statistics. *CA—A Cancer Journal for Clinicians* **49**: 33–64.

Pelusi, J. (1994). Case study: R.B., a single, 23-year-old Hopi woman presented with abnormal vaginal bleeding to the Indian Health Service Clinic. *Cancer Practitioner* **2**: 10.

Peretz, T., Baider, L., Ever-Hadani, P. and De-Nour, A.K. (1994). Psychological distress in female cancer patients with Holocaust experience. *General Hospital Psychiatry* **16**: 413–418.

Schraub, S. and Helary, J.P. (1991). [Unproven treatment in cancerology (in French).]. *Bulletin Cancer Paris* **78**: 915–920.

Shankar, A.D. (1997). Pilot Study: The influence of cultural components on breast cancer patients' perceptions of their support systems. *The Howard Journal of Communications* **8**: 101–111.

Shook, V. (1985). *Ho'oponopono: Contemporary Uses of a Hawaiian Problem-solving Process*. Honolulu: The East–West Center.

Soldavini, M.L., Meister, N.D., Giuliano, A., Volk, J., Robinson, J.W., Daeffler, R.J., Drake, J. and Burhansstipanov, L. (1994). R.B., a single, 23-year-old Hopi woman presented with abnormal vaginal bleeding to the Indian Health Service Clinic. *Cancer Practice* **2:** 10–15.

Stjernsward, J. and Teoh, N. (1993). Current status of the global cancer control program of the World Health Organization. *Journal of Pain and Symptom Management* **8:** 340–347.

Tamura, T. and Lau, A. (1992). Connectedness versus separateness: applicability of family therapy to Japanese families. *Family Process* **31:** 319–340.

Thomas, D.B. and Karagas, M.R. (1996). Migrant Studies. In D. Schottenfeld and J.F. Fraumeni (Eds), *Cancer Epidemiology and Prevention*. New York: Oxford University Press.

Triandis, H.C. (1994). *Culture and Social Behavior*. New York: McGraw-Hill.

Tseng, W.S. and Hsu, J. (1991). *Culture and Family*. New York: Haworth.

Yi, J.K. (1995). Acculturation, access to care and use of preventive health services by Vietnamese women. *Asian American and Pacific Islander Journal of Health* **3:** 31–41.

7

The Role of Japanese Families in Cancer Care

TOSHINARI SAEKI, TOMOYUKI MANTANI, SHIGETO YAMAWAKI
Department of Psychiatry and Neurosciences,
Hiroshima University School of Medicine, Hiroshima, Japan

YOSUKE UCHITOMI
Psycho-oncology Division,
National Cancer Center Research Institute East, Kashiwa, Japan

Family members of the cancer patient should be recognized as 'second-order patients,' because the diagnosis of cancer in a family member presents a frightening crisis to the whole family and all of the family members react in their characteristic ways. Nevertheless, Japanese medical oncologists seem to take it for granted that the family will be available as an extended agent of patient care. Moreover, the important cancer information is often selected, divided and dispensed to various family members. Therefore, in trying to protect themselves and the patient, many families reduce the communication process and create a 'conspiracy of silence,' which has already been well documented in Western literature.

In this chapter, we first address such specific patient–family–doctor relationships in Japan with the theoretical and research background. Second, two brief cases of Japanese families confronted with such a 'conspiracy of silence' are described. Third, we review the available Japanese literature referring to family issues in cancer care with a view to clarifying the central role of the family and developing a comprehensive approach to family evaluation and intervention. Finally, the future directions of empirical family studies in the field of Japanese psycho-oncology are discussed.

PATIENT–FAMILY–DOCTOR RELATIONSHIPS IN JAPAN

TRUTH TELLING ISSUES IN CANCER CARE

Surveys of bereaved families conducted by the Japanese Ministry of Health and Welfare (JMHW) (1992) showed that only 18.2% of family members who had cared for a terminally ill cancer patient (28.6% of the age-adjusted sample in 1994;

Cancer and the Family, 2nd Edn. Edited by L. Baider, C. L. Cooper and A. Kaplan De-Nour
© 2000 John Wiley & Sons, Ltd

Japanese Ministry of Health and Welfare, 1994) reported that the cancer patient was given the true diagnosis. Although a clear trend toward disclosure has been observed between the two surveys, 42.5% (43.8% in 1994) of caregivers reported that the patient might have suspected cancer, 25.1% (28.8% in 1994;) reported that patient was not aware of the diagnosis, and 12.6% (3.2% in 1994) had no idea whether the patient was aware of the diagnosis.

In Japan, the principle family members (e.g. spouse and children) are usually informed by the physician of the cancer patient's diagnosis, prognosis, and the treatment plan before the cancer patient is told the truth (Hattori et al., 1991). Then, the family member(s) decide whether the patient should be told, usually after discussions with other family members (e.g. the patient's siblings, uncles and aunts). The physician usually accepts the family's decision. At the time of the diagnosis, rapid treatment will probably be needed to improve the patient's chance of survival. Thus, most cancer patients who are not informed of the diagnosis probably suspect that they have cancer (Long and Long, 1982). Usually, the patient never says the word 'cancer' to his/her family or physician (Long and Long, 1982; Tsuji, 1990). Therefore, Japanese people seem to fear that disclosure of the truth would cause tension and distress among the family members, including the patient, and between the family and the physician, and that the patient may not accept the family's and physician's decision to withhold the cancer diagnosis.

This practice of family decision making is common in Japan and can be traced to the aspects of Japanese culture that guide interpersonal relations, which probably originated in the traditional agricultural society of Japan (Namihira, 1988). Group decision making is more common than an individual making his/her own decisions, because the sense of belonging to the family is strong. Cancer patients who are not informed of the diagnosis but who nevertheless suspect that they have cancer may accept the family's decision because they think that their family hopes to protect them from disappointment. In Japan, the rate of psychiatric morbidity (e.g. adjustment disorder with depressed mood) in cancer patients who knew the true diagnosis was higher than for those who did not know the truth (Hosaka et al., 1994) and a similar observation has been made in Indian society (Alexander et al., 1993). Thus, Japanese cancer patients may accept their family's decision to withhold the diagnosis in order to avoid distress and tension within the family and so that they can be informed about their own disease step by step, rather than all at once. The family may buffer the psychological impact of the cancer on the patient.

THE JAPANESE CUSTOM OF MOURNING FOR THE DEAD

Although the recent trend in Japan has been a move away from extended families toward a more nuclear family-based society, similar to that of the West, the relationships within the family remain closer than those of the West. Following the death of a loved one in Japan, the family members will gather together to mourn the deceased. As an observance of Bhuddist ritual, the family will carry out periodic services over a very long period of time (more than 30 years). This close relationship between the patient and family deserves further description.

First, with the date on which the patient has died counted as 'day 1', the family assembles and reads a mass for the repose of the deceased's soul on the 'first week', or the 6th day after death, with the '49th day' being 48 days after death and the '100th day' being the 99th day after death. On the same day each month and year as the day of death, referred to as the 'monthly' and 'yearly anniversary of death', respectively, a priest from the local temple in which the families' ancestors are entombed is often invited to the house to chant a prayer for the deceased. On the first anniversary of death, the family assembles and a mass reading for the repose of the soul of the deceased is performed, called the '*isshu-ki*'. Thereafter, with the year in which the patient died referred to as year 1, the third '*kai-ki*' (memorial service for the deceased) on the second anniversary is performed in the second year, a seventh *kai-ki* in the sixth year and similar periodic services are held on the thirteenth, seventeenth, twenty-third and twenty-seventh *kai-ki*. At such times, close family members meet and hold a gathering to remember the deceased. In many cases, a thirty-third *kai-ki* is held on the 32nd year after death and occasionally, a further fiftieth *kai-ki* is held in the 49th year after death, called the 'final service', when the services for the deceased patient conclude.

In today's Japan, in which the lifestyle since the end of the Second World War has rapidly become more and more Westernized, the fact that these special mourning rituals continue to be observed, extending as they do over a period of many years, may be seen as an extension of the Japanese custom of trying to protect the patient by shouldering as much of the psychological burden as possible. The family members try lightening the patient' burden by making various decisions related to cancer treatment. In one sense, by continuing the mourning services over a long period of time after the death of the patient, it is thought that the family as a whole are apologizing and showing repentance for possibly not being able to adequately support the deceased while he/she was still alive. However, these trends are contrary to the Western way of thinking, in which the patient's autonomy is paramount with regard to information about cancer and the method of treatment. In Japan, these Western ideals are quickly spreading among hospitals specializing in cancer treatment, with respect for the patient's autonomy and establishment of support systems for the family being important aspects of this trend.

BRIEF REPORTS OF FAMILIES IN DISTRESS

CASE 1: MR A, AGED 26, SINGLE MALE

The patient developed malignant lymphoma at the age of 25. He developed severe depression during the initial treatment and was referred to a psychiatrist. The depression was alleviated by administration of 150 mg amitriptyline, 100 mg maprotiline and 50 mg clomipramine by drip. Thereafter, a relatively stable mental state was maintained with only 100 mg maprotiline. At the time, the family was against informing the patient of the malignant lymphoma diagnosis, but during repetitive chemotherapy treatments, the patient guessed his own illness. Due to the stability of the depression and the patient's own strong wishes, the leading specialist treating the patient notified him of his condition. However, after notification, the patient refused chemotherapy and for the three months thereafter, only palliative pain control was administered. During this time, the parents, who were in favor of a more positive treatment regimen, became extremely upset. The mother at one point had to be treated for the same depression as the patient himself. However, the patient's attitude changed dramatically after meeting and hearing the pleas of a family friend whom he greatly respected, and thereafter the patient had a strong desire to survive the disease. He was admonished by his parents and once again began treatment, the ultimate result being complete remission.

CASE 2: MRS B, AGED 64, MARRIED WOMAN

The patient was diagnosed with stomach cancer at the age of 62, but was not informed of the type of disease. One year after surgery, liver metastasis was detected and the patient was referred to the University Hospital. Her condition was inoperable at that point, and radiotherapy alone was performed in hopes of giving her some quality of life. Her husband was deeply concerned over how to accommodate her during her remaining days, and as a result, he asked that she be notified that her prognosis was for 6 months. However, the patient was calm on hearing the news and stated that she wished to spend her remaining time together with her husband. After leaving the hospital, the two went on a second honeymoon to Miyazaki prefecture where they spent their original honeymoon. Soon after arriving back home, the patient's condition deteriorated and she was once again admitted to the University Hospital. Her symptoms were alleviated but her fear of dying worsened and she was subsequently referred to a psychiatrist. Through administration of small doses of benzodiazepine and her husband's emotional support, the patient eventually came to accept her impending death. She passed away shortly after thanking the hospital staff for enabling her to go on a second honeymoon and for allowing her to once again view the cherry blossoms of April. Later, the psychiatrist received a letter from the husband saying that he was now living with friends who had all participated in the monthly anniversary memorial services of her death. He appeared to be handling his grief well.

REVIEW OF THE LITERATURE

FROM DESCRIPTIVE STUDIES

Ueno et al. (1983) studied the psychological changes observed in the families of five terminally-ill cancer patients, and reported that the care of these families was enhanced by a natural exchange of information between the various family members. They reported that it was important to provide a medical environment wherein the families felt free to discuss the various problems that were troubling them.

Kashiwagi (1989), a psychiatrist at one of the leading hospices in Japan, stressed the importance of two points, based on his experience in the care of many terminally ill patients, as essential for the proper support of families by medical personnel: (a) listening to the family members' feelings, both in a receptive manner and in a quiet place, so as to ensure their privacy and allow them to fully express their feelings of sadness; (b) holding meetings with family members in an effort to help them come to accept the patient's death and not go into denial over it.

From their clinical experiments on palliative care procedures by psychiatrists and anesthesiologists, Ito et al. (1995) raised the following three points as potential dilemmas families face in palliative care: (a) the stress brought about by acting as a nursing assistant; (b) the psychological conflict related to notifying the patient of his/her illness; and (c) the hardship the family members face in coming to terms with the death. They indicated that taking the needs of the family into account, as well as those of the patient, and providing help to the family, are two closely related factors in the proper care of the patient.

In addition to the above reports, others have appeared, including a retrospective survey of bereaved family members of 12 patients, including six with cancer (Kawano, 1993), a questionnaire survey of family members of 40 cancer patients in an internal ward at the terminal stage treatment (Tsutsumi et al., 1994), reports of interviews with the bereaved family members of 25 cancer patients (Yokota et al., 1995), and case reports from the nurses' points of view. However, research in Japan has only recently begun to investigate the psychological aspects of cancer patients, and the number of reports that take the families of the patients into account are also very low. The greatest reason for this current state of affairs in Japan, where Western theoretical models and family therapies have only recently been introduced, is that our own theories and therapies are scarce and the methodology of family assessment is extremely limited (Saeki et al., 1998).

METHODOLOGY OF FAMILY ASSESSMENT

In terms of evaluating the functions of the entire family, standardized self-report questionnaires in use in Japan include the Japanese versions of the Family Adaptability and Cohesion Evaluation Scale III (FACES III), Family Environment Scale (FES) and Family Assessment Device (FAD).

FACES III is a simple self-report questionnaire consisting of 20 items and two subscales (Cohesion and Adaptability). Although it is easy to use, problems exist in that there is still discussion in the West as to the validity of the family theoretical model that forms the basis of this questionnaire. Although the Japanese version of FACES III has been standardized, a number of modified versions have been generated, leading to some confusion (Sadaki and Kayano, 1997).

FES comprises 90 items and 10 subscales. Although it is the most widely used self-report measure for family research in the West, some of the subscales in the Japanese version are not reliable (Saito et al., 1996) and for this reason it is still not widely used in Japan.

FAD, which is widely used in the West, comprises 60 items and seven subscales. The Japanese version of FAD has recently been standardized (Saeki et al., 1997, 1999) and we have confirmed the feasibility of FAD with the results of a preliminary study using FAD with families of breast cancer patients (Saeki et al., 1998). As it includes such a large number of items, FAD is problematic, but is nonetheless suitable for a detailed examination of family functioning.

These family assessment measures will likely prove important after empirical and international comparative studies are carried out relating to cancer patients and their families.

The Japanese version of the Parental Bonding Instrument (PBI), which assesses the raising of children by the parent as seen from the child's point of view, is available as a measure of the parent–child relationship. No standardized observer-rating scale of the family, and no measures for marital quality, family stress and coping, are currently being developed in Japan.

DIRECTIONS FOR FUTURE RESEARCH

In the Japanese psycho-oncology field, there is a pressing need to establish a proper methodology for family research. As the cultural background deeply influences the family state, the development of original Japanese methodology is preferable. However, if Japan is to enter international comparative studies, the most likely solution is to fully examine and then introduce a methodology established in the West and applicable to Japan. Accordingly, the empirical family studies using the previously described family assessment measures should be promoted as much as possible in the future.

Future research will require the accumulation of observational studies of psychological distress in the families of patients with each type of cancer. Furthermore, research of the spouses of breast cancer patients, to whom psychosocial factors are strongly related due to the length of time of the disease process, and research on the parents of children with cancer for whom grief is particularly deep, are also required. In today's Japan, it is not easy to continue the custom of mourning for the dead. However, considering the increased trend toward nuclear families, research into providing emotional support to the bereaved members of the deceased's family is important.

REFERENCES

Alexander, P.J., Dinesh, N. and Vidyasagar, M.S. (1993). Psychiatric morbidity among cancer patients and its relationship with awareness of illness and expectations about treatment outcome. *Acta Oncologia* **32**: 623–626.

Hattori, H., Salzberg, S.M., Kiang, W.P., Fujimiya, T., Tejima, Y. and Furuno, J. (1991). The patient's right to information in Japan: legal rules and doctors' opinions. *Social Science and Medicine* **32**: 1007–1016.

Hosaka, T., Aoki, T. and Ichikawa, Y. (1994). Emotional states of patients with hematological malignancies: preliminary study. *Japanese Journal of Clinical Oncology* **24**: 186–190.

Ito, J., Yagihashi, M. and Shimoyama, N. (1995). A supportive approach to the patient's family in palliative care. *Shinshin-Igaku* **35**: 235–240 (in Japanese with an English abstract).

Japanese Ministry of Health and Welfare (1993). FY 1992 report on the socio-economic survey of vital statistics: malignant neoplasms. Statistics and Information Department, Minister's Secretariat, Japanese Ministry of Health and Welfare, Tokyo, Japan (in Japanese).

Japanese Ministry of Health and Welfare (1995). FY 1994 report on the socio-economic survey of vital statistics; medical treatment for terminally ill patients. Statistics and Information Department, Minister's Secretariat, Japanese Ministry of Health and Welfare, Tokyo, Japan (in Japanese).

Kashiwagi, T. (1989). Role of psychiatrist in terminal case. *Clinical Psychiatry* **18**: 653–658 (in Japanese).

Kawano, H. (1993). Diseases after bereavement—bereavement stress and health disorders. *Shinshin-Igaku* **33**: 35–38 (in Japanese).

Long, S.O. and Long, B.D. (1982). Curable cancers and fatal ulcers: attitudes toward cancer in Japan. *Social Science and Medicine* **16**: 2101–2108.

Namihira, E. (1988). *Brain Death, Organ Transplantation, and Telling the Truth to Cancer Patients: Anthropological Studies on Death and Medical Care*. Tokyo: Fukutake Shoten.

Sadaki, T. and Kayano, J. (1997). The assessment of family functioning based on the Circumplex Model of marital and family system: A study of clinical usefulness of FACES scales. *Archives of Psychiatric Diagnostics and Clinical Evaluation* **8**: 125–135 (in Japanese with an English abstract).

Saeki, T., Asukai, N., Miyake, Y., Miguchi, M. and Yamawaki, S. (1997). Reliability and validity of the Japanese version of the Family Assessment Device. *Archives of Psychiatric Diagnostics and Clinical Evaluation* **8**: 181–192 (in Japanese with an English abstract).

Saeki, T., Kataoka, T., Saeki, M., Horiguchi, J., Dohi, K. and Yamawaki, S. (1998). Family functioning and mood states among patients with breast cancer: Feasibility of the Japanese version of the Family Assessment Device (FAD). In *Proceedings of The 13th Tokyo Institute of Psychiatry International Symposium 'Cutting-Edge Medicine and Liaison Psychiatry'*, Tokyo, Japan, pp. 91–92.

Saeki, T., Horiguchi, J. and Yamawaki, S. (1998). Family stress in palliative care. *Current Therapy* **16**: 1245–1248 (in Japanese)

Saeki, T., Yokoyama, T., Saeki, M., Asukai, N., Miyake, Y. and Yamawaki, S. (1999). Response bias on the Japanese version of the Family Assessment Device: Low correlation with social desirability and score disagreement between family members. *Archives of Psychiatric Diagnostics and Clinical Evaluation* **10**: 75–82 (in Japanese with an English abstract).

Saito, S., Nomura, N., Noguchi, Y. and Tezuka, I. (1996). Translatability of family concepts into the Japanese culture: Using the Family Environment Scale. *Family Process* **35**: 239–257.

Tsuji, S. 1990. Psychological aspects of dying patients. In Shi no Rinsho 1, *Japanese Society of Death and Dying* (Eds.). Ningen to Rekishi Sha, Tokyo, Japan, pp. 114–127. (in Japanese).

Tsutsumi, Y., Kashima, T., Nozoe, S. and Ushiyama, Y. (1994). Terminal care for malignant tumors and family members' impressions on it in a university hospital. *Shinshin-Igaku* **34**: 377–384 (in Japanese with an English abstract).

Ueno, I., Murata, K., Ohara, K. and Omachi, S. (1983). On the terminal care of the patients with cancer: a research based mainly on family study. *Seishin-Igaku* **25**: 1197–1206 (in Japanese).

Yokota, T., Tokashiki, A. and Ishizu, H. (1995). A study of present situation in terminal care for patients and their families and of families' health problems. *Shinshin-Igaku* **35**: 511–517 (in Japanese with an English abstract).

8

Beliefs about Cancer Causation and their Influence on Family Function

MARIA DIE-TRILL

Psycho-Oncology Unit, Hospital Universitario Gregorio Marañón,
and Universidad Complutense, Madrid, Spain

Beliefs and expectations about cancer are often characterized by defeat, despair, hopelessness, fear, and superstition. Powerful negative images of the disease exist and are frequently made by healthy as well as ill individuals. Because man responds not only to actual danger but also to the threats and symbols of danger, the negative meanings associated to cancer may adversely affect the individual's response to it. On the other hand, not infrequently, the clinician encounters patients and families who experience cancer as a positive changing point in their lives, an experience that has enabled and motivated them to make vital changes that have enhanced the quality of their lives. Kleinman (1986) suggests that quality of life in the context of health and sickness is directly associated with individual meanings attached to the experience of illness. Regardless of what cancer means to the patient and his/her family and how these beliefs are developed, they will influence the psychological response towards the illness and its treatment, they will alter the patient's interpersonal relationships, and they may influence adjustment to the medical experience. For example, the distress originated by the uncertainty of not knowing what has caused cancer, or by feeling unable to control it, may be alleviated by explanations of cancer based on self-blame or on blaming others, because they provide a means of avoiding the intolerable conclusion that no-one is responsible for the disease.

A concept of disease is incomplete unless it takes into account that a person is not only a biological organism but encompasses the realm of feeling and symbolic activities in thought and language. How a person experiences disease and the meaning attributed to it, and how this meaning influences his/her behavior and interaction with others, will be integral components of disease viewed as a 'total human response' (Lipowski, 1969).

This chapter addresses how and why individuals develop beliefs about cancer causation. The influence of causal beliefs in cancer on psychosocial adjustment and family function is also described, taking sociocultural factors into account.

Cancer and the Family, 2nd Edn. Edited by L. Baider, C. L. Cooper and A. Kaplan De-Nour
© 2000 John Wiley & Sons, Ltd

DEVELOPMENT AND DESCRIPTION OF
CAUSAL BELIEFS ABOUT CANCER

Medical science provides theoretical models of illnesses, which describe what a specific illness is, what it consists of, what are its symptoms and its causes, how it is prevented and recognized, how it is medically treated, why it affects some individuals and not others, and why not everyone responds to treatment in the same manner, among other factors. Due to limitations in medical knowledge and technology, medicine cannot always provide explanatory models for all illnesses. As a consequence, patients who suffer from them and their families will search for their own personal explanations in order to shape and give meaning to the illness experience. Beliefs held by individuals with cancer and their families are important to identify because they can influence participation in prevention and early detection activities, decisions about treatment, emotional responses, and sexual and family relationships.

Rokeach (1969) defined a 'belief' as a simple proposition, conscious or unconscious, inferred from what a person says or does, capable of being preceded by the phrase, 'I believe that'. Robbins (1987) emphasized the power of beliefs by reporting that they are the most powerful force in human behavior.

Beliefs about disease causation have been studied initially within the context of Kelley's (1967, 1971) attribution theory, which proposes that negative or unexpected events challenge one's sense of meaning. According to Kelley, people search for reasons (causal attributions) for the occurrence of events that threaten or modify their status. Causal attributions of illness have been described as reflecting both the 'cognitive processes by which an individual arrives at an explanatory belief, and also . . . the explanation itself' (Stoekle and Barsky, 1980, p. 224). In a culture such as ours, which emphasizes cause-and-effect relationships and justifies the administration of medical treatments based on causal explanations, our ignorance about cancer is difficult for patients and their families to accept (Bearison et al., 1993). Causal attributions in cancer facilitate people's understanding of the meaning of the illness and its treatment and their coping emotionally with it. In this respect, causal attributions may be important ways of understanding people's response to and adjustment to cancer. Research on causal attributions in cancer is scarce and focuses almost exclusively on the patient and not on the family, consequently limiting our understanding of how beliefs about cancer's origin influence family dynamics.

Several authors have demonstrated that the process of attributing causes occurs in individuals with serious illness as an initial attempt at gaining some control over their lives (Taylor et al., 1984; Michela and Wood, 1986). Causal attributions, as Kelley pointed out, have been described to occur in cases of life-threatening illnesss because patients and their families have a need to recover basic assumptions that are shattered by such situations (Janoff-Bulman and Frieze, 1983). An almost universal cognitive attempt at gaining some degree of mastery over cancer in order to explain and understand its origins and mechanisms was already described in the 1950s. It was even reported that as threats from illness increase in severity, individuals have an increasing need to develop beliefs about the causes of the illness (Bard and Dyk, 1956), a hypothesis that has not been totally supported by later research.

Causal beliefs about illness may range from scientifically valid ones to the most irrational, ilogical and even delusional (Mabry, 1964). Furthermore, the irrationality of the individual's beliefs about the illness was initially thought to increase in direct proportion to the seriousness of the illness (Bard and Dyk, 1956).

Causal attributions of illness have also been studied in the context of learned helplessness theory (Seligman, 1975). Both attribution and learned helplessness theories contend that loss of control can contribute to the development of feelings of anxiety, depression and withdrawal. However, tests of these relationships in cancer are limited and research on the efficacy of cancer patients' beliefs regarding personal control is inconclusive (Lowery et al., 1993). Rothbaum and colleagues (1982) argued that a strong belief in personal control may not be beneficial in situations that are largely uncontrollable, and that what is operative in most situations is a balance between a sense of personal (internal) control and control by others (external control). In this case, a diminished sense of one type of control would be compensated for by the strength in the other type.

Views about the cause of disease differ across cultures (Die-Trill, 1998). Health among Philippino immigrants is believed to be impaired by natural causes (heredity, pathogens, traumas), by inappropriate behavior (criticism, shame, social irresponsibility), by social punishment for improper behavior, or by supranatural causes (Anderson, 1983). Illness in Jamaica is believed to be caused by cold, gas, wind, heat, bile, blood imbalances or germs (Mitchell, 1983). Beliefs about disease causation in Uganda fall under the following categories: magical, supernatural, infectious and hereditary (Namboze, 1983). Cold, dirt, improper diet, 'low blood' ('low blood' is conceptually allied with anemia but may be terminologically confused with low blood pressure. Its symptoms are weakness, lassitude, fatigue, and 'falling out'), and improper behavior have been identified as causes of disease among lower-class black Americans (Snow, 1983). Disease in France and in Germany has been described as a failure of internal defenses, rather than as an invasion from without. Anglo-Saxons, on the contrary, are said to view disease as caused by an external force (Payer, 1990). Mexican–American patients have been described as passive recipients of disease: patients themselves are blameless for what happens to them, as disharmony is the work of witches or evil spirits (Kim, 1983).

Not infrequently, adult cancer patients blame themselves or others for their illness and interpret cancer as a form of punishment (Abrams and Finnesinger, 1953; Bard and Dyk, 1956; Chodoff et al., 1963; van den Borne et al., 1986; Houldin et al., 1996). Cancer patients have reported a variety of causal attributions about their disease, including: chance (Gotay, 1985; van den Borne et al., 1986; Lowery et al., 1993); stress (Taylor et al, 1984; Timko and Janoff-Bulman 1985; Dodd et al., 1985a,b); accumulation of physical discomfort and having 'too many children' or a 'bad personality' (Dodd et al., 1985b); physical factors (Dodd et al., 1985a); heredity (Linn et al., 1982); religion (Taylor et al., 1984); psychic problems and environmental pollution (Riehl-Emde et al., 1989); homosexuality (Price, 1993); and lifestyle (van den Borne et al., 1986). Late-stage cancer patients in the USA believed past behavior (e.g., smoking) was clearly associated with the development of cancer (Linn et al., 1982). Psychological and genetic factors were identified as causing cancer by almost 50% of a sample of Swiss oncology patients (Kesserling et al., 1986). Healthy Hispanics were found to have more misconceptions about causes of cancer than their Anglo-Saxon counterparts and more frequently identified sugar substitutes, bruises from cuts, microwave ovens, eating pork or spicy foods, and antibiotics as causing cancer (Perez-Stable et al. 1992). Breathing polluted air, using aluminum and lead utensils, and eating frozen foods have been described as causing cancer by healthy Chinese–American women (Mo, 1984). Baider and Sarell (1983) studied perceptions and causal attributions in Jewish Israeli women with breast cancer and described two distinct response patterns: the Western patients' orientation (science-oriented and active) and the Eastern patients' orientation (fatalistic and passive).

Clinical interviews reveal how beliefs about cancer and its treatment can increase anxiety levels and interfere with patient compliance and overall adjustment. For example, a 58 year-old woman with newly diagnosed colon cancer was referred to our Psycho-Oncology Unit for an evaluation after refusing treatment with chemotherapy. The patient's husband had died of cancer after several chemotherapy trials. Two other individuals whom she had met in the chemotherapy clinic during her husband's illness had also died after prolonged treatments with chemotherapy. The patient believed that the treatment she was being offered was a 'poison that has killed my husband and his hospital friends' and was obviously reluctant to receive it. Based on this and other observations, a descriptive study on causal attributions in cancer was carried out (Die Trill et al., 1998). The study's objectives were: (a) to identify the beliefs held by oncology patients and their families about the cause of cancer; and (b) to provide patient education and psychological interventions in order to correct misconceptions about cancer, improve patient compliance and reduce anxiety secondary to causal attributions. Sixty patients with cancer, aged 17–79 (mean age, 52.6 years; $SD = 13.5$) and 15 family members, who were referred to the Psycho-Oncology Unit for an evaluation of psychological symptoms, were asked what they believed to have caused the illness. Time since diagnosis ranged between 1 month and 10 years (mean, 19.24 months; $SD = 25.4$): cancer diagnosis, level of education and psychiatric diagnosis are shown in Table 8.1. Over 55% of the patients interviewed met DSM–IV criteria for a psychiatric diagnosis. Only 10% of patients made no causal attributions when asked what they believed had originated their cancer, and 11 (18.3%) of patients identified more than one causal attribution. Identified attributions were divided into two categories: internal or external, depending on the degree of control the patient was considered to have over the identified cause of his illness. More patients identified internal (64%) than external (36%) attributions and the former predominated in all age groups. Subtypes of attributions and the frequency with which they were identified can be seen in Table 8.2. Most attributions (83.5%) were made by patients within 24 months following diagnosis. All patients who made no causal attribution had been diagnosed within the 24 months previous to the study interview. These findings suggest that patients who make causal attributions do so upon diagnosis or shortly thereafter, while patients who do not engage in causal attributions initially, will tend not to do so later on during the course of their disease. We may hypothesize that two distinct groups of patients exist. One group needs to engage in a causal search for their cancer in order to cope with, and give meaning to, the chaos initially originated by a cancer diagnosis, its treatments, and their side-effects. A second group of patients use other coping strategies to confront the illness. There was no correlation between level of education and number or type of attributions made. Of the patients identifying more than one attribution, 72% identified attributions within the same category (internal vs. external). With respect to adjustment, among the patients diagnosed with

Table 8.1   Level of education, cancer diagnosis and DSM–IV psychiatric diagnosis in patients participating in a causal attributions study

	Frequency (%)
Level of education	
High school	32
College	28
Post-graduate studies	20
Unknown	20
Cancer diagnosis	
Breast cancer	35
Lung cancer	23
Gynecological cancer	10
Gastric cancer	5
Bladder cancer	5
Brain tumors	3.3
Lymphoma	3.3
Colon cancer	3.3
Sarcoma	3.3
Others	8.8
DSM–IV diagnosis	
Adjustment disorder with depressed and/or anxious mood	33.3
Major depression	18.3
Organic brain syndrome	3.33
Others (e.g., obsessive–compulsive disorder)	1.7
No psychiatric diagnosis	15
Unknown psychiatric diagnosis	28.3

Table 8.2   Classification of causal attributions and their frequencies

Type of attribution	Frequency (%)
External causal attributions	
Constitutional susceptibility (aging, genetics)	33.3
Environmental (nutrition, exposure to certain materials)	25
Trauma (physical injury)	25
Fate	12.5
Physical (inflammation)	4.2
Internal causal attributions	
Behavioral (dieting, drinking, smoking, overworking, scratching, others)	37.21
Affective (stress, suffering, disappointments, depressed affect, being 'grumpy')	37.21
Self-blame/punishment (revenge, course)	20.9
Cognitive (obsessions and thoughts about having cancer in the future)	4.65

adjustment disorders or major depressions, according to DSM–IV criteria, 72.5% identified internal causal attributions, whereas only 27.5% identified external attributions, suggesting that those that made external attributions were, overall, better adjusted, as pointed out in other studies. One-quarter of patients identified causal attributions embedded in their family relationships. Family histories in these cases often shaped patients' beliefs about cancer causation and were usually helpful to the patient in interpreting and giving meaning to their disease experience. Such was the case of 38 year-old, HL, who believed her lymphoma to be a consequence of the suffering associated to the recent loss of both her parents. Some patients reported divorce or marital problems to have caused their cancer. A 61 year-old male with gastric cancer believed that the distress caused by his daughter's marriage to a physically disabled individual had originated his disease. Suffering caused by the death of one sibling and the diagnosis of a chronic disease in another was identified by a 59 year-old patient as causing her breast cancer. Another 44 year-old female with ovarian cancer believed she had unconsciously caused her illness in order to 'reunite' herself with her daughter, who had died at the age of 10, 2 years earlier. Other patients identified curses or revenges by family members as the causes of their cancer. EJ was a 23 year-old female with lymphoma diagnosed one week after her marriage. Prior to getting married, EJ had been engaged to her husband's brother. This first relationship broke up after EJ discovered that her fiancé had been imprisoned, had lied to her about his employment status, and was a drug addict. EJ strongly believed that her illness was the result of a curse from her brother-in-law for not having married him but his sibling instead. VM was a bright, extravert, 35 year-old travel agent who was diagnosed with breast cancer. VM had known, since she was a child, that her father maintained an extramarital affair with a neighbor. Three months prior to her diagnosis, VM had confronted her father's lover about this affair and requested that she 'left her father alone.' A few weeks later the lover died of a chronic medical condition. VM believed her newly diagnosed cancer was the result of the dead woman's revenge. Results on interviews with family members will be presented in another section of this chapter.

Various factors may influence the development of beliefs about cancer: the individual's age; sex; personal and familial experience with cancer; socio-economic status; educational level; cultural and religious backgrounds; health and illness-related beliefs; social milieu (interpersonal relationships, employers, and mass media); site and extent of the disease; time since diagnosis; type of treatments administered, knowledge about cancer; and events that take place during an individual's and a family's lifetime. Beliefs about cancer causation are maintained despite medical or other technical information that contradicts them. For example, there exists a generalized belief that the proximity of waste-emitting industries to residential areas along the Mississippi River has adversely impacted the health of the residents, including increasing the rates of cancer. However, Lousiana Tumor Registry data do not support this widely-held belief of increased cancer rates (Fick et al., 1999).

Attributing a cause to cancer determines, in part, the modes of treatment that individuals seek when confronting the illness. Treatment of the 'immediate cause' of a disease (e.g., pathogens) may be sought at the same time that a healer who will deal with the 'ultimate cause' (e.g., bad luck) is consulted, because different medical systems are directed to different levels of cause (Clark, 1983).

Beliefs about cancer causation influence preventive behaviors as well (Die-Trill, 1998). Cultural values with respect to modesty and sexuality, especially in unmarried women, partly account for a Chinese lack of attention to breast health (Mo, 1992). Four out of five healthy adults in Australia believed that individuals can take steps to reduce their risk of cancer, including not smoking, dietary measures, and solar protection (Hill et al., 1991). Similar beliefs have been found among British (Cancer Relief Macmillan Fund, 1988) and other European communities (Commission of European Communities, 1987) suggesting an increased sense of control over health among members of these cultural groups. People who believe they can control their disease may be more likely to engage in unconventional treatments, which can be taken to an extreme, as in the case of visual imagery to control cancer (Die-Trill and Holland, 1993). On the other hand, cultures that ascribe supernatural or internal causes to cancer will most likely believe that there is little they can do to prevent or treat it, and will be more likely to adopt more passive attitudes during the course of the disease (Die-Trill, 1998).

Nielsen et al. (1992) have identified eight published and unpublished instruments used to assess beliefs about cancer, cancer prevention and cancer treatment within a variety of age groups and ethnic populations. Many of these instruments were at their initial phase of development at the time of the review and issues of validity or reliability were not addressed by some authors.

INCIDENCE OF CAUSAL ATTRIBUTIONS IN CANCER

The percentage of patients reported to engage in causal thinking about their illness varies significantly. It remains unclear whether variations in reported rates are the result of the manner in which the attribution question is asked, a function of the different illness populations, or the result of some other methodological limitation. Between 25% and 50% of women with gynecological and breast cancer reported having thought about the question, 'Why me?' (Gotay, 1985; Lowery et al., 1993). In a study of causal thinking and adjustment among women with varying stages of breast cancer, 65% of the sample initially reported having an idea or theory about the cause of their cancer. With probing, 95% eventually provided a theory (Taylor et al., 1984). Causal thinking has been associated with time since diagnosis: the more recent the diagnosis, the more patients were likely to report causal attributions (Lowery et al., 1993), results that were corroborated in our study (Die-Trill et al., 1998). Two theories were provided to explain this. First, that the intensity of the situation at the time of diagnosis may be sufficient to evoke such thinking, and that intensity subsides with time. Second, that at later stages of illness, patients do not recall having such thoughts, although such thoughts did occur.

A distinction must be made between patients and their family members who do not engage in causal thinking about their illness at all, and those who do engage in it but fail to identify specific causal attributions about it. The percentage of patients who make no causal attribution for their cancer, or who report not knowing what has caused the disease when asked, also varies significantly and ranges between 12% and 92% (Dodd et al., 1985a,b; Kesserling et al., 1986; Lowery et al., 1993; Bearison et al., 1993). Such wide variations may reflect not only methodological differences, but also differences in respondent's level of education, knowledge about cancer, and socio-cultural backgrounds, given that reported studies have been carried out in different cultural groups. One of the few causal attribution studies in cancer to include family members of oncology patients is that of Bearison and his colleagues (1993), who interviewed parents and caregivers of children with cancer. Among these, only 30% did not attribute a cause to their child's cancer when asked. In our study, only 20% of cancer patients' relatives interviewed did not attribute a cause to the patient's illness.

CAUSAL ATTRIBUTIONS AND PSYCHOSOCIAL ADJUSTMENT TO ILLNESS

Illness-related causal beliefs are thought to facilitate an individual's understanding of what is happening to him/her or a member of his/her family and to reduce ambiguity, uncertainty, and anxiety. However, research does not entirely support the assumption that adjustment is adversely affected in cancer patients that do not engage in causal thinking (e.g., Taylor et al., 1984). In addition, research rarely includes the patients' family members. It does however, provide evidence that the relationship between specific attributions and adjustment is quite complex (Lowery et al., 1987, 1993).

Guilt and self-blame related to illness have been described as maladaptive because they may interfere with positive coping during treatment (Abrams and Finesinger, 1953; Houldin et al., 1996). In some studies, patients who engaged in a search for causal attributions were found to have more affective problems and to be less optimistic than patients who did not engage in a causal search for their illness (Lowery and Jacobsen, 1985; Lowery et al., 1987). Other studies fail to show a relationship between adjustment and search for attributions on the origins of cancer (e.g., Lavery and Clarke, 1996). It has been hypothesized that patients who develop internal and controllable attributions for their illness will develop more negative affect in the face of failing health (e.g., 'I am sick because I have not taken care of myself') (Lowery et al., 1993, p. 38). Bearison et al. (1993) found that both pediatric cancer patients and their parents or caretakers who made external types of attributions coped significantly better than those who made internal kinds of attributions or accepted the physician's advice that the cause of the illness was unknown (no attribution). Not all research supports cause–adjustment relationships of this type (Turnquist et al., 1988). For example, no particular attribution has predicted adjustment in other studies (Taylor et al., 1984; Gotay, 1985; Lowery et al., 1993), although internal and external causal attributions have been significantly positively correlated with perceived control in lung cancer patients (Berckman and Austin, 1993).

Evidence with regard to causal beliefs, personal control, and adjustment is therefore inconclusive, and suggests the possibility that causal thinking may facilitate adjustment to cancer in some cases, may not have any effect on the illness experience in others, or may even have a negative influence on psychosocial adjustment to illness in some individuals.

CAUSAL ATTRIBUTIONS IN CANCER AND THE FAMILY

The nature and extent of family relationships have particular significance for perceived quality of life and life satisfaction generally, and more specifically, for the interpretation of physical malaise and subsequent treatment (Marshall, 1990). Hough et al. (1991) identified strategies used for coping with a mother's chronic illness by well- and poorly-adjusted families. Well-adjusted families were found to have constructed some positive meaning out of the illness experience. According to the authors, these families commonly reported a greater appreciation of life, of living in the here-and-now, and achieving a better balance between work and other aspects of one's life. Other positive meanings included a positive evaluation of competence and self-efficacy, and an increase in sensitivity and empathy with others. In contrast to the well-adjusted families, poorly-adjusted families reported no positive effects or meanings related to the illness experience. This negative view was so strong that it was extended to experiences that had the potential of being positive. Consistent with the stress and coping model, families who develop positive meanings from the illness experience report lower stress and higher levels of well-being. They are also seen as better adjusted by researchers (Shannon, 1996).

In addition to attributing meaning to the disease themselves, families may facilitate the patient's search for meaning. Taylor (1993) not only corroborated that adjustment to illness was associated with a clear sense of meaning in cancer patients, but found that married patients had significantly higher scores in the Purpose of Life Test than did single patients.

Ethnographic methods have been used to explore the process implemented by families to develop meanings to chronic illness (Seaburn et al., 1992). Through their discussions with families, the authors found that families faced with the task of giving meaning to the illness experience story-telling, narrative, and language that is transgenerational to develop meanings for current experiences. These meanings are then shaped to support the family's way of dealing with the demands of illness and can enhance how a family copes with the illness experience. The authors conclude with four basic ideas. The first is that families must give their illness experience meaning. For example, a family's view that illness is a challenge may bring order and direction to daily living. The second idea is that family meanings are passed from one generation to another and are continually evolving. These historical meanings can guide families and may contain spiritual, political, or cultural elements. The third idea is that story-telling is a vehicle through which families pass on illness meanings. Stories from the past create a structure for current experiences. The fourth and final idea is that meanings resulting from stories told by families provide influences and guides for daily functioning. Those families who construct meanings from stories of strength and triumph find chronic illness to be less burdensome. According to Patterson and Garwick's (1994) Family Adjustment and Adaptation Response (FAAR) Model, where the family is seen as attempting to maintain homeostasis through using its capabilities to meet its demands, family meanings are constructed on three levels that are dynamically inter-related. Situational meanings are the most concrete and can increase the family's perceived resources and competencies. Family identity defines boundaries and guides family relationships. The third and most abstract level is the family world view, relating to the family's orientation to the world and the way reality is interpreted. All three levels of meaning shape the family's response to the chronic illness.

As with individual patients, familial interpretations of cancer vary, depending on a number of factors, which include, but are not limited to: the family's experience with cancer and losses; knowledge about the disease; relationships and attachments within the family; degree of cohesion in the family; beliefs about health and illness that are transmitted from one generation to another; the patient's age and sex; and the family's religious beliefs and cultural background. Cancer may be seen by some family members as a stigma or as something shameful, a belief frequently held by siblings of pediatric patients; or it may be considered as more painful and distressing than other diseases. Such interpretations of the cancer experience will influence the family's behavior towards the patient and the illness. For example, the belief that cancer is infectious can lead to isolation of the patient, fear of sharing dishes or towels with him/her, withdrawal of physical contact, or to couples not sharing the same bed and avoiding sexual relationships. Cancer viewed as hereditary may lead to anxiety and anger towards the ill progenitor for fear that he/she may pass on the disease to future generations. Family members' actions can attest to the belief that the patient will die. For example, milestones in the family's life cycle may be accelerated in response to cancer, as occurs when children marry earlier than planned, or family visits increase in frequency or extend in time.

In the process of attributing meaning to an illness experience, families, like individual patients, engage in searches for causes that might explain the disease despite the fact that physicians tell them the cause is unknown. Perceptions of the cause of cancer differ according to the observer's relationship to the patient (Curbow et al., 1986). Several reasons account for such variations in perception. First, people view intimate others in a positive light, giving them credit but not the blame (Taylor and Koivumaki, 1976). Thus, family members are likely to be influenced by their emotional ties to the patient. Second, self-protection influences perceptions of cause. For instance, Dunkel-Schetter and Wortman (1982) suggested that strangers or acquaintances may blame the cancer patient in order to maintain their belief in a 'just world', while family members and health professionals may blame the patient to absolve themselves of guilt for not helping. Third, lay persons and health professionals may be differentially inclined to make causal attributions. Except during the initial diagnosis, family members and friends may have a greater need than helping professionals do to know why the patient was stricken with cancer— much like the cancer patients themselves.

In our descriptive study on causal attributions in cancer, we asked 15 oncology patients' first-degree relatives what they believed had caused the patients' illness (Die-Trill et al., 1998). All relatives had been referred to the Psycho-Oncology Unit for evaluation of psychological or psychiatric symptoms. Among the 80% of relatives identifying an attribution, almost half (41.6%) blamed themselves for the patient's cancer. Such was the case of MB, who held herself responsible of her 35 year-old daughter's death from a brain tumor. After the patient's death, MB had recurring thoughts of her daughter having frequent headaches as a child and not taking her to the physician because she was afraid that her neighbors and friends would think she was an incompetent mother if she had a sick child. RL was the husband of a 56 year-old woman who died of metastatic breast cancer. RL's first wife had also died of cancer, as had both his parents and two of his younger brothers. As the eldest of eight siblings, RL had taken care of his ill parents and brothers, as well as both his wives. After his second wife's death, RL feared he had caused cancer in those closest to him and was fearful of getting emotionally involved with anyone in case he 'transmitted' the disease. Affective attributions (e.g., sadness, disappointments, frustrations) and trauma (e.g., physical injury) were each identified by 25% of the patient's relatives. IM's mother believed that the cause of her 26 year-old son's leukemia was that his blood 'stirred up' after his girlfriend broke up with him. RT's sister strongly believed that the cause of the melanoma that killed her brother was having been hit by a ball during a soccer game. Only one relative in the study blamed the patient for his illness. TR believed her husband's lung cancer was a consequence of his frequent contacts with prostitutes during their married life. As can be seen by these case histories, familial beliefs about cancer are frequently interlaced with the family's history and relationships between its members. Our sample, in addition to being small, is biased in that only relatives with distress that requested psychological intervention were interviewed.

Familial causal attributions can also be influenced by the role that the patient has within the family. It is usually difficult for a family to understand why a well-adjusted individual who has never maintained problematic family relationships develops cancer. On the other hand, disease in a conflictive family member can be interpreted by the family in the context of the patient's past inappropriate behavior. Such was the case of DF, a 35 year-old male diagnosed with bladder cancer. DF's family was angry at him for having cancer. He was described as the 'black sheep' of the family, always causing trouble and difficulties for the family. DF had dropped out of school at an early age. He had initiated several jobs but never seemed to be able to maintain them. His relationship to his family was conflictive most of the time. He was blamed not only for having caused his disease by his past behavior, but also for the distress that he was now causing the family 'one more time' with his illness.

Familial beliefs about the cause and prognosis of cancer and the efficacy of its treatments may either aid the patient in achieving optimal psychological recovery or may interfere with his/her adjustment. Families may be better adjusted when their attributions for the causes of cancer are similar to those held by the patients themselves. Similarity in beliefs may facilitate family cohesion, which in turn will ease the process of adjustment to the illness. Bearison et al. (1993) hypothesized that children and their parents would be expected to make similar kinds of causal attributions to childhood malignancies. In their study, parents of children with cancer coped significantly better when they matched their ill child with regard to whether they make a causal attribution for their cancer. Gotay (1985) studied causal attributions in early and advanced-stage cancer patients and their mates, their level of adjustment and the relationship between attributions and adjustment. Attributions here were not found to be significant predictors of adjustment. It was suggested that not making strong causal attributions may be adaptive for cancer patients and their families.

Not only do familial attributions about cancer's origins influence patient adjustment, patient's beliefs about the cause of their disease can also influence the family's coping with the illness, and may even interfere significantly with the survivor's bereavement after the patient dies. JL, a 65 year-old woman with metastatic breast cancer, blamed her daughter FT for her illness and imminent death, because FT had left the family home years earlier, against the patient's will, in order to initiate her studies. JL lay in her hospital bed days before dying, repeatedly telling her daughter that had she stayed taking care of her, the patient would now be healthy. FT requested psychological treatment two years after her mother's death for a complicated bereavement. PL had difficulties in working through her grief in response to her husband's death due to cancer. PL was a physician and believed she should have been able to prevent her husband's death by using her medical knowledge. NR was a 68 year-old woman married to a man diagnosed with paranoid schizophrenia who used to lock her up at home daily upon going to work in order for her 'not to have contact with other men'. During the couple's 40 years of marriage, her husband frequently and falsely accused NR of behaviors she had not engaged in. Upon denying them, her husband would threaten her: 'If you are lying to me, may you die of cancer', to which NR usually responded: 'You are the one who will die of cancer because I am not the one lying'. NR's husband died years later of colorectal cancer, which she believed to have caused herself with her angry remarks. Three years after the death, NR had persisting feelings of guilt and a complicated bereavement reaction. Blame-focused views of illness are not only theoretically suggestive but practically significant in terms of their impact on treatment and family dynamics. Any effort to establish liability and accountability for disease can constrain patient or family control over medical choice and the therapeutic process and may further complicate adjustment to the illness. Attributing health responsibility to family members reduces individual control, because it is the family that is held liable. Paradoxically, patient accountability (e.g., lifestyle) also limits control over the health process, since sickness and sick role status serve as indices that patients are irresponsible. In reality, health problems are multicausal and complex and it is extremely unwise and counterproductive to lay blame at any one source for a given health problem (Finnerman and Bennet, 1995).

DISCUSSION

Causal thinking about cancer is not part of the response of every patient or family to the disease. However, given the misconceptions that individuals hold about the origins of cancer and their influence on the illnesss experience, causal attributions are important to identify in both patient and family members. The clinician should attempt to elicit the patients' and families' belief models with simple, straightforward questions, and to formulate the physician's model in terms the individual can understand. Patient, family and physician models should be compared in order to identify contradictions and to engage in a negotiation towards shared models related to cancer (Kleinman et al., 1977). Perceptual schemata used in perceptions of cancer are amenable to change, based on access to increased information and to added experience (Rounds and Zevon, 1993). It is recommended that interventions to alter misconceptions related to the causes of cancer include these two components. Awareness of cultural and social issues is crucial in guiding this process.

Research on causal beliefs in families of cancer patients is scarce and provides contradicting evidence on the relationship between causal beliefs and psychosocial adjustment. Differences in the measurement of causal attributions, and of psychosocial adjustment to illness, may account for conflicting results. In addition, many other questions remain unanswered. At what point in time during the course of the illness do families engage in the search for causes of the disease? Do familial causal attributions persist in time? Can family events modify causal attributions identified during the initial stages of the disease? What types of families engage in searches for causal attributions when confronting cancer? What are the differences between these families and those who do not engage in such cognitive processes? Individual and family preferences, as well as coping styles, need to be taken into account in order to identify patients and families who may benefit from engaging in causal thinking processes when confronting cancer. In addition, familial beliefs about cancer causation are frequently interlaced with a family's history, experience with the disease, and relationships among its members. These variables, too, should be taken into account in future studies in order to understand the process of identifying attributions to cancer and their role in patient and family adaptation to the illness.

REFERENCES

Abrams, R.D. and Finnesinger, J.E. (1953). Guilt reactions in patients with cancer. *Cancer* **6**: 474–482

Anderson, J.N. (1983). Health and illness in Pilipino Immigrants. *Western Journal of Medicine* **139**: 811–819

Baider, L. and Sarell, M. (1983). Perceptions and causal attributions of Israeli women with breast cancer concerning their illness: The effects of ethnicity and religiosity. *Psychotherapy and Psychosomatics* **39**(3): 136–143

Bard, M. and Dyk, R.D. (1956). The psychodynamic significance of beliefs regarding the cause of serious illness. *Psychoanalytic Review* **43**: 146–162.

Bearison, D.J., Sadow, A.J., Granowetter, L. and Winkel, G. (1993). Patients' and parents' causal attributions for childhood cancer. *Journal of Psychosocial Oncology* **11**(3): 47–61

Berckman, K.L. and Austin, J.K. (1993) Causal attribution, perceived control, and adjustment in patients with lung cancer. *Oncology Nursing Forum* Jan–Feb; **20**(1): 23–30.

Cancer Relief Macmillan Fund (1988). *Public Attitudes to and Knowledge of Cancer in the UK*. London: Cancer Relief Macmillan Fund.

Chodoff, P., Friedman, S.B. and Hamburg, D.A. (1963). Stress, defenses and coping behavior: observations in parents of children with malignant disease. Presented at the meeting of the American Psychiatric Association, St. Louis, MO

Clark, M. (1983). Cultural context of medical practice. *Western Journal of Medicine* **139**(6): 806–810.

Commission of European Communities (1987). *Survey: Europeans and the Prevention of Cancer*. Brussels: Commision of the European Comunities.

Curbow, B., Andrews, R.M. and Burke, T.A. (1986). Perceptions of the cancer patient: causal explanations and personal attributions. *Journal of Psychosocial Oncology* **4**(1/2): 115–134

Die-Trill, M. (1998). The patient from a different culture. In J. Holland (Ed.), *Psycho-Oncology* (pp. 85–866). New York: Oxford University Press.

Die-Trill, M., Gomez Lazareno, J.A., Amodeo, S. and Calvo, F. (1998). Beliefs about cancer causation in oncology patients. Paper presented at the 4th International Congress of Psycho/Oncology, Hamburg, Germany. September 3–6.

Die-Trill, M. and Holland, J. (1993). Cross-cultural differences in the care of patients with cancer. A review. *General Hospital Psychiatry* **15**: 21–30.

Dodd, M.J., Ahmed, N.T., Lindsey, A.M. and Piper, B.F. (1985a). Attitudes of patients living in Egypt about cancer and its treatment. *Cancer Nursing* **8**(5): 278–284

Dodd, M.J., Chen, S., Lindsey, A.M. and Piper, B.F. (1985b). Attitudes of patients living in Taiwan about cancer and its treatment. *Cancer Nursing* **8**(4): 214–220.

Dunkel-Schetter, C. and Wortman, C.B. (1982). The interpersonal dynamics of cancer: problems in social relationships and their impact on the patient. In H.S. Friedman and M.R. DiMatteo (Eds), *Interpersonal Issues in Health Care* (pp. 69–100). New York: Academic Press.

Fick, A., Thomas, S.M., Williams, D.L. and Hayden, J. (1999). Perception of cancer and its causes among 'Industrial Corridor' residents: the LMRICS Planning Project. Lower

Mississippi River Interagency Cancer Study. *Journal of Louisiana State Medical Society* **15**(4): 182–188.

Finnerman, R. and Bennet, L.A. (1995). Guilt, blame and shame: responsibility in health and sickness. *Social Science and Medicine* **40**(1): 1–3.

Gotay, C.C. (1985). Why me? Attributions and adjustment by cancer patients and their mates at two stages in the disease process. *Social Science and Medicine* **20**(8): 825–831

Hill, D., White, V., Borland, R. and Lockburn, J. (1991). Cancer-related beliefs and behaviors in Australia. *Australian Journal of Public Health* **15**(1): 14–23.

Hough, E.E., Lewis, F.M .and Woods, N.F. (1991). Family response to mother's chronic illness: case studies of well and poorly adjusted families. *Western Journal Nursing Research* **13**: 568.

Houldin, A.D., Jacobsen, B. and Lowery, B.J. (1996). Self-blame and adjustment to breast cancer. *Oncology Nursing Forum* **23**(1): 75–79.

Janoff-Bulman, R. and Frieze, I.H. (1983). A theoretical perspective for understanding reactions to victimization. *Journal of Social Issues* **39**(2): 1–17.

Kelley, H.H. (1967). Attribution theory in social psychology. In D. Levine (Ed.), *Nebraska Symposium on Motivation*, Vol. 15. Lincoln: University of Nebraska Press.

Kelley, H.H. (1971). *Attribution and Social Interaction*. Morristown, NJ: General Learning Process.

Kesserling, A., Dodd, M.J., Lindsay, A.M., and Strauss, A.L. (1986). Attitudes of patients living in Switzerland about cancer and its treatment. *Cancer Nursing* **9**(2): 77–85.

Kim, S.S. (1983). Ethnic elders and American health care: a physician's perspective. *Western Journal of Medicine* **139**(6): 885–891.

Kleinman, A. (1986). Culture, the quality of life and cancer pain: anthropological and cross-cultural perspectives. In V. Ventafridda, S. van Dam, R. Yancik and M. Tamburini (Eds), *Assessment of Quality of Life and Cancer Treatment* (pp. 43–50). Amsterdam: Elsevier Science.

Kleinman, A., Eisenberg, L. and Good, B. (1977) Culture, illness and care: clinical lessons from anthropological and cross-cultural research. Unpublished report.

Lavery, J.F. and Clarke, V.A. (1996). Causal attributions, coping strategies, and adjustment to breast cancer. *Cancer Nursing* **19**(1): 20–28.

Linn, M.W., Linn, B.S. and Stein, S.R. (1982). Beliefs about causes of cancer in cancer patients. *Social Science and Medicine* **16**(7): 835–839.

Lipowski, Z.J. (1969) Psychosocial aspects of disease. *Annals of Internal Medicine* **71**: 1197–1206.

Lowery, B.J. and Jacobsen, B.S. (1985). An attributional analysis of chronic illness outcomes. *Nursing Research* **34**: 82–88.

Lowery, B.J., Jacobsen, B.S. and DuCette, J. (1993) Causal attribution, control and adjustment to breast cancer. *Journal of Psychosocial Oncology* **10**(4): 37–53.

Lowery, B.J., Jacobsen, B.S. and McCauley, K. (1987). On the prevalence of causal search in illness situations. *Nursing Research* **36**: 88–93.

Mabry, J.H. (1964). Lay concepts of etiology. *Journal of Chronic Diseases* **17**: 371.

Marshall, P.A. (1990). Cultural influences on perceived quality of life. *Seminars in Oncology Nursing* **6**(4): 278–284.

Michela, J. and Wood, J. (1986). Causal attributions in health and illness. *Advances in Cognitive–Behavioral Research and Therapy* **5**: 179–235.

Mitchell, M.F. (1983). Popular medical concepts in Jamaica and their impact on drug use. *Western Journal of Medicine* **139**(6): 841–846.

Mo, B. (1984). Black magic and illness in a Malaysian Chinese community. *Social Science and Medicine* **18**(2): 147–157.

Mo, B. (1992). Modesty, sexuality and breast health in Chinese–American women. *Western Journal of Medicine* **157**: 260–264.

Namboze, J.M. (1983). Health and culture in an African society. *Social Science and Medicine* **17**: 2041.

Nielsen, B.B., McMillan, S. and Diaz, E. (1992). Instruments that measure beliefs about cancer from a cultural perspective. *Cancer Nursing* **15**(2): 109–115.

Patterson, J.M. and Garwick, A.W. (1994).   The impact of chronic illness on families: a family systems perspective. *Annals of Behavioral Medicine* **16**: 131.

Payer, L. (1990).   Borderline cases: how medical practice reflects national culture. *The Sciences* **Jul/Aug**: 38–42.

Perez-Stable, E.J., Sabogal, F., Otero-Sabogal, R. et al. (1992).   Misconceptions about cancer among Latinos and Anglos. *Journal of the American Medical Association* **268**(22): 3219–3223.

Price, J.H. (1993).   Perceptions of colorectal cancer in a socioeconomically disadvantaged population. *J Community Health* **18**(6): 347–362.

Riehl-Emde, A., Buddeberg, C., Muthny, F.A., Landolt-Ritter, C., Steiner, R. and Richter, D. (1989).   Causal attributions and coping with illness in patients with breast cancer. *Psychotherapie, Psychosomatik, Medizinische Psychologie* **39**(7): 232–238.

Rokeach, M. (1969).   *Beliefs, Attitudes and Values*. San Francisco, CA: Jossey-Bass.

Rothbaum, F.,Weisz, J. and Snyder, S. (1982).   Changing the world and changing the self: a two-process model of perceived control. *Journal of Personality and Social Psychology* **42**: 5–37.

Rounds, J.B. and Zevon, M.A. (1993).   Cancer stereotypes: a multidimensional scaling analysis. *Journal of Behavioral Medicine* **16**(5): 485–495

Seligman, M. (1975).   *Helplessness*. New York; W.H. Freeman.

Seaburn, D., Lorenz, A. and Kaplan, D. (1992).   The transgenerational development of chronic illness meanings. *Family Systems Medicine* **10**: 385.

Shannon, C. (1996) Dealing with stress: families and chronic illness. In C. Cooper (Ed.), *Handbook of Stress Medicine and Health* (pp. 321–336). New York: CRC Press.

Snow, L.F. (1983).   Traditional health beliefs and practices among lower class Black Americans. *Western Journal of Medicine* **139**(6): 820–828.

Stoekle, J.D. and Barsky, A.J. (1980) Attributions: uses of social science knowledge in the 'doctoring' of primary care. In L. Eisenberg and A. Kleinman (Eds) *The Relevance of Social Science for Medicine* (pp. 23–240). Boston: D. Reidel.

Taylor, E.J. (1993).   Whys and wherefores: adult patient perspectives of the meaning of cancer. *Seminars in Oncology Nursing* **11**(1): 32–40.

Taylor, S. and Koivumaki, J.H. (1976).   The perception of self and others: acquaintanceship, affect, and actor–observer differences. *Journal of Personality and Social Psychology* **33**: 403–408.

Taylor, S.E., Lichtman, R.R., and Wood, J.V. (1984).   Attributions, beliefs about control, and adjustment to breast cancer. *Journal of Personality and Social Psychology* **46**(3): 489–502.

Timko, C. and Janoff-Bulman, R. (1985).   Attributions, vulnerability, and psychological adjustment: the case of breast cancer. *Health Psychology* **4**(6): 521–544.

Turnquist, D., Harvey, J. and Andersen, B. (1988).   Attributions and adjustment to life-threatening illness. *British Journal of Clinical Psychology* **27**: 55–65.

van den Borne, H.W., Pruyn, J.F.A. and de Meij, K. (1986).   Help given by fellow patients. In B.A. Stoll and A. Weisman (Eds). *Coping with Cancer Stress* (pp. 103–111). Boston: Martinus Nijhoff.

Section III
PSYCHOLOGICAL INTERVENTIONS WITHIN THE FAMILY

9

Preventing Affective Disorders in Partners of Cancer Patients: An Intervention Study

CAROLYN PITCEATHLY and PETER MAGUIRE

CRC Psychological Medicine Group, Christie Hospital NHS Trust,
University of Manchester, Manchester, UK

Research has identified the importance of partners' support for cancer patients' psychological adjustment to the illness and the adverse impact that cancer can have on partners. The severity of that impact may limit partners' effectiveness as a support for patients. So, partners have continued to interest researchers. Clinical levels of psychological disorder have been less studied, although psychological difficulties of sufficient severity to be diagnosed as affective disorders have cost implications for the family and society, as well as for the individual sufferer (Haddad et al., 1996).

This chapter describes a concerns-focused intervention currently being offered to the partners of cancer patients at the Christie Hospital, Manchester, in the context of a randomized, controlled trial. The aim is to prevent affective disorders amongst partners and the study is ongoing. The intervention was developed from previous work—early studies with partners and our own study of risk factors for affective disorders. These studies and their contribution to the theoretical framework of the intervention are discussed. Case studies are described to show how the intervention works in practice and to illustrate partners' responses to it. Our experiences are then compared with those of other intervention studies and the implications discussed.

BACKGROUND

Early studies highlighted the importance of families' and, in particular, partners' support for patients' adjustment to cancer (Lichtman et al., 1987; Northouse, 1988). They described partners' commitment to that support role (Vess et al., 1988) and their conviction that being supportive meant being strong and positive (Zahlis and Shands, 1991). Studies also identified the impact of the illness for partners. Partners, like patients, have fears and concerns about the illness and patients' survival (Northouse, 1989; Coe and Kluka, 1990). In addition, they worry about their ability

Cancer and the Family, 2nd Edn. Edited by L. Baider, C. L. Cooper and A. Kaplan De-Nour
© 2000 John Wiley & Sons, Ltd

to support patients emotionally and help them with their distress (Coe and Kluka, 1990; Zahlis and Shands, 1991). The illness brings disruptions to partners' daily lives and personal relationships (Vess et al., 1988; Northouse, 1989) and, although the illness brings many couples closer (Lichtman, 1987; Omne-Ponten et al., 1993), for some it creates strain and distance (Zahlis and Shands, 1991). In particular, some couples hold back from sharing their feelings about the illness with each other (Zahlis and Shands, 1991; Pistrang and Barker, 1992). Whilst most partners appear to cope well with the demands of the cancer predicament, a substantial minority have difficulties and these may become prolonged (Maguire, 1980; Oberst and Scott, 1988).

FACTORS RELATED TO ADJUSTMENT DIFFICULTIES

Sociodemographic Factors

Some studies have found no relationship between sociodemographic variables and psychological adjustment (Cassileth et al., 1985; Given et al., 1993; Northouse et al., 1995; Glasdam et al., 1996) but others have found a link.

Results are not consistent. Some studies show that female caregivers report more adjustment difficulties (Wellisch et al., 1983; Siegel et al., 1991). However, Baider et al. (1989) found that husbands of colon patients were more distressed than wives, although this finding was not replicated in a subsequent study with a mixed cancer population (Baider et al., 1996).

In Oberst et al.'s (1989) study, carers of lower social status and those with less education reported higher harm/loss and threat appraisal scores, while younger carers viewed the illness as less benign. Vess et al.'s (1985) study found evidence that, for families with children, families with adolescent children (or older) made role adjustments more easily.

Medical Factors

Disease and treatment factors such as recurrent disease (Given and Given, 1992), adjuvant treatment (Northouse et al., 1995), cancer site (Baider and De-Nour, 1988), and symptom distress (Northouse et al., 1995) have been associated with poorer adjustment. Cassileth et al. (1985) found that caregivers' psychological well-being worsened when patients were receiving active treatment, compared with follow-up care, and deteriorated still further when treatment was palliative.

Not all studies have identified medical factors as significant. Keller et al. (1996) found no relationship between illness stage, disease site, or performance status and spouse distress.

Patient–Partner Relationship

Studies have shown a consistent relationship in adjustment to illness, between groups of patients and partners (Northouse and Swain, 1987; Oberst and Scott, 1988), and within couples (Baider and De-Nour, 1984, 1988; Cassileth et al., 1985; Omne-Ponten et al., 1995). These findings suggest that patient–spouse interactions influence adjustment. In a study with breast cancer patients and spouses, Hannum et al. (1991) found that the way husbands coped predicted their wives' distress better than the women's own coping behaviors.

However, longitudinal studies have found differences in patients' and partners' adjustment. Oberst and Scott's (1988) study with bowel and genito-urinary patients and partners found that distress changed over time and in different temporal patterns. In Given and Given's (1992) study with caregivers (mostly partners) of patients with recurrent and new disease, levels of depression amongst patients decreased over a 6-month period but caregiver levels increased in both groups.

Members of a couple may behave in a complementary way when one partner's distress is extremely high. Lee Walker's (1997) study with breast patients and husbands found that when the fear of recurrence or emotional distress scores were high for one spouse, scores were not elevated for the other. Similarly, in Hannum et al.'s (1991) study, both members of a couple did not report extreme distress simultaneously.

Reports of the comparative severity of difficulties experienced by patients and partners have varied. While some studies have shown equivalent levels of distress (Northouse and Swain, 1987; Keller et al., 1996; Baider et al., 1996), others have found more distress amongst patients (Cassileth et al., 1985) or amongst partners (Keitel et al., 1990).

Gender differences have been noticed in the influence that one partner has on the other's adjustment. Northouse et al. (1995) and Hannum et al. (1991) suggested that breast cancer patients were more influenced by their hubands' adjustment than husbands were influenced by wives, but in Keller et al.'s (1996) study with a mixed cancer population, male partners' distress was almost exclusively accounted for by wives' distress and female partners' distress was moderated by other factors.

Marital Relationship/Informal Support

Feeling supported by a partner within an intimate relationship appears to help partners as well as patients to adjust (Hoskins et al., 1996; Lee Walker, 1997). Lewis et al. (1989) focused on fathers of school-age children whose wives were diagnosed with breast disease. Spouses' depression was related to lower levels of marital adjustment. Keller et al. (1996) did not find a relationship between marital quality and couple distress overall but couples who reported dissatisfying relationships were more distressed than those who were most satisfied with their marriages.

It is not exclusively patients' support that has been identified in relation to partners' adjustment. Hoskins et al.'s (1996) prospective study found that support from adults other than patients, particularly close interpersonal and family relationships, predicted husbands' emotional adjustment. Keller et al. (1996) also found that support from outside the family moderated female partners' distress.

COMMUNICATION

Studies with patients have shown positive benefits for illness adjustment, mood and role functioning when patients have an opportunity to share concerns and there is open communication with the family (Spiegel et al., 1983; Lichtman et al., 1987; Vess et al., 1985). Glasdam et al. (1996) studied spouses of patients from a wide range of disease groups. Those scoring above the threshold for affective disorder (HADS) were more likely to have problems they had never talked about.

Conversely, Hannum et al. (1991), Keller et al. (1996), and Lee Walker (1997) found no relationship between distress and open communication. In Lee Walker's study, spouses' fear of recurrence was related to more communication, suggesting that whilst confiding may be protective, it may also be a response to difficulty, hence the null finding overall. Whilst not identifying any benefits for adjustment from communication, both male and female spouses in Keller et al.'s (1996) study felt that it was more difficult to share painful feelings and thoughts than patients did.

Formal Support/Information

Both patients and partners have highlighted the importance of receiving adequate information and support from medical staff in enabling them to adjust to their illness and treatment (Wellisch et al., 1978; Vess et al., 1988; Northouse, 1989). Keller et al. (1996) found that the amount of information spouses received was not related to their distress. More than a quarter of the spouses in the sample felt additionally burdened by being involved in decision-making. These spouses were not specific by gender or age, leading the authors to conclude that spouses should be asked for their preferences on information and participation.

Burden of Care, Role Change and Appraisal

Difficulty with life roles (Hoskins et al., 1996) and the perception of more illness and caregiving demands (Lewis et al., 1989; Oberst et al. 1989) have been associated with poorer emotional adjustment, depression and stress appraisal. Partners' perceptions of illness demands are inevitably a subjective assessment, so the associations identified can only truly confirm the relationship between negative appraisal and adjustment difficulties, well established by the coping literature (Lazarus, 1993). This relationship has been consistently confirmed. Given et al. (1993) found that caregivers' psychological adjustment and their reports of the impact of the illness on their health and daily schedules was better predicted by the carers' levels of optimism than by patients' depression or physical dependencies; Hannum et al. (1991) found that husbands' psychological adjustment was related to patients' optimism and their own denial, and Northouse et al. (1995) found that husbands reported less emotional distress and fewer role adjustment problems when they were more hopeful. In Keller et al.'s (1996) study, spouse distress was related to the subjective illness experience, i.e. the way patients perceived their physical status, but not to objective medical data. Finally, Keitel et al. (1990) found that spouses who appraised surgery for cancer as stressful had higher depression and anxiety scores.

A wide range of measures has been used in the studies reviewed to assess both outcomes (adjustment) and the dependent variables. This may have contributed to inconsistent findings and illustrates the risk of drawing conclusions or generalizing findings beyond the focus and function of the measures used.

INTERVENTION STUDIES

Based on this literature a number of interventions have been designed to help partners, couples or families adjust (Goldberg and Wool, 1985; Sabo et al., 1986; Derdiarian, 1989; Ward et al., 1991; Walsh-Burke, 1992; Carter and Carter, 1994; Toseland et al., 1995 and Blanchard et al., 1996; Horowitz et al., 1996). These intervention studies have differed in the disease groups involved, the style of interventions offered and the outcomes aimed for.

Carter and Carter (1994)

Carter and Carter reported on the rationale and method used to provide traditional psychotherapy to 125 breast patients and half of their husbands. Problems prompting referrals from health professionals or patients included relationship or psychological difficulties. Husbands were offered five sessions of individual or conjoint therapy, dependent on the therapist's assessment of which was more suitable. The criteria for the decisions made are clearly described. The benefits of the intervention were assessed by the therapists, who concluded that traditional therapy can be used with cancer patients and spouses but is only suitable when the process of recovery 'is confounded by intrapsychic or interpersonal problems.'

Walsh-Burke (1992)

Walsh-Burke offered a weekend retreat program for families to promote open communication and social support. Of a convenience sample of 14 families recruited, only seven completed all the questionnaires. Questionnaires developed specifically for the study included measures of problems, coping strategies and frequency of communication. Families were offered workshops conducted by 'oncology professionals', aimed at enhancing communication about illness-related feelings and concerns. Although the results suggested that couples' frequency of communication had increased, problem scores had also increased.

Sabo et al. (1986)

Sabo et al. offered a 'multi-session' men's discussion group with two facilitators to 24 husbands of mastectomy patients The aim was to encourage communication and self-disclosure to aid the men's adjustment and their effectiveness as support for their wives. Of the 24 men who responded to advertisements, six agreed to join the group. The men completed a self-report instrument that included measures of frequency of verbal communication about mastectomy, self-esteem and depression. For those who attended the group, communication about the mastectomy with their wives increased but there were no other effects on the measures used.

Horowitz et al. (1996)

Horowitz et al. described a support group for spouses of brain tumor patients. The rationale for setting up the group was that these spouses had extraordinary stresses to cope with. Not only is the prognosis for the patients poor but profound personality and behavioral changes take place as the disease progresses.

The aim of the group was to help spouses 'sustain themselves physically and emotionally' and to provide education about symptom management. The multi-disciplinary neuro-oncology team ran the group and selected 10 spouses initially, who met with the team, identified their needs and requested a regular meeting. The team assessed potential new members. Spouses were not referred to the group if they were likely to challenge the group process or find the group situation overwhelming or threatening. Twenty spouses were actively involved, with an average of 10 spouses at each meeting. The group met fortnightly for 90 minutes over an 18-month period. The first 30 minutes were devoted to education and information and the remaining time, led by the social worker and psychiatrist, focused on the spouses' emotional needs.

Evaluation of the group was a subjective assessment by the leaders. They felt that the group met the spouses' illness-related needs for social support.

RANDOMIZED, CONTROLLED STUDIES

Four randomized, controlled studies are reported. The descriptions of the studies and their results, here, focus on the effects of intervention for the spouses or partners in the samples.

Derdiarian (1989)

The theoretical basis for this controlled intervention was Lazarus's (1993) proposal that information seeking is a primary mode of coping for individuals facing new situations. Previous research had shown that information needs pertain to personal, family and social concerns as well as the disease and that both patients and spouses need similar types and amounts of information. Male cancer patients and spouses were offered information, referral, counselling and follow-up care individualized to the couples' needs or routine information, referral, counselling and follow-up care. The hypothesis was that patients and spouses receiving individualized care would be more satisfied with the information received and cope better with the diagnosis and its implications. Subjects were newly diagnosed, male patients with partners, aged between 25–55 years. The patients and partners completed an information needs assessment instrument Derdiarian Needs Assessment Instrument (DINA) and Satisfaction scale before receiving either the individualized program based on their responses to the DINA (intervention group), or the routine care program (control). Five to ten days later, subjects completed the measures again. After intervention, patients and spouses reported less need for information and greater satisfaction with information. There was no change in either information needs or satisfaction for patients and partners in the control group.

Goldberg and Wool (1985)

Goldberg and Wool's study examined a psychotherapeutic intervention (involving 12 sessions of counselling) offered to the significant key others (SKOs) of lung cancer patients. All the patients in the study were counseled. Forty-eight SKOs were randomized to intervention or the control group, most of whom were spouses. There was no provision to ensure that the intervention and control groups were comparable e.g. for gender or distress, at baseline. The intervention aimed to assist the SKO fulfill five specified support functions. The final stage of the intervention dealt with the SKOs problems, affect, grief, and coping activities. SKOs were assessed at recruitment into the study, and 8 and 16 weeks later, using the Profile of Mood Scale (POMS) and the Psychosocial Adjustment to Illness Scale (PAIS) to measure emotional and social functioning, respectively. Results were limited to the 23 SKOs who completed all the assessments. No differences were found between the control and intervention groups. A major reason was that patients and partners were adjusting reasonably well at inception into the study, so there was little room for change.

Toseland et al. (1995) and Blanchard et al. (1996)

Toseland et al. and Blanchard et al. reported on a randomized controlled study offering a problem-solving intervention aimed at helping spouses cope with distress. Improvements in perceived health, psychological well-being and social support were anticipated for spouses who received the intervention. Spouses' anxiety and stress and their coping behaviors were measured. Benefits were anticipated for patients' psychological well-being and perceived social support when spouses received intervention.

Patients were recruited if 3 months from initial diagnosis and not eligible for hospice care. Of 346 spouses eligible for the study, 109 (25%) agreed to participate. Subjects were assessed at baseline (Time 1), after the 6-week intervention (Time 2) and 6 months after baseline (Time 3). The analysis focused on the 66 partners who remained in the study at Time 3, 19% of the potential sample. Equal numbers of male and female spouses were recruited. Spouses were randomized to intervention or control.

A standardized intervention protocol, 'Coping with Cancer' (CWC), was used. The intervention was carried out by an oncology social worker who offered six 1-hour sessions. The intervention focused on identifying problems, generating solutions, discussing and carrying out action plans and evaluating the plans. Action plans targeted reappraisal, use of formal and informal supports and changing coping responses.

The spouses in the intervention group showed no greater improvement in any of the measures compared with the control group. However, patients whose spouses received intervention were less depressed at follow-up ($p < 0.01$). In discussing the absence of an intervention effect for spouses, the authors highlighted that the spouses felt that they were coping with their most pressing problems, even though the level of depression in the sample was higher than community norms. They acknowledged the paradox of offering a problem-solving intervention to individuals who perceive that they are coping with their problems.

Ward et al. (1991)

Ward et al. examined the effects of social support and communication on patients' self-esteem. Ninety-nine patients (65% compliance) undergoing chemotherapy were randomized to one of three information-giving conditions: standard information about chemotherapy; enhanced information about how to cope with side effects and maintain self-esteem; and enhanced information given in the company of their partners. Enhanced information only had a positive effect on patients' self-esteem when given in the company of the partner. Although the study did not measure outcomes for partners, it is important in confirming partners' role in promoting patients' adjustment. It highlights the importance of giving partners appropriate information to enable them to perform their support role effectively and, as in Blanchard et al.'s (1996) study, it indicates that interventions with partners can produce tangible benefits for patients.

Most of these studies were limited by small and unrepresentative samples, poor compliance, the use of non-standardized questionnaires, subjective assessment of outcomes and the lack of controls. None identified a sample of partners at risk of adjustment difficulties. Although the studies based their interventions on the literature, reasons for the context in which the intervention was offered were not usually given. The high refusal and drop-out rates suggest that partners in the populations studied either did not perceive intervention as necessary or found it unacceptable. Where intervention effects were measured, they frequently showed limited benefit. Helpfully, the randomized controlled studies with partners (Goldberg and Wool, 1985; Toseland et al., 1995; Blanchard et al., 1996) reported fully on their methods, their interventions and the problems encountered. Derdiarian's (1989) early study showed benefits for couples. It had a clear conceptual basis in coping theory and the intervention was tailored to meet the individual needs identified by both patients and partners in the sample.

AFFECTIVE DISORDERS AMONGST PARTNERS OF CANCER PATIENTS

None of the studies or interventions reviewed used standardized psychiatric interviews to determine the extent to which the partners developed clinically significant affective disorders (anxiety or depression). When health service resources are scarce, investment in preventive intervention is unlikely unless demonstrable gains can be predicted. Partners who develop a clinical disorder are a potential demand on health care resources and unlikely to provide effective support for patients. So, a successful intervention would offer tangible benefits. Identifying risk factors for more serious adjustment difficulties offers a basis for defining the type of preventive intervention that might be effective and the optimal time to intervene. For these reasons, a retrospective study was conducted to identify the prevalence of affective disorders among partners of cancer patients and to determine whether specific factors contributed to their development (Haddad, 1994).

Methods

Partners were interviewed approximately 2 years after the patients' initial cancer diagnoses. Trained interviewers used a semi-structured interview to ask about partners' experiences and partners completed a Concerns Checklist (Devlen, 1984—adapted); the Psychiatric Assessment Schedule (Dean et al., 1983) was administered and psychiatric morbidity was diagnosed according to DSM III–R criteria (American Psychiatric Association, 1980).

Results

Of 225 partners approached, 168 (75%) agreed; 118 (70%) were male and 50 (30%) female. A heterogeneous group of cancer diagnoses were included, although 86 (51%) were partners of breast cancer patients.

Prevalence of Affective Disorder

Twenty (12%) of 168 partners developed an affective disorder (major depression, generalized anxiety disorder, adjustment disorder) in the 26 months following the patients' cancer diagnosis. Eight of the 20 partners had not sought any help.

Factors Associated with Disorder

The likelihood of developing an affective disorder was related to female gender, lower social class and having a history of affective disorder prior to the cancer. For those partners reporting role and relationship changes since the cancer, disorder was associated with having a negative view of at least one of those changes and having experienced a major change in at least one of the life domains explored.

There was also a link with feeling dissatisfied with information about illness and treatment. Overall, satisfaction with information was high: 82% of partners were satisfied with the information they received about the illness and treatment, but 35% of partners had received most of their information from the patient, confirming Derdiarian's (1989) and Keller's (1996) conclusions, that partners have different needs and so information should be individually tailored.

A partner was three times more likely to develop an affective disorder if his/her patient spouse had developed a similar disorder since the cancer diagnosis. Partners' disorder usually followed the patients'.

Partners who had developed an affective disorder reported having more unresolved concerns at interview. While there was good agreement between the concerns of patients and partners, partners were more likely to be concerned about the level of emotional distress in the patient than patients themselves. The results confirm the consistent findings in the literature of the relationship between patients' and partners' adjustment and their difficulties with the emotional support role.

THE ROLE OF CONFIDING

Our finding that whether or not partners confided their concerns or talked about role changes was not related to the development of affective disorder was surprising, but was consistent with our patient study (Harrison et al., 1994). It suggests that, as identified in the literature, there may be situations where confiding illness-related concerns to a partner is unnecessary or unhelpful and that adaptive communication patterns may be specific to individual couples (Chekryn, 1984; Ward et al., 1991; Hannum, 1991; Gotcher, 1992). The partners confirmed Keller et al.'s (1996) finding that partners do not share their feelings with others. At each stage of the illness from early symptoms onwards, at least one-third of the partners said they had not shared their fears or negative feelings with either the patient or anyone else.

COPING

Finding that partners who developed a disorder appraised more illness demands or difficulties and were dissatisfied with the information given is consistent with other work (Lewis et al., 1989; Oberst et al., 1989; Wellisch et al., 1978) and with the coping literature (Lazarus, 1993). For example, Beck and Clark (1988) reported that anxious or depressed individuals demonstrate a bias in information processing. They overestimate the degree of threat associated with a situation and selectively emphasize negative information. Individuals who fail to cope are likely to perceive their situation as more difficult, to underestimate both their own coping resources and their available supports and to abandon coping efforts prematurely. Failure to cope reinforces the belief that problems are unmanageable and a negative cycle of coping is established (Parle et al., 1996).

The coping literature also affords a model for understanding the relationship between adjustment and patient–partner confiding. In their study of coping amongst 603 cancer patients, Dunkel-Schetter et al. (1992) found that less emotional distress was associated with utilizing social support, focusing on the positive, and distancing. A partner who is 'being positive' may be meeting his/her own coping needs, and this behaviour may be perceived by the patient as supportive or in conflict with his/her need for social support. The helpfulness of patient or partner communication (or lack of it) may depend on how the behavior is appraised by the other partner.

DEVELOPING AN INTERVENTION

Because of the significance of undisclosed and unresolved concerns in both patients and partners, our intervention seeks to focus on eliciting partners' concerns and determining the extent to which they have attempted to resolve them. Thus, at the first interview partners are invited to share their previous illness experiences and to identify their current concerns about the patient's illness and treatment. On the basis of the concerns and difficulties identified, the focus for further sessions is made explicit and agreed with the partner. Subsequent sessions define the problems identified in more detail and explore ways of resolving difficulties, whether by problem solving or cognitive reappraisal. The partner's understanding of the patient's illness and view of the patient's response is explored. Particular emphasis is placed on any communication difficulties identified by the partner, whether these are with the patient, medical staff, or other confidants. Effective coping and valuable support resources, both formal (e.g. medical and nursing staff) and informal (e.g. family and friends), are acknowledged. While the aim of this intervention is to prevent affective disorders among partners, we anticipate that it will also facilitate patients' adjustment.

The intervention sample comprises partners of patients referred to our psychiatric service because they are suffering from a major depressive illness, generalized anxiety disorder or adjustment disorder. Such partners have a one in four chance of developing an affective disorder. Eligible partners are being randomized to an intervention or a control group. The intervention offered is up to six 1-hour sessions delivered at approximately 2-week intervals. The number of sessions is tailored to the needs of the partner to maximize study compliance and generalizability of the intervention to other settings. The number of sessions is consistent with other brief, focused therapies (Greer et al., 1992) and with our experience in piloting the intervention.

The intervention is given on an individual basis, since evidence from the literature and our own studies indicated that many partners do not disclose their true concerns and feelings to the patients (Keller et al., 1996). Interventions are delivered by a social worker or psychiatrist, since we seek to demonstrate that the intervention can be used effectively by health professionals from different backgrounds.

THE PARTNERS' RESPONSE.

Partners currently in the study have responded to the first intervention session in one of the following ways:

1. The partner identifies concerns and coping difficulties at the first session and the partner and intervener agree the focus for further sessions (up to six).
2. The partner completes the first intervention session, does not identify outstanding concerns or has concerns but feels he/she is coping effectively. No further sessions are planned and the partner is given a contact number.
3. The partner identifies concerns and coping difficulties at the first session but refuses further sessions.

The following case studies demonstrate the process of the intervention in the context of each of the three responses.

CASE STUDY 1

The partner identifies concerns and coping difficulties at the first session and the partner and intervener agree the focus for further sessions (up to six).

The patient, Mrs A, had received treatment for breast cancer. Eight months after her original diagnosis, when all treatment had finished, she was referred to the psychiatric service and diagnosed as having a major depressive disorder. Mr A was recruited to the study.

Intervention Session 1

At the first assessment interview Mr A was concerned about the possible recurrence of his wife's illness and the prospect of losing her. He was also concerned about losing his elderly father, to whom he was close, and about the level of stress in his work. Mr A experienced panic attacks twice a week, when he had difficulty breathing, had palpitations and feared that he would die. He felt very tense and anxious most of the time. He traced the onset of these problems to the time of his wife's cancer diagnosis. Mr A identified the main source of his anxiety as work stress.

Intervention Sessions 2–6

The remaining five sessions of the intervention focused on this concern. The explicit task was to understand and explore the thoughts and concerns that were generating his anxiety. Mr A worked as a maintenance technician on a busy production line. He was an experienced engineer but new to this job. The thought behind his anxiety was that he might be unable to mend a machine when he was called to do so. Such a failure threatened his view of himself as a skilled technician. He also feared that, because wages were dependent on the level of production, the machine operator would become frustrated and lose her temper with him. Further exploration of these ideas demonstrated that it was inappropriate to associate failure to mend a machine with professional incompetence. The fear that the operator would lose her temper was unrealistic when seen in the context of his work experience but was understandable in the light of much earlier experiences. Having explored the cognitions associated with his anxiety, we planned behavioral strategies to reduce the likelihood of the feared events occurring and to deal with them if they should arise. After three sessions, Mr A was generalizing the ability to challenge his own anxiety-provoking thoughts to situations in his daily life, but this did not substantially reduce his feelings of anxiety and tension, particularly at work. We then focused specifically on those feelings, brainstorming cognitive and behavioral strategies that had helped in the past or that might work in his current situation. These ranged from self-instruction (e.g. 'I can mend this machine and even if I can't, how much does it matter') and taking more exercise to acknowledging that this was an inherently stressful job and looking to change it.

The Conclusion

After six sessions Mr A no longer suffered panic attacks and he judged his level of tension and anxiety to be 50% less than before the intervention. His problem-solving skills had been effectively generalized to those concerns that were not a focus in the sessions. He said that he had reflected on the prospect of his father's death and, although he knew that he would be very distressed, he felt that he would cope. He had talked with his wife about her illness and felt they had a common and, for himself, a more positive view.

Partner's Evaluation of the Intervention

Mr A's assessment of the intervention effect was that he had felt lost and swamped by his feelings before it. Afterwards he felt that he had a perspective on the direction he wanted to take in his life and a sense of being in control.

CASE STUDY 2

The partner completes the first session, does not identify outstanding concerns or has concerns but feels he/she is coping effectively. No further sessions are planned. The partner is given a contact number.

The patient, Mrs B, was diagnosed with Hodgkin's disease. The diagnosis was unexpected and given very abruptly to Mrs B alone. She had young children and recent family history of terminal cancer. Mrs B was referred to the psychiatric service by her clinician during her course of chemotherapy and diagnosed with a major depressive disorder. Mr B was recruited to the intervention study.

Intervention session 1

Mr B was devastated by his wife's diagnosis and angry about the way it was given. He coped by 'thinking things through' and looking for information from medical staff in whom he had confidence. He had survived serious illness a few years earlier and felt he had learned to cope with painful realities by facing them and then finding ways to deal with the difficulties. Many of his own experiences with doctors had been good. He felt that this helped him not to generalize his lack of confidence in the first doctor to other medical staff responsible for his wife's care. He was very distressed by the impact of the chemotherapy and its side effects on his wife but coped by reminding himself that it was helping her. He felt more positive about the illness because she was responding well to treatment. The couple talked openly about the illness and their concerns and Mr B had friends who made explicit their willingness to listen to his worries, especially those that he might not feel able to share with his wife.

The Conclusion

Mr B felt that although he had concerns about the future, these were realistic, he was coping, had adequate support and did not need further intervention.

Partner's Evaluation of the Intervention

Mr B felt that it had been useful to reflect on his experiences and to recognize that he was coping. He felt it was particularly important to know that if he needed help in future, there was a service available, specifically for partners.

CASE STUDY 3

The partner identifies concerns and coping difficulties at the first session but refuses further sessions.
    The patient, Mrs C, had received treatment for bowel cancer. Mrs C was referred to the psychiatric service by her clinician after 5 months of adjuvant chemotherapy treatment and diagnosed with a major depressive disorder. Her husband, Mr C was recruited to the intervention study.

Intervention Session 1

At the assessment interview, Mr C described his shock at his wife's cancer diagnosis. She had been suffering from bowel problems for some time but neither he nor his wife had suspected cancer. His initial fear was that she would die. The couple were more positive as treatment plans were made, but Mrs C was very anxious before her surgery that she might be given a colostomy. Although this did not happen, Mrs C had some problems with infections following the surgery and her recovery was slow. When she started adjuvant treatment she became moody and irritable. Mr C coped with his wife's irritability by being patient and trying to avoid arguments. Mr C understood that his wife's mood problems were a response to the stress of the illness but felt that they put a strain on their relationship. His wife's mood had continued to deteriorate and she accused him of being uncaring and unsupportive.

Mrs C was always accompanied to hospital appointments by her sister because Mr C felt he could not take time from work to be with her. When he returned home after work, Mrs C wanted her husband to be with her, but Mr C continued to maintain his evening job at a local pub. He explained that he needed to keep working for financial reasons. Following further exploration of his motives, he was asked, 'Is there any other reason why you spend so much time away from home?' Mr C acknowledged that he was still very fearful about his wife's illness, in particular that the treatment might not work and he might lose her. He coped by trying to maintain his life as close to normal as possible. He avoided visiting the hospital or spending time with his wife when she was physically unwell after treatment because this brought him too close to the reality of her illness.

Mr C was hurt by his wife's criticism of him but could see that his behavior might seem uncaring to her. He was concerned about his wife's health and her low mood but his main concern was the continuing deterioration in their relationship. He coped by not thinking about his fears and worries and did not share them with anyone.

The Conclusion

Mr C did not feel that he could explain his behavior to his wife in terms of his need to cope with his own fears and distress because this would mean acknowledging those realities with her and this would be too painful for him. He recognized that his way of coping was contributing to their relationship problems but chose not to continue with the intervention.

Partner's Evaluation of the Intervention

Mr C felt that he it had been helpful to talk about his difficulties but could not bear to reflect on the situation or his feelings further.

SUMMARY

Positive Responses to the Intervention—The Benefits Gained

This intervention offers all partners an opportunity to identify their concerns, to make the effectiveness of current coping strategies explicit and to identify the formal and informal supports that are available. For partners who are coping well, the intervention acknowledges and confirms effective coping but gives the partner a brief experience of professional intervention. As a result, such intervention may become an additional support resource, a 'safety net' for the future.

For partners who identify coping deficits, the intervention gives an opportunity to explore and practice alternative strategies and find ways to resolve or reduce the impact of problems and to identify and use other formal and informal supports more effectively.

Negative Responses to the Intervention—The Benefits Gained

There are partners who find the intervention unacceptable because it challenges their established ways of coping. For partners who use avoidance or distancing strategies, the intervention allows the benefits and limitations of this way of coping to be made explicit. As a result, the option to consider other strategies in the future, with or without professional help, becomes available.

CONCLUSIONS

The study is ongoing, so we cannot make predictions about the effectiveness of the intervention in preventing affective disorders amongst partners. One hundred and thirty (76%) of the 170 partners eligible for recruitment so far have agreed to join the study. This level of compliance suggests that the timing of the intervention, when the patient is diagnosed with an affective disorder, is theoretically appropriate and relevant from the partner's perspective.

From baseline data we are able to confirm that we have identified a group of partners who have adjustment difficulties. The median baseline General Health Questionnaire (GHQ) score for the 130 partners in the study is 7, and 77 (59%) partners scored 5 or above, the accepted cut-off for psychological morbidity.

Our experience so far suggests that the decision to make the number of intervention sessions negotiable was valid. Some partners find that participating in the intervention beyond the initial session is not consistent with their coping. We have suggested that there may be benefits from the intervention for these partners. There is also potential for the intervention to have a negative impact if pursued without regard for the partners' preferred coping style (Ward et al., 1991).

The intervention focuses on the partners' main concern(s). No effort is made to focus on the patient–partner relationship or a partner's effectiveness as the patient's support unless the partner identifies these issues as problems. If the partner does not identify concerns, or all issues are resolved before completing six sessions, the intervention terminates. This is consistent with Blanchard et al.'s (1996) conclusion that there is nothing to be gained from offering a problem-solving intervention to partners who are not experiencing problems.

It is our experience that some partners find the intervention inappropriate at specific times in the illness trajectory. Although the protocol requires that patients recruited to this study should be expected to survive the 1-year study period, some patients have become seriously ill and died much sooner. If partners are involved in the intervention when the patient's illness becomes critical, some have asked for the intervention to lapse or 'go on hold'. Taking time to reflect on the situation or themselves appears to be inconsistent with the partners' need to 'hold things together' and focus exclusively on caring for the patient. One partner failed to take up the intervention for this reason but found the intervention helpful after the patient's death. This is consistent with the view that coping style is not exclusively a trait characteristic. Effective coping is specific to the nature of the situation or to the stage in the course of a situation as it evolves (Lazarus, 1993).

Partners in the study have valued the freedom to express negative feelings and thoughts that they are reluctant to share with family and friends (Keller, 1996). This has confirmed our decision to interview partners alone, particularly for the initial session. However, the frequency with which relationship and support problems are highlighted has raised the possibility that conjoint sessions might be helpful and appropriate for some couples. This is consistent with the Carter and Carter's (1994) perspective that the intervention should be tailored to meet the nature of the problem.

At present there are two limitations apparent in the intervention. The timing of the intervention is based on the finding from our earlier study (Haddad, 1994) that partners are at risk when the patient has developed an affective disorder. This is not evidence that the best time to intervene with partners is when that disorder has developed and been identified. The GHQ scores reported by partners at their initial assessment interview show high levels of distress and for some partners the intervention comes too late to prevent the development of disorder. A second limitation is that female patients are more frequently referred to the psychiatric service and so the majority of our partners are male (n=95; 73%). As our initial study identified that female partners are more likely to develop disorders, this point of intervention is limiting access to the partners who are most at risk.

This study has addressed some of the difficulties encountered by other authors when offering intervention to partners. The study targets partners at risk of developing psychiatric problems and offers a theoretically-based intervention, tailored to meet individual needs. Most importantly, the style and timing of the intervention is acceptable to the majority of partners and their patient spouses.

REFERENCES

American Psychiatric Association (1980). *Diagnostic and Statistical Manual of Mental Disorders (DSM–III)*, 3rd edn. Washington D.C: American Psychiatric Association.

Baider, L., De-nour, A.K. (1984). Couples reactions and adjustment to mastectomy: a preliminary report. *International Journal of Psychiatry in Medicine* **4**: 265–277.

Baider, L. and De-Nour, A.K. (1988). Adjustment to cancer: who is the patient—the husband or the wife? *Israel Journal of Medical Science* **24**: 631–636.

Baider, L., Perez, T. and De-Nour, A.K. (1989). Gender and adjustment to chronic disease. A study of couples with colon cancer. *General Hospital Psychiatry* **11**: 1–8.

Baider, L., Kaufman, B., Peretz, T., Manor, O., Ever-Hadani, P. and De-Nour, A.K. (1996). Mutuality of fate: adaptation and psychological distress in cancer patients and their partners. In Baider, L., Cooper, C.L. and De-Nour, A.K. (eds) *Cancer and the Family*. Chichester: Wiley.

Beck, T. and Clark, D.A. (1988). Anxiety and depression: an information processing perspective. *Anxiety Research* **1**: 23–36.

Blanchard, C.G., Toseland, R.W. and McCallion, P. (1996). The effects of a problem-solving intervention with spouses of cancer patients. *Journal of Psychosocial Oncology* **14**: 1–21.

Carter, C.A. and Carter, R.E. (1994). Some observations on individual and marital therapy with breast cancer patients and spouses. *Psychosocial Oncology* **12**: 65–81.

Cassileth, B.R., Lusk, E.J., Strouse, T.B., Miller, B.S., Brown, L.L. and Cross, P.A. (1985). A psychological analysis of cancer patients and their next-of-kin. *Cancer* **55**: 72–76

Chekryn, J. (1984). Cancer recurrence: personal meaning, communication, and marital adjustment. *Cancer Nursing* **7**: 491–498.

Coe, M. and Kluka, S. (1990). Comparison of concerns of clients and spouses regarding ostomy surgery for treatment of cancer: Phase II. *Journal of Enterostomal Therapy* **17**: 106–111.

Dean, C., Surtees, P.G. and Sashidharan, S.P. (1983). Comparison of research diagnostic systems in an Edinburgh community sample. *British Journal of Psychiatry* **142**: 247–256.

Derdiarian, A.K. (1989). Effects of information on recently diagnosed cancer patients' and spouses' satisfaction with care. *Cancer Nursing* **12**: 285–292.

Devlen, J. (1984). *Psychological and social aspects of Hodgkin's disease and non-Hodgkin's lymphoma*. Doctoral thesis, University of Manchester, Manchester, U.K.

Dunkel-Schetter, C., Feinstein, LG., Taylor, S.E. and Falke, R.L. (1992). Patterns of coping with cancer. *Health Psychology* **11**: 79–87.

Given B. and Given CW. (1992). Patient and family caregiver reaction to new and recurrent breast cancer. *Journal of the American Medical Women's Association* **47**: 201–206 and 212.

Given, C.W., Stommel, M., Given, B., Osuch, J., Kurtz, M.E. and Kurtz, J.C. (1993). The influence of cancer patients' symptoms and functional states on patients' depression and family caregivers' reaction and depression. *Health Psychology* **12**: 277–285.

Glasdam, S., Jensen, A.B., Madsen, A.L. and Rose, C. (1996). Anxiety and depression in cancer patients' spouses. *Psycho-Oncology* **5**: 23–29.

Goldberg, R.J. and Wool, M.S. (1985). Psychotherapy for the spouses of lung cancer patients: assessment of an intervention. *Psychotherapy and Psychosomatics* **43**: 141–150.

Gotcher, J.M. (1992). Interpersonal communication and psychosocial adjustment. *Journal of Psychosocial Oncology* **10**: 21–39.

Greer, S., Moorey, S., Baruch, D.R., Watson, M., Robertson, B.M., Mason, A., Rowden, L., Law, M.G. and Bliss, J.M. (1992). Adjuvant psychological therapy for patients with cancer: a prospective randomised trial. *British Medical Journal* **304**: 675–680

Haddad, P. (1994) *Affective disorders amongst partners of cancer patients.* MD Thesis, University of Manchester. U.K.

Haddad, P., Pitceathly, C. and Maguire, P. (1996). Psychological morbidity in the partners of cancer patients. In Baider, L., Cooper, C.L. and De-Nour, A.K. (eds) *Cancer and the Family.* Chichester: Wiley.

Hannum, J.W., Giese-Davis, J., Harding, K. and Hatfield, A.K. (1991). Effects of individual and marital variables on coping with cancer. *Journal of Psychosocial Oncology* **9**: 1–20.

Harrison, J., Maguire, P., Ibbotson, T., Macleod, R. and Hopwood, P. (1994). Concerns, confiding and psychiatric disorder in newly diagnosed cancer patients: a descriptive study. *Psycho-Oncology* **3**: 173–179.

Horowitz, S., Passik, S.D. and Malkin, M.G. (1996). 'In sickness and in health': a group intervention for spouses caring for patients with brain tumours. *Journal of Psychosocial Oncology* **14**: 43–56.

Hoskins, C.N., Baker, S., Budin, W., Ekstrom, D., Maislin, G., Sherman, D., Steelman-Bohlander, J., Bookbinder, M. and Knauer, C. (1996). Adjustment among husbands of women with breast cancer. *Journal of Psychosocial Oncology* **14**: 41–68.

Keitel, M.A., Zevon, M.A., Rounds, J.B., Petrelli, N.J. and Karakousis, C. (1990). Spouse adjustment to cancer surgery: distress and coping responses. *Journal of Surgical Oncology* **43**: 158–153.

Keller, M., Heinrich, G., Sellschop, A., Beutel, M. (1996). Between distress and support: spouses of cancer patients. In Baider, L., Cooper, C.L., De-Nour, A.K. (eds), *Cancer and the Family.* Chichester: Wiley.

Lazarus, R.S. (1993). Coping theory and research: past, present and future. *Psychosomatic Medicine* **55**: 234–24

Lee Walker, B. (1997). Adjustment of husbands and wives to breast cancer. *Cancer Practice* **5**: 92–98.

Lewis, F.M., Woods, N.F., Hough, E.E., Bensley, L.S. (1989) The family's functioning with chronic illness in the mother: the spouse's perspective. *Social Science and Medicine* **29**: 1261–1269.

Lichtman, R.R., Taylor, S.E. and Wood, J.V. (1987). Social support and marital adjustment after breast cancer. *Journal of Psychosocial Oncology* **5**: 47–74.

Maguire, G.P. (1980). The repercussions of mastectomy on the family. *International Journal of Family Psychiatry* **1**: 85–503.

Northouse, L.L. (1988). Social support in patients' and husbands' adjustment to breast cancer. *Nursing Research* **37**: 91–95.

Northouse, L.L. (1989). The impact of breast cancer on patients and husbands. *Cancer Nursing* **12**: 276–284.

Northouse, L., Dorris, G. and Charron-Moore, C. (1995). Factors affecting couples' adjustment to recurrent breast cancer. *Social Science and Medicine* **41**: 69–76.

Northouse, L. and Swain, M. (1987). Adjustment of patients and husbands to the initial impact of breast cancer. *Nursing Research* **36**: 221–225.

Oberst, M. and Scott, D. (1988). Postdischarge distress in surgically treated cancer patients and their spouses. *Research in Nursing and Health* **11**: 223–233.

Oberst, M.T., Thomas, S.E., Gass, K.A. and Ward, S.E. (1989). Caregiving demands and appraisal of stress among family caregivers. *Cancer Nursing* **12**: 209–215.

Omne-Ponten, M., Holmberg., L., Bergstrom, R., Sjoden, PO. and Burns, T. (1993). Psychosocial adjustment among husbands of women treated for breast cancer; mastectomy vs. breast-conserving surgery. *European Journal of Cancer* **29A**: 1393–1397

Omne-Ponten, M., Holmberg, L., Sjoden, P.O. and Bergstrom, R. (1995). The married couple's assessment of the experience of early breast cancer—a longitudinal interview study. *Psycho-Oncology* **4**: 183–190.

Parle, M., Jones, B. and Maguire, P. (1996). Maladaptive coping and affective disorders among cancer patients. *Psychological Medicine* **26**: 735–744.

Pistrang, N. and Barker, C. (1992). Disclosure of concerns in breast cancer. *Psycho-Oncology* **1**: 183–192.

Sabo, D., Brown, J. and Smith, C. (1986). The male role and mastectomy: support groups and men's adjustment. *Journal of Psychosocial Oncology* **4**: 19–31.

Siegel, K., Raveis, V.H., Mor, V. and Houts, P. (1991). The relationship of spousal caregiver burden to patient disease and treatment-related conditions. *Annals of Oncology* **2**: 511–516.

Speigel, D., Bloom, J.R. and Gottheil, E. (1983). Family environment as a predictor of adjustment to metastatic breast carcinoma. *Journal of Psychosocial Oncology* **1**: 33–44.

Toseland, R.W., Blanchard, C.G. and McCallion, P. (1995). A problem solving intervention for caregivers of cancer patients. *Social Science and Medicine* **40**: 517–528.

Vess, J., Moreland, J. and Schwebel, A. (1985). An empirical assessment of the effects of cancer on family role functioning. *Journal of Psychosocial Oncology* **3**: 1–16.

Vess, J.D. Jr, Moreland, J.R., Schwebel, A.I. and Kraut, E. (1988). Psychosocial needs of cancer patients: learning from patients and their spouses. *Journal of Psychosocial Oncology* **6**: 31–51.

Walsh-Burke, K. (1992). Family communication and coping with cancer: impact of the we can weekend. *Journal of Psychosocial Oncology* **10**: 63–81.

Ward, S., Leventhal, H., Easterling, D., Luchterhand, C. and Love, R. (1991). Social support, self-esteem and communication in patients receiving chemotherapy. *Journal of Psychosocial Oncology* **9**: 95–116

Wellisch, D.K., Jamison, K.R. and Pasnau, R.O. (1978). Psychosocial aspects of mastectomy: II. the man's perspective. *American Journal of Psychiatry* **135**: 543–546.

Wellisch, D.K., Fawzy, F.I., Landsverk, J., Pasnau, R.O. and Wolcott, D.L. (1983). Evaluation of psychosocial problems of the home-bound cancer patient: the relationship of disease and the sociodemographic variables of patients to family problems. *Journal of Psychosocial Oncology* **1**: 1–15.

Zahlis, E.H. and Shands, M.E. (1991). Breast cancer: demands of the illness on the patient's partner. *Journal of Psychosocial Oncology* **9**: 75–93.

10

Psychosocial Adaptation Following Treatment: A Family Systems Perspective on Childhood Cancer Survivorship

JAMIE OSTROFF and STEPHANIE ROSS
Memorial Sloan–Kettering Cancer Center, New York, USA

PETER STEINGLASS
Ackerman Institute for the Family, New York, USA

Having a child with cancer is one of the most stressful experiences that a family can encounter. The diagnosis of cancer typically results in an arduous course of aggressive treatments, numerous painful medical procedures, several lengthy hospitalizations, and debilitating side effects. Cancer clearly poses extraordinary practical and emotional challenges to the entire family with the impact of cancer on the family, changing as a function of the course of the disease (Chesler and Barbarin, 1987).

However, due to advances in early detection and treatment modalities, survival rates for many types of childhood cancer have improved dramatically. For example, acute lymphocytic leukemia, the most common type of childhood cancer, has a five-year survival rate of 80% (American Cancer Society, 1998), and Hodgkin's disease, most commonly diagnosed during adolescence, has a 5-year survival rate of 81% (American Cancer Society, 1998). Thus, many types of childhood cancer that were once considered to be universally fatal illnesses now have good prognoses for long-term survival.

While these survival rates are certainly encouraging, these changes in the nature of childhood cancer have introduced new issues for patients and their families. As survival rates have improved, a growing body of research has documented the long-term effects of many modern cancer treatments. These physical disabilities can include cognitive impairment, learning disabilities, infertility, attenuated growth, persistent immunodeficiency, cardiopulmonary defects, as well as a heightened risk of a secondary cancer (Byrd, 1985; Green, 1993; Meadows and Silber, 1985). Along

---

Cancer and the Family, 2nd Edn. Edited by L. Baider, C. L. Cooper and A. Kaplan De-Nour

with the risk of medical late effects, the threat of disease recurrence further underscores the chronic nature of childhood cancer and the associated ambiguity experienced by cancer survivors and their families. As the population of cancer survivors increases, we are witnessing a new phase of coping with cancer—an off-treatment survivorship phase encompassing a distinct set of psychosocial issues. Making a successful transition from an active treatment phase to an off-treatment, survivorship phase represents an important goal of overall adaptation to childhood cancer.

In this chapter, we undertake two main tasks related to a discussion of the off-treatment, survivorship phase. First, we briefly review the major issues faced by childhood cancer survivors and describe potential patient, family and medical team factors associated with differential adequacy of psychosocial adaptation to childhood cancer survivorship. Second, we describe a family-oriented intervention—a Multiple Family Discussion Group (MFDG)—designed to help facilitate a more successful transition of adolescent cancer patients and their families from the active treatment phase to the off-treatment phase. This MFDG intervention represents a direct clinical extension of the family systems concepts we describe in the second section of the chapter.

PSYCHOSOCIAL ADAPTATION FOLLOWING TREATMENT OF CHILDHOOD CANCER

PSYCHOLOGICAL ADJUSTMENT OF CHILDHOOD CANCER SURVIVORS

The psychosocial implications of surviving childhood cancer have become an active area of research. Cancer survivors are not only at risk for recurrence of their original disease, but may develop a second malignancy, experience delayed toxic effects of their treatment, or suffer from a range of social and psychological consequences of their experiences as a cancer patient (Zeltzer, 1993). Fortunately, most studies of long-term survivors of childhood cancer have found adequate overall psychosocial functioning and a clear absence of severe psychopathology (Fritz et al., 1988; Kazak and Meadows, 1989; Smith et al., 1991; Teta et al., 1986). The few studies that have compared childhood cancer survivors to healthy peers typically find no significant differences in global psychosocial functioning. These findings demonstrate the overall resiliency of childhood cancer survivors.

However, many studies have found specific areas of psychosocial difficulty. For instance, Koocher et al. (1981) found that nearly half of their sample of young adult survivors of childhood cancer reported adjustment problems of low self-esteem, social isolation and school or work difficulties directly related to persistent fears of illness recurrence. Similarly, while reporting global psychological adjustment, cancer survivors have also described persistent illness-related concerns, negative body image and somatic preoccupation (Fritz et al., 1988; Greenberg et al. 1989; Madan-Swain et al., 1994; Mulhern et al., 1989). Several studies have found that childhood cancer survivors may also experience delays in achieving normative developmental milestones, such as leaving their parental home, getting married or obtaining full-time employment (Byrne et al., 1989; Lansky et al., 1986; Teta et al., 1986).

Most recently, the constellation of intrusive thoughts about illness and deliberate avoidance of illness reminders have been summarized as post-traumatic stress disorder (PTSD) responses (Kazak et al., 1992). Indeed, PTSD symptoms are common among childhood cancer survivors (Kazak et al., 1997, 1999) and are even more frequent among their parents (Manne et al., 1998), who have been found to display more posttraumatic stress symptoms than parents of healthy children (Barakat et al., 1997). Pelcovitz et al. (1998) found that the mother's PTSD status was highly associated with PTSD risk in adolescent cancer survivors. In our studies of adolescent cancer survivors (Ostroff et al., 1989; Smith et al., 1991), we have found that survivors experience both areas of vulnerability (e.g. emotional distress, persistent intrusive thoughts about their illness and treatment, concerns about body image and dating) as well as resiliency (school achievement, social competence, positive self-concept).

In summary, these findings convey both the weight of the stresses imposed by childhood cancer and the strength and resiliency that these survivors demonstrate. The task of health care providers is to develop psychosocial services that meet the specific needs of this growing patient population. Recent evidence of the high incidence of post-treatment post-traumatic stress and other psychosocial after-effects of cancer, and the reciprocal influence of symptoms among family members, highlight the need for post-treatment interventions for cancer survivors and their families.

FACTORS ASSOCIATED WITH POST-TREATMENT ADJUSTMENT OF CHILDHOOD CANCER SURVIVORS

As illustrated in the previous review of the psychosocial issues pertinent to the off-treatment phase of cancer, it is clear that there is no universal psychological response to completing cancer treatment. This variability in post-treatment adjustment leads to important questions about what factors may facilitate and impede coping with these issues. It is important to identify key factors that influence post-treatment adjustment that are targeted to the specific needs of survivors and their families. Our work and that of others has begun to examine several potential components of this coping process.

PATIENT FACTORS

Individual factors pertaining to the nature and severity of the disease and its treatment have been explored. In general, patients who have an excellent prognosis for long-term survival (e.g., early stage of disease, certain types of cancer) and who receive treatments that are shorter in duration and less toxic, as evidenced by fewer acute side effects and less physical disability, report the least amount of psychosocial difficulties (Cella et al., 1987; Greenberg et al., 1989; Koocher et al., 1981; Spinetta and Deasy-Spinetta, 1981). More recently, Kazak et al. (1992) have hypothesized that these findings may be explained by considering that the greater the trauma during the acute phase of illness, the greater the likelihood of post-traumatic stress responses following treatment completion. The age at which a child is diagnosed with cancer has been shown to be an important factor in long-term psychosocial adjustment, with adolescents reporting more psychosocial difficulties than younger children (Koocher et al., 1981). Presumably, the juxtaposition of adolescence, with its hallmark tasks of establishing independence from parents and beginning to prepare for future adult roles and relationships, and the diagnosis of a life-threatening chronic illness represent a 'poor fit' because of the demands and restrictions imposed by cancer. Finally, the amount of time since treatment completion appears to have a complex influence on post-treatment coping. While hypothesized to be important, the cross-sectional nature of previous work has not provided a clear understanding of the temporal process of coping with the chronic phase of cancer. On the one hand, patients and their families are delighted to complete the rigorous treatment. However, in the period shortly after treatment, patients may continue to experience treatment side effects, such as fatigue and weight loss, while persistent concerns about disease recurrence may temper their enthusiasm at this early stage of treatment completion. In one of the few published longitudinal studies, psychosocial adjustment generally improved over time (Kupst and Schulman, 1988).

FAMILY FACTORS

We are just beginning to understand the impact of surviving cancer on families and how family context might facilitate or impede childhood cancer survivors' post-treatment adjustment (Kazak, 1989; Kazak and Nachman, 1991; Kupst, 1993; Overholser and Fritz, 1990). Not surprisingly, the diagnosis and treatment of cancer takes its toll on the entire family. Non-patient family members experience considerable emotional, interpersonal, physical and financial strain related to the ongoing demands of medical care and the uncertainty of outcome (Chesler and Barbarin, 1987). Cancer taxes family resources and poses a significant risk of psychosocial impairment for the entire family.

Family members often claim that they do not stop to think about the ordeal they have been through until the initial crisis of diagnosis and the active phase of treatment are completed. Certainly, cancer remains an indelible memory for families, as evidenced by several reports of post-traumatic stress responses among the parents of childhood cancer survivors (Kazak et al., 1992; Manne et al., 1998). In our work, families, particularly mothers, repeatedly report a high degree of psychological distress, intrusive thoughts about the illness, and persistent fears of an uncertain future. While many families state that the experience of cancer has resulted in increased closeness, these persistent feelings of emotional distress may also strain relationships within the family (e.g., marital, sibling, parent–child).

Families are given minimal guidance about how to make the transition from the active phase to the off-treatment, survivorship phase of cancer. For many families, this transition is challenging in that, for months or even years, the acute illness and the demands of cancer treatment have virtually governed daily family life. Families often report that typical responsibilities (e.g., job duties, community involvement) and routines (e.g., extracurricular activities, leisure time, holidays) have been either suspended or greatly altered during the active phase of treatment. Reintegrating non-illness activities, routines, priorities, and goals is a vital reorganization task that involves flexibility and accommodation to the changing demands of cancer. Families engage in this re-entry process while simultaneously remaining on guard for disease recurrence or late complications of the treatment. Understandably, it may be quite challenging to balance the ongoing demands of an illness with an unpredictable course while maintaining efforts to meet the broader needs of family members.

Financial issues are also imminent for many families coping with cancer's aftermath. The rise of managed care and concurrent federal and state healthcare cut-backs have incited a host of potential financial issues. Many families will face financial problems resulting from overwhelming medical bills long after their child's cancer has been deemed 'cured'. Lack of insurance benefits, high deductibles and co-pays, and lack of reimbursement for experimental procedures, can all contribute to sizable debt. Time away from work and unproductive time caused by the distraction of facing a major medical crisis may also have a devastating financial impact. Months and years after aggressive treatment ends, when memories should seemingly begin to fade, insurance disputes and financial strain may serve as constant reminders of the cancer. Financial issues are also one of the leading causes of marital distress; distress that resonates with the entire family system, impeding healthy family functioning. Because of cuts in public and private health care systems, families may have had limited access to mental health or supportive services during the crisis phase of the illness, leaving many issues unprocessed and hence unresolved.

In our work with families, we have encountered four challenges experienced by most families who are entering the survivorship phase of childhood cancer. First, many normative family needs typically continue to be subordinated to the perceived needs and requirements of the illness. An illness-focused response, which was essential and adaptive during the acute phase, becomes less adaptive as the cancer moves into remission. The developmental, practical and emotional needs, not only of other family members but also of the patient, are often minimized or neglected as cancer concerns continue to dominate family life (even though no medical rationale may exist for such concerns). As a consequence, there is a predictable build-up of stress, frustration and poor communication within the family. Families who remain organized around the illness may disrupt normative development. Balancing the ongoing needs of the chronic phase of cancer with the broader developmental needs of the family is hypothesized to be a key ingredient in facilitating post-treatment psychosocial adjustment.

Second, within-family emotional and behavioral coalitions that developed during the intensive treatment phase continue to shape family life well into the off-treatment phase. In particular, coalitions formed between one parent (usually mothers) and ill children, bonds that invariably exclude spouses and other children, remain in place even though they are no longer practically necessary (during the hospitalization phase they may have been put in place as a logical response to the logistical demands of supporting the patient through highly demanding treatment protocols). This continued exclusion and isolation of other family members in turn leads to divisive and destructive family interactions.

Third, these patterns of family response are adhered to rigidly. The family finds it difficult, if not impossible, to change the ways it handles the illness, even if the current coping strategies are dysfunctional. It is as if the family believes that any adjustments to the precarious structure of its coping with the illness will bring the whole house down (e.g., monitoring of physical symptoms as signs of illness recurrence). For example, in our work with adolescent cancer survivors, we have observed that typically well-intended, continued parental vigilance often restricts teenagers' efforts to resume social activities following the completion of treatment. Families often report that it is difficult to switch from 'living day-to-day' to a stance that allows for an orientation towards future planning. These examples of illness-governed roles and routines are especially difficult to change because of their adaptability in an earlier phase of cancer treatment. In another case, a parent who has deftly managed a complex health care system and nurtured an ill child may hesitate to establish a non-illness role which provides an equal measure of security, purpose, and pride. Several studies have suggested that a family's ability to change and adjust to the changing demands of cancer may be most predictive of long-term adjustment (Kazak and Meadows, 1989; Kupst and Schulman, 1988).

Fourth, the rigidity of family coping style is sustained, in part, by the family's relative isolation from friends and extended family. Feelings of stigmatization and anger, not only about being a cancer 'victim' but also about how friends and extended family may have avoided them during the acute phase of the illness, all contribute to the family's continuing sense of being different and of being isolated from others. Many 'cancer families' feel that 'normal' families who have not experienced childhood cancer simply will not understand the practical demands and shifting emotions they face daily. Several studies have concluded that an openness in family communication about illness concerns and a supportive social network facilitates post-treatment adjustment (Kupst and Schulman, 1988; Koocher et al., 1981; Rait et al., 1992; Spinetta and Deasy-Spinetta, 1981).

MEDICAL TEAM FACTORS

The ways in which health care providers influence post-treatment adjustment have been largely unexplored. In sharp contrast to the treatment protocol that families are instructed to follow during the active phase of cancer treatment, guidelines for post-treatment medical care are often perceived by families to consist of little more than 'watch and wait'. To a family that has come to depend on the knowledge, technical skill and security provided by their physician, this post-treatment protocol offers little guidance, comfort or reassurance. In an attempt to console anxious families, the health care team may convey a unilateral message of definitive treatment completion ('all's well, it's over'). However, one-sided optimism betrays a family's potent fears of recurrence and realization of the chronic nature of cancer. While it is appealing for families to embrace the notion that the illness is over, the awareness of the risks of recurrence and long-term effects of treatment contributes to the ambiguity experienced by families.

Little is known about how to best prepare families for the off-treatment, survivorship phase of cancer. Health care providers can and should play a supportive role in helping families to establish realistic expectations for survivorship. The task of health care professionals is to foster the family's acquisition of relevant coping skills, ultimately leading to greater independence and competence in dealing with the ongoing stress of cancer. The family's satisfaction with the quality of medical care provided and the relationship with their health care providers has been found to be related to long-term psychosocial adjustment (Koocher et al., 1981).

In summary, the above review strongly suggests: (a) that the transition from the active treatment to the off-treatment phase of childhood cancer poses myriad challenges for both patients and their families; and (b) that *both* patient and family factors play a significant role as determinants of successful adaptation to the off-treatment phase. In combination, these two conclusions also suggest that cancer treatment centers would be well advised to implement programs specifically geared to childhood cancer survivors and their families. In the next section, we will describe one such intervention, the Multiple Family Discussion Group (MFDG), designed specifically to help children with cancer and their families to negotiate the transition from the active phase to the off-treatment phase of cancer.

THE ACKERMAN/MEMORIAL SLOAN–KETTERING MULTIPLE FAMILY DISCUSSION GROUP PROGRAM

RATIONALE FOR THE MFDG PROGRAM

As we noted above, because of the dramatic improvement in long-term prognosis of patients with childhood cancers, the medical and psychological concomitants of survivorship have taken on new import. Given the rigors of active treatment, the continuing uncertainty that accompanies remission, and the potential for the development of serious treatment side effects, it is not surprising that fears of recurrence, death, and other health-related anxieties are nearly universal experiences for patients and their families following the completion of cancer treatment. Many cancer treatment centers have therefore established 'long-term follow-up' clinics and have instituted educational programs for patients and parents who are thirsty for information about such issues as the sequelae of radiation therapy, fertility, and prevention of relapse.

However, as we have also discussed, many of the factors that seem to predict successful adaptation to survivorship are psychological and include parameters of family as well as individual functioning. We would argue that the weight of evidence points to the *primacy* of family factors in determining functionality/dysfunctionality of post-treatment psychosocial adaptation. A strong case can be made that programs and services aimed at facilitating successful familial psychosocial adaptation during the transition from the active treatment to the off-treatment phases of childhood cancer management should be designed to include families as well as patients. The familial impact of the off-treatment survivorship phase differs, in many respects, from the active treatment phase and demands specifically tailored interventions. While the active treatment phase often resembles a crisis state, anxiety regarding disease recurrence, physical or cognitive limitations, periodic clinic visits, and other factors reminiscent of other chronic medical conditions frequently characterize the off-treatment phase. While there exist numerous support groups focused on cancer treatment issues, very few specifically address the numerous psychosocial issues relevant to cancer survivorship and almost none target entire families.

Post-treatment interventions that specifically target the emotional needs of childhood cancer survivors and their families are clearly indicated. Kazak et al. (1999) designed and implemented a 1-day family group intervention program for adolescent survivors of childhood cancer, their parents, and siblings. All participants reported that the intervention was helpful and standardized measures indicated decreases in both anxiety and post-traumatic stress symptoms. The positive outcome of this intervention is encouraging in that it demonstrates the feasibility and efficacy of the multiple-family group format, while concurrently emphasizing the clinical utility of providing services geared specifically toward cancer survivors and their families. It is this perspective that has guided our efforts to design and implement a family-focused intervention specifically geared to facilitate successful off-treatment adjustment of patients with childhood cancers.

The intervention—the Ackerman/Memorial Sloan–Kettering Multiple Family Discussion Group program (MFDG)—is a short-term (six weekly sessions), psycho-educationally-oriented family-focused intervention. An adaptation of an MFDG originally designed for chronic illness families (Gonzalez et al., 1989), the program brings together up to four families per group, including the child with cancer, to discuss cancer-related family problems in a structured discussion format. Although led by two trained group leaders, the program is grounded in the notion that families who share a common problem—the presence of a very serious medical condition—are best able to help each other to understand maladaptive coping patterns and to propose alternative methods of handling illness-related problems. The group is specifically geared toward issues relevant to the survivorship phase.

CONCEPTUAL MODEL UNDERLYING THE MFDG

Structural Issues

Because of its unique structure—the conjoint meeting of four to six families including the index patients—the MFDG operates on two distinct levels. On the *intrafamily* level, the MFDG works like a single family intervention. With the help of trained group leaders, family members can talk among themselves in new ways, clarify their dissatisfying patterns of behavior and try alternative strategies. Therapists can use some of the techniques typically associated with individual family therapy, such as 'reframing' of a particular family's problem. The MFDG sessions are often the first time both 'patient' and 'non-patient' family members will have extensive discussions together about the impact of the medical condition on the family, where they are able to hear each other's perspectives.

On the *interfamily level*, the MFDG permits family members to more readily observe and understand their own attitudes and behaviors by comparing themselves with other families. These interfamily interactions and observations are often the most direct and profound level on which the MFDG operates. The group abounds in 'useful analogies'. Within single families there are no useful analogies, that is, there is (at most) one father, one mother, one big brother, one little sister, etc. In the presence of several other families, each person finds at least one (and often several) other person who shares his/her position or viewpoint within the family.

Further, with childhood cancer as the focus of the current program, the useful analogies multiply. Patients empathize with other patients, and 'well' family members share their feelings and perspectives on the influence of cancer on family life. Agreements and disagreements across families challenge each family's sense of isolation and singularity in their response to the illness condition. Further, interfamily connections made among group members provide each member with support. This is particularly important with regard to the index patient. With the patient receiving support from other patients, 'well' family members feel freer to express their own feelings and concerns without fear of upsetting or harming the patient.

In addition to useful analogies, the multiple family format offers participants the opportunity to observe members of their own families interact with others in ways that are different from their typical intrafamily positions, attitudes, and tones of voice. Within single families, members can become quite entrenched in repetitive, negatively reinforcing interactions, particularly related to the illness. When family members are seen to respond differently than expected, the opportunity is initiated to reorganize family patterns of response. For instance, in one MFDG session a greater sense of intrafamily empathy was observed when a mother poignantly explained her fear of illness recurrence in response to an adolescent from *another* family complaining about how overprotective his parents continued to be.

Family Regulation and Development

Thus, one aspect that provides the MFDG with its therapeutic impact is its structure. However, it is also important to underscore that our version of an MFDG relies on a clearly delineated conceptual model of family functioning (especially the interface between family and medical illness) for its design. Two concepts have been central in this regard: (a) family regulatory mechanisms as described in family systems theory (Steinglass, 1987; Steinglass et al., 1987); and (b) a developmental approach to illness course (Reiss and Kaplan De-Nour, 1989; Rolland, 1987; Stein and Jessup, 1982), a conceptual model that places illnesses like cancer within a life course framework, one that helps us understand why coping with cancer may call for fundamentally different adaptational styles at different phases in its course (e.g., the diagnostic phase, the active treatment phase, the survival phase).

When challenged by a serious medical illness, most families react by trying to gain mastery over the situation (Cole and Reiss, 1993; Rolland, 1993). Typically, adaptive mechanisms include a heightening of what we are calling family regulatory behaviors (Imber-Black et al., 1988; Wood, 1993). However, it is also the case that once these adaptive mechanisms are put into place, they can take on a life of their own. For example, organizing daily routines around illness-related needs (e.g., special diet, limitation of physical activities, hypervigilant behavior) can easily become a semi-permanent way of life, even though the acute crisis has long since passed and these behaviors are no longer medically necessary. Thus, in examining issues associated with transitions from one illness phase to another, one factor to track is whether family regulatory behaviors are also shifting in synchrony with changing illness needs and demands (Reiss et al., 1993; Wynne et al., 1992).

This is the very situation being faced by most childhood cancer families as they move into the off-treatment transition. One way of understanding the difficulties these families experience in successfully negotiating this phase is that they remain stuck in an 'acute phase' behavioral style, a style characterized by hyper-regulation (rigidity) of daily life and a 'day-to-day' mentality. What is required is a return to a more balanced posture between stability and growth, but most families need help in effecting this change.

However, in order to engage families in a discussion of these highly abstract issues, they must be brought down to earth, personalized via concrete examples or illustrative metaphors. Further, because our MFDG model is such a time-limited one (only six sessions), it is also necessary to focus the discussion on a fixed number of concepts that will bring these more abstract family systems and illness course constructs alive. We have focused on three main sets of constructs, all of which are parameters of family functioning that serve to regulate family life.

The first set of constructs describe ways in which families develop shared and implicit views of their social world. Variously called 'family world views' (Ransom et al., 1992) or 'family paradigms' (Reiss, 1981), the notion here is that families, over time, develop shared ideas (hypotheses) about how their social world operates and how the family should cope with these external environmental characteristics. One family might develop a shared view of the world as masterable, best approached with an open and continuously changing perspective, an exciting place in which to live. Another family might see the world as largely unfathomable, as potentially hostile and alien, as a place that calls for extreme caution and a steady and unchanging course based on long tradition.

These shared views of the external environment in turn would, then, play an important role in shaping behavior whenever the family is interacting with its social world. For example, the nature of family paradigms might in turn provide the guidelines for the assumptions families bring to their interactions with health care systems. From the vantage point of the physician or nurse, these differences would then translate into whether the family was perceived as cooperative, compliant, receptive to medical information, etc. (a 'good family'), or suspicious, combative, unduly demanding, unappreciative, etc. (a 'bad family').

A second set of constructs focus not so much on how the family construes its environment, but rather on how the family sees *itself* in relation to its larger world. Variably called the family's *'identity'* (Steinglass et al., 1987) *'sense of coherence'* (Antonovsky and Sourani, 1988), these constructs refer to a family's shared values and priorities, that is, the way the family might think about itself and describe itself to outsiders. A particularly important point here is that most families tend to pick a delimited number of themes around which to organize their identities, and these themes in turn play major roles in shaping family behavior.

For our purposes, the construct of family identity is useful because it is not uncommon for a family challenged by an illness like childhood cancer to actually reorganize itself around the medical condition as one of its central themes or priorities. This process is almost universal during the acute phase of the illness; however, this reorganization often persists long after the acute crisis has resolved. In such instances, the family not only continues to be illness-focused, it actually develops an identity built around illness-related experiences, demands and priorities. In the language of family systems theory, such a family has become skewed in the direction of hyper-regulation, and has become organized around a priority of defending itself against an outside force (cancer), rather than being able to return to more normative family issues (e.g. individuation of adolescents within the family).

For some medical conditions, this process is hard to avoid in that the realistic demands of the illness make other options difficult to pursue. For example, an illness such as end-stage renal disease, or a traumatic spinal cord injury, carries with it extremely time-consuming and expensive treatment consequences to which the family must somehow attend. But for childhood cancer, once the active treatment phase has ended, there are few mandatory demands the illness places on the family. Thus, we can assume that a family that continues to organize its behavior around cancer issues well into the survivorship phase is doing so largely for psychological, not medical, reasons.

Put another way, we can assume that one of the consequences of *all* medical illnesses for families is a need to bring increased order and regularity to daily life. However, for most illnesses this over-regulation of family life in the service of illness management is a temporary need. Once the illness has stabilized, a more balanced pattern of illness/non-illness activities can be restored. If that rebalancing process does not occur, we can conclude that the family has become 'stuck' around illness issues. A metaphor that helps to bring this phenomenon alive is to think about cancer as having *invaded* family life, and as a consequence created a *distortion* or imbalance in family priorities. It is this invasion/distortion process that the MFDG-intervention is designed to redress.

CONTENT AND STRUCTURE OF THE MFDG MEETINGS

Because the MFDG is designed as a short-term, focused intervention, each of its six sessions has a specific purpose and agenda. Although somewhat of an over-simplification, one way to describe how our MFDG intervention is structured is as a series of exercises designed: (a) to introduce families to the core constructs of our model of cancer and the family (family identity, family coping style, the developmental view of illness, etc.); (b) to suggest a series of useful metaphors that help illustrate these constructs and facilitate engagement with these issues; and (c) by manipulating the structure of the group, to encourage each family member to adopt multiple perspectives on the issues at hand.

Toward these overall aims, the six MFDG sessions are divided into the following three components (Illness Impact, Family Development and Family–Illness Integration), each with distinct goals:

1. Illness Impact component (two sessions):
   Identify cancer-related family issues and perspectives.
   Facilitate connections between participants occupying analogous family, developmental, and illness roles.
2. Family Development component (three sessions):
   Organize shared experiences and issues into categories and metaphors useful for further group work, with particular focus on the metaphor of 'keeping the illness in its place,' as a vehicle for transition to the off-treatment phase of cancer.
   Describe and clarify the family's view of the impact of cancer on family life, via the construction of art montages visually representing pre- vs post-cancer 'families'.

Family-by-family presentation of their montages to the group, followed by feedback from other group members.

Abstract (reframe) each family's 'story' about their montages (their 'cancer story'), with emphasis on core family values that have either been maintained or derailed by the intrusion of cancer into their lives.

Each family discusses specific post-treatment goals/issues and explores strategies for achieving these aspirations.

3. Family–Illness Integration component (one session):

Have group members bring to the final session representative 'physical reminders' of the illness. Use these reminders to describe and clarify to the group the impact of illness-related positive and negative feelings on family interaction and coping responses.

Also use this discussion to 'normalize' many of the family feelings being described, especially the intense affect generated by the uncertainty surrounding cancer prognosis.

Devise a family ritual for each family in the group that might serve symbolically to help the family to 'find an appropriate place' for the cancer experience in the family's life, thereby helping facilitate the family's transition to an 'off-treatment coping style'.

In addition to the content issues, the MFDG derives its impact from the use of a particular type of structural intervention the 'group-within-a-group' intervention—specifically designed to take advantage of the multi-level, multi-role composition of the group. At several points over the six sessions, group leaders divide the larger MFDG into two subgroups—a smaller subgroup that is asked to carry on a discussion around a specific stimulus question; and a larger subgroup that acts as an observing team. Subsequently, this 'observing team' is asked to comment on what they have seen and heard, a discussion that is in turn 'observed' by the other subgroup. Figure 10.1 illustrates the three phases of the group-within-a-group process.

This procedure of structuring the group discussion around a series of small groups, observed and responded to by the remaining members, is a core feature of the MFDG program. The purpose is to highlight the differing illness-related points of view and experiences of various family members and the analogous roles—developmental, family and illness——across families that provide supportive connections within the group. In highlighting shared perspective across families, differing attitudes and feelings are objectified and deintensified within families.

To facilitate the development of contrasting perspectives, whenever subgroups are formed during the meeting, each co-leader remains identified with his/her part of the group throughout the remainder of this part of the discussion. Each co-leader encourages interaction between members of his/her subgroup and organizes and summarizes the subgroup's ideas, feelings and impressions.

The following excerpt, taken directly from our treatment manual*, details the instructions given to group leaders about how to initiate the group-within-a-group that is formed during the first MFDG session:

---

*A treatment manual has been written that describes, in detail, the content of each MFDG session, along with instructions for group leaders about how to structure the meetings.

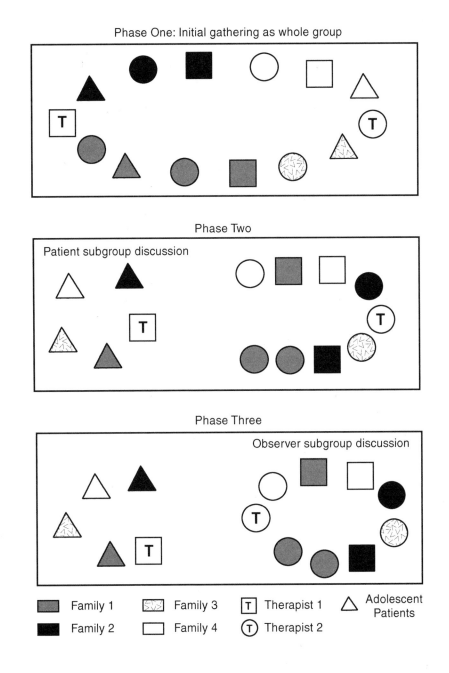

Figure 10.1 Structured schema of the group-within-group format of the MFDG. Circles=females; squares=males; triangles=adolescent patients.

To begin the discussion of the impact of cancer on family life, one of the group leaders asks the patient member from each family to meet with him/her for a smaller group discussion. Chairs are traded and rearranged so that the subgroup is spatially clearly demarcated. Subgroup members are then asked to talk with one another about the impact cancer has on them and on family life. The stimulus question to be used to focus the discussion is '*What is it like for you in your family to have been diagnosed with and treated for cancer?*' Other non-patient group members, along with the remaining co-leader, listen without interruption to the ensuing discussion.

In structuring this first subgroup discussion, co-leaders should make the structure and different roles clear to group members. It is helpful to say (subgroup co-leader, as he/she sits down with the patient subgroup), '*We're gong to talk just with each other during this part of the meeting as if the others weren't here.*' The observer co-leader might also reinforce this format by saying, '*We're going to listen during this part. But while we listen, it's important to pay attention also to our own thoughts and reactions for discussion later.*'

When the subgroup finishes its discussion, the co-leader might say '*A number of important ideas and feelings have come up here. It's our turn to sit back and listen to the impressions of others.*' The other (observer) co-leader would at this point say to his/her group, '*What thoughts or feelings come to mind as you listened to what the patient family numbers had to say?*'

The emphasis throughout this part of the session should be on discussion between the group members within each subgroup and on encouraging both similar and contrasting points of view. Families should become increasingly aware of differing perspectives within families and that the family as a group must take these differing viewpoints and feelings into account. On the other hand, the co-leaders should discourage cross-group discussion, because such exchanges will interfere with the structural intervention intended by organizing members along illness-role lines rather than by families.

SELECTION AND TRAINING OF DISCUSSION GROUP LEADERS

The MFDG program provides for the co-leadership of the discussion groups by two trained group leaders. The large number of people (10–20) usually participating in each group, as well as the multiple levels (intrafamily, interfamily, between patients and well members) on which interactions, both verbal and non-verbal, occur are more effectively monitored and constructively utilized with two co-therapists present. Optimally, all group leaders should have had training and practice in family and group therapy, as well as some experience working with medically ill patients and their families. Group leaders should possess an attitude of genuine interest in the families' experiences and a respect for their ongoing efforts to cope with the continuing legacy of cancer. We have found that the MFDG is easily learned and applied by health care providers from a number of different disciplines.

EFFICACY OF MFDGS

Recent anecdotal data (Steinglass, 1998) suggests that multiple-family discussion groups are content-relevant, helpful in initiating discussion of the cancer experience among family members, and enable families with similar cancer experiences to share their struggles with one another. Previous groups have had low drop-out rates despite families' initial hesitation about the time commitments required for group participation (Steinglass, 1998). We are currently in the process of implementing several empirical studies of MFDGs that will provide further qualitative information regarding their efficacy.

BARRIERS TO IMPLEMENTATION

While family-focused post-treatment services designed to meet the specific needs of childhood cancer survivors and their families represent a logical extension of comprehensive psychosocial care, there are several barriers for the delivery of these services. First, the off-treatment, survivorship phase of cancer has only recently been recognized as encompassing a unique set of psychosocial issues. Patients and families often find that psychosocial support services that were helpful during an earlier phase of cancer treatment may no longer seem as relevant (e.g., how to deal with acute side effects of treatment) and may even serve to exacerbate traumatic memories (e.g., meeting newly diagnosed cancer patients in a support group). Second, in comparison with the expected rigors of active treatment, families may perceive post-treatment psychosocial services to be unnecessary 'extra' expenditures of time and financial resources. Third, families may not take advantage of post-treatment services out of a desire not to appear vulnerable. In addition, some families may demonstrate a well-intentioned desire to protect each other from further emotional strain by declining participation in post-treatment family support programs. In fact, in our research, many families report that talking about persistent cancer-related concerns becomes a taboo subject of conversation after completion of treatment.

We believe that this subtle message of non-disclosure inadvertently contributes to the ambiguity of cancer survivorship and the isolation often experienced by family members. Health care providers may also introduce impediments for post-treatment psychosocial care. In an effort not to dampen the celebratory aspect of completing cancer treatment, health professionals may be reluctant to emphasize the potential for long-term physical and psychosocial sequelae of cancer. Thus, families typically complete treatment uncertain about what to expect during the off-treatment, survivorship phase. Finally, given scarce resources and limited staffing for specialized psychosocial services, priority is often given to crisis intervention delivered during the diagnostic, active and terminal phases of treatment.

While many of the barriers to implementation are emotional in nature, there are also several pragmatic issues that may constrain family participation in post-treatment programs such as the MFDG. The most challenging practical aspect of initiating a post-treatment intervention is participant recruitment. While participants in multiple family groups (e.g., Kazak et al., 1999; Steinglass, 1998) have overwhelmingly reported positive experiences, there are pragmatic constraints that may preclude family participation. In an era where both parents often work outside of the home and children participate in a myriad of extracurricular activities, for some families finding the time to commit to any activity for six consecutive weeks is deemed an impossible task. However, for many families, simply engaging in an activity together, whether it is therapy or some other task, has therapeutic benefits. Although offering post-treatment MFDGs in community settings would alleviate travel for many families, the relatively low prevalence of childhood cancer limits the number of eligible participants in a given community. As many families face financial problems related to medial expenses, the cost of psychotherapeutic intervention may also be prohibitive for some potential participants. If possible, fees for the intervention should be set according to a sliding-scale to help defer the cost to families. Steinglass (1998) suggests that the best strategy for eliminating recruitment problems for MFDGs would be to empirically demonstrate their efficacy through field trials and incorporate them as standard components in medical treatment protocols.

SUMMARY

It has been estimated that by the year 2000, one in 900 adults between the ages of 16 and 34 will be a survivor of a childhood cancer (Meadows et al., 1993). In recognition of the magnitude of this growing population of childhood cancer survivors and the multiple physical and psychosocial challenges they face, it has been recommended that greater effort be devoted to managing the medical late effects of cancer treatment and developing ways to promote the optimal psychosocial adjustment of childhood cancer survivors (Chesler et al., 1993; Reaman et al., 1993). Based on our clinical experience and research findings, we strongly advocate incorporating family members into the delivery of post-treatment services for childhood cancer survivors. The overall rationale for this approach is two-fold: cancer has a profound impact on family life, and family patterns seem critical to childhood cancer patients' full recovery from the ordeal of cancer.

Despite emotional and pragmatic obstacles, provision of support and information is needed to ensure the maintenance of emotional growth and development and reintegration to school, peer group and work settings (Barbarin, 1987; Robison, 1993). Continuation of the family–patient–health care provider collaboration is essential for gradual recovery from the active phase of cancer treatment and preparation for the psychosocial and physical challenges of the off-treatment, survivorship phase. Post-treatment interventions have the added benefit of engaging families who, due to practical or emotional constraints, did not receive psychosocial services during the diagnostic or crisis phases of cancer treatment. Given the demonstrated impact of childhood cancer on the family (e.g. Chesler and Barbarin, 1987; Rait et al., 1992), post-treatment interventions have the potential to reach families who may have previously unmet, yet critical needs. Supportive care, delivered in ways that respect family health and seek to promote optimal coping with the long-term issues of survivorship, is needed. We must also plan and deliver post-treatment psychosocial care that assists families in their efforts to integrate the persistent demands of cancer into family life while maintaining a balance with other family developmental needs.

REFERENCES

American Cancer Society (1998). *Cancer Facts and Figures.* Atlanta, CA: American Cancer Society.

Antonovsky, A. and Sourani, T. (1988). Family sense of coherence and family adaptation. *Journal of Marriage and the Family* **50**: 79–92.

Barakat, L.P., Kazak, A.E., Meadows, A.T., Casey, R., Meeske, K. and Stuber, M.L. (1997). Families surviving childhood cancer: a comparison of posttraumatic stress symptoms with families of healthy children. *Journal of Pediatric Psychology* 22: 843–859.

Barbarin, O.A. (1987). Psychosocial risks and invulnerability: a review of the theoretical and empirical bases of preventive family-focused services for survivors of childhood cancer. *Journal of Psychosocial Oncology* 5(4): 25–41.

Byrd, R. (1985). Late effects of treatment of cancer in children. *Pediatric Clinics of North America* 32: 835–857.

Byrne. J., Fears, T., Steinhorn, S. et al. (1989). Marriage and divorce after childhood and adolescent cancer. *Journal of the American Medical Association* 263(19): 2693–2699.

Cella, D., Tan, C., Sullivan, M., Weinstock, L., Alter, R. and Jow, D. (1987). Identifying survivors of pediatric Hodgkin's disease who need psychological interventions. *Journal of Psychosocial Oncology* 5(4): 83–96.

Chesler, M. and Barbarin, O. (1987). *Childhood Cancer and the Family*. New York: Bruner/Mazel.

Cheesier, M.A., Heiney, S.P., Perrin, R. et al. (1993). Principles of psychosocial programming for children and cancer. *Cancer* 10: 3210–3212.

Cole, R.E. and Reiss, D. (1993). *How do Families Cope with Chronic Illness?* Hillsdale, NJ: Erlbaum.

Fritz, C.K., Williams, J.R. and Amylon, M. (1988). After treatment ends: psychosocial sequelae in pediatric cancer survivors. *American Journal of Orthopsychiatry* 58(4): 552–561.

Gonzalez, S., Steinglass, P. and Reiss, D. (1989). Putting the illness in its place: discussion groups for families with chronic medical illnesses. *Family Process* 28: 69–87.

Green, D.M. (1993). Effects of treatment for childhood cancer on vital organ systems. *Cancer* 10: 3299–3305.

Greenberg, H.S., Kazak, A.E. and Meadows, A.T. (1989). Psychologic functioning in 8- to 16-year-old cancer survivors and their parents. *Journal of Pediatrics* 114(3): 488–493.

Imber-Black, E., Roberts, J. and Whiting, R. (Eds) (1988). *Rituals in Families and Family Therapy*. New York: Norton.

Kazak, A. (1989). Families of chronically ill children: a systems and socio-ecological model of adaptation and challenge. *Journal of Consulting and Clinical Psychology* 57: 25–30.

Kazak, A.E., Barakat, L.P., Meeske, K., Christakis, D., Meadows, A., Casey, R., Penati, B. and Stuber, M.L. (1997). Post-traumatic stress, family functioning, and social support in survivors of childhood leukemia and their mothers and fathers. *Journal of Consulting and Clinical Psychology* 65: 120–129.

Kazak, A.E. and Meadows, A.T. (1989). Families of young adolescents who have survived cancer: social-emotional adjustment, adaptability, and social support. *Journal of Pediatric Psychology* 14(2): 175–191.

Kazak, A.E. and Nachman, C.S. (1991). Family research on childhood chronic illness: pediatric oncology as an example. *Journal of Family Psychology* 4(4): 462–483.

Kazak, A.E., Simms, S., Barakat, L., Hobbie, W., Foley, B., Golomb, V. and Best, M. (1999). Surviving Cancer Competently Intervention Program (SCCIP): a cognitive-behavioral and family therapy intervention for adolescent survivors of childhood cancer and their families. *Family Process* 38: 175–191.

Kazak, A.E., Stuber, M., Torchhinsky, M., Houskamp, B., Christakis, D. and Kasiraj, J. (1992). Post-traumatic stress in childhood cancer survivors and their parents. Annual Meeting of the American Psychological Association, Washington, DC.

Koocher, C.P., OMalley, J.E. and Foster, D.J. (1981). The special problems of survivors. In C.P. Koocher and J.E. O'Malley (Eds), *The Damocles Syndrome* (pp. 112–129). New York: McGraw-Hill.

Kupst, M.J. (1993). Family coping. *Cancer* 10: 3337–3341.

Kupst, M.J. and Schulman, J.L. (1988). Long-term coping with pediatric leukemia: a six-year follow-up study. *Journal of Pediatric Psychology*, 13(1): 7–22.

Lansky, S.B., List, M.A. and Ritter-Sterr, C. (1986). Psychosocial consequences of cure. *Cancer* 58: 529–533.

Madan-Swain, A., Brown, R.T., Sexson, S.B., Baldwin, K., Pais, R. and Ragab, A. (1994). Adolescent cancer survivors. Psychosocial and familial adaptation. *Psychosomatics* **35**(5): 453–459.

Manne, S., DuHamel, K., Gallelli, K., Sorgen, K. and Redd, W. (1998). Post-traumatic stress disorder among parents of pediatric cancer survivors; diagnosis, co-morbidity and utility of the PTSD checklist as a screening instrument. *Journal of Pediatric Psychology* **23**: 357–366.

McDaniel, S., Hepworth, J. and Doherty, W. (Eds) (1992). *Medical Family Therapy: A Biopsychosocial Approach to Families with Health Problems*. New York: Basic Books.

Meadows, A.T., Nesbit, M.E., Strong, L.C., Nicholson, H.S., Green, D.M., Hays, D.M. and Lozowski, S.L. (1993). Long-term survival. *Cancer* **10**: 3213–3215.

Mulhern, R.K., Wasserman, A.L., Friedman, A.G. and Fairclough, D. (1989). Social competence and behavioral adjustment of children who are long-term survivors of cancer. *Pediatrics* **83**(1): 18–23.

Ostroff, J., Smith, K. and Lesko, L. (1989). Promotion of mental health among adolescent cancer survivors and their families. *Proceedings of the Mental Health Services for Children and Adolescents in Primary Care Settings*. A NIMH Research Conference, 1989, New Haven, CT.

Overholser, J.C. and Fritz, C.K. (1990). The impact of childhood cancer on the family. *Journal of Psychosocial Oncology* **8**(4): 71–85.

Pelcovitz, D., Libov, B.G., Mandel, F., Kaplan, S., Weinblatt, M. and Septimus, A. (1998). Post-traumatic stress disorder and family functioning in adolescent cancer. *Journal of Traumatic Stress* **11**: 205–221.

Rait, D.S., Ostroff, J.S., Smith, K., Celia, D.F., Tan, C. and Lesko, L.M. (1992). Lives in a balance: perceived family functioning and the psychosocial adjustment of adolescent cancer survivors. *Family Process* **31**: 383–397.

Ransom, D.C., Fisher, L. and Terry, H.E. (1992). The California Family Health Project: II Family world new and adult health. *Family Process* **31**: 251–267.

Reaman, C.H., Bonfiglio, J., Krailo, M. et al. (1993). Cancer in adolescents and young adults. *Cancer* **10**: 3206–3209.

Reiss, D. (1981). *The Family's Construction of Reality*. Cambridge, MA: Harvard University Press.

Reiss, D. and Kaplan De-Nour, A. (1989). The family and medical team in chronic illness: a transaction and developmental perspective. In C. Ramsey Jr (Ed.), *Family Systems in Medicine*. New York: Guilford.

Reiss, D., Steinglass, P. and Howe, G. (1993). The family's organization around the illness. In R.E. Cole and D. Reiss (Eds.), *How Do Families Cope with Chronic Illness?* (pp. 173–214). Hillsdale, NJ: Lawrence Erlbaum Associates.

Robison, L.L. (1993). Issues in the consideration of intervention strategies in long-term survivors of childhood cancer. *Cancer* **10**: 3406–3410.

Rolland, J.S. (1987). Chronic illness and the life cycle: a conceptual framework. *Family Process* **26**: 203–221.

Rolland, J.S. (1993). Mastering family challenges in serious illness and disability. In F. Walsh (Ed.), *Normal Family Processes*, 2nd Edn. New York: Guilford.

Smith, K., Ostroff, J., Tann, C. and Lesko, L. (1991). Alterations in self-perceptions among adolescent cancer survivors. *Cancer Investigation* **95**(5): 58–8

Spinetta, J.J. and Desy-Spinetta, P. (Eds) (1981). *Living with Childhood Cancer*. St Louis, MO: C.V. Mosby.

Stein, R.E. and Jessup, D.J. (1982). A non-categorical approach to chronic childhood illness. *Public Health Report* **1970**: 354–362.

Steinglass, P. (1987). A systems view of family interaction and psychopathology. In T. Jacob (Ed.), *Family Interaction and Psychopathology: Theories, Methods, and Findings*. New York: Plenum.

Steinglass, P., Bennett, L.A., Wolin, S.I. and Reiss, D. (1987). *The Alcoholic Family*. New York: Basic Books.

Steinglass, P. (1998). Multiple family discussion groups for patients with chronic medical illness. *Family, Systems and Health* **16**: 55–70.

Teta, M.J., Del Po, M.C., Kasl, S.V., Meigs, J.W., Meyers, M.H. and Mulvihill, J.J. (1986). Psychosocial consequences of childhood and adolescent cancer survival. *Journal of Chronic Diseases* **39**(9): 751–759.

Wood, B. (1993). Beyond the psychosomatic family: a biobehavioral family model of pediatric illness. *Family Process* **32**: 261–278.

Wynne, L.C., Shields, C.C. and Sirkin, M. (1992). Illness, family theory, and family therapy: conceptual issues. *Family Process* **31**: 3–18.

Zeltzer, L.K. (1993). Cancer in adolescents and young adults psychosocial aspects: long-term survivors. *Cancer* **10**: 3463–3468.

11

A Model of Family-Centered Intervention during Palliative Care and Bereavement: Focused Family Grief Therapy (FFGT)

DAVID W. KISSANE

Department of Medicine, St Vincent's Hospital and Peter MacCallum Cancer Institute, University of Melbourne, Victoria, Australia

A FAMILY VIGNETTE

Divorce had ended a marriage of 20 years between a couple with three daughters, but the mother's terminal illness 18 years later led to resolution of unfinished business from that marital breakdown. Her eldest daughter had been most distressed as a teenager, but her mother's bitterness prevented consolation. This mother knew intuitively that something remained amiss. An invitation to sort this out before she died was provided as the result of a process of screening for their family functioning. Both her current and former husbands were able to join the four women in family meetings. Each member's perspective of the marital breakup was shared as the family retold their story. Enhanced understanding developed with greater acceptance and forgiveness. The mother's role was affirmed with gratitude. Reminiscence helped celebrate her life while the family prepared for her loss. It was a model of family-centered care that created the opportunity for this family to resolve its unfinished business.

The family is inevitably involved in care-provision when a progressive and life-threatening illness affects one of its members. They are challenged to cope with the distress accompanying the illness and then their subsequent bereavement. There has been growing awareness over recent years that treatment of the whole family is the optimal approach to be adopted by a palliative care service (Cassileth and Hamilton, 1979; Northouse, 1984; Rait and Lederberg, 1989; Bluglass, 1991; Baider et al., 1996; Lederberg, 1998). Maintaining continuity of care into bereavement maximizes support for the whole family.

Cancer and the Family, 2nd Edn. Edited by L. Baider, C. L. Cooper and A. Kaplan De-Nour
© 2000 John Wiley & Sons, Ltd

Before exploring notions of family-centered care, we need to know something about the degree and type of psychosocial morbidity that can occur in the family of a cancer patient. The rate of psychological distress found among patients receiving palliative care is certainly higher than in a general cancer population (Derogatis et al., 1983; Kaasa et al., 1993; Pinder et al., 1993). In an Australian sample, we found significant distress in 50% of patients during palliative care (Kissane et al., 1994a). Not all of these were formally diagnosed with a psychiatric disorder, rates of depression, for example, generally lying in the 10–20% range (Chochinov et al., 1995). The distress experienced during palliative care is more broadly composed of existential suffering, grief, fear, and unhappiness, as well as psychiatric disorders.

Rates of psychological distress for spouses have ranged between 18% and 35% (Buckley, 1977; Plumb and Holland, 1977; Maguire, 1981; Gotay, 1984; Ell et al., 1988; Northouse, 1989), including a rate of 35% in our Australian sample (Kissane et al., 1994a). Moreover, this distress endured for up to 18 months in longitudinal studies (Ell et al., 1988; Northouse, 1989). While in some, there has been a close correlation between the psychological status of the patient and spouse, others found personal vulnerability in the spouse (Ell et al., 1988) or the perceived degree of social support (Goldberg et al., 1984; Ell et al., 1988) to be more predictive of psychological morbidity.

Only a few studies have involved offspring or more distant family members (Cassileth et al., 1985; Ell et al., 1988; Vess et al., 1985, 1988), but in our Australian sample, one-quarter of offspring exhibited significant distress (Kissane et al., 1994a). We found that offspring carried greater hostility ($p < 0.01$) than their parents on the Brief Symptom Inventory (Derogatis and Spencer, 1982). The burden of care for adult offspring with children of their own, anticipatory grief or the pattern of communication in the family could explain this greater level of anger. Children may receive less information about the illness and its treatment, despite medical expectations that understanding would be transmitted through the family. Similarly, Vess and colleagues (1985, 1988) found behavioral changes in 39% of children in their studies of younger families. The anger carried by the offspring of patients receiving palliative care points to the need for family-centered care. Clearly, distress reverberates throughout the family as members become tangled up in a web of emotion and conflict (Kissane, 1994a).

However, we require both conceptual and practical methods of classifying families if we are to systematically adopt a model of family-centered care. Historically, one approach has been to conceptualize families in terms of the phases of illness they must negotiate (Giacquinta, 1977; Northouse, 1984; Rait and Lederberg, 1989); another stressed the family's needs or the associated burdens it experienced (Cassileth and Hamilton, 1979; Adams-Greenly and Moynihans, 1983; Bluglass, 1991); a third focused on the family's developmental stage (Carter and McGoldrick, 1980; Eisenberg et al., 1984). While each of these methods contributed to our understanding of the family, what proved predictive of how a family coped over time was their pattern of relating together and functioning as a unit (Kissane et al., 1994b, 1996a, b). This provided us with an empirically derived approach to family-centered care.

OUR STUDIES OF FAMILY FUNCTIONING DURING PALLIATIVE CARE AND BEREAVEMENT

Employing a longitudinal design to study adult families caring for a dying parent, we used cluster analysis to define a typology of how they functioned (Kissane et al., 1994b). They were followed across 13 months of bereavement (670 individual responses from 115 families) to confirm the temporal utility of our classification (Kissane et al., 1996a, b). Five types of family emerged, based upon members' perceptions of their cohesiveness, expressiveness and conflict resolution. Two classes appeared well-functioning: one-third were classified as '*Supportive*,' characterized by high levels of cohesiveness, and one-fifth as '*Conflict Resolvers*,' in whom effective communication and cohesion provided the wherewithal to tolerate differences of opinion and resolve conflict constructively. There were low levels of psychosocial morbidity among these well-functioning families.

In contrast, two classes of families were clearly dysfunctional: '*Hostile*' families were distinguished by high conflict, low cohesiveness and poor expressiveness; '*Sullen*' families reported moderate levels in these three domains—their anger was more muted, but they carried the highest rates of clinical depression. During palliative care, 15% of families bore one of these maladaptive patterns, but this rate rose to 30% at 6 weeks post-bereavement before gradually returning to 15% by 13 months post-death. High rates of psychosocial morbidity occurred among members of these dysfunctional families.

The final class of family was termed '*Intermediate*', between one-third to one-fifth by proportion, and they exhibited moderate cohesiveness, but were still prone to psychosocial morbidity. Their functioning lay in between the well-functioning and more dysfunctional groupings. Moreover, they tended to become more dysfunctional with the stress of bereavement, before eventually returning to their former status 13 months post-death. This class of family appeared particularly suited to preventive intervention.

Our method of classifying families by their functioning proved predictive of individual psychosocial outcome for their membership over time (Kissane et al., 1996b). Sullen families not only experienced the most intense grief, but also were at greatest risk of depression. Intermediate families merged with the more dysfunctional pair in displaying reduced overall social adjustment, as well as decreases in domains of housework, social and recreational functioning. Intermediate families also made low use of rules by which their family lived, and were the least ambitious for achievement by their members. Our sample reflected the multicultural nature and social diversity of Australian families; 34% of patients were born overseas.

Impressively, Supportive families expressed high levels of grief without adverse consequences, ostensibly because their cohesiveness facilitated sharing of distress, while at the same time fostering mutual consolation and caring. This confirmed the clinical observation that adaptive families grieve successfully together (Kissane and Bloch, 1994). Further observation of family coping style (via the Family Crisis Oriented Personal Evaluation Scale; McCubbin et al., 1985) showed that well-functioning families made regular use of coping strategies, while Hostile families used these the least. Thus, the latter's disruptive style of relating—poor communication and high conflict—was matched by their inability to avail themselves of social support, use community resources, or seek spiritual support. On these dimensions, they contrasted with Sullen families, who, as if in recognition of their distress, did seek support, both spiritual and social, and made use of community resources. Hence, we found in our studies that use of these coping strategies distinguished the two most dysfunctional classes; Hostile families appeared impervious to help, whereas Sullen families searched for the assistance they sensed they needed.

These significant findings of the association between family functioning and outcome of grief are supported by clinical observation. Thus, Munson (1978) first highlighted family conflict as a factor in the non-resolution of grief, while Vollman and colleagues (1971) differentiated cohesive families with supportive social networks from families that were closed and socially isolated in their experience of grief. Similar differences between adaptive and maladaptive patterns were described in younger families following the death of a child (Davies et al., 1986).

This conceptual method of classifying families according to their functioning empowers us to differentiate adaptive families from that group with greater need. We ought to respect the potential of well-functioning families to grieve effectively. On the other hand, when families are at some risk because their functioning is Hostile, Sullen or Intermediate in nature, preventive intervention appears worthwhile, indeed, warranted. Our model permits screening of families to recognize those in need.

SCREENING FOR FAMILIES AT GREATER RISK

The Family Relationships Index is a 12-item, self-report scale that can be extracted from the short form of the Family Environment Scale (Moos and Moos, 1981), a well-validated questionnaire whose predictive capacity has been supported by its use in extensive research (Moos, 1990). We recommend that family members be individually screened, including children above the age of 12 (who can easily read this questionnaire). A family is deemed at risk if one or more respondents score 9 or less out of 12, or less than 4 on cohesiveness (see Table 11.1). The latter rule is included because reduced cohesiveness is the most sensitive predictor of poor outcome in our model. In screening all available family members, we attempt to understand what the major 'family environment' is, through inspection of scores to

Table 11.1 Typology of families

Family type	Defining FRI* scores	Percentage membership of family class across the phases of care in the Melbourne family grief studies		
		Palliative care	Early bereavement	Late bereavement
Supportive	12	33	28	34
Conflict resolvers	10–11	21	25	22
Intermediate	8–9	31	17	24
Sullen	5–7	9	18	7
Hostile	0–4	6	12	13

*FRI=Family Relationships Index (Moos and Moos, 1981)

discern which aspect is particularly problematic, e.g. cohesion, conflict or expressiveness. On the other hand, averaged family scores are not considered, as this approach would eliminate some of the more subtle aspects of family functioning reflected in notions like 'symptom bearer' or 'scapegoat' (see Rolland, 1984, 1987). Although our typology has been confirmed on both individual perceptions and hierarchically, using the whole family as the unit of analysis (Kissane et al., 1996a), we prefer to base assessments on the perceptions of individuals, whose insight into their family might otherwise be overlooked if mean scores were used. Screening several members takes effort, but is manageable if they are met as a group and provides more complete understanding of the family.

FOCUSED FAMILY GRIEF THERAPY (FFGT): A MODEL OF INTERVENTION FOR PALLIATIVE CARE

Having developed from empirical observation this method of recognizing families most in need, an intervention was developed via a brainstorming process with colleagues, recorded in a manual and piloted (Kissane et al., 1998), before being thoroughly tested through a randomized, controlled trial with 100 families to confirm its effectiveness. According to this model of intervention, therapy progresses through five phases (Table 11.2): assessment; agreement about concerns or issues; focused treatment; consolidation; and termination. Its broad features are outlined below.

GOALS OF FFGT

To fulfill the objective of improving family adjustment during palliative care and thus reduce bereavement morbidity, the model concentrates on enhancing family functioning, particularly cohesiveness, conflict resolution and expression of thoughts and feelings. Grief, however, is an indispensable dimension of this work. We promote the sharing of grief within the family, in the process inextricably enhancing functioning.

Our therapy is time-limited, brief, and focused. The strengths of members are particularly affirmed, so that these are harnessed to empower them to face the challenge of relevant change. At the same time, we accept the limits of the exercise by not getting drawn into overambitious work with complex families or delving into long-standing personality problems. In practice, the family determines who participates, so that the therapist works with whatever configuration can be accessed. Should a key member elect not to attend, one draws confidence from the knowledge that has accumulated in family therapy that change in one part of the family system is likely to influence others and that benefits tend to percolate throughout the whole system (Hoffman, 1981; Selvini Palazzoli, 1983; Campbell et al., 1991).

Importantly, at no stage do we label families as 'pathological' or 'dysfunctional'. The therapist simply indicates that he/she is interested in working with families to help them assist their sick relative. We state that in our experience families do benefit by coming together for meetings in which we review concerns and work together.

Table 11.2   The course of focused family grief therapy

1.   Assessment (story of illness, family functioning and genogram)
2.   Engagement through identification of issues or concerns
3.   Focused treatment (grief, problem solving, conflict resolution)
4.   Consolidation (affirmation of change in family functioning)
5.   Termination (with future orientation)

ASSESSMENT PHASE OF FFGT

The family is invited to tell their story of illness, promoting expression of feelings and clarifying the understanding and concerns of members as this proceeds. Circular questioning (Tomm, 1988) reveals patterns of interaction and specifically exposes communication processes, supportive endeavors, roles, traditions and sources of conflict. A genogram is routinely constructed (often in a second session) to identify the family structure and patterns of relating across generations (McGoldrick and Gerson, 1985). Previous occasions of loss and bereavement are closely considered, with an emphasis on customary coping patterns.

Throughout this assessment, the therapist needs to avoid acting judgmentally. He/she also strenuously avoids 'siding' with particular family members, thus preserving his/her neutrality. Moreover, the strengths and assets of the family are identified and affirmed. This leads the therapist to a balanced perspective from which he/she can endorse these strengths as a potential means to grapple with identified concerns.

Towards the end of the assessment, the family is invited to prioritize their primary issues or concerns. This is a crucial step in facilitating the family assuming responsibility for aspects they would like to change. Successful engagement of the family in ongoing work depends on their recognition of this list of concerns. These become the basis for future focused sessions. The therapist ensures that the basic goals of our model in promoting cohesiveness, conflict resolution and expressiveness are attended to as appropriate within this list of concerns.

THE FOCUSED TREATMENT IN FFGT

Once a therapeutic alliance has been forged through the assessment phase (usually 1–2 sessions), the ongoing frequency of sessions varies from weekly to fortnightly to monthly in accordance with the family's needs. On each occasion, the therapist reviews the family's progress and agreed focus. Affirmation is a core feature of this review (Allman et al., 1992), including recognition of the advantages of any growing cohesiveness. Praise from the therapist is likely to reinforce the family's efforts at supporting each other.

Problem solving is a key strategy used to guide the family in their work on concerns. Through exploring antecedents and consequences, the therapist helps members arrive at preferred solutions to issues, without imposing his/her own. The family become increasingly adept at observing their patterns of functioning, thus being empowered to make choices that were not previously apparent to them.

Where long-established resentment has dominated interactions, conflict becomes more challenging to resolve. A family pattern of criticizing and blaming others may have been transmitted from generation to generation. Making overt this pattern of relating as an entrenched 'script' (Byng-Hall, 1988, 1991) may enlighten the family and empower them to move to a new style of more adaptive functioning. Furthermore, members may be unaware of the expectations they impose on others, causing frustration and disappointment that could otherwise be avoided.

In this setting of grief, where loss may be perceived as grossly unfair, clarification of the source of anger is important. Whenever rage leads to a maladaptive outcome, it needs to be checked and redirected (Kissane, 1994b). In particular, family members may need to better understand and respect differences that exist between them. The strength that comes from diversity warrants acknowledgment. In this manner, tolerance is fostered as members acknowledge differences in interests, temperament and style. From time to time, families may need to consider the role of forgiveness. It can empower them to come together at a pivotal moment when they sense the threat of loss. The dying person may be a powerful influence if he/she spurs the family to relate more tolerantly and compassionately.

COMMON THEMES THAT ARISE DURING FFGT

A series of predictable concerns recur among families receiving therapy (Table 11.3). These include the delivery of instrumental care, the emotional challenge of suffering, altered access and intimacy, the process of farewell, the experience of death, cultural and religious practices, needs of particular family members, including children, historical influences on the family, and the final pain of separation. These common themes can be flexibly discussed during the middle phase of therapy.

Care Provision

Research has demonstrated a range of unmet needs in carers, including the provision of information (Wright and Dyck, 1984; Tringali, 1986; Schofield et al., 1998), emotional support (Northouse, 1984; Stetz, 1987; Woods et al., 1989; Wingate and Lackey, 1989; Hileman and Lackey, 1990; Schofield et al., 1998), practical help with physical care (Tringali, 1986; Kristjanson and Ashcroft, 1994; Watson, 1994; Schofield et al., 1998), guidance about coping strategies (Klagsburn, 1994; Given and

Table 11.3   Common themes that arise in FFGT

---
1. Care provision for ill member
2. Suffering
3. Intimacy
4. Discussing death
5. Saying goodbye
6. Good death or disappointment
7. Culture and religion
8. Needs of younger children
9. Past history and its influences
10. Grief of bereavement

Given, 1996; Schofield et al., 1998), and recognition of altered roles and choices (Schofield et al., 1998).

Any sense of burden may be problematic if it induces guilt and avoidant behaviors (Given et al., 1993). To lessen burden, the domiciliary palliative care team engages volunteers to provide respite. Moreover, fatigue can be eased through a comprehensive appraisal of carer needs (Jensen and Given, 1991). The conduct of a family meeting in the home may be pivotal in permitting expression of these issues. The opportunity commonly arises for offspring to reassure their parents about the gratification they receive in returning some of the love and care they received during childhood (Hinton, 1994).

In Australia, Schofield and colleagues (1998) surveyed carers and identified five predictors of burden: resentment, family conflict, depression, close relationship with the patient or, alternatively, anger directed at him. Furthermore, social support, anger, coping difficulties, and unclear medical diagnoses influenced carer resentment. Some 38% of carers reported problems with coping, one-third reported health concerns, and over half reported unmet needs. Yet only 12% received counseling. During this period of caring, families experienced greater compassion, but tension was also common. Feelings of resentment, conflict and love could coexist. Overall, one-quarter of the families in their study reported disagreement among members.

When roles can be flexibly taken up and certain tasks shared, there will be reduced burden consequent upon teamwork (Given and Given, 1994). Many of the everyday tasks, exemplified by housework, shopping, and transport, can be sorted out through problem solving during a family meeting, while the family grows in mutual understanding through discussion.

Migrants need more assistance in organizing social services, communicating with others and seeking financial support (Schofield et al., 1998). Otherwise, they will utilize fewer respite services. They are worthy targets of a family intervention. We have found that cultural difference within a family merits reflection, challenging therapists to understand and draw strength from the richness within these traditions.

Suffering

The modern family can be ill-prepared through its lack of historical experience with death and dying (Cherny et al., 1994). They struggle with the commitments of working couples, uncertainty, and helplessness (Kissane, 1998). Furthermore, our community carries an unconscious expectation that all suffering can be relieved, a myth perpetuated by modern medicine (Callahan, 1995). Frank discussion about the illness and its treatment can help to ameliorate suffering, while also tempering any unrealistic expectations (Ferrell et al., 1991a, b, c).

Occasionally, families will be concerned about loss of dignity in their dying relative. Personal perceptions are critical here. Frailty develops slowly for the patient, permitting adjustment over time. Onlookers lose sight of this gradual process, perceiving indignity through identification with their perception of the plight of their relative. Caution about such interpretations is warranted; discussion in a family meeting can helpfully clarify the reality of a patient's quality of life, in the process easing any associated suffering of family members (Ferrell et al., 1991b).

Intimacy

Frank communication of reactions to the illness may pre-empt abhorrence about bodily disfigurement, odor and surgical dressings. Some families grow closer as a result of the challenge of cancer (Bloom, 1982; Neuling and Winefield, 1988), but others get stuck in awkwardness and avoidance (Reiss et al., 1993). Prior patterns of intimacy, comfort, and support can be fostered during this time if information is shared to promote understanding and teamwork (Griffith and Griffith, 1994).

Discussing Death

Despite the inevitability of death, it is often unwelcome, and its pending reality denied. Avoidant mechanisms may be perpetuated by one or more dominant family members, sometimes influenced by a cultural attitude towards truth telling (Gotay, 1996). In a family meeting, one can enquire about prognosis and its understanding by different relatives, thus opening up discussion of death (Wellisch et al., 1978). Commonly, one member will openly reveal his/her expectation of death, bringing expression of anticipatory grief into the family circle. While some might protectively prefer to avoid the sadness that follows, directly naming and normalizing their grief may help the family to communicate about these matters (Ringler et al., 1981; Acworth and Bruggen, 1985; Buckman, 1993).

Depending upon the closeness of death, a balance may need to be struck between anticipatory grief and the living out of life remaining (Parkes, 1998). Excessive premature grief may mar this final phase. On the other hand, life satisfaction can be generated by reminiscence and lead to increased acceptance of pending loss (Yalom, 1980). If this choice between grief and continued embracement of life are pointed out, the family is empowered to more reflectively pace themselves through this experience, generally adjusting their position according to the physical condition of the dying member.

Saying Goodbye

Although individuals regularly perceive this to be a final act, in practice it evolves gradually as a temporal process (Hinton, 1981). The major components of this farewell include review of the nature of relationship with the ill family member, affirmation of the contribution of each person, completion of unfinished business and expression of gratitude for the good times shared (Meares, 1981). A parent can be encouraged to share hopes and wishes for his/her children, acknowledging delight in their success. Since affirmations may be poignantly remembered for years to come, encouragement of their expression is worthwhile in these family sessions.

The tasks involved in saying goodbye can be easily postponed by well-intentioned families, motivated to protect their dying member from distress. Guidance is distinctly helpful so that families do not misjudge the time remaining for this farewell.

Good Death or Disappointment

News of the death usually reaches the therapist via the multidisciplinary palliative care team. The family is invariably appreciative of his/her expression of sympathy at this time. We have found that telephone contact and attendance at the funeral, when this is possible, greatly strengthens the therapist's alliance with the family.

Not all events will go smoothly for families, particularly if symptoms have been distressing and not easily controlled (Portenoy et al., 1994). Complex factors influence this experience (Bass and Bowman, 1990). Sense of failure, meaninglessness, lack of fulfillment, and alienation from others may especially contribute to guilt and disappointment. It is helpful to acknowledge such emotional pain, listening quietly to the story involved (Grobe et al., 1996).

At times, criticism and anger may reverberate through the family and be easily displaced onto undeserving scapegoats. Disappointment may signify underlying ambivalence over relationships and unresolved longer-term issues (Freud, 1917; Klein, 1940). Wise clinicians sustain continuity of care over time, providing opportunities for review and gradual working through of these issues. In the interim, however, they can be left with the knowledge and burden of an unhappy death, all the more distressing when the ideal of a good death had been ardently sought. Rural general practitioners may feel particular discomfort about the outcome of death when mixing socially with the bereaved in their local communities. Open discussion with these families does much to ameliorate distress.

Cultural Issues and Religious Practices

Rituals and customary behaviors, often prescribed by religious tradition, provide a structure that can guide the family through this stressful time (Eisenbruch, 1984a, b; Rosenblatt et al., 1993). Such practices have arisen across centuries as cultural groups have sought to help their bereaved. A clinician's respect for ritual conveys sensitivity about spiritual aspects of life; endorsement of their value can clarify potential benefit for those less certain (Imber-Black, 1991).

When doctors, nurses or therapists attend a funeral service, they communicate their personal reaction about the loss to the bereaved. This can be a source of significant consolation. Furthermore, the personal grief work of these care providers facilitates their adaptation and closure of relationship with the deceased, while powerfully signaling interest in and ongoing availability to the survivors (Vachon, 1995). In FFGT, we do not perceive a significant boundary violation to occur when the therapist does attend a funeral, given the therapeutic benefits that flow from this practice, but there is an appropriate point following the formal ceremony when the therapist should sensitively and sensibly withdraw.

Younger Children

Parents can be understandably caught up in their own distress. Discussion of the needs of younger children will help clarify the support they receive (Nelson et al., 1994). Honest communication about the illness and its effects helps the child to cope. Moreover, clarification of a child's thoughts allays misunderstanding about the cause of illness and death (Sawyer et al., 1993). Family sessions during bereavement, in which children draw and paste photographs into scrapbooks as personal memoirs of their dead parent, focus attention specifically on their grief. Occasionally, the plight of children belonging to a dying single parent warrants careful discussion and planning (Compas et al., 1996).

Historical Issues Influencing the Family

Numerous past experiences influence the family's pattern of relating and coping (Sales et al., 1992). Separation and divorce, bereavement, psychiatric disorder, employment difficulty, residential and financial stress, disappointment about lifestyle choice and unresolved conflict could hamper progress in improving family functioning (Bloch et al., 1994). Recognition and acknowledgment of transgenerational patterns can empower adoption of new choices for relating together. Care providers need patience and wisdom in setting goals, sometimes limiting these to modest and realizable realities (Zabora and Smith, 1991).

The Grief of Bereavement

Eventually death ensues, bringing that period of intense grief to the family. As the pain of separation grows, the time of maximal risk for more vulnerable members arrives (Raphael, 1984; Parkes, 1998). Loneliness is especially prominent in more dysfunctional families. Where the therapist has established a strong alliance with the family, he/she will be well placed to sustain support during this difficult phase. Through creating a forum in which members come together and review their progress, the capacity of the family to comfort and care for its members in distress is nurtured (Kissane et al., 1998). By modeling the sharing of emotions in a family meeting, we can guide the family to enhanced communication, which fosters understanding and greater cohesion to the benefit of all involved.

Australian families currently live in an era in which religion and ritual are perceived to be less relevant, yet our Melbourne grief study showed that funeral and anniversary memorials were widely practiced. A religious funeral rite was used by 77% of families, while 88% commemorated the anniversary, with spouses supported by family or friends in 86% of these cases. Overall family coping was found in regression analyses to be the most significant correlate of bereavement outcome in terms of psychological morbidity and social adjustment of individual family members (Kissane et al., 1997). Attention to the family is imperative in any setting of death or dying.

CONSOLIDATION AND TERMINATION OF FFGT

With engagement of the family occurring during palliative care, therapy is continued across the early months of bereavement, sustaining support over this stressful time (Coyle, 1989). As progress is achieved with adaptive grief and enhanced family functioning, the interval between sessions is increased in recognition of the gains. Usually by approximately 6 months post-death, the therapist and family reach a point where consideration can be given to ending therapy. Before doing so, members are invited to consider any residual concerns.

The theme of loss is rekindled by discussion about ending therapy, the therapist becoming a metaphor for the deceased family member. Disclosure of feelings about termination will model an adaptive approach to mourning. The family is invited to consider its future needs, reviewing priorities for its members. Alongside celebration of the gains made by the family in its functioning, they are reminded that old issues are likely to recur, thus needing continued attention in the months ahead. However, a message of confidence in the family's ability to maintain the changes that it has introduced is emphasized (Walsh, 1996), reinforcing their likelihood to take responsibility for this in an ongoing manner.

CHALLENGES IN THE DELIVERY OF FFGT

We have encountered a range of issues that present difficulties for therapists engaged in FFGT. These include the engagement of more reluctant family members, setting realistic limits to therapeutic goals, delivering therapy in the family home, sustaining the focus of the endeavor, and living with the uncertainty of prognosis.

PROBLEMS WITH ENGAGEMENT

When a family's difficulties have been long-standing and entrenched, well exemplified by our Hostile class of families, they can be very difficult to engage in therapy. Indeed, Hostile families are the most challenging as, by their very nature, they reject services. Nonetheless, news of terminal illness serves as powerful motivation for a family to come together. Thus, the phase of palliative care provides the best chance of gathering the family together. If a therapist is able to engage the family during this time, he/she can usually extend his/her work into bereavement. But if this opportunity is missed, resistance to attend family sessions can be prominent post-death.

Given that our model is preventive and by invitation, before definite clinical problems have necessarily emerged, we respect the wishes of those who do not want to participate. Care needs to be taken that we do not label these families, or predict difficulties for them, but rather allow the experience to unfold naturally over time.

LIMITS TO POSSIBLE THERAPEUTIC GOALS

Given that our model is time-limited, we endeavor to sustain the focus on family functioning and grief. From time to time, individual members are encouraged to seek personal assessment and care, when their needs exceed the focus of our objective. Long-standing differences between specific family members may be acknowledged to lie beyond the scope of this therapy, thus generating pragmatic limits to what we strive to achieve. The homeostatic pull towards the status quo is strong (Selvini Palazzoli, 1983); at times resistance to change may warrant acceptance.

THERAPY IN THE FAMILY HOME

Use of a neutral setting, exemplified by the therapist's office, places family members on equal terms, and is generally encouraged. Fractured families with a prominent history of conflict gain particular advantage from a neutral location. Sometimes, however, disability in the patient, such as cancer-induced paraplegia, prominent frailty or closeness to death will necessitate therapy being located in the patient's home. Families are generally appreciative of the therapist's willingness to come to them, such home visitation being commonly mirrored by domiciliary nurses and the family's general practitioner. Importantly, this approach permits therapy to continue during a critical time of illness.

Prior to commencing therapy in the home, the therapist needs to negotiate rules to both protect and empower the subsequent course of therapy. These include agreed times to commence and finish each session, selection of room, attention to seating arrangements, avoidance of interruptions by blocking telephone calls and rescheduling visitors, and deferment of refreshments. Therapists need to be assertive in ensuring that seating arrangements are advantageous rather than passively accepting unsuitable furniture placement. Failure to routinely and actively enunciate these guidelines prior to each session will lead to unnecessary interruptions, distraction, and resistance or avoidance during therapy.

The clinical state of the dying person poses particular difficulties, since features such as frailness, cognitive disturbance or other dimensions of illness may interfere with concentration and possible involvement for the whole session. The family group may move between the patient's bedroom and lounge, ensuring sufficient time is shared with the patient before continuing the session in a more suitable location. Fortunately, many of these hurdles evident in the home are surmountable, leaving the family grateful that therapists are willing to travel to them.

SUSTAINING FOCUS DURING THE THERAPY

Issues identified to be of concern to the family need to be made explicit and resummarized by the therapist at each session, so that the focus on family functioning is maintained. Over several months, it is striking how much happens that commands attention in families. Pregnancies, relationship breakdown, alcohol abuse, employment problems, infidelity, secrets, and accidents all occur. Families may want to talk about these events. The therapist's skill is required to monitor family functioning as stories unfold, always endeavoring to focus on its strength or vagary. Otherwise a crisis for any one individual in the family could distract from issues of importance to the family as a whole.

LIVING WITH THE UNCERTAINTY OF PROGNOSIS

Family therapists do not always have precise clinical knowledge about each cancer. They are thus in a similar position to the family in living with uncertainty as to when death might actually occur. Sometimes therapists are surprised by the variable course of illnesses encountered. Discussion with the treatment team is actively encouraged to clarify expectations regarding prognosis.

In our randomized, controlled trial, one entry criterion has been a prognosis of less than 6 months, a requirement often mirrored by domiciliary palliative care services in Australia. Time and again, the prognosis has proved to be an underestimate, tempting some of our therapists to conjecture that their therapy is life-sustaining. Indeed, work done with the family prior to death strengthens coping and adaptation during bereavement. A reflective reader might ask, why not engage families when they first present to a cancer service? Sometimes this is wise, but as a generalization, treatment for early stage cancer tends to be more individually focused, the family being more readily drawn into care once progression of disease and sense of potential loss come to the fore (Bluglass, 1991; Lederberg, 1998).

SPECIFIC THERAPIST INTERVENTIONS

Our model does not involve complex therapeutic interventions, such as paradoxical or split messages delivered by family therapy teams working with a one-way mirror (Campbell et al., 1991). What then are the significant therapeutic steps that we consider important within this model? First, the building of a good therapeutic alliance is vital, as this models the nature of relationships encouraged within the family. Second, in acknowledging family strengths, the therapist utilizes praise and affirmation. Third, by reaching agreement over identified problems, named in sessions as 'issues' or 'concerns', a form of 'contract' is negotiated in which the family decide to work in partnership with the therapist on these identified issues. Thereafter, problem solving becomes the mainstay of treatment, providing the means of the family taking responsibility for their own solutions.

Fortunately, the bringing of the family together invites openness of communication, which, as members self-disclose, trust, and support each other, naturally serves to enhance cohesion. Techniques that also help in brief or focal therapy include the ability to summarize and prioritize, use of circular and reflexive questioning (Tomm, 1988), and appropriate encouragement of expression of feelings, as in guided grief therapies (Paul and Grosser, 1965). Flexibility in therapists is important to ensure they are responsive to families' needs. Sometimes the choice between promoting expression of grief or respecting denial is challenging. Fortunately, over time, important issues recur, inevitably providing further opportunity to intervene differently if needed.

The write-up of a formulation of the family and its functioning following the assessment sessions ensures reflection, with appropriate hypothesis generation about family dynamics. Our therapists bring these formulations to peer group supervision, thus supporting each other as they grapple to understand their families more fully. Transgenerational patterns of relationship emerge repeatedly during our discussion of a family's genogram, empowering developmental understanding of significant individuals. Formulation is critical to identification of the focus of therapy. A further, helpful feature of supervision has been reflection on the therapist's personal reaction to each family. Identification of both positive and negative countertransference has assisted maintenance of neutrality and clarified occasional sources of therapist confusion.

ILLUSTRATIVE FAMILIES THAT OUR TEAM HAS TREATED

THE FAMILY WITH ADOPTED CHILDREN

A focus on openness of communication assisted this family (Figure 11.1) to tolerate ambivalence and pull more closely together. Both daughters had been adopted. The elder had been a rebellious child, was rejected on reunion with her biological mother, and entered a lesbian relationship in adult life. The younger had a more turbulent adolescence, including deliberate self-harm episodes, but found her biological mother accepting and went on to marry and reproduce.

Their adoptive father was dying from advanced prostate cancer, irritable in his grief and burdensome through demands on his wife. He tended to be critical and controlling, much like his wife's mother. His wife suffered from low self-esteem and a tendency to depression. She had found acceptance of her daughter's homosexuality difficult. However, she now felt better supported by her girls as she strove to care for her husband. Their joint efforts as parents in trying to create a happy home for their daughters had taught them to tolerate their ambivalence towards each other. Affirmation of their efforts at closeness, while acknowledging that they carried mixed feelings, helped this family to build greater tolerance and begin to successfully grieve a sad loss.

THE FAMILY WITH AN ALCOHOLIC FATHER

The parents of this family (Figure 11.2) provided mutual comfort for each other, despite childhood deprivation in their past, which restricted their range of coping

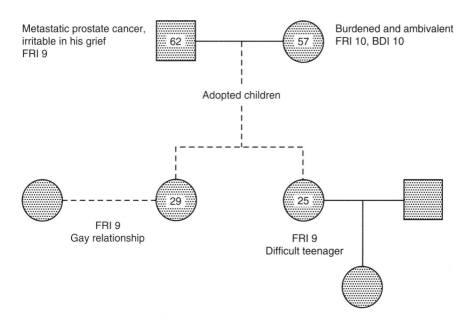

Figure 11.1   Intermediate family with reduced expressiveness. FRI=Family Relationships Index; BDI=Beck Depression Inventory (short form, where BDI > 5 suggests caseness for depression); squares=males; circles=females; number within symbols=age at assessment

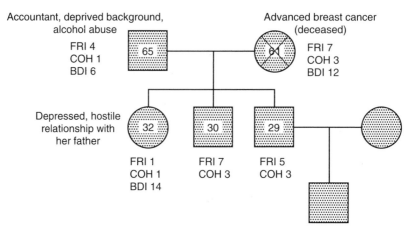

Accountant, deprived background, alcohol abuse
FRI 4
COH 1
BDI 6
65

Advanced breast cancer (deceased)
FRI 7
COH 3
BDI 12

Depressed, hostile relationship with her father
32
FRI 1
COH 1
BDI 14

30
FRI 7
COH 3

29
FRI 5
COH 3

Figure 11.2 Sullen family with high expressed emotion. FRI=Family Relationships Index; COH=Cohesiveness; BDI=Beck Depression Inventory (short form, where BDI>5 suggests caseness for depression); symbols as in Figure 11.1

responses. The father was an intelligent and religious man, but 10 years in an orphanage had left him with a limited capacity to respond to the needs of others. He drank heavily and was critical of his children. His wife had developed more gentleness of manner through her grandmother, although her own mother was blunt and emotionally unavailable. Her family of origin had lived amid much poverty, but her strength of character nurtured her own family until her unwelcome death from cancer.

This family's grief was intense and devastating. The therapist sustained a 'holding' function across 18 months post-death, linking a family cast centrifugally onto lonely paths. The widower walked long distances and drank away the pain of his terrible loss. 'It feels like a flood and I have to swim through it, and I cry and feel ashamed of this.' Again, he despaired, 'My uselessness. A timeless life. I am withered up. I have nothing. I think of suicide.' He eventually turned to travel and study to rebuild his world.

His three children maintained contact with him, but more constructively with each other. His daughter tried to be encouraging and arranged family gatherings, but she was often too critical of his drinking for compatible harmony. His elder son provided more steadfast support and gradually took up the mother's role. He guided his sibs and coaxed his sister through her crises. This family's tendency to criticize its members caused pain, yet sustained drive and determination. Their mourning was complicated by depression, yet they declined referrals for individual assistance, sustaining their alliance with our therapist. Gradually the pain of grief eased as they struggled forward in search of better lives.

Our therapist carried considerable anxiety for this family as she encountered their conflict, rage, anguish and despair. Her role as container of emotionality was prominent, and, in turn, she debriefed through peer supervision. In the end, she helped hold this wounded family together, sustaining some cohesion, limiting conflict and empowering members to remain productive in their workplace and relationships with others. Two of the three children improved their relationships with partners; holidays became enjoyable; their mother's love and determination survived in them.

Simple, outcome measures monitoring mood and social functioning seem inadequate in evaluating the complexity of a family like this. Their stage seemed set for considerable morbidity. Clearly, ill-health and maladaptive grief ensued, but a conviction remained with us that this therapy was effective in preventing greater calamity and distress. A needy family such as this (Sullen type) clearly profits beneficially from FFGT.

THE FAMILY BURDENED BY DOUBLE CANCER

Intense grief was found in a family in which both mother and one daughter suffered from cancer (Figure 11.3). These provided both opportunity and burden. The parents came from quite opposite backgrounds—the mother's family was very close, while the father migrated and lost all contact with his. Curiously, when their two daughters grew up, the elder moved interstate for several years. She was perceived as the 'black sheep of the family,' while her sister achieved academically and bonded closely to her mother.

The younger daughter developed breast cancer, then her mother became ill with lung cancer. The threat of these illnesses drew the family closer. In therapy, a greater sense of reconciliation was developed with the elder daughter. The therapist invited the sons-in-law to join the circle of support created by family meetings. Further time was taken exploring ways of creating memories for the grandchildren. Eventually, a creative outcome became evident despite the challenge of illness.

THE FAMILY WITH A DEPRESSED ADOLESCENT

The youngest son in this family, (Figure 11.4) whose mother had leukemia, told our research staff he planned to suicide. He was his mother's confidant, but struggled

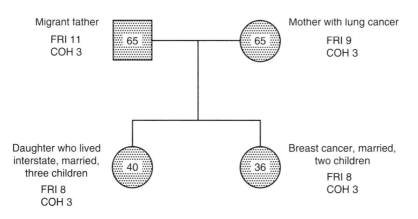

Figure 11.3   Intermediate family burdened with two cancers. FRI=Family Relationships Index; COH=Cohesiveness; Symbols as in Figure 11.1

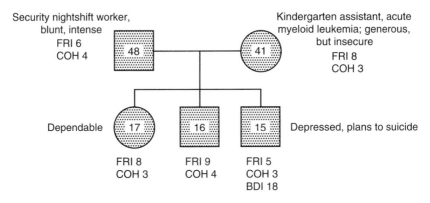

Figure 11.4   Sullen family with a depressed adolescent.
FRI=Family Relationships Index; COH = Cohesiveness; BDI = Beck Depression Inventory (short form, where BDI > 5 suggests caseness for depression)

with low self-esteem. The parents' marriage had always been conflictual, but this was partly avoided by the father working nights. He came from a violent family affected by wartime experiences, while her family of origin provided the 'idealized' model. When the father became angry, his wife became depressed.

The therapist asked the youngest child's permission to talk about his responses to the questionnaires. His parents had been unaware of his suicidality. As a symptom bearer, he drew his family together with concern. He kept a diary that, thereafter, he discussed weekly with his father.

The mother died from complications of bone marrow transplantation. The father appeared absent through working nightshifts; the family, sad and angry. The sessions brought the family together to share their grief, the father receiving support and help to focus his energies again in the direction of his children. The early bereavement period remained traumatic, with the youngest son still the symptom bearer. However, as the painful year unfolded, a gradual sense of resolution developed.

DISCUSSION

Families come from a wide range of cultural and social backgrounds. Despite this diversity, recurring patterns of behavior occur that have permitted development of a practical classification of families, providing a conceptual means to proceed with a systematic model of family-centered care. Such a clinical approach, as outlined in this chapter, enables families at increased risk of morbid outcome to be targeted and preventively assisted with FFGT.

There are a number of predictable issues or concerns that families grapple with during palliative care, death and bereavement. If we can respond to these through family-centered care, we can reduce substantial psychosocial morbidity, to the greater benefit of family members and our broader community.

Previous studies of family interventions with grieving families (Lieberman, 1978; Williams and Polak, 1979; Rosenthal, 1980; Black and Urbanowicz, 1985, 1987) have offered hope but yielded inconsistent outcomes. Importantly, they did not target families at risk. Our model addresses this and provides a means of directing limited resources to the more vulnerable. It recognizes the family group as the most available and natural source of social support, and strives to maximize its functioning to enhance the effectiveness of this support. By increasing cohesiveness, opening communication channels and enhancing problem solving to reduce conflict, we can facilitate a supportive environment that fosters evolution of stronger bonds between family members. This approach echoes that intuitively followed by traditional, extended families in former years. As we extend our work through a controlled trial to determine more exactly its efficacy, we are excited by its prospect as a definitive model of family-centered care during terminal illness and bereavement.

ACKNOWLEDGMENTS

The author gratefully acknowledges the work of research assistants, Maria McKenzie and Imogen O'Neill, family therapists, Kate Cogan, Barbara Donnelly, Ester Elbaz, Rose Heard, Marilyn Kenny, Rochelle Nitzan, Anna McDowall, Penny Sanderson, Carmel Spottiswood, Anne Strong and Judith Zuliani, and senior collaborators, Sidney Bloch and Dean McKenzie. This research has been funded by The Bethlehem Griffiths Research Foundation, The Australian Rotary Health Research Fund and the National Health and Medical Research Council of Australia.

REFERENCES

Acworth, A. and Bruggen, P. (1985).   Family therapy when one member is on the death bed. *Journal of Family Therapy* **7**: 379–385.
Adams-Greenly, M. and Moynihans, R. T. (1983).   Helping the children of fatally ill parents. *American Journal of Orthopsychiatry* **53**: 219–229.
Allman, P., Bloch, S. and Sharpe, M. (1992).   The end-of-session message in systemic family therapy: a descriptive study. *Journal of Family Therapy* **14**: 69–85.
Baider, L., Cooper, C.L. and De-Nour, A.K. (Eds)(1996).   *Cancer and the Family*. Chichester: Wiley.
Bass, D.M. and Bowman, K. (1990).   The transition from caregiving to bereavement: the relationship to care-related strain and adjustment to death. *Gerontologist* **30**: 35–42.
Black, D. and Urbanowicz, M.A. (1985).   Bereaved children—family intervention. In J. Stevenson (Ed.), *Recent Research in Developmental Psychopathology*. Oxford: Pergamon.
Black, D. and Urbanowicz, M.A. (1987).   Family intervention with bereaved children. *Journal of Child Psychology and Psychiatry* **28**: 467–476.
Bloch, S., Hafner, J., Harari, E. and Szmukler, G.I. (Eds)(1994).   *The Family in Clinical Psychiatry*. Oxford: Oxford University Press.
Bloom, J. R. (1982).   Social support, accommodation to stress and adjustment to breast cancer. *Social Science and Medicine* **16**: 385–392.
Bluglass, K. (1991).   Care of the cancer patient's family. In M. Watson (Ed.), *Cancer Patient Care, Psychological Treatment Methods*. Cambridge: British Psychological Society and Cambridge University Press.
Buckley, I.E. (1977).   *Listen to the Children: Impact on the Mental Health of Children of a Parent's Catastrophic Illness*. New York: Cancer Care Inc. and National Cancer Foundation.
Buckman, R. (1993).   Communication in palliative care: a practical guide. In D. Doyle, G. W. C. Hanks and N. McDonald (Eds), *Oxford Textbook of Palliative Medicine*. Oxford: Oxford University Press.

Byng-Hall, J. (1988). Scripts and legends in families and family therapy. *Family Process* **27**, 167–180.

Byng-Hall, J. (1991). Family scripts and loss. In F. Walsh and M. McGoldrick (Eds), *Living Beyond Loss: Death in the Family*. New York: Norton.

Callahan, D. (1995). Frustrated mastery: the cultural context of death in America. *Western Journal of Medicine* **163**: 226–230.

Campbell, D., Drayzer, R. and Crutchley, E. (1991). The Milan System approach to family therapy. In A.S. Gurman and D. Kniskern (Eds.), *Handbook of Family Therapy Vol. II*. New York: Brunner/Mazel.

Carter, E.A. and McGoldrick, M. (1980). *The Family Life Cycle: A Framework for Family Therapy*. New York: Gardner Press.

Cassileth, B.R. and Hamilton, J. N. (1979). The family with cancer. In B.R. Cassileth (Ed.), *The Cancer Patient: Social and Medical Aspects of Care*. Philadelphia: Lea and Febiger.

Cassileth, B.R., Lusk, E. J., Strouse, T.B., Miller, D.S., Brown, L.L. and Cross, P.A. (1985). A psychological analysis of cancer patients and their next-of-kin. *Cancer* **55**: 72–76.

Cherny, N.I., Coyle, N. and Foley, K.M. (1994). Suffering in the advanced cancer patient: a definition and taxonomy. *Journal of Palliative Care* **10**: 57–70.

Chochinov, H.M., Wilson, K.G., Enns, M., Mowchun, N., Lander, S., Levitt, M. and Clinch, J.J. (1995). Desire for death in the terminally ill. *American Journal of Psychiatry* **152**: 1185–1191.

Compas, B.E., Worsham, N.L., Ey, S. and Howell, D.C. (1996). When Mom or Dad has cancer: II. Coping, cognitive appraisals, and psychological distress in children of cancer patients. *Health Psychology* **15**: 167–175.

Coyle, N. (1989). Continuity of care for the cancer patient with chronic pain. *Cancer* **63**: 2289–2293.

Davies, B., Spinetta, J., Martinson, I., McClowry, S. and Kulenkamp, E. (1986). Manifestations of levels of functioning in grieving families. *Journal of Family Issues* **7**: 297–313.

Derogatis, L.R. and Spencer, P. M. (1982). *Administration and Procedures. BSI Manual-I*. Baltimore, MD: Clinical Psychometric Research.

Derogatis, L.R., Morrow, G.R., Fetting, J., Penman, D., Piasetsky, S., Schmale, A.M., Henrichs, M. and Carnicke, C.L.M. (1983). The prevalence of psychiatric disorders among cancer patients. *Journal of the American Medical Association* **249**: 751–757.

Eisenberg, M.G., Sutkin, L.C. and Jansen, M.A. (Eds.) (1984). *Chronic Illness and Disability through the Life Span: Effects on Self and Family* New York: Springer.

Eisenbruch, M. (1984a). Cross-cultural aspects of bereavement I: a conceptual framework for comparative analysis. *Culture, Medicine and Psychiatry* **8**: 283–309.

Eisenbruch, M. (1984b). Cross-cultural aspects of bereavement II: ethnic and cultural variations in the development of bereavement practices. *Culture, Medicine and Psychiatry* **8**: 315–347.

Ell, K., Nishimoto, R., Mantell, J. and Hamovitch, M. (1988). Longitudinal analysis of psychological adaptation among family members of patients with cancer. *Journal of Psychosomatic Research* **32**: 429–438.

Ferrell, B.R., Ferrell, B.A. and Rhiner M. (1991a). Family factors influencing cancer pain management. *Journal of Postgraduate Medicine* **67**: 9.

Ferrell, B.R., Rhiner, M. and Cohen, M.Z. (1991b). Pain as a metaphor for illness. Part 1: Impact of pain on family caregivers. *Oncology Nursing Forum* **18**: 1303–1309.

Ferrell, B.R., Cohen, M.Z. and Rhiner, M. (1991c). Pain as a metaphor for illness. Part II: Family caregivers management of pain. *Oncology Nursing Forum* **18**, 1315–1321.

Freud, S. (1917). Mourning and melancholia. In J. Strachey (Ed. and Trans.), *The Complete Psychological Works*, Standard Edition Vol. 14: 243–258. New York: Norton, 1976 (original work published 1923).

Giacquinta, B. (1977). Helping families face the crisis of cancer. *American Journal of Nursing* **77**: 1585–1588.

Given, C.W., Stommel, M., Given, B.A. et al. (1993). The influence of cancer patients, symptoms and functional state on patient's depression and family caregivers' reaction and depression. *Health Psychology* **12**: 277–285.

Given, B.A. and Given, C.W. (1994). Family home care for individuals with cancer. *Oncology* **8**: 77–88.

Given, B.A. and Given, C.W. (1996). Family caregivers' burden from cancer care. In R. McCorkle, M. Grant, M. Frank-Stromberg and S.B. Baird (Eds), *Cancer Nursing—A Comprehensive Textbook*. Philadelphia: Saunders.

Goldberg, R.J., Wool, M.S., Glicksman, A. and Tull, R. (1984). Relationship of the social environment and patients' physical status to depression in lung cancer patients and their spouses. *Journal of Psychosocial Oncology* **2**: 73–80.

Gotay, C.C. (1984). The experience of cancer during early and advanced stages: the views of patients and their mates. *Social Science and Medicine* **18**: 605–613.

Gotay, C.C. (1996). Cultural variation in family adjustment to cancer. In L. Baider, C.L. Cooper and A. Kaplan De-Nour (Eds), *Cancer and the Family*. Chichester: Wiley.

Grobe, M.E., Iistrup, D.M. and Ahmann, D.L. (1996). Skills needed by family members to maintain the care of an advanced cancer patient. *Cancer Nursing* **19**: 371–375.

Hileman, J.W. and Lackey, N.R. (1990). Self-identified needs of patients with cancer at home and their caregivers: a descriptive study. *Oncology Nursing Forum* **17**: 907-9-13.

Griffith, J.L. and Griffith, M.E. (1994). *The Body Speaks: Therapeutic Dialogues for Mind–Body Problems*. New York: Basic Books.

Hinton, J. (1981). Sharing or withholding awareness of dying between husband and wife. *Journal of Psychosomatic Medicine* **25**: 337–343.

Hinton, J. (1994). Can home care maintain an acceptable quality of life for patients with terminal cancer and their relatives? *Palliative Medicine* **8**: 183–186.

Hoffman, L. (1981). *Foundations of Family Therapy*. New York: Basic Books.

Imber-Black, E. (1991). Rituals and the healing process. In F. Walsh and M. McGoldrick (Eds), *Living Beyond Loss: Death in the Family*. Boston: Allyn and Bacon.

Jensen, S. and Given, B. (1991). Fatigue affecting family caregivers of cancer patients. *Cancer Nursing* **14**: 181–187.

Kaasa, S., Malt, U., Hagen, S., Wist, E., Moum, T. and Kvikstad, A. (1993). Psychological distress in cancer patients with advanced disease. *Radiotherapy and Oncology* **27**: 193–197.

Kissane, D.W. (1994a). Grief and the family. In S. Bloch, J. Hafner, E. Harari and G.I. Szmukler (Eds), *The Family in Clinical Psychiatry*. Oxford: Oxford University Press.

Kissane, D.W. (1994b). Managing anger in palliative care. *Australian Family Physician* **23**: 1257–1259.

Kissane, D.W. and Bloch, S. (1994). Family grief. *British Journal of Psychiatry* **164**: 728–740.

Kissane, D.W., Bloch, S., Burns, W.I., McKenzie, D.P. and Posterino, M. (1994a). Psychological morbidity in the families of patients with cancer. *Psycho-Oncology* **3**: 47–56.

Kissane, D.W., Bloch, S., Burns, W.I., Patrick, J.D., Wallace, C.S. and McKenzie, D.P. (1994b). Perceptions of family functioning and cancer. *Psycho-Oncology* **3**: 259–269.

Kissane, D.W., Bloch, S., Dowe, D.L., Snyder, R.D., Onghena, P., McKenzie, D.P., and Wallace, C.S. (1996a). The Melbourne family grief study, I: perceptions of family functioning in bereavement. *American Journal of Psychiatry* **153**: 650–658.

Kissane, D.W., Bloch, S., Onghena, P., McKenzie, D.P., Snyder, R.D. and Dowe, D.L. (1996b). The Melbourne family grief study, II: psychosocial morbidity and grief in bereaved families, *American Journal of Psychiatry* **153**: 659–666.

Kissane, D.W., Bloch, S. and McKenzie, D.P. (1997). Family coping and bereavement outcome. *Palliative Medicine* **11**: 191–201.

Kissane, D.W., Bloch, S., McKenzie, M., McDowall, A.C. and Nitzan, R. (1998). Family grief therapy: a preliminary account of a new model to promote healthy family functioning during palliative care and bereavement. *Psycho-Oncology* **7**: 14–25.

Kissane, D.W. (1998). Models of psychological response to suffering. *Progress in Palliative Care* **6**: 197–204.

Klagsburn, S. C. (1994). Patient, family and staff suffering. *Journal of Palliative Care* **10**: 14–27.

Klein, M. (1940). Mourning and its relationship to manic-depressive states. *International Journal of Psycho-analysis* **21**: 125–153.

Kristjanson, L.J. and Ashcroft, T. (1994). The family's cancer journey: a literature review. *Cancer Nursing* **17**: 1–17.

Lederberg, M.S. (1998). The family of the cancer patient. In J. Holland (Ed.), *Psychooncology*. New York: Oxford University Press.

Leiberman, S. (1978). Nineteen cases of morbid grief. *British Journal of Psychiatry* **132**: 159–163.

Maguire, P. (1981). The repercussions of mastectomy on the family. *International Journal of Family Psychiatry* **6**: 485–503.

McCubbin, H., Larsen, A. and Olson, D. (1985). Family crisis oriented personal evaluation scales. In D. Olson and H. McCubbin (Eds), *Family Inventories,* Revised Edn. St. Paul, Minneapolis, MN: Family Social Science.

McGoldrick, M. and Gerson, R. (1985). *Genograms in Family Assessment*. New York: Norton.

Meares, R. (1981). On saying goodbye before death. *Journal of the American Medical Association* **246**: 1227–1229.

Moos, R.H. and Moos, B.S. (1981). *Family Environment Scale Manual*. Palo Alto, California: Consulting Psychologists Press.

Moos, R.H. (1990). Conceptual and empirical approaches to developing family-based assessment procedures: resolving the case for the Family Environment Scale. *Family Process* **29**: 199–208.

Munson, S.W. (1978). Family structure and the family's general adaptation to loss. In D.J.Z. Sahler (Ed.), *The Child and Death*. St. Louis, MO: C.V. Mosby.

Nelson, E., Sloper, P., Charlton, A., et al. (1994). Children who have a parent with cancer. *Journal of Cancer Education* **9**: 30–36.

Neuling, S.J. and Winefield, H.R. (1988). Social support and recovery after surgery for breast cancer. Frequency and correlates of supportive behaviors by family, friends and surgeon. *Social Science Medicine* **22**: 385–392.

Northouse, L. (1984). The impact of cancer on the family. *International Journal of Psychiatry in Medicine* **14**: 215–242.

Northouse, L. (1989). A longitudinal study of the adjustment of patients and husbands to breast cancer. *Oncology Nursing Forum* **16**: 511–516.

Parkes, C.M. (1998). *Bereavement. Studies of Grief in Adult Life,* 3rd Edn. Madison, CT: International Universities Press.

Paul, N.L. and Grosser, G.H. (1965). Operational mourning and its role in conjoint family therapy. *Community Mental Health Journal* **1**: 339–345.

Pinder, K.L., Ramirez, A.J., Black, M.E., Richards, M.A., Gregory, W.M. and Rubens, R.D. Psychiatric disorders in patients with advanced breast cancer: prevalence and associated factors. *European Journal of Oncology* **29**A: 524–527.

Plumb, M.M. and Holland, J. (1977). Comparative studies of psychological function in patients with advanced cancer 1. Self-reported depressive symptoms. *Psychosomatic Medicine* **39**: 264–276.

Portenoy, R. K., Thaler, H. T., Kornblith, A.B. et al. (1994). Symptom prevalence, characteristics and distress in cancer population. *Quality of Life Research* **3**: 183–189.

Rait, D. and Lederberg, M.S. (1989). The family of the cancer patient. In J.C. Holland and J.H. Rowland (Eds), *Handbook of Psychooncology*. New York: Oxford University Press.

Raphael, B. (1984) *The Anatomy of Bereavement: A Handbook for the Caring Professions*. London: Hutchinson.

Reiss, D., Steinglass, P. and Howe, G. (1993). The family's organization around the illness. In R.E. Cole and D. Reiss (Eds), *How Do Families Cope with Chronic Illness?* Hillsdale, NJ: Erlbaum.

Ringler, K.E., Whitman, H. H. and Gustafson, J.P. (1981). Technical advances in leading a cancer patient group. *International Journal of Group Psychotherapy* **31**: 329–344.

Rolland, J.S. (1984). Toward a psychosocial typology of a chronic and life-threatening illness. *Family Systems Medicine* **2**: 245–263.

Rolland, J.S. (1987). Chronic illness and the life-cycle: a conceptual framework. *Family Process* **26**: 203–221.

Rosenblatt, P.C. (1993). Cross-cultural variation in the experience, expression, and understanding of grief. In D.P. Irish, K.F. Lundquist and V.J. Nelson (Eds), *Ethnic Variations in Dying, Death and Grief: Diversity in Universality*. Washington: Taylor and Francis.

Rosenthal, P.A. (1980). Short-term family therapy and pathological grief resolution with children and adolescents. *Family Process* **19**: 151–159.

Rubens, R.D. (1993). Psychiatric disorders in patients with advanced breast cancer: prevalence and associated factors. *European Journal of Oncology* **29**: 524–527.

Sales, E., Schulz, R. and Biegel, D. (1992). Predictors of strain in families of cancer patients: a review of the literature. *Journal of Psychosocial Oncology* **10**: 1–26.

Sawyer, M.G., Antoniou, G., Toogood, I., Rice, M. and Baghurst, P.A. (1993). A prospective study of the psychological adjustment of parents and families of children with cancer. *Paediatric Child Health Watch* **29**: 352–356.

Schofield, H., Bloch, S., Herrman, H., Murphy, B., Nankervis, J. and Singh, B. (1998). *Family Caregivers. Disability, Illness and Ageing*. St. Leonards: Allen and Unwin.

Selvini Palazzoli, M. (1983). The emergence of a comprehensive systems approach. *Journal of Family Therapy* **5**: 165–177.

Stetz, K.M. (1987) Caregiving demands during advanced cancer. The spouse's needs. *Cancer Nursing* **10**: 260–268.

Tomm, K. (1988). Interventive interviewing: part III. Intending to ask lineal, circular, strategic or reflexive questions? *Family Process* **27**: 1–15.

Tringali, C.A. (1986). The needs of family members of cancer patients. *Oncology Nursing Forum* **13**: 65–70.

Vachon, M.L. (1995). Staff stress in hospice/palliative care: a review. *Palliative Medicine* **9**, 91–122.

Vess, J.D., Moreland, J.R. and Schwebel, A.I. (1985). An empirical assessment of the effects of cancer on family role functioning. *Journal of Psychosocial Oncology* **3**: 1–16.

Vess, J.D., Moreland, J.R., Schwebel, A.I. and Kraut, E. (1988). Psychosocial needs of cancer patients: learning from patients and their spouses. *Journal of Psychosocial Oncology* **6**, 31–51.

Vollman, R.R., Ganzert, A., Picher, L. and William, W.V. (1971). The reactions of family systems to sudden and unexpected death. *Omega* **2**: 101–6.

Walsh, F. (1996). The concept of family resilience: crisis and challenge. *Family Process* **35**: 261–82.

Watson, M. (1994). Psychological care for cancer patients and their families. *Journal of Mental Health* **3**: 453–461.

Wellisch, D.K., Mosher, M.B. and Van Scoy, C. (1978). Management of family emotion stress: family group therapy in private oncology practice. *International Journal of Group Psychotherapy* **28**: 225–231.

Williams W.V. and Polak, P.R. (1979). Follow up research in primary prevention: a model of adjustment in acute grief. *Journal of Clinical Psychology* **35**: 35–45.

Wingate, A.L. and Lackey, N.R. (1989). A description of the needs of non-institutionalized cancer patients and their primary care givers. *Cancer Nursing* **12**: 28–33.

Woods, N.F., Lewis, F.M. and Ellison, E.S. (1989). Living with cancer. Family experiences. *Cancer Nursing* **12**: 28–33.

Wright, K. and Dyck, S. (1984). Expressed concerns of adult cancer patient's family members. *Cancer Nursing* **7**: 371–374.

Yalom, I.D. (1980). Death and psychotherapy. In I.D. Yalom (Ed.), *Existential Psychotherapy*. New York: Basic Books.

Zabora, J.R. and Smith, E. D. (1991). Family dysfunction and the cancer patient: early recognition and intervention. *Oncology* **5**: 31–38.

Section IV
THE CHILD'S PERCEPTION
OF A PARENT'S ILLNESS

12

Blowing Away the Myths about the Child's Experience with the Mother's Breast Cancer

FRANCES MARCUS LEWIS, LYNN C. BEHAR,
KATHRYN HOEHN ANDERSON, MARY ELLEN SHANDS,
ELLEN H. ZAHLIS, EMILY DARBY, and JANET A. SINSHEIMER
Department of Family and Child Nursing, University of Washington School of Nursing,
Seattle, WA, USA

In 1999, an estimated 175 000 women in the USA will be diagnosed with breast cancer (American Cancer Society, 1999). Although the parity status of these women is unknown, an estimated 25% of them will be in their child-rearing years. Assuming one to two children per household, this means that between 43 000–86 000 children will have a mother newly diagnosed with breast cancer in the USA. These numbers are substantial underestimates: breast cancer is an international illness, not a disease limited to the USA. When we expand to include children from mothers of other countries, well over 100 000 children will be potentially impacted with the diagnosis of breast cancer in their mother.

To date, children of mothers with breast cancer have been treated with benign neglect (Lewis, 1997). They have been under-represented in the research literature and under-served by health care services. This is true for children of mothers with cancer of any type as well as for children whose mothers have breast cancer. Although children are members of the diagnosed mother's household, the mother's well-being, not the child's, is the priority for the family. This is especially true during the acute phase of diagnosis and treatment.

In the past decade there has been a gradual awareness of cancer as a family experience, as contrasted to it as a solo patient's diagnosis. This perspective was heralded by early theoretical papers by Litman (1974), Litman and Venters (1979) and Parkes (1975b). But only recently has family level research in cancer evolved in the research programs of a small group of scientists (alphabetical): Compas (Compas et al., 1994, Welch et al., 1996); Germino (1984); Given and Given (1992); Gotay (1984); Hilton (1993, 1996; Hilton and Elfert, 1996); Lewis (Armsden and Lewis,

Cancer and the Family, 2nd Edn. Edited by L. Baider, C. L. Cooper and A. Kaplan De-Nour
© 2000 John Wiley & Sons, Ltd

1993, 1994; Issel et al., 1990; Lewis and Hammond, 1996; Lewis et al., 1989, 1993, 1996); Northouse (Northouse, 1992; Northouse and Swain, 1987); and Wellisch et al. (1991, 1992). Within this literature, there are only two published studies of the mothers' report of the children's experience with the mother's cancer exclusive of the current investigative team's work (Hymovich, 1993; Lichtman et al., 1984). Except for Lewis' work, the studies involved mothers with breast cancer of mixed stages (Lichtman et al., 1984) or involved parents with cancer of mixed types (Hymovich, 1993; Compas et al., 1994, 1996). Except for a retrospective interview study (Lichtman et al., 1984) and our work, none of the studies involved interviews with children of mothers with breast cancer.

The absence of information and research data is the breeding ground for myths and misunderstandings. These myths, not facts, have the potential to dominate both the clinician's and the scientist's views of what it is like for children to have a mother with breast cancer. The goal of this chapter is to replace myth with fact. More specifically, the purpose of this chapter is to expose myths that exist about children and their experience with maternal breast cancer. Children include 8–19 year-olds who are living in the home with the diagnosed mother (The data base for younger children is small and yields unreliable results. Although younger children are important, we have insufficient data from which to comment). Data that challenge these myths are provided from research studies that have been completed by the investigative team (Lewis, 1992–1996, 1995–1999, 1995–1997, 1995–1998, 1996–1999; Lewis and Woods, 1986–1990; Lewis et al., 1983–1986).

There are three sections to this chapter. The first section contains a description of the assumptions about families that are held by the investigative team. Second, myths are identified and challenged on the basis of data obtained from our completed research. Third, recommendations are made for needed services and programs for children whose mother is diagnosed with breast cancer. These recommendations derive from research data obtained to date.

FAMILIES AS NURTURANT SYSTEMS OF CARE FOR CHILDREN:
OUR ASSUMPTIONS

The background for understanding the impact of maternal illness on the child and the need to attack prevailing myths is based firmly in the science of family dynamics and the role the family plays in the development and adjustment of children. The family is one of the basic societal structural units (Curran, 1983), the fundamental unit of health care (Anderson and Tomlinson, 1992; Litman, 1974; Litman and Venters, 1979), and the primary unit interacting with the broader social environmental system (Ell and Northen, 1990). For children, the family provides physical and emotional care, and forms the baseline environment for behavior, thoughts, and feelings (Friedman, 1998). The quality of family relationships and interactions directly influence child and family development (Gottman, 1999) and may determine the success or failure of a child's life (Friedman, 1998). Minuchin (1974) summarizes the role of the family as 'the matrix of its members' sense of identity, of belonging and of being different. The family's chief task is to foster its member's psychosocial growth and well-being throughout their life in common.' (Minuchin, 1974, p. 3).

Families are systems that nurture, sustain, and socialize children. As *nurturant*, family members attend to and respond to the children's feelings, concerns, and fears. Attentiveness includes focused time and interactions with the child whose priority is the child and the child's thoughts and feelings. Families act to *sustain* the children by establishing structures that protect them from physical elements, including both emotional and physical danger (weather, noise, deflammatory experiences). They also sustain the children by creating and maintaining routines and predictable environments in which the child is able to developmentally evolve (Armsden and Lewis, 1993). Families *socialize* the children (Berger, 1967; Parsons, 1954). This socialization involves the inculcation of both societal norms and family values. Such socialization reinforces what is valued; it reciprocates the behavior of the child with behavior of other family members (Berger, 1967). Socialization also involves education and mentoring. The family teaches the child about life, about normative and non-normative transitions, and it supports the child through such transitions (Parkes, 1971, 1975a,b; Lewis, 1993). The family also assists the child to gain the skills necessary to function in the world both within and outside the family.

When a mother is diagnosed with a potentially life-threatening illness like breast cancer, research evidence challenges the family's ability to achieve their child-focused goals. Evidence is that these assumptions are not consistently upheld in the everyday behavior of family members. As such, these assumptions become myths. Seven myths are of particular relevance; see Table 12.1.

DATA-BASED CHALLENGES TO THE MYTHS

The investigative team has completed multiple cross-sectional as well as large-scale, longitudinal hypothesis-testing studies with families whose child-rearing mothers were diagnosed with breast cancer (Lewis et al, 1989, 1993; Lewis and Hammond, 1992, 1996; Woods and Lewis, 1995). Two clinical trial intervention studies have also been completed, one involved married and one single mothers with breast cancer (Lewis, 1992–1996, 1995–1999). In addition, multiple case-intensive interview studies have been completed with child-rearing mothers and their children (Behar, 1999; Lewis, 1996–1999; Lewis et al., 1996; Shands et al., 2000; Zahlis, 1999; Zahlis and Lewis, 1998). Finally, multiple secondary analyses have been conducted on the above

Table 12.1   Myths about the child's experience with maternal breast cancer

Myth 1	Families understand the child's experience with the mother's breast cancer
Myth 2	Families are able to assist the child through the mother's breast cancer
Myth 3	Children feel comfortable talking with their parent(s) about the breast cancer
Myth 4	The mother's mood and anxiety are filtered and managed without affecting the child
Myth 5	Children are able to interpret the breast cancer in the least distressful ways on their own
Myth 6	Compromised parenting in one parent can be compensated by the parenting practices of the other parent
Myth 7	Tension in the marriage from the illness is a private matter between the diagnosed mother and her spouse

Table 12.2 Data-based papers on children with mothers with breast cancer completed by the investigative team

Reference	Title	Journal
Armsden and Lewis, 1994	Behavioral adjustment and self-esteem among school-age children of mothers with breast cancer	*Oncology Nursing Forum*
Behar, 1999	Getting through it alone: a descriptive study of the experiences of single mothers with breast cancer and adolescent children	Unpublished doctoral dissertation, University of Washington
Darby and Lewis, 2000	Maternal breast cancer and adolescent adjustment: a test of the 'faucet hypothesis'	Under review
Issel, Ersek, and Lewis, 1990	How children cope with mother's breast cancer	*Oncology Nursing Forum*
Lewis, 1996	The impact of breast cancer on the family: lessons learned from the children and adolescents	In Baider, Cooper and De-Nour (Eds), *Cancer and the Family* 1st Ed
Lewis, 2000	Risk and protective factors of children's functioning with maternal breast cancer: a discriminant analysis	Under review
Lewis and Hammond, 1992	Psychosocial adjustment of the family to breast cancer: a longitudinal analysis	*Journal of the American Medical Women's Association*
Lewis, Hammond and Woods, 1993	The family's functioning with newly diagnosed breast cancer in the mother: the development of an explanatory model	*Journal of Behavioral Medicine*
Lewis and Hammond, 1996	The father's, mother's, and adolescent's functioning with breast cancer	*Family Relations*
Lewis and Hammond, 1999	Breast cancer in a mother: an identification of risk and protective factors for the school age child	Paper presented at the meeting of The Fifth National Conference on Cancer Nursing Research, Newport Beach, CA
Lewis and Zahlis, 2000	The child's attribution model of the mother's breast cancer	Under review
Lewis, Ellison and Woods, 1985	The impact of breast cancer on the family	*Seminars in Oncology Nursing*

(Continued)

Table 12.2 (*Continued*)

Reference	Title	Journal
Lewis, Woods, Hough and Bensley, 1989	The family's functioning with chronic illness in the mother: the spouse's perspective	*Social Science and Medicine*
Lewis, Zahlis, Shands, Sinsheimer and Hammond, 1996	The functioning of single women with breast cancer and their school-aged children	*Cancer Practice*
Shands, Lewis and Zahlis, 2000	The mother's and child's interactions about mother's breast cancer: an interview study	*Oncology Nursing Forum*
Shands, Sinsheimer and Lewis, 2000	Coaching couples experiencing early stage breast cancer: an analysis of their stated concerns	Under review
Woods and Lewis, 1995	Women with chronic illness: their views of their families' adaptation	*Health Care for Women International*
Zahlis and Lewis, 1998	Mothers' stories of the school-age child's experience with the mother's breast cancer	*Journal of Psychosocial Oncology*
Zahlis, 1999	When mom has breast cancer: sources of distress in school age children	Paper presented at the meeting of the Fifth National Conference on Cancer Nursing Research, Newport Beach, CA
Zahlis, 2000	The child's worries about the mom's breast cancer	Under review

data bases in order to test additional hypotheses about the child's functioning with maternal breast cancer (Behar, 1999, Darby and Lewis, 2000; Lewis and Hammond, 1999). Data from these studies will be used to challenge the myths about the child's experience with the mother's breast cancer. See Table 12.2 for a summary of the completed studies involving diagnosed mothers and their children by the research team.

MYTH 1—FAMILIES UNDERSTAND THE CHILD'S EXPERIENCE WITH THE MOTHER'S BREAST CANCER

The child's experience with the mother's breast cancer is essentially uncharted. Not until very recently have scientists attempted to systematically document what families know or understand about the child's experience with the mother's illness. Research evidence is that family members, including mothers, do not always know what the child is going through because of the breast cancer (Zahlis and Lewis, 1998). In a retrospective study of 26 mothers referencing 36 school-age children, the majority of mothers stated that they did not know what their child wondered or worried about during the acute period of diagnosis or treatment (Zahlis and Lewis, 1998). Results from another interview study with mothers revealed that they commonly relied on the child's questions as the stimulus to talk about the cancer (Shands et al., 2000). When the child was silent, withdrawn, or did not ask questions, some mothers did not initiate discussion. This mother's statements are illustrative:

> We haven't really discussed (the breast cancer). We really haven't talked a lot about it. I didn't want to push anything. I didn't want to say anything. I didn't want to scare her, and I kind of thought that maybe when she was ready, she would ask me questions. I don't want to push it on her...I'm not hiding it. If she wants to know, when she asks, then we will discuss it.

Mothers offered many examples of the child's not understanding what was happening or the mother not being able to correctly interpret what was happening to their child (Zahlis and Lewis, 1998). As this mother shared, 'She didn't really ask questions. And I thought that she understood what was going on...but she really didn't...'. Another mother offered:

> We were talking about chemotherapy and the ramifications of cancer. And I remember that he (12 years) just literally exploded and was very upset and tearful...didn't know how to express himself...didn't know how to ask questions. Didn't know what was going to happen. Just didn't understand any of what was going on or why it was happening (Zahlis and Lewis, 1998).

MYTH 2—FAMILIES ARE ABLE TO ASSIST THE CHILD THROUGH THE MOTHER'S BREAST CANCER

Evidence is mixed on the ability of the family to assist the child with the mother's breast cancer. During the acute phase of the breast cancer, mothers are in 'survival mode' (Lewis et al., 1996). They want to help their child but are often too distressed, too symptomatic, or too taxed to be able to parent in the ways they want. Mothers of children have explicitly expressed difficulty in knowing what to say or how to help the child deal with the impact of the cancer (Zahlis and Lewis, 1998). Mothers report that they want to parent the child in helpful ways about the cancer but claim they do not know how to talk to the child about the cancer in ways that avoid further upsetting the child (Zahlis and Lewis, 1998). Evidence is that the mothers are especially concerned about being able to respond to their children's emotional needs, particularly when those needs are in competition with the mother's abilities in the moment (Lewis et al., 1996). As one mother shared, 'I was aware of the fact that the kids' emotional needs had to take second place to mine and that was hard. With the fatigue, I just didn't have enough energy to listen' (Lewis et al., 1996). Mothers reported they did not want to tell the child what the cancer was or wanted the breast cancer to be over and not to dwell on it. Mothers also offered that they did not feel confident that they could allay the child's concerns and some mothers reported they were unable to deal with their child's emotional state (Zahlis and Lewis, 1998).

In an interview study of 81 children, trained nurses conducted confidential interviews in the homes of children whose mother had been diagnosed with breast cancer an average of 2.5 years previously (Issel et al., 1990). Children were asked four questions, including what the family did on a day-to-day basis that made it easier for the child to handle the mother's illness, as well as who helped the children cope with what was happening. One-third of the younger children aged 6–12 and a quarter of the older children aged 13–20 said they *talked with their mother about her illness* (Issel et al., 1990). This meant that 66.6% of the young children and 75% of the older children did not state that they talked to their mother about the cancer (Issel et al., 1990). When asked *who helped them cope with the mother's cancer*, 89% of the younger children claimed that their mother, father, or parents helped them. In contrast, only 63% of the older children made the same claim. This meant that 11% of the younger children and 37% of the older children did not report that anyone helped them deal with their mother's breast cancer (Issel et al., 1990). When asked *what the family did that helped the children cope*, 25% of the younger children and 15% of the older children stated that the family did nothing to help them.

In studies in which there is evidence that the mothers interacted with their child about the cancer, the content and form of that interaction raises concerns about its developmental appropriateness (Shands et al., 2000; Zahlis and Lewis, 1998). In the previously noted Zahlis and Lewis (1998) study, mothers detailed the ways they told the child about the diagnosis, including disclosure of overly charged information and details in their attempt to be 'honest' and to 'not hide anything' from the child. With rare exceptions, the mothers said they did not plan in advance what was said to the child about the diagnosis and often told the child about the diagnosis during the height of their own fear and anxiety. The intensity of the diagnostic moment is illustrated in this mother's report:

> *She (9 years old) was here the day that I got the phone call that I found out about the breast cancer and everybody was hysterical. She heard me talking to my doctor and she went outside screaming* (Zahlis and Lewis, 1998).

In another interview study of 19 mothers who had 30 school-age children, results revealed that mothers primarily used a biomedical–talk–teach–tell model to interact with their child about the breast cancer (Shands et al., 2000). During interactions with the child, mothers did not give evidence of systematically checking on the children's understanding of what was told to them, did not elicit the child's concerns, and exposed the child to emotionally laden or potentially frightening images, words or experiences. The following message from one mother illustrates how she described the cancer to her 8 year-old son:

'It (cancer) was a group of bad cells that if allowed to grow could cause...well, I think I did mention that it could be fatal' (Shands et al., 2000). A mother of a 10-year-old girl offered: 'I just told her that I was seriously ill.' One mother offered, 'We've told them that the doctors said the prognosis is very good, between 95 and 97% are non-returns.' A mother of 12 and 9 year-old boys shared, 'I told them I didn't plan to (die)...but that some people did.' In this same study, in an attempt to be helpful, mothers talked with daughters about their chance of also getting breast cancer. One mother of a 10 year-old daughter told her daughter, 'Well, you know you might be some day (sic). You know, you might have it, too.' A mother told her 10 year-old daughter that '...*she would have to be very cautious in the future to check herself like momma does and did.*'

Interaction with the child about the cancer can include talking about it and accompanying the mother to medical appointments (Shands et al., 2000). In the same study by Shands et al. (2000), some children accompanied their mothers to treatment and were shown physical changes in their mothers' bodies. Mothers reported that their children viewed their surgical scar, tattoos or prosthesis. Remarks by the mother of 10 and 7 year-old girls indicated her receptiveness to providing such experiences for them: '*Whenever they wanted to look at the scar or the prosthesis, I was always open to that.*' Another mother of 12 and 9 year-old boys made a similar statement: '*They wanted to look at the scar and they wanted to see the tattoos from the radiation breast treatments, so I let them look at them.*'

Evidence is that parents may not prioritize assisting their children with the breast cancer even when given the opportunity to do so. Instead, research evidence is that marital pairs experiencing the acute phase of breast cancer chose other issues on which to receive professional coaching assistance (Lewis and Zahlis, 1997). In a recently completed intervention study with couples in which the woman had breast cancer (Lewis, 1992–1996), rarely did couples identify helping the children as an area of their concern. When invited by professional coaches to work through a cancer-related issue of highest concern to them, in only three out of 234 completed intervention sessions did the couples request assistance in helping their child with the mother's cancer (Shands et al., 2000). What couples chose to work on instead were issues related to tension in their relationship, which they attributed to the breast cancer (Shands et al., 2000). The relative absence of requests for assistance for the children suggested three things: possibly the couples had already handled the child-related issues; or couples were unaware that their children had any issues; alternatively, during the acute phase of the mother's disease, the couples' interpersonal issues, not their children's issues, assume highest priority. We hypothesize that the latter two explanations are likely.

Single mothers may be at particular risk for challenges in assisting their child with the illness. In a completed multi-method study, 22 single compared to 104 married mothers with breast cancer scored significantly lower on parenting quality based on scores on a standardized measure of parenting (Lewis et al., 1996). Further analysis revealed that the sources of social support identified by the single women revealed a pattern of over-reliance on their children for support. This over-reliance occurred even though the network size and quality of social support were comparable for the single compared to married mothers (Lewis et al., 1996). Evidence was that the single mothers viewed their children as major sources of their feeling liked or loved; that their children were those with whom the single women confided about their illness; and that their children were the single mother's source of assistance when they needed immediate help (Lewis et al., 1996). It was as if the children were the parents of the diagnosed mother, not the other way around. One single mother of a 17 year-old daughter offered these words:

> *I just want her to be there for me... if I had a rough day. Maybe I do expect her to be the other adult. I think I expect some emotional support for me... I want her to feel what I'm going through... it's hard as a single mom.*

In a recently completed multiple-occasion interview study of diagnosed single mothers with adolescent children, several mothers gave reasons why they could not or did not talk with their adolescents about their cancer (Behar, 1999). They claimed they did not know what to say, did not think they were good communicators, thought that the adolescents would come to terms with the cancer in their own time, or found it difficult to find sufficient family time to schedule such exchanges (Behar, 1999). In data from this same study, there were many examples of the child parenting or being expected to parent or support the diagnosed mother (Behar, 1999). This pattern is reflected in the words of the following mother, whose 17 year-old son was having difficulty maintaining his grades at school and whose score on the Child Behavior Checklist (Achenbach) was borderline for the clinical range. Note how her son shifts his life in order to try to 'be there' for his mother:

> *[My son] went to school and talked to all of his counselors and changed a bunch of classes around because he feels that it's more important for him to be where I can connect with him when necessary ... He's the one that's still at home and he feels an obligation, which is okay, you know, because it's all part of growing. But I found I felt a little guilty about that because he's still a kid, you know. But that's okay, too. Kids have to face hardships too, and he told me, he says 'Mom, you spoil me, you know, you spoil me, so just let me do what I have to do, too.' It's kind of funny because now he's taking on the role of helping out financially ... Which is fine. He seems to be enjoying it, so okay, fine. I don't have a problem with that. He's working extra time and that's why he did it.*

There were repeated examples in the single mothers' reports that they expected or wanted their adolescent to be unconditional sources of support for them when they experienced distress from the breast cancer. Often mothers expected the adolescents to figure out and respond to the mother's needs, even when such needs went unspoken (Behar, 1999). In this same study, one mother reported crying with her adolescents, telling them that she needed to be loved and needed them to physically show their love by touching and listening and 'letting her carry on.' Another mother talked about expressing her despair to the children, telling them everything she was feeling, and how alone she felt. One mother relied on her children to cradle her when she was despairing; here are the words of this mother of a 14 year-old daughter and a 13 year-old son.

> *I tried a few things with the kids, uh, just to be with them and cry in front of them, and tell them they don't have to do anything, you know, just, uh, just to love me. And they'd put their arms around me and just let me cry or whatever, and it was wonderful. Wonderful.*

Unknown are the consequences, either short- or long-range, of this behavior for these adolescents.

MYTH 3—CHILDREN FEEL COMFORTABLE TALKING WITH THEIR PARENT(S) ABOUT THE BREAST CANCER

Children are not always forthcoming with their questions, worries or concerns about the breast cancer. Data obtained from confidential interviews with the children reveal that children do not want to add to the burdens of their ill mother or to the family, both of whom children see as already pressured by the illness. Instead, there is evidence that children may hold back or conceal their thoughts, fears, and feelings in an attempt to protect their mother or to not cause more tension in their relationship with her (Issel et al., 1990).

In the most recently completed interview study by the team, children who were 8–12 at the time of their mother's diagnosis discussed what it was like for them to talk with their mother or other parent about the cancer (Lewis, 1996–1999; Zahlis, 2000). When asked what, if anything stopped them from talking more to their mom about the cancer, a 12 year-old child said, *'I didn't want to upset her. I didn't want to, you know, like make her cry or anything.'* A child who was 8 at the time of his mother's diagnosis worried that talking would forever cause a disconnection between him and his mother:

> *It'd be like you'd lost contact. It's like you ... like ... they built a moon base, and then they lost contact with earth. It's like you can see it so close, yet so far? I was just afraid that I would upset her so bad or something, that she'd just would never talk to me again.*

When the children were asked how it was to talk to their mom when she was having a hard time because of the breast cancer, children reported that it was difficult (Zahlis, 2000). They wanted to connect over the illness but worried that it would make the mother feel worse. One child's words are revealing: *'It was hard ... very hard ... I knew that she was feeling worse than I was. And I didn't want to make her feel any worse'* (Zahlis, 2000). Another child offered: *'I tried not to mention it and stuff, 'cause I didn't want to upset her. And I didn't want to make her feel awkward.'* Another child offered that he did not want to get his mother worried, *'It's like I wanted to be the one who was worrying about it. I wanted her to get better ...'*

In an ideal world, children can turn to the non-ill parent to assist them to make sense of and interpret what is happening (Amato and Ochiltree, 1986). An ideal world, however, is not always reality during the acute phase of the mother's breast cancer. Some children worried about their father and knew that he needed help dealing with the cancer, but did not know how or what to say or do. Here are the words of a 12 year-old child.

> *The other thing was with my dad. I wanted to help. I don't know, it was just really hard for him as well ... Well, we had our neighbors, but there was no one really that he could talk to. And I thought that I could have helped in that way. But ... I don't know. It's hard to open lines of communication when you're ... when that kind of thing is going on. So, I didn't really do that ... I don't think that I'm really a great communicator, and I don't think that he is either. And so, it was kind of hard for me to ... cause I think that sometimes he ... he might stuff it as well. And so I just wondered, but I couldn't go ... I didn't feel comfortable doing anything about it, so I just didn't.*

MYTH 4—THE MOTHER'S DEPRESSED MOOD AND ANXIETY ARE FILTERED AND MANAGED WITHOUT AFFECTING THE CHILD

An estimated 25–33% or more of women who are diagnosed with breast cancer score in the clinical range on measures of depressed mood, anxiety, or both (Lewis, 1997; Darby and Lewis, 2000). (These rates vary depending on measurement methods, time since diagnosis, marital stress of the diagnosed mother, among other variables.)

Research evidence is that maternal negative mood impinges on the household and continues over time as a negative influence, even as illness-related pressures diminish and tension in the marital dyad decreases (Lewis and Hammond, 1992). Research evidence from interviews with children revealed that not only did they worry about the mother getting upset with them if they talked about the breast cancer, but they learned to filter out 'negative' talk. They told the mother about positive things to keep from introducing topics that could negatively affect the mother (Zahlis, 2000).

Maternal depressed mood may be particularly elevated in single mothers diagnosed with breast cancer. In a study comparing depression in single compared to married mothers, results revealed that 36.4% of the single mothers but only 16.8% of the married mothers were depressed, based on scores on a standardized measure, the Center for Epidemiological Studies Depression Scale (CES-D) (Lewis et al., 1996). Another point of clinical relevance is a score of 10 or more on the CES-D Scale. Results revealed that 59.1% of the single compared to 39.6% of the married mothers scored at that level (Lewis et al., 1996). When the proportion of single and married mothers with scores above the clinical cut-off point were examined over time, results were again remarkable: on three separate occasions at 4-month intervals, depression levels were significantly higher for the single women compared to the married women with breast cancer (Lewis et al., 1996).

To test the predictive and discriminating power of the mother's depressed mood on the child's level of functioning, secondary analyses were completed on data obtained from 82 mothers with recently diagnosed early stage breast cancer (Stages 0, 1, 2) and their 82 school-age children (Lewis and Hammond, 1999). Maternal depressed mood was measured by the CES-D and child functioning was measured by Achenbach's Child Behavior Checklist (CBCL) and Harter's Social/Peer Acceptance Scale. Results revealed that the mother's level of depressed mood was able to correctly classify 73.17% of the 'normal' and 'abnormal' grouped cases on the total score of the CBCL, 74.39% on the Internalizing score (CBCL) and 79.27% on the Externalizing score (CBCL). The mother's level of depressed mood, together with child anxiety, correctly classified 68.29% of the 'normal' and 'abnormal' grouped cases of children on the Social/Peer Acceptance Scale (Harter) (Lewis and Hammond, 1999).

MYTH 5—CHILDREN ARE ABLE TO INTERPRET THE BREAST CANCER IN THE LEAST DISTRESSFUL WAYS ON THEIR OWN

Our evidence is that children work to interpret and make sense out of what is happening to them and to their family because of the breast cancer. Their explanations sometimes contain frightening images as well as partial or total misunderstandings about the cancer, including the biology of the disease (Lewis, 1996–1999; Lewis and Zahlis, 1999; Zahlis, 2000). Our evidence is that children, like adults, typically equate the diagnosis of breast cancer in their mother with a 'death' sentence. Every child in the most recently completed child interview study feared that his/her mother would die from the cancer (Zahlis, 2000).

Our own team has begun to posit that standardized measures of child functioning are insensitive to the child's personal experiences with the mother's breast cancer. That is, these measures fail to successfully index the intensity of experience, as well as the domains of the experience, that are reflected in the data we have obtained through interviews with the children. We now hypothesize that at least a proportion, if not the majority, of children living with a seriously ill parent experience disenfranchised grief (Lewis and Sinsheimer, 2000). 'Disenfranchised grief' is defined as a sense of loss that is socially unrecognized or unacknowledged, with a limited capacity for the griever to mourn (Doka, 1989). In particular, the child's loss is not always recognized and the child as a griever can go unnoticed (Doka, 1989; Kauffman, 1989).

The earliest suggestive evidence of disenfranchised grief is derived from the first study involving children of mothers with breast cancer, the Family Impact Study (Lewis et al., 1983–1986). Mothers in this study were a median of 35.28 months since time of diagnosis. Data obtained from confidential child-focused interviews were divided into three age groups in order to describe the children's cancer-related concerns (Lewis et al., 1985). Children 6–10 years old were fearful about the integrity of the family and about the future. They also expressed feelings of sadness, fear, loneliness, and anxiety. Some children worried whether their mother's cancer would return. Children 10–13 years old talked about the disruption or change that their mother's illness caused in their own lives, such as being expected to do more household chores, assume more responsibility, or get along better with other household members. The adolescents talked about being pulled simultaneously in two directions: wanting to help their mothers more and wanting to spend more time in individual activities (Lewis et al., 1985).

MYTH 6—COMPROMISED PARENTING IN ONE PARENT CAN BE COMPENSATED BY THE PARENTING PRACTICES OF THE OTHER PARENT

Clinicians and therapists want to believe in the compensatory power of a two-parent household. In the ideal world, one parent's parenting practices are able to compensate for the compromised parenting of the other parent. The research evidence is mixed in breast cancer: parenting by each parent has significant effects on the child's functioning and there is some suggestive evidence that compensatory parenting may be an effective predictor of higher functioning in the child (Darby and Lewis, 2000).

To assess the effects of compensatory parenting, data were obtained from adolescents using standardized questionnaires to measure parenting quality: (adolescent report), Inventory of Parent and Peer Attachment, as well as adolescent functioning; the Child Behavior Checklist (CBCL); and Rosenberg's Self-Esteem Scale (Darby and Lewis, 2000). Prior to analysis, the sample was stratified into three groups based on the adolescent's report of the quality of his/her relationship with each parent: (a) adolescents with a poor relationship with neither parent; (b) adolescents with a poor relationship with one parent; (c) adolescents with a poor relationship with both parents. Results on parenting quality revealed statistically significant effects on both adolescent self-esteem and anxiety (Darby and Lewis, 2000).

The results provided support for the compensatory parenting hypothesis. When adolescents reported poor parenting from both parents, there were statistically significant deleterious effects on the child's self-esteem and anxiety. When adolescents reported compromised parenting from one but not both parents, the adolescents' level of adjustment was higher than it was for adolescents who reported poor parenting in both parents. Finally, adolescent adjustment was highest when adolescents reported high parenting quality from both parents. Separate analyses by mother and father revealed that although the parenting practices of both parents were statistically significant, the father's parenting practices were statistically more significant than the practices of the mother on both adolescent self-esteem and anxiety (Darby and Lewis, 2000).

MYTH 7—TENSION IN THE MARRIAGE FROM THE ILLNESS IS A PRIVATE MATTER BETWEEN THE DIAGNOSED MOTHER AND HER SPOUSE

Tension in the marriage of women diagnosed with breast cancer has diffuse, negative effects on the household. This is a substantiated claim in every study of families with breast cancer completed by our research team (Lewis, 1998). As such, marital tension is a family matter, not a private matter between the diagnosed partner and her spouse.

The first evidence of the negative effects of illness-related tension in the marriage surfaced in the Family Impact Study, which included three chronic illness groups, one of which consisted of families with maternal breast cancer (Lewis et al, 1989; Woods and Lewis, 1995). Later evidence of deleterious effects in the acute phase of the mother's breast cancer occurred in a study involving 80 mothers diagnosed with breast cancer, their 8–12 year-old school age children, and husbands (Lewis et al., 1993). Instead of coping with the illness, results revealed that family members were coping with the couple's level of marital tension related to the illness (Lewis et al., 1993). Heightened levels of marital tension negatively and significantly impacted the quality of the parent–child relationship, the family member's coping behavior, and the overall functioning of the household (Lewis et al., 1993). These study results suggested that an escalating positive or deviation-amplifying feedback loop was operating (Broderick and Smith, 1979), in which worsening conditions in the marriage resulted in less effective coping, diminished parenting quality, decreased child functioning, and compromised household functioning (Lewis et al., 1993).

NEEDED ELEMENTS FOR PROGRAMS AND SERVICES

The family affects an illness and the illness affects the family simultaneously (Campbell, 1986). The most important considerations for families and illness are how the illness experience affects cherished family relationships (Rolland, 1994), the individual lives of family members, and the life of the household (Anderson and Valentine, 1998; Lewis, 1999). Programs and services need to: assist the family to sustain the family as a nurturant system of care for the children; balance the illness-work of the family with the family's life as a family (Lewis, 1999); and enhance the quality of connections between family members. Such programs and services will help protect the family as it works to integrate the cancer into everyday routines, while simultaneously maintaining the family's life as a family (Lewis, 1999). Four program goals are needed for new services. These program goals and related recommendations follow.

ASSIST THE FAMILY TO BE RESPONSIVE TO THE CHILD: ENGAGE THE CHILD'S VIEW

Family-focused services need to assist the family to engage with the child's view of the breast cancer. Family members need to help listen—deeply listen—to what the child is experiencing. Without knowledge of the child's view, we have no assurance that the child will be comforted. In fact, we fear that the child will be forced to experience disenfranchised grief because of the absence of engagement (Lewis and Sinsheimer, 2000).

Counsel the family on ways to interact with the child so that he/she is able to disclose fears, concerns, or worries about the cancer. Assist the family to know how to listen calmly to the child and to hold back from prematurely comforting him/her about the disease, particularly before the child has had an opportunity to fully describe what it is like for him/her to experience the illness.

Work with the family to develop comfortable ways to interpret the illness and its impact on the family. If not assisted, the child may develop frightening images and misattributions about what is happening because of the breast cancer.

Parents may need concrete behavioral tips on ways to successfully interact with the child about the cancer, particularly if there is strain in the parent–child relationship, if the parent is highly symptomatic, for example from fatigue or nausea or vomiting; or when the child is quiet or withdrawn. Ideally, the ill parent needs to be fully present for the child when the child is with him/her (Armsden and Lewis, 1993). Being physically present but emotionally absent may be all that is possible, but the hypothesis is that such a superficial level of connection may not be as beneficial to the child as a connection which is punctuated by emotional connection. Private times between the ill parent and the child can be created and preserved, even if they are 10 minutes a day. One mother creatively used her time with each of her three young daughters, even during the most symptomatic time of the mother's medical treatment. She gave each of three daughters 10 minutes of their own 'snuggling' with her at the end of each day, even when the mother was so ill that she could only snuggle them in her own bed.

Children are often very sensitive to even subtle changes in their environment and will likely be aware of parental preoccupation with illness-related concerns and symptoms (Armsden and Lewis, 1993). The child will need assistance in understanding these matters. Parents might be able to help the child by labeling their own emotions and commenting on their own behavior to the child. It is difficult, even for older children or adolescents, to understand others' emotions when they are concurrently experiencing their own emotions and threats to their mothers' well-being (Armsden and Lewis, 1993).

ASSIST THE FAMILY TO BALANCE THE ILLNESS-WORK OF THE FAMILY WITH THE FAMILY'S LIFE AS A FAMILY

Family-focused services need to create a cognitive map of the illness for the family. This is not a map about the biological facts about the cancer, it is a map of the impact of the illness on the family. The map will include the processes through which family members go as they work to integrate the illness into the family's everyday life (Anderson and Valentine, 1998). It will also identify the work of the family to balance its cancer-related work with their life as a family (Lewis, 1999).

Hold a family meeting in the early phase of the mother's diagnosis during which a family-focused provider (nurse, social worker, patient educator, mental health counselor) sits face-to-face with family members to do two primary things: (a) *to answer questions about the impact of the illness on the family*; and (b) to *normalize the processes of adjustment for the family.*

Let the family know that families are unique but that they also experience common concerns and feelings when a mother is diagnosed with cancer. Help them identify their concerns and feelings. Will mom die? What will happen to our family now? Will we be able to do what we were going to do as a family before mom got the cancer? Will we be OK? What will happen to my plans to do what I was going to do before mom was diagnosed?

Help each member talk through his/her views and questions. Identify for them the diverse as well as common ways families experience the mother's cancer. Let them know that fears and concerns about the mother's well-being can be talked about; that bad or sad thoughts do not cause bad things in the family; and that they all deserve to be heard and supported. Let them know that they can work up a plan, as a family, to develop routines and activities that will help both the mother and the family get through the illness together.

Talk to them about the importance of keeping part of their week for family time that is not related to the illness. Assist them to explore specific operational ways that they can maintain members' and the household's <u>non</u>-illness related activities and routines. Successful functioning of the family involves the family in rearranging their routines and daily work in ways that accommodate to the demands of the illness, while still maintaining time and energy for family life that is not illness-related (Lewis, 1999).

STABILIZE COMFORTABLE HOUSEHOLD ROUTINES AND PATTERNS

Children, even adolescents, draw substantial comfort from predictable environments. All of us do! When life-threatening illness 'hits' the mother, the child's and the adolescent's world can symbolically fall apart. Creating predictable routines and patterns creates comfort zones for the children.

Engage the children in planning and deciding about that which can and should be stabilized (Armsden and Lewis, 1993). Invite them to be co-creators of the plan; even young children have the ability to contribute to such a plan. For the younger school-age child (8–12), such an invitation is consonant with their developmental goals for self-agency and industry (Putnam, 1992; Wells and Stein, 1992). For adolescents, such an invitation is consistent with their need for heightened autonomy and self-direction (Remschmidt, 1994). Working out a joint plan also helps them be full participants in linking the illness experience with their ongoing life plan (Armsden and Lewis, 1993).

ASSIST MOTHERS WITH THEIR DEPRESSED MOOD AND ANXIETY

Research results provide evidence of the importance of assessing the mother's level of depressed mood and linking her to additional resources as needed. The goal of such assessment is not to label the mother or to automatically initiate pharmacological intervention. The diagnosed mother is not the problem; her sources of depressed mood are the problem (Lewis et al., 1996).

Evidence from our research is that depressive mood produces an accentuated negative view of the illness and causes families to function less effectively as a family unit (Lewis and Hammond, 1992). The bottom line is that we need to triage clinically depressed mothers into additional service and support programs. These mothers deserve systematic attention.

CONCLUDING REMARKS

Despite the studies completed to date, research for families experiencing breast cancer in the mother is in its infancy and programs and services are sorely lacking. A review of the past 15 years of published papers in the *Journal of Psychosocial Oncology* yielded only descriptions, not scientific evaluations, of programs. There is more guidance offered to children whose parent is dying than children whose parent is diagnosed with a serious medical illness (Adams-Greenly, 1984; Adams-Greenly and Moynihan, 1983; Bourne and Meier, 1988; Heiney et al., 1995).

Families as families have been given short shrift. Families are forgotten by provider systems, even though an occasional nurse, counselor, or other health professional provides the rare exception. Health care systems are instead geared to managing the disease of the patient, not the healing of the family. Families are valued by members of the health care team, but as context, not as foreground. *Valuing the family is not the same as SERVICING the family* (Lewis, 1998).

When a patient is put on a Taxol (paclitaxel) protocol, there are certain minima that must occur. We have no such minima for families whose mother is diagnosed with cancer (Lewis, 1998). What needs to be the minimum is a family-focused program that involves three levels of service: minimum, intermediate, and case-intensive (Lewis, 1998). *Minimum service* involves contact with the family by a trained professional or volunteer who introduces the family to pre-developed program materials. These materials include videotapes, instructional booklets, web sites, information bases, and other audio or printed materials. The goal of the professional or trained volunteer is to offer minimum interpretation of these materials and to help the family member(s) be informed consumers. High-functioning families would be the best consumers of such materials. *Intermediate service* involves the minimum service component plus *a professional coach*. Trained professionals, nurses, social workers, patient educators, and mental health counselors work with the family to help them enact and behaviorally integrate new skills and strategies to manage the impact of the cancer (Lewis and Zahlis, 1997). The third level of service involves *case-intensive* service for highly distressed families (Lewis, 1998). Such a service refers the family for intensive counseling or therapy. Families for case-intensive services would include severely disrupted families who were unable to manage what was happening to them and who were unable to behaviorally utilize educational materials or a professional coach. Rarely would this intensive service be needed if psycho-educational services were available.

In the ideal, the family is a haven for warmth, support, love, and acceptance (Friedman, 1998). The experience of mutuality, intimacy, and reciprocity in families is critical to maintaining meaningful family relationships and relationships with others in the larger world. These emotional bonding characteristics allow the child to feel safe, to experience trustfulness, and facilitate attachment (Bowlby, 1977), identification (Turner, 1970), and responsiveness in interpersonal interactions. The family's experience with breast cancer has the potential to disrupt the intimacy, warmth, and reciprocity of the family members' relationships.

Health care providers need to generate a *prescription for healing the family* (Lewis, 1998). This is not current practice. Current practice is to exorcise the breast cancer through surgery and to ablate its potential growth through radiation, chemotherapy, and hormone therapy. A prescription is needed for helping the family in ways that restore their wholeness and vitality as well as minimize illness-related distress. It is interesting that a mother who is diagnosed with a fractured femur has a rehabilitation program recommended to her. There is nothing comparable for families and children dealing with breast cancer. Nothing. Nothing is not good enough.

ACKNOWLEDGEMENTS

Research reported in this chapter was sponsored by the National Institutes of Health (National Center for Nursing Research RO1-NR-01000; Division of Nursing RO1-NU-01000; National Institute for Nursing Research RO1-NR-01435; and the National Cancer Institute RO1-CA-55347); the American Cancer Society; the intramural research program at the University of Washington; the Center for Women's Health Research, University of Washington; the Susan G. Komen Breast Cancer Foundation, Puget Sound Affiliate; the Oncology Nursing Foundation; and the Dorothy S. O'Brien Special Projects Fund, Cancer Lifeline.

The authors acknowledge members of the Family Functioning Research Team, including: Nancy F. Woods, RN, PhD; Edith E. Hough, RN, EdD; Mary A. Hammond, PhD; Sandra Adams Motzer, RN, PhD; Gail Houck, RN, PhD; and (alphabetical): Gay C. Armsden, PhD; Maggie W. Baker, RN, MSN; Connie Bellin, RN, FNP; Maryanne Bletscher, MS; Sue Bodurtha, RN, MN; Maryanne Bozette, RN, PhD; Patricia Buchsel, RN, MN; Patricia Carney, RN, PhD; Rob Carroll, RN, MS; Susan Casey, RN, MS; Barbara Bean Cochrane, RN, PhD; Rochelle Crosby, RN, PhD; Lisa W. Deal, RN, MN, MPH; Cindy Dougherty, RN, PhD; Mary T. Ersek, RN, PhD; Aileen Fink, RN, MN; Sharon C. Firsich, RN, MN; Rebecca Fiser, RN, MN; Melissa Gallison, RN, PhD; Jane Georges, RN, PhD; Mel R. Haberman, RN, PhD; Lisa E. Hales, AA; Kathleen Halvey, RN, BSN, MN; Blanche Hobs, RN, MN; L. Michele Issel, RN, PhD; Gail Kieckhefer, RN, PhD; Huei-Fang Chen, RN, MSN; Sallie Davis Kirsch, RN, MN, PNP; Katherine Klaich, RN, PhD; Judy Kornell, RN, MN; Colleen Lucas, RN, MN; Katryna McCoy, RN, BSN; Jean Moseley, RN, MN; Ingrid R. Nielsen, RN, MN; Sandy O'Keefe, RN, MN; Nancy Packard, RN, PhD; Aileen Panke, RN, MN; Mary Patterson, RN, OCN; Debby Phillips, RN, MS; Janet Primomo, RN, PhD; Connie V. Rousch, RN, MN;

Marguerite Samms, RN, MN; Terri Forshee Simpson, RN, PhD;, Joanne Solchaney, RN, MSN; Lillian B. Southwick, PhD; Rebecca Spirig, CNS; Kathleen Stetz, RN, PhD; Viva J. Tapper, RN, MN; Maye Thompson, RN, MN; Susan Turner, RN, MN; Lynn Wheeler, MSN, WHCNP; Bernice Yates, RN, PhD; and Gretchen Zunkel, RN, PhD.

REFERENCES

Adams-Greenly, M. (1984). Helping children communicate about serious illness and death. *Journal of Psychosocial Oncology*, **2**(2): 61–72.

Adams-Greenly, M. and Moynihan, R. (1983). Helping the children of fatally ill parents. *American Journal of Orthopsychiatry*, **53**: 219–229.

Amato, P.R. and Ochiltree, G. (1986). Family resources and the development of child competence. *Journal of Marriage and Family* **48**: 47–56.

American Cancer Society (1999). *Cancer Facts and Figures 1999*. Atlanta, GA: American Cancer Society.

Anderson, K.H. and Tomlinson, P.S. (1992). Family Health System as an emerging paradigm in nursing. *Image: Journal of Nursing Scholarship* **24**(1): 57–63.

Anderson, K.H. and Valentine, K.L. (1998). Establishing and sustaining a Family Nursing Center for families with chronic illness: the Wisconsin experience. *Journal of Family Nursing* **4**(2): 127–141.

Armsden, G.C. and Lewis, F.M. (1993). The child's adaptation to parental medical illness: theory and clinical implications. *Patient Education and Counseling* **22**: 153–165.

Armsden, G.C. and Lewis, F.M. (1994). Behavioral adjustment and self-esteem among school-aged children of mothers with breast cancer. *Oncology Nursing Forum* **21**: 9–45.

Behar, L.C. (1999). Getting through it alone: a descriptive study of the experiences of single mothers with breast cancer and adolescent children. Unpublished doctoral dissertation, University of Washington.

Berger, P.L. (1967). *The Sacred Canopy: Elements of a Sociological Theory of Religion*. New York: Doubleday.

Bourne, V. and Meier, J. (1988). What happens now? A book to be read to children who have lost a loved one. *Oncology Nursing Forum* **15**(1): 81–85.

Bowlby, J. (1977). The making and breaking of affectional bonds. *British Journal of Psychiatry* **133**: 201–210.

Broderick, C. and Smith, J. (1979). The general systems approach. In W.R. Burr, R. Hill, F.J. Nye and I.L. Reiss (Eds), *Contemporary Theories about the Family* Vol. 2 (pp. 112–129). New York: Free Press.

Campbell, T.L. (1986). Family's impact on health: a critical review. *Family Systems Medicine* **4**: 135–332.

Compas, B.E., Worsham, N.L., Epping-Jordan, J.E., Grant, K.I., Mireault, G., Howell, D.C. and Malcarne, V.L. (1994). When mom or dad has cancer: markers of psychological distress in cancer patients, spouses and children. *Health Psychology* **13**: 507–515.

Compas, B.E., Worsham, N.L., Ey, S. and Howell, D.C. (1996). When mom or dad has cancer. II. Coping, cognitive appraisals, and psychological distress in children of cancer patients. *Health Psychology* **15**: 167–175.

Curran, D. (1983). *Traits of a Healthy Family*. San Francisco, CA: Harper & Row.

Darby, E. and Lewis, F.M. (1999). Breast cancer and adolescent adjustment: a test of the 'faucet hypothesis.' (manuscript submitted for review).

Doka, K.J. (1989). Disenfranchised grief. In K.J. Doka (Ed.), *Disenfranchised Grief: Recognizing Hidden Sorrow* (pp. 3–9). Lexington, MA: Lexington Books.

Ell, K. and Northen, H. (1990). *Families and Health Care: Psychosocial Practice*. New York: Aldine de Gruyter.

Friedman, M.M. (1998). *Family Nursing: Research, Theory and Practice* (4th Edn). Stamford, CT: Appleton and Lange.

Germino, B.B. (1984). Family members' concerns after cancer diagnosis. Unpublished Doctoral dissertation, University of Washington, Seattle, WA.

Given, B. and Given, C.W. (1992). Patient and family caregiver reaction to new and recurrent cancer. *Journal of the American Medical Women's Association* **47**(5): 201–206.

Gotay, C.C. (1984). The experience of cancer during early and advanced stages: the views of patients and their mates. *Social Science and Medicine* **18**: 605–613.

Gottman, J.M. (1999). *The Seven Principles for Making Marriage Work*. New York: Crown.

Heiney, S.P., Dunaway, N.C. and Webster, J. (1995). Good grieving—an intervention program for grieving children. *Oncology Nursing Forum* **22**(4): 649–655.

Hilton, B.A. (1993). Issues, problems and challenges for families coping with breast cancer. *Seminars in Oncology Nursing* **9**(2): 88–100.

Hilton, B.A. (1996). Getting back to normal: the family experience during early stage breast cancer. *Oncology Nursing Forum* **23**(4): 605–614.

Hilton, B.A. and Elfert, H. (1996). Childrens' experiences with mothers' early breast cancer. *Cancer Practice* **4**(2): 96–104.

Hymovich, D.P. (1993). Child-rearing concerns of parents with cancer. *Oncology Nursing Forum* **20**(9): 1355–1360.

Issel, L.M., Ersek, M. and Lewis, F.M. (1990). How children cope with mother's breast cancer. *Oncology Nursing Forum* **17**(Suppl. 3): 5–13.

Kauffman, J. (1989). Intrapsychic dimensions of disenfranchised grief. In J.K. Doka (Ed.), *Disenfranchised Grief: Recognizing Hidden Sorrow* (pp. 26–29). Lexington, MA: Lexington Books.

Lewis, F.M. (1992–1996). Family Home Visitation Program: The Nurse as Coach. RO1-CA-55347. Funded by National Cancer Institute, National Institutes of Health.

Lewis, F.M. (1993). Psychosocial transitions and the family's work in adjusting to cancer. *Seminars in Oncology Nursing* **9**(2): 127–129.

Lewis, F.M. (1995–1997). The School-age Child's Experience with the Mother's Breast Cancer. Funded by Cancer Lifeline, Dorothy S. O'Brien Special Projects Fund.

Lewis, F.M. (1995–1998). Enhancing the Single Woman's Adjustment to Breast Cancer (pilot study). Funded by Oncology Nursing Society/Sigma Theta Tau Award.

Lewis, F.M. (1995–1999). Promoting Adjustment in Single Women with Breast Cancer. RO1-NR-04135. National Institute of Nursing Research, National Institutes of Health.

Lewis, F.M. (1996). The impact of breast cancer on the family: lessons learned from the children and adolescents. In L. Baider, C.L. Cooper and A. Kaplan De-Nour (Eds), *Cancer and the Family*, (pp. 265–281). Chichester: Wiley.

Lewis, F.M. (1996–1999). The School-age Child's Experience with Breast Cancer: An Uncharted Journey. Funded by University of Washington School of Nursing Intramural Research Funding Program.

Lewis, F.M. (1997). Behavioral research to enhance psychosocial adjustment and quality of life after cancer diagnosis. *Preventive Medicine* **26**(5): S19–S29.

Lewis, F.M. (1998). Family-level services in oncology nursing: facts, fallacies, and realities revisited. *Oncology Nursing Forum* **25**(8): 1377–1388.

Lewis, F.M. (1999). The relational model of functioning with cancer: a family-focused framework for nursing practice. In C. Miaskowski and P. Buchsel (Eds), *Cancer across Health Care Sites* (pp. 319–331). St. Louis, MO: Mosby Year Book.

Lewis, F.M. (2000). Risk and protective factors of children's functioning with maternal breast cancer: a discriminant analysis. (manuscript under review).

Lewis, F.M., Ellison, E.S. and Woods, N.F. (1985). The impact of breast cancer on the family. *Seminars in Oncology Nursing* **1**(3): 206–213.

Lewis, F.M. and Hammond, M.A. (1992). Psychosocial adjustment of the family to breast cancer: a longitudinal analysis. *Journal of the American Medical Women's Association* **47**(5): 194–200.

Lewis, F.M. and Hammond, M.A. (1996). The father's, mother's and adolescent's functioning with breast cancer. *Family Relations* **45**: 456–465.

Lewis, F.M. and Hammond, M.A. (1999). Breast cancer in a mother: an identification of risk and protective factors for the school age child. Paper presented at the Fifth National Conference on Cancer Nursing Research, Newport Beach, CA.

Lewis, F.M., Hammond, M.A., N.F. (1993). The family functioning with newly diagnosed breast cancer in the mother: the development of an explanatory model. *Journal of Behavioral Medicine* **16**: 351–370.

Lewis, F.M. and Sinsheimer, J.A. (2000). Disenfranchised grief in children: the hidden experience with maternal breast cancer (manuscript under review).

Lewis, F.M. and Woods, N.F. (1986–1990). Family Functioning in Chronic Illness. RO1-NR-01000. Funded by National Institutes of Health, Center for Nursing Research.

Lewis, F.M., Woods, N.F. and Ellison, E.S. (1983–1986). Family Impact Study: The Family and Cancer. RO1-NU-01000. Funded by National Institutes of Health, Division of Nursing.

Lewis, F.M., Woods, N.F., Hough, E.E. and Bensley, L.S. (1989). The family's functioning with chronic illness in the mother: the spouse's perspective. *Social Science and Medicine* **9**: 1261–1269.

Lewis, F.M. and Zahlis, E.H. (1997). The nurse as coach: a conceptual framework for clinical practice. *Oncology Nursing Forum* **26**: 1695–1702.

Lewis, F.M. and Zahlis, E.H. (1999). The child's attribution model of the mother's breast cancer (manuscript under review).

Lewis, F.M., Zahlis, E.H., Shands, M.E., Sinsheimer, J.A. and Hammond, M.A. (1996). The functioning of single women with breast cancer and their school-aged children. *Cancer Practice* **4**: 15–23.

Lichtman, R.R., Taylor, S.E., Wood, J.V., Bluming, A.Z., Dosik, F.M. and Leibowicz, R.L. (1984). Relations with children after breast cancer: the mother–daughter relationship at risk. *Journal of Psychosocial Oncology* **2**: 1–19.

Litman, T.J. and Venters, M. (1979). Research on health care and the family: a methodological overview. *Social Science Medicine* **13A**(4): 379–385.

Litman, T.J. (1974). The family as a basic unit in health and medical care: a social-behavioral overview. *Social Science Medicine* **8**(9–10): 495–519.

Minuchin, S. (1974). *Families and Family Therapy*. Cambridge, MA: Harvard University Press.

Northouse, L. and Swain, M.A. (1987). Adjustment of patients and husbands to the initial impact of breast cancer. *Nursing Research* **36**(4): 221–225.

Northouse, L.L. (1992). Psychological impact of the diagnosis of breast cancer on the patient and her family. *Journal of the American Medical Women's Association* **47**(5): 161–164.

Parkes, C.M. (1971). Psychosocial transitions: a field for study. *Social Science and Medicine* **5**: 101–115.

Parkes, C.M. (1975a). Psycho-social transitions: comparison between reactions to loss of a limb and loss of a spouse. *British Journal of Psychiatry* **127**: 204–210.

Parkes, C.M. (1975b). The emotional impact of cancer on patients and their families. *Journal of Laryngology and Otolaryngology* **89**(12): 1271–1279.

Parsons, T. (1954). *Essays in Sociological Theory*. New York: Free Press.

Putnam, N. (1992). Seven to ten years: growth and competency. In S. Dixon and M. Martyin (Eds), *Encounters with Children: Pediatric Behavior and Development* (pp. 329–338). St. Louis, MO: Mosby Year Book.

Remschmidt, H. (1994). Psychosocial milestones in normal puberty and adolescence. *Hormone Research* **41**(2): 19–29.

Rolland, J.S. (1994). *Families, Illness, and Disability: An Integrative Treatment Model*. New York: Basic Books.

Shands, M.E., Lewis, F.M. and Zahlis, E.H. (2000). Mother and child interactions about the mother's breast cancer: an interview study. *Oncology Nursing Forum*.

Shands, M.E., Sinsheimer, J.A. and Lewis, F.M. (1999). Coaching couples experiencing early stage breast cancer: an analysis of their stated concerns (manuscript submitted for review).

Turner, R.H. (1970). *Family Interaction*. New York: Wiley.

Welch, A.S., Wadsworth, M.E. and Compas, B.E. (1996). Adjustment of children and adolescents to parental cancer. Parents' and children's perspectives. *Cancer* **77**(7): 1409–1418.

Wellisch, D.K., Gritz, E.R., Schain, W., Wang, H.J. and Siau, J. (1991). Psychological functioning of daughters of breast cancer patients. Part I: Daughters and comparison subjects. *Psychosomatics* **32**: 324–335.

Wellish, D.K., Gritz, E.R., Schain, W., Wang, H.G. and Siau, J. (1992). Psychological functioning of daughters of breast cancer patients. Part II: Characterizing the daughter of the breast cancer patient. *Psychosomatics* **33**: 171–179.

Wells, R. and Stein, M. (1992). Seven to ten years: the world of the elementary school child. In S. Dixon and M. Martin (Eds), *Encounters with Children: Pediatric Behavior and Development* (pp. 317–326). St. Louis, MO: Mosby Year Book.

Woods, N.F. and Lewis, F.M. (1995). Women with chronic illness: their views of their families' adaptation. *Health Care for Women International* **16**: 135–148.

Zahlis, E.H. and Lewis, F.M. (1998). The mother's story of the school age child's experience with the mother's breast cancer. *Journal of Psychosocial Oncology* **16**(2): 25–43.

Zahlis, E.H. (1999). When mom has breast cancer: sources of distress in school age children. Paper presented at the meeting of The Fifth National Conference on Cancer Nursing Research, Newport Beach, CA., February.

Zahlis, E.H. (2000). The child's worries about the mom's breast cancer (manuscript under review).

13

Correlates of Self-Esteem Among Children Facing the Loss of A Parent to Cancer

KAROLYNN SIEGEL, VICTORIA H. RAVEIS and DANIEL KARUS

Joseph L. Mailman School of Public Health, Columbia University, New York, USA

Children with a chronically ill parent confront a variety of stressors that present multiple, ongoing adaptational challenges. Furthermore, the number of young children and adolescents facing these challenges is relatively large, given the prevalence of diseases such as cancer, arthritis, multiple sclerosis, diabetes, and heart conditions among young and middle-aged adults. Yet there has been a surprising paucity of research on these children's long and short-term psychosocial adaptation and the factors that predict such adjustment (Worsham et al., 1997). What work has been carried out, however, has shown that their self-esteem is frequently adversely impacted.

In a study comparing self-esteem among adolescents (aged 12–18) of parents suffering from depression, arthritis or no physical or mental illness, Hirsch et al. (1985) found that those with ill parents reported lower self-esteem than those with well parents. Interestingly, no significant differences were found between those with depressed or arthritic parents. Armsden and Lewis (1994) compared 6–12 year-olds whose mothers had breast cancer with children whose mothers had diabetes and those whose mothers had fibrocystic breast disease. While the children of mothers with breast cancer scored better than children in the non-cancer illness groups on behavioral adjustment, they scored the lowest of all three groups on self-esteem, although their scores were similar to those in the diabetes group and significantly different only from the fibrocystic breast disease group. Further, Armsden and Lewis found the negative self-ratings of the children of mothers with breast cancer to be relatively stable over an 8-month period. Similarly, Siegel and her colleagues (1992) found that the children of cancer patients with advanced disease had significantly lower self-esteem and social competence, as well as higher anxiety and depression than normal controls.

A number of mechanisms have been hypothesized to account for the erosion of children's self-esteem in the context of parental illness (Armistad, et al., 1995;

Cancer and the Family, 2nd Edn. Edited by L. Baider, C. L. Cooper and A. Kaplan De-Nour

Armsden and Lewis, 1994; Reiss et al., 1993; Issel et al., 1990). One potential explanation is that as the parents cope with illness-treatment-related demands, they are likely to have less time and energy to devote to their children. Their emotional accessibility may also diminish as they become absorbed in dealing with the psychological ramifications of the diagnosis, illness and treatments. Unfortunately, children may interpret these changes in the parents' availability and attention as a rejection or punishment (Armsden and Lewis, 1994), misperceptions which can reinforce a prevalent fantasy of young children of ill parents—the belief that they are in some way responsible for ill parents' disease or suffering. Since all children at some time harbor angry and destructive feelings toward their parents, it is understandable that the inability (especially among younger children who engage in magical thinking) to distinguish between the wish (for harm) and the deed can lead to feelings of culpability for the parent's illness, guilt, self-recrimination, and a loss of self-esteem.

Further, varying levels of depressed mood in the ill and well parent associated with the illness and its sequelae are common (Siegel et al., 1996; Northouse, 1992; Baider and Kaplan DeNour, 1984) and may lead to social withdrawal from others, including their children. In addition, depression in the mother or father tends to impair parenting. Depressed parents are less communicative, more irritable, and more coercive (Goodman and Brumley, 1990; Panaccione and Wahler, 1986). These changes in the parent's behavior again may be assumed by children to be evidence of their parent's disinterest and rejection, which may account for the finding that children of depressed parents have lower self-esteem (Hirsch et al., 1985; Politano et al., 1992).

A number of other illness-related changes in the family environment may also lead to children's diminished self-esteem. These include an increase in both family and marital conflict associated with having to adjust to the reallocation of roles and responsibilities brought about by the family's reorganization around the illness (Lewis, 1996). All family members, but especially the children, may resist and resent these changes, which are stressful, can disrupt peer involvements, and are often perceived as unfair. Unfortunately, children's responses to these changes will often include disruptive and uncooperative behavior. When parents fail to recognize these behaviors as stress reactions they may become angered by their children's seeming selfishness and lack of cooperation, further exacerbating parent–child conflict. This conflict is likely to diminish children's self-esteem as they misinterpret the parents' anger as a form of criticism and rejection. Further, under the numerous stresses of the situation, parents are also likely to become less patient, less willing to reason with children, and less tolerant of disruptive or oppositional behavior, which may in fact be motivated by the child's need for the parent's attention. Out of a need to feel in control of some aspect of their life, parents may become stricter in their discipline and more punitive. This action may serve to again further enhance conflict and cause children to perceive a loss of love and support, thereby diminishing their self-esteem. Increased marital conflict can also distract parents' attention from their children as they seek to negotiate their own relationship (Lewis, 1986).

It has also been suggested that the self-esteem of young children of breast cancer patients may suffer because they internalize the negative changes in self-worth that their ill mothers may suffer as a result of the dependency, impaired role functioning, and disfigurement brought about by their disease (Armsden and Lewis, 1994). The inability, especially among young children, to fully differentiate themselves from the mother could conceivably contribute to such a process.

While the explanations discussed above for the negative impact of a parent's illness on children's self-esteem are plausible and persuasive, to a large extent they rely on speculation, extrapolation, or anecdotal evidence. The purpose of the analyses presented below is to extend our understanding of the mechanisms through which a parent's illness can lead to negative changes in children's self-esteem by empirically investigating the impact of several variables on two manifestations of self-esteem—trait self-esteem and state self-esteem. The data come from a sample of children of cancer patients with advanced disease and a poor prognosis.

METHODS

Study children were from families who participated in a longitudinal investigation assessing the efficacy of a preventive intervention program designed to facilitate the adjustment of school-aged children to the terminal illness and subsequent death of a parent. Potentially eligible families were located through a review of hospital records at a major urban comprehensive cancer center, to identify terminally ill patients with an expected survival time of 4–6 months, who were married with dependent children. Participation was limited to families who were intact (i.e. two-parent households) with at least one child in the household between the ages of 6 and 16 and whose members were fluent in English. Eligible families were randomly assigned to either the intervention program or the no-treatment control group.

Families completed three research interviews: a pre-death interview, conducted during the final months of the parent's illness; and two post-death interviews, conducted 6 and 14 months after the parent's death. Both the well/surviving parent and the participating child(ren) (hereafter referred to as 'study children') completed separate, private, face-to-face research interviews conducted by a trained mental health clinician. All interviews were held at the family's home. The individual interviews with the surviving parent and study children ranged from 1.5 to 2.0 hours each in duration. Study participation was preceded by obtaining written informed consent from the well parent and written assent from the children.

Findings presented in this chapter are based on data from the pre-death interview. Since the pre-death interviews were conducted prior to initiation of the intervention for families in the intervention group, families from both the intervention and control groups are included in these analyses to increase the statistical power of the sample. The analyses presented were limited to children whose parent actually died within one year of the pre-death interview, to ensure that they reflected the experiences of children whose parents were indeed in the terminal stages of their illness. Analyses were further restricted to children whose interview included a measure assessing their perceptions of the quality of parenting they received from the well parent. Unfortunately, this measure was not included at the beginning of the study. Thus, the findings presented in this chapter are based on data obtained from a total of 119 children, weighted by the reciprocal of the total number of children from the family included in these analyses, to reflect the fact that the children came from 77 different families. Weighted data were used to prevent overweighting the effect of families with more than one study child or the unique situational factors affecting the family as a whole.

MEASURES

The analyses presented below utilized data obtained from three sources—interviews with the well parent, interviews with the study children, and data abstracted from the ill parent's medical records. Described below are the measures utilized in the regression analyses. Whenever appropriate, the reliability of multi-item measures for the present sample, as assessed by Cronbach's alpha, is presented.

DURATION OF ILLNESS

The *Number of Days from Cancer Diagnosis to Interview* was computed based on the date the surviving parent reported the deceased parent was first diagnosed with cancer. For children in 10 families, who had either not yet been born or were under 4.5 years of age at the time of the ill parent's cancer diagnosis, the value of the measure was set to the interval in days from when the child turned 4.5 years of age and his/her interview. This modification was made for these children to estimate the length of time the children might have had either an understanding or the ability to understand/appreciate the impact their parent's illness may have had on the household.

CHARACTERISTICS OF THE WELL PARENT

Included in the regression analyses were gender (*Well Parent—Female*) and educational attainment (*Well Parent Graduated from College*). *Well Parent's Psychological Distress* was assessed through self-reports using the General Severity Index (GSI) of the Brief Symptom Inventory (BSI), a 53-item symptom inventory which is a shortened version of the Symptom Check List 90–R(34). Respondents rated each item using a five-point scale reflecting the range of distress associated with that item, from 'not at all' (0) to 'extremely' (4). The BSI consists of both global measures of psychological distress and measures for each of nine primary symptom dimensions. GSI is the most sensitive of the global measures reflecting all nine dimensions assessed by the BSI (Derogatis and Spenser, 1982). The GSI is computed as the average of all 53 item scores. Reliability among parents in the present sample was high (Cronbach's alpha=0.96). To control for gender differences in scores found in normative samples, GSI scores were converted into gender-specific T-scores prior to their inclusion in the regression analyses. Since gender-specific T-scores control for the fact that women tend to report more distress than men, the T-scores included in these analyses represent the well parent's level of depressive distress relative to levels reported by a normative sample of the same gender.

CHARACTERISTICS OF THE STUDY CHILD

The regression models presented include gender (*Study Child—Female*) and age (*Age 12–16*) as independent variables. In addition, as part of their interview, children were asked whether they had experienced any of 28 life events in the past year. Seven of the events reflected the study child's experience of *Other Losses/Rejection in Past Year* besides those potentially associated with his/her parent's illness and the threat the illness represented. A count representing the total of the number of such events (potential range 0–7) reported by the child, was included in the analyses to control not only for the direct threat to children's self-esteem posed by these losses, but also to control for the fact that such losses may render children particularly vulnerable or sensitive to the perceived/feared loss of the ill parent. Events included in this count were: the departure of a friend to another school; the extended absence/departure of teacher; spending less time with friends; a good friend(s) moved away; an upsetting break-up with a girlfriend or boyfriend; the end of a good friendship; and/or failure to be picked for a school/other activity for which she/he tried out.

The children completed a 45-item measure developed for this study to assess their *Perceptions of Parenting Provided by the Well Parent*. Individual items asked children the degree of consistency with which the well parent engaged in various parenting behaviors related to general communication, supportiveness, reliability, and attentiveness. Responses to individual items ('Never', 'A little of the time', 'A lot of the time', and 'Almost always') were coded 0–3, with higher scores indicating a more favorable perception on the part of the child. The summary measure was computed by summing individual item scores, and then dividing the total by 135, to make the potential range for the measure 0–100. Reliability of the measure in the present sample was high (Cronbach's alpha=0.90).

The children also reported on their symptoms of *State Anxiety*, completing either the State–Trait Anxiety Inventory for Youths (STAIY) (Spielberger et al., 1983), if they were 12 or older, or the State–Trait Anxiety Inventory for Children (STAIC), if they were 11 or younger (Spielberger et al., 1973). Both measures contained 230 items tapping state anxiety (e.g. 'how you feel right now'), that is, temporary elevations in anxiety, such as those that occur after a stressful event. Scale scores were computed by summing the scores for the 20 state anxiety items. Reliability for both measures was high in this sample: Cronbach's alpha was 0.89 for the STAIC and 0.91 for the STAIY.

Since the State Anxiety scale of the STAIY comprised four-point items (coded 1–4), raw scale scores for the measure could range 20–80, with higher scores indicating greater anxiety. However, the State Anxiety items for the STAIC comprised three-point items (coded 1–3); consequently raw scale scores for this measure could range from 20–60. To maximize statistical power and facilitate discussion, all STAIC and STAIY scores were converted to age- and gender-specific linear T-scores. The use of T-scores allowed us to aggregate the data across age groups (children aged 6–11 who completed the STAIC and children aged 12–17 who completed the STAIY) and to compare the levels of anxiety reported by this sample of children with those reported for normative samples. By definition, a T-score of 50 was assigned to children with a raw scale score equal to the mean score of children of the same age and gender in the normative sample. Furthermore, each increment of 10 points in T-scores represented a difference of one standard deviation in raw scores among children of the appropriate age and gender in the normative sample.

SELF-ESTEEM

Study children completed two measures of self-esteem—the 25-item Self-esteem Inventory—Short Form (SEI) (Coopersmith, 1984) and the Negative Self-esteem Scale (CDI-NSE), a five-item subscale of the Children's Depression Inventory

(Kovacs, 1992). Whereas the SEI asks the child to assess self-esteem in general (i.e., as a trait), the CDI-NSE is phrased to assess negative self-esteem in the recent past (i.e. the child's present state). Both measures are described in further detail below.

Trait self-esteem was assessed with the SEI, a 25-item scale, to evaluate the respondent's attitudes toward him/herself in those areas of experience (i.e. social, academic, family, and personal) which are most likely to interact with children's self-esteem. For each item, the child is asked to indicate whether the statement is 'usually' either 'like me' or 'unlike me' Responses indicative of higher self-esteem are coded 4, while those indicative of lower self-esteem are coded 0. Scores for individual items are summed to yield the overall score (potential range 0–100). Reliability of the measure in the present sample was quite high (Cronbach's alpha=0.79).

State self-esteem was assessed with the Children's Depression Inventory (CDI) (Kovacs, 1992), a 27-item self-report inventory of symptoms of depression experienced in the recent past. For each item, the child chooses which of three statements best describes his/her feelings 'in the past 2 weeks'. The values assigned to each response are then summed to yield scores for a total summary scale and five subscales: negative mood, interpersonal problems, ineffectiveness, anhedonia, and negative self-esteem. The negative self-esteem subscale (CDI-NSE) is comprised of five items which assess: optimism/pessimism; self-like/self-hatred; level of suicidal ideation; positive/negative body image; and feeling loved/unloved. Although the CDI-NSE is usually coded such that higher scores reflect greater levels of negative self-esteem, for the purposes of the present analyses we reverse-coded the measure for comparability with the SEI. Reliability of the measure in the present sample was high (Cronbach's alpha=0.67).

In order to provide the reader with a sense of the scores of study children relative to other children, scores for both measures were also converted into appropriate gender-specific percentile scores. Whereas the percentile scores for the CDI-NSE were based on information provided by the authors of the scale and derived from their normative sample (Kovacs, 1992), the percentile scores for the SEI are based on data from a large normative sample of children who completed the full SEI (Coopersmith, 1984).

In the remainder of this chapter we describe the levels of self-esteem reported by children with a parent having terminal cancer, and compare the congruence of their reports on the two different self-esteem measures. We also assess the salience and relative importance of variables and constructs suggested by previous research as correlates of psychological adjustment among such children as correlates of each self-esteem measure.

RESULTS

SAMPLE

Table 13.1 shows the sociodemographic characteristics of the study sample. The sample comprised boys and girls equally, nearly four-fifths (79%) of whom were white. The mean age of the children at the time of the interview was just under 11 years (mean=10.7; SD=2.9). Nearly four-fifths (78%) of the children reported experiencing at least one loss/rejection in the past year (mean=1.7; SD=1.4), with 26% of the children reporting three or more such events. On average, children's perceptions of the quality of the parenting provided by the well parent was quite high. Their average score on the measure was 70.2 (SD=14.9) out of a maximum score of 100, with none of the children scoring less than 26. The study children did not report high levels of anxiety compared to normative samples of children. The mean T-score of study children on the State Anxiety scale of the STAI was 52.3 (SD=12.4).

Well parents were disproportionately female (57%), and had a mean age of just under 42 years (mean=41.7; SD=6.1). Less than two-fifths (38%) had graduated from college. On average, the well parents reported high levels of psychological distress. The mean T-score of parents for the GSI in the present sample (mean=60.9; SD=10.2) was over one standard deviation above that of the normative sample (Derogatis and Spenser, 1982). Nearly two-thirds of the parents (64%) met the criteria for caseness on the overall BSI.

In 20% of families, the study child was the only child present, 40% had two children (including children who did not participate in the study), 27% had three children, and only 13% reported four or more children present (mean=2.4; SD=1.0). The mean length of time between the ill parent's cancer diagnosis (or the child becoming 4.5 years of age) and the child's interview was approximately 2 years (mean=736.7 days, SD=669.6 days). This period of time was less than 1 year for 30% of the children, 1–2 years for 22%, and over 2 years for the remaining 40%. The average length of time between the interview and the parent's death was a little over 3 months (mean=134.9 days; SD=107.1 days), with 35% interviewed less than 2 months (2–60 days), 31% interviewed 2–6 months (61–183 days) prior to the death, and the remaining 34% interviewed 6–12 months (184–345) prior to the death.

SELF-ESTEEM

Prior to their inclusion in multivariate analyses, preliminary analyses were conducted to determine the face validity of regarding the SEI and CDI-NSE as, respectively, trait and state measures of the same concept. Table 13.2 presents the mean scores of children on both measures. The bivariate correlation between the SEI and CDI-NSE was high ($r=0.623$; $p<0.001$), but well below identity. On average, the percentile scores of children on the SEI were close to those reported for children in the normative sample (mean percentile score=48.4; SD=29.9). On the other hand, as one might expect given their parent's illness, scores for the children on the CDI-NSE were appreciably lower (mean percentile score=42.6, SD=26.1). Overall, whereas 56% of study children had a percentile score of 50 or less on the SEI, 68% had such a score on the CDI-NSE. These results are consistent with the hypothesis that the parent's illness may be adversely impacting the self-esteem of children, at least during the terminal phase of the illness.

Also, given the assumption that the SEI is measure of self-esteem as a trait, and the CDI-NSE assessed a more transient state, one would expect that children who scored low on the SEI to also score low on the CDI-NSE; while scores of children who reported high levels of self-esteem on the SEI would be more likely to range from low to high depending on the child's current circumstances. Indeed, in the present sample, whereas 81% of the children with a percentile score of 50 or lower on the SEI also had a percentile score of 50 or less on the CDI-NSE; the analogous figure among children with a percentile score above 50 on the SEI was only 50%.

Table 13.1 Sample and family characteristics

	(%)	Mean (SD)
Study child		
Gender		
Male	50	
Female	50	
Race/ethnicity		
White	79	
Other/mixed	21	
Age		10.7 (2.9)
7–11	60	
12–16	40	
Experience of losses/rejection outside family in past year		1.7 (1.4)
0	22	
1	27	
2	25	
3 or more	26	
Perceptions of parenting	—	70.2 (14.9)
1–25	—	
26–50	10	
51–75	50	
76–100	40	
State anxiety (T-score)		52.3 (12.4)
Well-parent		
Gender		
Male	43	
Female	57	
Age		
29–39	37	
40–44	35	
45–61	25	
Educational attainment	62	
Did not graduate college		
College graduate	38	
Psychological distress (T-score)		60.9 (10.2)
Family characteristics		
Number of children in household (including study child)		2.4 (1.0)
1	20	
2	40	
3	27	
4 or more	13	
Number of days from cancer diagnosis to interview[a]		736.7 (669.6)
42–365		
	38	
366–731	22	
732–3054	40	
Number of days from interview to death of ill parent		134.9 (107.1)
2–60	35	
61–183	31	
184–345	34	

[a]Or days from age 4.5 years, whichever was later.

Table 13.2   Scores of study children from self-esteem measures

	Mean (SD)
Trait self-esteem (SEI)	
Raw score	65.6 (18.9)
Percentile score (gender-specific)	48.4 (29.9)
State self-esteem (CDI-NSE[a])	
Raw-score	8.4 (1.7)
Percentile score (gender- and age-specific)	42.6 (26.1)

[a]Scores reverse-coded for comparability with trait measure.

Predictors of Self-esteem

Multivariate regression analysis was used to determine the relative importance of several potential correlates of the child's reported trait and state self-esteem. Among the predictors included in these analyses were: the number of days from the initial cancer diagnosis to the interview of the study child (converted to its natural log in order to allow for the skewed distribution); three variables relating to the well parent (gender, whether she/he had graduated from college, and psychological distress); and five variables relating to the study child (gender, age, their perception of the experience of parenting provided them by the well parent, and state anxiety). Table 13.3 presents the zero-order correlations between both self-esteem measures and the independent variables included in the regression models, as well as the results of the regression models themselves.

Predictors of Trait Self-esteem   Overall, the model predicting trait self-esteem explained 42.9% of the variance in the children's SEI scores ($F(9, 59)=4.974$; $p<0.01$). The child's experience of losses/rejection outside the family ($B=-4.346$; beta$=-0.325$; $p=0.004$), his/her perceptions regarding the quality of parenting by the well parent ($B=0.317$; beta$=0.250$; $p=0.023$), and being 12 years or older ($B=9.166$; beta$=0.240$; $p=0.027$) were the only significant predictors of the trait measure. The model predicts that, all other things being equal, older children will report higher levels of trait self-esteem, as will children who perceive the quality of the parenting provided by the well parent more favorably. On the other hand, the model suggests that, all other things being equal, lower levels of trait self-esteem were likely to be reported by children who had experienced losses and/or rejection outside the family in the past year. In addition, although not statistically significant at $p<0.05$, the model also suggests that the child's level of self-esteem might also be somewhat inversely related to the well parent's reported level of psychological distress ($B=-0.340$; beta$=-0.185$; $p=0.086$) and the child's state anxiety ($B=-0.300$; beta$=-0.197$; $p=0.095$).

Predictors of State Self-esteem   Overall, the model explained 39.7% of the variance in the children's T-scores for state self-esteem ($F(9, 59)=4.354$; $p<0.001$). The child's experience of losses/rejection outside the family in the past year ($B=-0.435$; beta$=0.003$) and the level of anxiety reported by the child ($B=0.044$; beta$=-0.315$; $p=0.011$) were the only significant predictors of state self-esteem. The model

Table 13.3 Summary of regression analyses for models predicting children's trait self-esteem (SEI) and state negative self-esteem (CDI subscale).

Variable	Trait self-esteem (SEI)			State self-esteem (CDI-NSE)		
	r	B	beta	r	B	beta
Natural log (number of days from cancer diagnosis to interview)	-0.094	-0.963	-0.058	-0.150	-0.249	-0.163
Well parent:						
Female	0.165^+	5.633	0.149	0.108	0.065	0.018
Graduated from college	-0.037	0.885	0.023	-0.201^*	-0.379	-0.106
Psychological distress	-0.224^*	-0.340	-0.185^+	-0.193^*	-0.020	-0.116
Study child:						
Female	0.169^+	-5.772	-0.154	0.157^+	-0.652	-0.188^+
Age 12–16	0.177^+	9.166	0.240^*	0.007	-0.043	-0.012
Experience of losses/ rejection outside family in past year	-0.400^{***}	-4.346	-0.325^{**}	-0.433^{***+}	-0.435	-0.351^{**}
Perceptions of parenting	0.330^{**}	0.317	0.250^*	0.181^+	0.004	0.035
State anxiety	-0.397^{***}	-0.300	-0.197^+	-0.444^{***}	-0.044	-0.315^{**}
Constant		$88.820^{***}(24.115)$			14.886^{***} (2.295)	
R^2		0.429			0.397	
Adjusted R^2		0.343			0.306	

$^+p \leqslant 0.10$; $^*p \leqslant 0.05$; $^{**}p \leqslant 0.01$; $^{***}p \leqslant 0.001$.

predicted that, all other things being equal, lower self-esteem will be reported by children who experience losses/rejection outside the family in addition to their parent's illness. The model also suggests that, after controlling for the other variables included in the model, the level of children's self-esteem is significantly and inversely correlated with their current level of anxiety. It is also interesting to note that, although not statistically significant at $p \leqslant 0.05$, children's state self-esteem appeared to be somewhat lower for girls ($B=0.652$; beta$=0.188$; $p=0.087$).

Interaction Effects

To explore whether there were significant interactions between various independent variables included in the regression models for trait and state self-esteem, both models were re-estimated using a series of cross-product terms. Tests were made to determine whether there were statistically significant interaction effects: (a) between the age of the study child and the gender of the well parent; (b) between the age of the study child and his/her perceptions of the quality of the parenting provided by the well parent; (c) between the age of the study child and his/her experience(s) of loss/rejection outside the family; (d) between the gender of the study child and the gender of the well parent; and (e) between the age of the study child and the gender of the study child. In addition, it seemed possible that there might be a three-way interaction between the age and gender of the study child and the gender of the well parent. However, none of these interaction terms significantly increased the explanatory power of the models presented in Table 13.3 when added to the equation predicting either trait self-esteem or state negative self-esteem.

DISCUSSION

The analyses presented suggest that many children facing the impending death of a parent to cancer experience diminished self-esteem. Although the percentile scores of children on the trait self-esteem were close to those reported for children in the normative sample, the state self-esteem scores were appreciably lower, suggesting that the terminal illness of their parent was adversely impacting on the child's current self-image. Further support for this supposition is provided by the finding that a large proportion of children who scored high on the trait self-esteem measure scored low on their state self-esteem score. This suggests that the manifestations of problematic adjustment to the impending death of a parent may be complex and require incorporating measures that permit assessment of reactive states as well as more enduring traits. Failure to include both types of measures may have implications for the accurate estimation of the prevalence of problematic adjustment among children prior to the death of a parent and the identification of children who might be at risk of poor adjustment following the death of the parent.

It is notable that in addition to the children's diminished levels of self-esteem, reports of the children's current circumstances suggest problems in multiple domains. The children's state anxiety levels were elevated, their well parents exhibited high levels of psychological distress, and the children reported one or more losses/rejection in the past year. These findings are disturbing because they suggest that, should these current circumstances persist, the children may be particularly vulnerable when faced with having to deal with the additional adaptational challenges that will be imposed by the subsequent loss of their parent.

The analyses also indicated that a number of mechanisms that have anecdotally been postulated as contributing to the erosion of children's self-esteem in the context of parental illness do have an impact. The levels of self-esteem (both state and trait) reported by the bereaved children in the sample were found to be highly correlated with the experiences of losses/rejection outside the family in the past year. These events may have had a more adverse impact because they occurred in conjunction with the myriad stresses and changes that are likely to have transpired in the children's households as a consequence of the illness progression and its treatment (e.g., alterations in family lifestyle, absence or withdrawal of the ill parent from family functions, preoccupation of the well parent with illness-related care-giving responsibilities and household economic changes; Christ et al., 1993; Siegel et al., 1992).

The child's perception of the well parent's parenting was also significantly correlated with trait self-esteem. Those children who more favorably judged the quality of their well parents' parenting reported higher levels of trait self-esteem, even after controlling for other potentially important factors. As noted above, with illnesses such as cancer, it is not uncommon for the well parent to become increasingly absorbed in dealing with the various illness- and treatment-related demands. He/she is also likely to be confronting the psychological ramifications of the spouse's terminal illness. Our data suggest that, to the extent to which these demands cause their children to view their parenting less favorably, their children's psychological functioning can also be adversely impacted.

Other significant coefficients in the regression models merit further comment. State anxiety was significantly correlated with trait self-esteem and suggestive of a relationship with state self-esteem. Since the children in the study exhibited elevated anxiety levels, the correlation of anxiety with diminished self-esteem is a concern. Their elevated anxiety may be an essential component in the initiation of the anticipatory mourning process. If so, it could be viewed as a temporary elevation, which mourning itself would ultimately alleviate. It is also possible that the children's elevated anxiety levels are transient and primarily a reflection of the upheavals of the terminal stage of the illness. In this case, a reduction in anxiety may follow a settling of the turmoil in their family life, even if the settling is the result of the death of the parent.

Age of the study child was also found to be significantly correlated with trait anxiety, with younger children reporting lower self-esteem levels. It is possible that developmental or maturational differences may render younger children more vulnerable than older ones to the stresses associated with the myriad changes in the family system that occur with the serious illness of a parent. As discussed above, Armsden and Lewis (1994) have suggested that the self-esteem of young children of breast cancer patients may suffer because of their inability to fully differentiate themselves from their mothers, so that, as a consequence, they internalize the illness-related negative changes in self-worth that their ill mothers undergo. Their more limited cognitive development may also lead to erroneous beliefs and misconceptions concerning their role in either the etiology or progression of their parent's illness.

There was some indication that girls' self-esteem might be more vulnerable to serious illness in the family. This potential relationship may be due to either innate factors (e.g., greater emotional vulnerability) or to situational factors related to parental illness (e.g., the illness may result in increased household responsibilities for girls, which adversely impacts their psychological well-being). These results are notable, given the fact that the state self-esteem scores were converted to percentile scores that controlled for gender and age differences found among children in the community.

Because self-esteem has been shown to buffer the link between stressors and psychological symptoms in children and adolescents (Kliewer and Sandler, 1992), its erosion in children during the period preceding the death of their parent from cancer is concerning. Our data suggest the need for interventions targeting processes that would enhance or preserve children's self-esteem during the terminal and post-death period as a way of alleviating their distress. While children could likely benefit from access to professional intervention during the period of their parent's terminal illness, in reality they remain a largely hidden population. This is because children, especially young ones, do not routinely accompany their parents to medical treatments and are often not permitted in their parent's hospital rooms. Many parents try to protect them from the seriousness of the illness during this stressful time, often by removing them, from the situation, for example, by sending them to spend time with relatives or friends (Siegel et al., 1990). In our work with bereaved families, we have found that a strategy of indirectly targeting the children through intervening with their well parents is an effective means of reaching the children. Through such an approach, clinicians can enhance parents' awareness of their children's special needs and strengthen their parenting skills, thereby increasing the likelihood that help will be available to the children as they need it (Siegel et al., 1990). Such a strategy may be particularly fruitful in preserving children's self-esteem, especially in light of our finding that children's favorable judgment of the quality of their well parents' parenting was significantly correlated with the children's state and trait self-esteem levels. Thus, supporting parental functioning may result in the child's perceptions that he/she is being adequately cared for. This in turn might help preserve self-esteem as a protection against depression.

An important aspect of the present analysis is that the sample consisted of 'normal' children, i.e., children not referred for professional intervention. Our results, therefore, are more likely to reflect the normal range of reactions that children exhibit during the stressful period of a parent's terminal illness than results based on the experiences of a clinic or referred sample. Another important feature is that the children's psychological functioning was assessed through self-report measures. Many of the earlier studies of children's reactions to stressful life events relied on the parents' reports of their children's affective states. Such reports can be unreliable, in part because the well parents' own illness-related distress can compromise their ability to reliably inform on their child's psychological functioning (Brody and Forehand, 1986). Investigators have generally found a weak relationship between a child's self-report and a parent's rating of his/her child's depression and self-esteem (Doerfler et al., 1988; Kazdin et al., 1983; Lewis, 1996; Weissman et al., 1980).

Broad generalizations of findings from the present analysis must, of course, be limited for a number of reasons. For example, the families participating in this study were predominantly white and middle or upper class, and this may have impacted on the children's adjustment process. The experiences of children from other ethnic and/or socio-economic groups may have yielded a different profile of vulnerability factors. Additional studies need to be conducted with more ethnically and socio-economically diverse samples.

The relatively small number of cases available for these analyses precluded the reliable estimates of separate models for subgroups. Given the significance in the models of age as a predictor of trait self-esteem, and the suggestive trend that gender may be a correlate of state self-esteem, if analyses were possible for subgroups defined by these variables (e.g., gender, developmental stage) or combinations thereof (e.g., adolescent girls), additional significant predictors of state or trait self-esteem may emerge for specific groups of children. Such an approach, however, would necessitate either a larger sample size or a study targeting children of a specific developmental stage or restricted to a specific gender.

Finally, this study focused on families with a parent who was terminally ill with cancer. Other disease situations may yield a different set of consequences. Some findings from other work suggest that children whose parents are suffering from cancer fare less well than those whose parents have another illness (Armsden and Lewis, 1994). However, further exploration of the factors that predict children's psychosocial adaptation in other illness situations is still needed.

ACKNOWLEDGEMENTS

This work was supported in part by a grant from the National Institute of Mental Health (MH41967). The authors would like to thank Karen Faber for her assistance in the review and preparation of this chapter.

REFERENCES

Armistead, L., Klein, K. and Forehand, R. (1995). Parental physical illness and child functioning. *Clinical Psychology Reviews* **15**: 409–422.

Armsden, G.C. and Lewis, F.M. (1994). Behavioral adjustment and self-esteem among school-age children of mothers with breast cancer. *Oncology Nursing Forum* **21**: 39–45.

Baider, L. and Kaplan De-Nour, A. (1984). Couples reactions and adjustment to mastectomy. *International Journal of Psychiatry in Medicine* **14**: 265–276.

Brody, G.H. and Forehand, R. (1986). Maternal perceptions of child maladjustment as a function of the combined influence of child behavior and maternal depression. *Journal of Consulting and Clinical Psychology* **54**: 237–240.

Christ, G., Siegel, K., Freund, B., Langosh, D., Henderson, S., Sperber, D. and Weinstein, L. (1993). Impact of parental terminal cancer on latency-age children. *American Journal of Orthopsychiatry* **63**: 417–427.

Coopersmith, S. (1984). *Self-esteem Inventories*. Palo Alto, CA: Consulting Psychologists' Press.

Derogatis, L.R. and Spenser, P.M. (1982). *The Brief Symptom Inventory (BSI) Administration Scoring and Procedures Manual-1*. Baltimore, MD: Clinical Psychometric Research.

Doerfler, L.A., Felner, R.D., Rowlinson, R.T., Raley, P.A. and Evans, E. (1988). Depression in children and adolescents. *Journal of Consulting and Clinical Psychology* **56**: 769–772.

Goodman, S.H. and Brumley, H.E. (1990). Schizophrenic and depressed mothers: relational deficits in parenting. *Developmental Psychology* **26**: 31–39.

Hirsch, B.J., Moos, R.H. and Reischel, T.M. (1985). Psychological adjustment of adolescent children of a depressed, arthritic, or normal parent. *Journal of Abnormal Psychology* **94**: 154–164.

Issel, L.M., Erseck, M. and Lewis, F.M. (1990). How children cope with their mother's breast cancer. *Oncology Nursing Forum* **17**: 5–13.

Kazdin, A.E., French, N.H., Unis, A.S. and Esveldt-Dawson, K. (1983). Assessment of childhood depression. *Journal of the American Academy of Child Psychiatry* **22**: 157–164.

Kliewer, W. and Sandler, I.N. (1992). Locus of control and self-esteem as moderators of stressor-symptom relations in children and adolescents. *Journal of Abnormal Child Psychology* **20**: 393–411.

Kovacs, M. (1992). *Children's Depression Inventory*. North Tonawanda, NY: Multi-Health Systems.

Lewis, F.M. (1996). The impact of breast cancer on the family: lessons learned from the children and adolescents. In L. Baider, C.L. Cooper and A. Kaplan De-Nour. *Cancer and the Family*. Chichester: Wiley.

Northouse, L.L. (1992). Psychological impact of the diagnosis of breast cancer on the patient and her family. *Journal of the American Women's Association* **47**: 161–164.

Panaccione, V.F. and Wahler, R.G. (1986). Child behavior, maternal depression, and social coercion as factors in the quality of child care. *Journal of Abnormal Child Psychology* **14**: 263–278.

Politano, P.M., Stapleton, L.A. and Correll, J.A. (1992). Differences between children of depressed and non-depressed mothers: locus of control, anxiety and self-esteem: a research note. *Journal of Child Psychology and Psychiatry* **33**: 451–455.

Reiss, D., Steinglass, P. and Howe, G. (1993). Family environment as perceived by children with a chronically ill parent. *Journal of Chronic Diseases* **38**: 301–308.

Siegel, K., Mesagno, F.P. and Christ, G. (1990).   A prevention program for bereaved children. *American Journal of Orthopsychiatry* **60**: 168–175.

Siegel, K., Mesagno, F.P., Karus, D., Christ, G., Banks, K. and Moynihan, R. (1992).   Psychosocial adjustment of children with a terminally ill parent. *Journal of the Academy of Child and Adolescent Psychiatry* **31**: 327–333.

Spielberger, C.D., Edwards, C.D., Lushene, R.E., Montouri, J. and Paltzek, D. (1973).   *STAIC Preliminary Manual.* Palo Alto, CA: Consulting Psychologists' Press.

Spielberger, C.D., Gorsuch, R.L., Lushene, R., Vagg, P.R. and Jacobs, G.A. (1983).   *Manual for the State–Trait Anxiety Inventory (Form Y).* Palo Alto, CA: Consulting Psychologists' Press.

Weissman, M.M., Orvaschel, H. and Padian, N. (1980).   Children's symptoms, and social functioning self-report scales. *Journal of Nervous and Mental Disease* **168**: 736–740.

Worsham, N.L., Compas, B.E. and Ey, S. (1997).   Children's coping with parental illness. In S.A. Wochik, I.N. Sandler et al. (Eds), *Handbook of Children's Coping: Linking Theory and Intervention. Issues in Clinical Child Psychology.* New York: Plenum.

A Different Normal: Reactions of Children and Adolescents to the Diagnosis of Cancer in a Parent

ANDREA FARKAS PATENAUDE

Dana-Farber Cancer Institute and Harvard Medical School, Boston, MA, USA

One of the first thoughts that occurs to parents who are diagnosed with a malignancy is concern for the impact the cancer will have on the lives of their children ('What will this do the kids?'). In the USA an estimated 1,221,800 new cases of cancer were diagnosed in 1999 (American Cancer Society, 1999). One in 51 women and one in 61 men under age 39, and one in 11 women and one in 12 men aged 40–59 develop cancer in the USA (American Cancer Society, 1999). Many of these patients have school-age children. Despite the primacy of parental concern, there are still few resources to guide parents with cancer in their interactions with and planning for their children through the period of diagnosis and treatment. Although Rosenfeld et al. (1983) identified intervention with children of cancer patients as 'almost virgin territory', ideal for primary prevention research, the literature in this area remains minimal. Thirteen years later, Lewis (1996) characterizes as 'benign neglect' the medical profession's consideration for the emotional impact on children and adolescents of their mother's breast cancer. Guidance to parents with cancer at the time of diagnosis or during the course of their treatment about their children's well-being remains the exception. Medical professionals are necessarily focused on the treatment of the cancer and the immediate well-being of their patients. Doctors and even researchers often omit consideration of the impact of cancer and cancer treatment on the children in the family and the corresponding effects of the children's well-being on their parents.

Why is this such a neglected area? The answer reflects the emotional and practical stresses of the circumstances. Despite much progress societally in openness about illness (Kubler-Ross, 1987), we nonetheless shy away from painful communication with children. Uncertainty about what children understand about illness and how best to present the material is intensified by an understandable avoidance of the shock, fear, and directness of children's responses (Hoke, 1997). Parents may fear that they cannot be as solid, articulate, and certain about the path and outcome of

Cancer and the Family, 2nd Edn. Edited by L. Baider, C. L. Cooper and A. Kaplan De-Nour
© 2000 John Wiley & Sons, Ltd

the disease to their children as they would like to be. They find it difficult to emphasize hope for the future while also being honest about the inherent uncertainty of the situation. Discussions with children are often postponed until more medical information is available. However, because certainty is never possible, these discussions sometimes do not happen at all or do not occur in a thoughtful or consistent manner. It is often only after the treatment is finished that parents hear of the fears, anger, and loneliness that the child experienced.

Research on the population of children with a parent who has recently been diagnosed with cancer is difficult, since access to the children during the stressful period of diagnosis and treatment is limited. Parents often do not want the child to see the ill parent nauseous, sedated, or in pain. The well parent may also not be able simultaneously to oversee children and to minister to the needs of her/his husband or wife who is receiving chemotherapy. Hence, young or school-age children are often not brought to the clinic or hospital. Researchers (and institutional review boards!) are reluctant to intrude on families in the midst of a crisis. There is often not the leisure to explain the rationale for the research to the children, to acquire their assent, or to carefully introduce the researchers. It is especially challenging, then, to develop an ethically and scientifically acceptable methodology in this field which does not unreasonably add to the burdens of the families of newly-diagnosed cancer patients.

Due largely to the amazing resilience of children, the majority appear to cope with the changes parental illness brings about. For many, the experience of parental illness is an emotional, but transitory, stressor (Lewis, 1990). For others, it is a deeply felt trauma which shapes much of the future (Buckley, 1977). This chapter will focus on the reactions of children and adolescents to cancer diagnosis and treatment in a parent. Our aim is to describe what children of different ages are likely to focus on and how they may interpret the illness in their parent and the resulting changes in family life. We will focus on communication about medical and emotional matters, on normal fears and typical questions, and on the management of emotion, social support and resilience, utilizing the literature in this and related areas. We will review ways to identify children whose coping may indicate a need for additional professional input.

PRESENTING A DIAGNOSIS

One of the main rationales offered for a failure to talk to children is confusion about what they would understand of the complex information presented to a patient at diagnosis. Indeed, children, especially young children, do not understand details about tumor markers, surgical options, etc. They are, however, focused on the basic questions of whether the treatment will succeed, whether their needs will be met and by whom, whether the treatment will change their parents emotionally and physically, and how the structure of life will change. Interestingly, the majority of questions posed by young children mirror the basic concerns of their parents about the disease and treatment. Self-observation by the parent of what primary questions they most wanted answered by medical professionals can serve as a guide for anticipating the questions their children are likely to have.

Sometimes parents think they can 'spare' their children by not telling them about their cancer diagnosis. Trying to hide a serious diagnosis such as cancer from one's children is usually not possible. Even children as young as 3 or 4 quickly sense a change in the tone of family communication and events. As research showed in the 1960s when it was thought that children who had cancer should be protected from that information, when asked, the children not only knew that they were ill, but most often knew the name of their disease and the prognosis (Waechter, 1968). Since the developmental tasks of childhood involve modeling adult behavior, children are close observers of how things work in a family and, thus, are quick to note change. Without proferred explanations, children are often confused about the exact *reason* for the changes they perceive. Their anxiety is aroused by noticing an unexplained change and is exacerbated when they feel they do not get direct answers to the questions they pose to adults about why the change has occurred. They, like adults, often invent rationales or explanations when none exist for things they do not understand.

Secrecy has detrimental effects on children. Long-term exposure to family secrets is associated with learning problems (Brodie, 1967). Secrecy negatively rewards children for their inborn and essential curiosity, by giving them information which is false, and thus, not useful in their attempts to integrate the world around them. When they feel they are being left out of important family discussions, even young children experience tension and distrust. Thus, attempts at sparing children by failing to communicate basic facts about the diagnosis do not usually achieve their desired end.

This does not mean that all information or fears about a cancer diagnosis or illness should immediately be shared with the child. Newly-diagnosed parents often need time to come to terms with the diagnosis and to be able to speak the word 'cancer' in relation to themselves before they feel ready to discuss the illness with their children. Time may also be needed for parents to talk together and come to a consensus about how and when to tell the children about the diagnosis and how to continue to share information with them. However, because children are so quick to pick up clues, it is helpful to give them some idea of the events which are unfolding. Many children report knowing something was wrong before being informed by their parents of the diagnosis of cancer. If the ill parent is not able to engage in discussions with the children, then the other parent or a close family friend can give the children at least some idea of what the issues are which are affecting the emotional climate in the family. Information can be offered in steps, allowing the children time to integrate the information that their parent may be seriously ill.

STAGES IN CHILDREN'S UNDERSTANDING OF ILLNESS

Understanding how children at different developmental stages think about illness may help in formulating an approach to discussions with the children in a family where a parent has recently been told he/she has cancer.

CHILDREN AGED 2 AND UNDER

These children will respond mostly to separation from parents and to the emotional tension they perceive viscerally. Holding the child, allowing the child to see the ill parent, and trying to plan interactions between child and parent when the parent is more rested and available will help reassure the child. Verbal explanation will be of little use. The relative ignorance of the illness by the child and his/her persistence with normal tasks may be of help to the parent as distraction from concerns about treatment and illness. On the other hand, the ill parent may have little patience for the needs of the very young child. A particularly affecting change in this age group may be the necessity for sudden weaning of a young child because of the mother's need to begin cancer treatment. As expected, this may be difficult for both mother and child and both may require patience and support. The child's irritability and difficulty in understanding what is perceived as a rejection should be responded to with reassurance in tone and word. Concrete presentation of a gift or toy may help to convey the message that rejection or lack of caring did not motivate this change.

CHILDREN AGED 3–6

'(Cancer) is an illness that takes over a lot of you.' That's how a 6-year-old child described the illness her mother had. Children in this age group have primitive concepts of illness, often centering on contagion theories. Hence, it is important to reassure pre-school-age or young school-age children that they are not themselves at risk for cancer by being close to their ill parent. Children of this age group also tend to have quite concrete expectations about short-term treatments (bandages, creams, pills) as ways to cure illness. Their time frame is short; they are likely to believe that the parent's illness should be gone within a few weeks and may be frustrated by the continuing needs for treatment and family focus on the ill parent. Routines are quite important at this age, and maintenance of normal schedules (naps, school, play groups), is advisable, if at all possible.

CHILDREN AGED 7–13

Latency-age children have both abstract and concrete concerns about the illness. They are well aware of the seriousness of a cancer diagnosis. Exposure to television shows and appeals for money from cancer funds provide often heart-rending and frightening messages about cancer as a 'killer', and concern for the vulnerability of their parent will be pre-eminent in children during this developmental period. They will want to know if Mommy or Daddy will be 'all right' and will want to know in some detail about the illness and treatment plan. They may attach guilt about their own behavior to the parent's diagnosis and wonder if the 'stress' of caring for them contributed to the parent's developing cancer. Children may strive to be 'very good' to avoid troubling their parents, only to find that the strains in the family and the absence of the usual attention from the sick parent leads them to outbursts of anger or frustration, which, in turn, they feel very guilty about. Appreciation for their efforts and good behavior, acceptance of their failures, and assurance that they are as loved as before the parent was ill, may help to re-balance the emotions of latency-age children. Information is often useful to school-age children. Brochures or other printed material about cancer, available from the Cancer Society or hospital, may provide them with the basis for a school report or other way of proudly revealing their new 'expertise'. Continuation in activities, like sports teams, clubs, musical groups, etc., may provide distraction. They may require reassurance that it is not selfish of them to enjoy themselves in such activities while their parent is sick, but, rather, that all members of the family will seek distractions when possible from the burdens of cancer. If there are outside supports in school or through a religious institution, team, neighborhood, or extended family, informing adults in these groups about the illness and empowering them to talk with the child may be useful in offering a second source of support, especially when both parents are preoccupied with the patient's treatment or emotional needs. It is important to share with the child information about who has been informed about the parent's illness, both so that the child does not needlessly worry about how to inform these people and so that he/she is not surprised by expressions of concern for his/her parent.

ADOLESCENTS

As children enter adolescence, the subtlety of their concerns increases, with worry about genetic predisposition, embarrassment about the parent's physical appearance, and conflict about how to develop independence at a time when family cohesion may be mandated by the demands of the disease and treatment. While some research suggests that adolescence is the period during which children are most vulnerable to illness in their parents (Compas et al., 1996), other work finds that adolescents' greater capacity for intellectualization and abstraction and their ability to seek social support make them less at risk than younger children (Christ et al., 1994). The range of reactions to parental illness among adolescents varies considerably from sexual acting-out, diminished school performance, over-identification and somatization (Wellisch, 1985), to sudden maturity. Adolescents seek to be like their friends; something as major and public as a parent's illness spotlights the child and the family in ways which are often associated with inferiority, being 'unlucky' and 'uncool'. Adolescents' resentment of their ill parent and wish to hide the parent's infirmities or signs of illness may lead to painful conflict between the adolescent and the parent, who is him/herself in need of reassurance about his/her appearance. Adolescents also often resent the focus on the ill parent and the interpretation of difficulties in family relationships or in the adolescent's performance as attributable to the parent's illness. Nonetheless, fears for the health of a parent and feelings about the impact of the illness are often preoccupying and distance the adolescent from the more age-appropriate concerns of his/her peers, e.g. dating, sports, clothes, etc. Physical restrictions on the adolescent may be increased as he/she is needed more for the care of younger children or performance of household chores or, even, for emotional support of the parents. Discussion with friends may be awkward, since the friends may not know whether 'bringing the subject up' will make the adolescent think about the parent's illness, which might be upsetting. Even close friends often do not know how or how often to ask about the health of the ill parent. However, failure to ask about the ill parent may be viewed by the adolescent as a sign that his/her friend doesn't care or doesn't recognize the centrality of these issues. This lack of communication can further isolate the teenager, just when support would be most welcome.

For some adolescents, a private meeting with their parent's doctor may be useful to allow them to ask questions they may be afraid to ask their parents, to feel that they are seen as mature members of the family, and to know that nothing is being hidden from them. This is a highly individual decision; some adolescents want to completely avoid the world of the hospital and would be very frightened by having such a session arranged without their approval. The value of such a meeting is, obviously, affected by the style of the physicians involved and their willingness to talk directly with the adolescent.

YOUNG ADULTS

Although not the prime focus of this chapter, it should be noted that the telling of adult children, especially young adults, is not less difficult for a parent than the telling of younger children. Depending on the age, style and family constellation, adult children may react to the news with positive offers of help and support and may in reality became a mainstay of social and practical support for the ill parent, or they may react in ways which emphasize their own continuing need for parental attention and nurturance, more like the adolescents they recently were. Wellisch et al. (1996) offer a broad overview of the impact on adult daughters of breast cancer in their mothers.

PREPARING PARENTS FOR TALKING TO THEIR CHILDREN

When parents are ready to talk to their children, it is useful to anticipate issues that may arise in the conversation. Ideal presentation of the information (often not possible) would include planning for a time when parents and children are not exhausted, when the family can be uninterrupted and the conversation can be open-ended. Parents need to consider whether to tell all their children together or separately, taking into consideration the varying abilities to understand medical information, the coping styles of the children, and the support they provide for each other. Parents should also discuss who will impart the information and what words will be used. Much anxiety focuses on whether or not to use the word 'cancer'. While avoidance of the word puts children at risk for hearing it first inadvertently, in the long run, it is not the words used that are crucial. If a parent is not yet comfortable enough to use the word 'cancer', another word, such as 'tumor', can be substituted in the initial conversation. Eventually it should be clarified that the child understands that tumors are cancers. Otherwise, their introduction to the word 'cancer' may be when it is used to them by another child, or a well-meaning adult, or when they overhear their parent on the telephone. If that occurs, the children will feel misled and the trust in parents to honestly inform them of the status of their ill parent will be diminished.

WHAT CHILDREN WANT TO KNOW

Interestingly, research has shown no difference in the perceived seriousness or stressfulness of a parent's cancer for children aged 6–10, adolescents, or young adults (Compas et al., 1996). This implies that children of all ages comprehend the fact that a major event is occurring in their family which is upsetting to them. How their parents and others react and how well they communicate to their children (Hoke, 1996) are major factors in determining the later impact of the illness on children.

Anticipation of the question their children may pose in response to being given the diagnosis may help the parents to be less shocked and distressed during the actual conversations with their children. Parents should consider and rehearse, if necessary, how they will answer the nearly inevitable question, 'Are you going to die?'. They should also plan how they might handle seeming lack of interest in their offspring, a not infrequent means of coping for overwhelmed children or adolescents. Parents should anticipate that they may observe and experience strong emotion in their children and themselves, as these discussions are often a touchstone for parents who have previously contained much of the fear and sadness connected to the diagnosis. In turn, the experience of seeing their parents upset is likely to set off tears in children of all ages. Parents can be comforted that such emotion is in keeping with the seriousness of the diagnosis and simply corroborates for the children what they have sensed, that a diagnosis of cancer is a serious and threatening event. The children will simultaneously require reassurance that their parent will be receiving strong treatment and/or surgery to combat the serious illness he/she has and that the children will be advised of the parent's progress. The hopes of the doctors and of the parents for cure or remission should be accurately conveyed.

There are a set of normal questions and fears which children are likely to bring up in a discussion of the parent's diagnosis. These may be phrased differently by children of different ages and are unlikely to be asked all at one time. They include: 'Will Mom/Dad die?'; 'How did (the parent) get it?'; 'Did I do anything to make this happen?'; 'Did (the parent) do anything to make this happen?'; 'Does this mean that I will get cancer too (either soon or when I am older)?'; or, for younger children: 'Will I get cancer if I get near Mommy/Daddy?'; 'Will (the other parent) get cancer?'; 'Will life ever be normal again?' (often asked by inquiring about specific plans, e.g. 'Who will take me to soccer practice?'; or 'Will Daddy be well by my birthday?').

A good plan for the discussion of the diagnosis is for the parent who is to inform the children to make a brief statement about what has occurred and then to invite a dialogue with the child or children about what they know about cancer, what they want to know, etc., giving the children ample opportunity to voice their questions. It is also useful to ask children to restate what they think they have been told, sometimes by saying something like, 'How would you tell Jack (a best friend) about this when you see him?' Misconceptions can often be discovered and corrected this way, even among older children. Children should certainly be encouraged to ask questions which arise later; some families even try to set up a set time during the week to review what has happened and to discuss again the basic issues. If questions arise that the parent can't answer, the child can be told that the doctors will be asked, but that sometimes even they do not know all the answers.

IMPACT ON THE CHILD

The impact that cancer in a parent has on an individual son or daughter is a function of many characteristics of the situation. The age of the child, the course of the illness, the relationship between the child and each of his/her parents, the marital relationship, openness in the family, warmth and social support available from within the family and from sources in the extended family and community, the financial situation and the kind of role-sharing which characterizes the family unit will all affect the nature and extent of the child's stress during the period of the parent's illness and treatment. Research suggests that it is the child's perceptions of the stressfulness of the situation, rather than objective measures of the stage of the illness or the prognosis, that determines his/her distress level (Compas et al., 1996).

Children, especially adolescents, are often asked to assume parental roles during this period. Depending on the emotional climate between parents and children and the child's maturity, these tasks may be perceived by the child or adolescent as a useful way for him/her to make a real contribution to reducing the burden on the family or may be perceived as a cause for anger and frustration at limitations on the adolescent's freedom imposed by the illness.

The emotional dynamics within a family may change with the diagnosis of cancer. Some families become more rigid in response to the stress of illness, while others experience change in the emotional balance and individual roles. If, in one family, the mother, for example, is the parent who talks regularly and openly with the children about their emotions and her own and she is the ill parent, the children may find themselves without their usual emotional outlet. Unused to talking with the father and reluctant to add to his distress, yet too worried to talk directly with their mother, given her vulnerable physical condition, the children may turn to friends, teachers, coaches, or a relative, if they are available (Braithwaite and Gordon, 1992). If there is no outlet for the child, he/she may try to distance him/herself from his/her emotions through avoidance. The latter stance has been shown repeatedly to be a non-adaptive coping strategy (Carver et al., 1993).

In some families, the emotional balance between the parents may also have been altered, and either the well or the ill parent may seek solace by talking more about his/her feelings than usual with one of the children. This can be a burden on the child, but one he/she may be reluctant to complain about, knowing that the parent is so stressed.

GENDER

Not surprisingly, research has shown that the emotional distress is greatest on a child when the parent of the same sex is ill. Compas et al. (1994) found that adolescent girls, the most distressed of all groups of children and young adults whose parent is ill, were most distressed when their mother was ill. Adolescent boys were also more distressed when their father was the cancer patient. Wellisch et al. (1992) also retrospectively found that women who had been adolescents at the time their mother was diagnosed with breast cancer were more distressed than women who had been younger at the time their mother became ill. More research is needed on the cause of this association, but we can speculate that a contributing factor is the threat to the growing identification of the adolescent. Witnessing the physical and emotional vulnerability of their same-sex parent may make them more hesitant to accept the changes in their own maturing bodies. Other factors that may contribute to the burdens on adolescent girls include changes in the previously discussed emotional balance within the family and the concurrent stressor of shifting family roles.

Pressure may be greater on the adolescent to fill the role of the ill parent when it is the parent of the same sex who is ill.

MAINTAINING NORMALCY/SOCIAL SUPPORT

There is for many parents and children a recognition that the life of the family is unalterably changed by the parent's illness. There is also, however, despite the seeming contradiction, a strong desire on the part of both children and parents for life to be as normal as possible during the course of the parent's treatment. One child referred to the new reality as, 'a different normal', a revised set of expectations about family activities. Daily events, previously taken for granted, such as parental attendance at a school play or Little League game, will take on new charged meaning, both in the case that a parent can be there, or in the more likely case, right after diagnosis, that a parent will not be able to attend. While keeping children in their daily routines as much as possible is helpful, how possible that is often depends on how much social support is available to the family and what form it takes.

It is well documented that the healthy parent, the spouse of the patient, experiences psychological stress at levels which are similar to that of the patient following the diagnosis of cancer (Baider et al., 1996; Lewis et al., 1989; Lichtman et al., 1988; Northouse et al., 1991). Besides worry about his/her wife or husband, the healthy spouse often assumes new roles of nurse, transporter, intermediary with medical staff, etc. as well as new roles in maintenance of the household. In addition, the healthy spouse has his/her own emotions to cope with, which can include anger and irritability. The children, who may realize they have little direct role in getting their parent well may believe that their role is to help both their parents to feel better, often an impossible task. The well parent may be too exhausted to offer even usual levels of nurturance or may be dealing with his/her own overburdened feelings through avoidance. Sometimes, care of the patient necessitates that even the well spouse is not at home. In some cases, travel with the patient to a distant city where specialized treatment may be available is necessary. Hence, it becomes critical for the children of cancer patients to have sources of physical and emotional support outside of the immediate family.

Family, friends, babysitters, and community members can fill some of the parental roles, but it is not always easy for parents to accept or ask for such help. Children are willing to accept some individuals as substitutes in parental activities (although they would still much prefer their parent to attend), but find others unacceptable or unhelpful. The parents, often especially the well parent, may be caught in a stressful position. They must learn to be direct in asking friends for services the family needs. For some parents who are used to being care-givers themselves, it is difficult to change roles. Some 'hardy individualists' find it hard to accept help of any kind. The position in which both the healthy and the ill parent find themselves highlights their helplessness. It confronts them with the fact that the diagnosis of cancer has forced them to give priority to the health of the spouse with cancer, even over some of the most treasured activities of parenthood. Children often compound the burdens on the parent by expressing dissatisfaction with the arrangements, a statement of how much they would prefer their parents' presence. It may be easier if the child can be given a choice about who takes them to the baseball game or whose house they spend the night at, but this is not always possible. Some older children with close friends may actually be pleased, at least initially, at the opportunity for 'school night' sleepovers at friends' homes. Some adolescents come close to moving out of their own house completely, preferring to remain at the house of a friend rather than facing the 'different normal' at home.

SPECIAL ISSUES

DIVORCE AND SINGLE PARENTING

While this chapter has been written largely about families in which two parents, one ill with cancer and the other healthy, are available for the support of the children, this is clearly not always the existing circumstance. With an increasing number of divorced families and families in which a single parent is raising children, we must also consider the issues when the family constellation includes one primary parent or two parents sharing custody of their children. In both of these circumstances, the likelihood is increased that the children will need to be physically relocated from their usual environment or pattern of stay with parents for at least some proportion of the time the treatment of the ill parent is ongoing. As noted above, the normalcy of the child's usual routine is a source of strength for them. Relocation, even if it simply means a changing percentage of time in one parent's house, can upset the child's sense of constancy. In some more extreme cases, relocation is necessary to an aunt or grandparents in a different city, with uncertainty about how long the relocation is for. These can be very difficult adjustments for a child to make, especially if they mean that the child is only rarely able to be with his/her own parent and to observe the changes brought by illness, treatment, and recovery. Nonetheless, even such radical changes are greatly affected by the ability of the relatives who are serving as interim parents to continue to inform the child of events, to discuss the child's views and questions, and to make every effort to keep dialogue alive (through letters, pictures, etc.) between the child and the ill parent. Both parent and child need the continuation of that connection between visits.

In these circumstances, worry about the survival of the ill parent may be intensified by questions about what his/her death would mean in terms of the custody of the children. While these are long-term issues in most cases that do not need to be decided at time of diagnosis, they will nonetheless occur to both parents and children. In some families these issues may have been prepared for and a plan is in place; in others, new discussion about these matters may stir emotions. Useful discussion about preferences may occur for some families; in other families the ill parent may not be up to such consideration. The most important immediate issue for the children is the provision of a plan which allows for consistency in their care during the period of diagnosis and treatment with a plan for return to the parent. An issue often overlooked is that the return of the child to his/her normal living arrangement, while usually long-awaited and desired, is accompanied by some fears about whether the parent is able to care for him/her now, what would occur if the parent became ill again, etc. A transition period should be anticipated and the issues discussed in anticipation of reconciliation.

OTHER STRESSORS

Unfortunately, the existence of a major stressor, like the diagnosis of cancer in a parent, is sometimes not the only ongoing family issue that causes stress on the children. Illness in a grandparent, divorce, developmental disability or ongoing academic problems, drug or alcohol abuse in parents or in adolescents, unemployment, or even rare events like a house fire or illness in both parents, can confound the experience of parental illness. Children's sense of what is financially and emotionally abnormal in a family may generate guilt about their angers and wishes for normalcy when others in the family seem very burdened. It may be harder for relatives to step in to provide support if stressors elsewhere in the family have precedence. It may be especially important for medical professionals to be aware of concurrent stressors which may complicate the situation and challenge the coping abilities of parents and children.

HEREDITARY DISPOSITION

Children will naturally begin to wonder whether their parent's having cancer means that they will also develop cancer, either in the near future or when they reach the same age their parent was at the time of diagnosis. Compounding this, there is much talk in the media currently about hereditary predisposition for certain forms of cancer. It is important to reassure children that only 5–10% of cancer is thought to be hereditary (American Cancer Society, 1997). However, there are some families in which hereditary disposition is identified. In these families where such reassurance cannot be offered, the children may have special concerns about the implications for themselves of the hereditary cancer predisposition which has been found in their family. It would be important to determine what exactly the child is concerned about regarding the hereditary risk. Depending on the issue and the age of the child, the parent can offer more or less detailed reassurance about the opportunities for close surveillance, genetic testing, and anticipated advances in cancer diagnosis and treatment by the time the children become old enough to be at risk for cancer due to the hereditary predisposition. They may remind the child of the 50% chance that they have not inherited the parental mutation and of the fact that, in most cases, not all of the mutation carriers develop cancer. Consultation with a genetic counselor may be useful for older adolescents.

RESILIENCE

Resilience has been noted by Garmezy and others (Haggerty et al., 1994; Werner and Smith, 1982) as a quality which allows some individuals to overcome difficult life circumstances and to avoid development of adverse personality development. Factors conducive to resilience in children are the presence of a supportive caregiving environment and a social network that engenders trust in others, provides information, and reinforces competence (Wills et al., 1996). Resilience in families affected by cancer in a parent is seen in reports of increased interpersonal closeness and greater sense of competence among parents and children (Weihs and Reiss, 1996). Distress is normal, however, during a period of threat; cancer in a parent threatens children at the core of their existence. When there are caring adults with whom a child can communicate about the difficult feelings (guilt, anger, rejection, frustration, jealousy, etc.) during the time a parent is sick, there is increased likelihood that the child will emerge from that experience without negative emotional sequelae.

INDICATORS THAT MORE HELP IS NEEDED

Because distress (tears, clinginess, irritability, etc.) and even depression are normal when parents are ill and often themselves depressed, it is often difficult for parents to know when their child's reaction indicates a need for professional help. As a rule of thumb, if the child seems like a different child, is withdrawn and isolated or manic and constantly busy, if his/her academic performance dramatically shifts, if he/she does not appear to have friends, it is likely that he/she is in distress and outside help should be considered. It should be remembered that children's emotions change rapidly during childhood and especially adolescence, and that parental illness may be only one of a number of stressors the child is responding to. Parents should try not to blame themselves for the child's problems, but rather should have a low threshold for getting a professional evaluation of the child's distress. In a crisis like family illness, reassurance from a professional or help with the problems can relieve stress and allow parents to feel that someone else is sharing the responsibility for monitoring the child's functioning. Children may be reluctant to talk to a mental health professional, although sometimes the mantle of the illness and the possibility that others in the family may be seeing a social worker, psychologist, or psychiatrist can help to normalize seeking help during a crisis. Some children may prefer to be seen at the cancer treatment center, others may want the privacy of a therapist's office outside the medical setting.

IMPACT ON THE PARENT WITH CANCER

Bloom and others (1991) have shown that family interaction is a major variable in the prediction of distress in the cancer patient, second only to coping style in predicting how difficult the experience of cancer is: 'Good family interaction can help cancer patients adjust to diagnosis, treatment and rehabilitation' (Bloom, 1996). How well the children fare during a parent's cancer treatment is a major factor influencing family interaction. Family interaction, in turn, affects access to social support from sources outside the family. It may be easier to see that parental adjustment has a major role in the adjustment of a child patient to his/her leukemia (Kupst and Schulman, 1988) than to recognize that children's well-being affects their ill parent. But parents who are patients are at least as likely to be influenced by the well-being of their children during the period when they, the adult cancer patients, are involved in cancer treatment.

The role of stress and social support as illness mediators is much studied (Lazarus, 1982; Spiegel et al., 1989; Wortman, 1984). Stress on a parent with cancer comes from many sources, but the parents' perceptions of how much their children are affected by the illness and how supportive the children are can be major factors in determining the stress on both the ill parent and the healthy spouse. Thus, interactions designed to aid the children of cancer patients are likely to have beneficial, preventive effects on the children, improve family interaction and have primary effects on the well-being of the patient. Given this, it is all the more important that the methodological problems of studying children of cancer patients be overcome so that interventions to reduce stress on all family members can be designed, tested, and integrated into standard care for cancer patients.

NEED FOR MORE RESEARCH

Better understanding of the factors contributing to stress on the children of cancer patients, especially the burdens on adolescent girls, would be useful in the development of targeted interventions. Evaluation research will be needed to determine the best ways of helping children of different ages, genders, and cultural background to cope with serious parental illness while maintaining progress towards maturity. Hospital, school, and community-based intervention projects (potentially with links between them) may help to reduce the methodological challenges in serving family members in a crisis. Within hospitals, families would be well served by the provision of psycho-educational interventions for parents, family-centered support services, and counselors trained to talk with children about parental illness. Patient-to-patient networks can help to provide a context for parents to understand the range of reactions children have to the stress of parental illness and to learn of approaches other families have used to cope with this issue. School- or community-based programs can bring together groups of children whose parents are ill for discussions about the experience, minimizing the sense of isolation and differentness which troubles many such children. Research is needed to define which aspects of family interaction are most difficult for families to mediate in the course of illness, and whether adaptive cognitive and behavioral coping strategies can be taught in the midst of family crisis. We need to understand what the best ways are of supplying information about the illness to children of different ages, and in what ways the long-term development of children whose parent has had cancer (career choice, intimacy, etc.) has been influenced by the illness experience. Research could also elucidate ways to screen children in these families, to detect maladaptive coping patterns, and to offer reassurance to the majority of parents whose children will emerge resilient from the experience. Reassurance about the well-being of their children could reduce stress on the ill parent and supporting spouse. Also, developing targeted interventions for children of divorced or single parents would be useful, as well as defining how siblings can help support each other through this period. Finally, it is essential to find ways to raise the awareness of physicians and other medical specialists to family issues, especially those related to the well-being of children in the families of their patients. Physician attention to the intertwining emotional needs of parents and children is necessary to alter the climate of 'benign neglect' which has characterized this area. Mental health clinicians and researchers must work with physicians to implement useful, easily-accessed interventions that can reduce the stress on all members of a family where a parent has cancer.

REFERENCES

American Cancer Society (1997). *Cancer and Genetics: Answering Your Patients' Questions.* Atlanta, GA: American Cancer Society.

American Cancer Society (1999). *Cancer Facts and Figures—1999.* Atlanta, GA: American Cancer Society.

Baider, L., Kaufman, B., Peretz, T., Manor, O., Ever-Hadani, P. and Kaplan De-Nour, A. In L. Baider, C.L. Cooper and A. Kaplan De-Nour (Eds), *Cancer and the Family* (pp. 173–186). Chichester: Wiley.

Bloom, J.R. (1996). Social support of the cancer patient and the role of the family. In L. Baider, C.L. Cooper and A. Kaplan De-Nour (Eds), *Cancer and the Family* (pp. 53–73). Chichester: Wiley.

Bloom, J.R., Kang, S.H. and Romano, P. (1991). Cancer and stress: the effects of social support as a resource. In C. Cooper and M. Watson (Eds), *Cancer and Stress: Psychological, Biological, and Coping Studies* (pp. 95–124). New York: Wiley.

Braithwaite, R.L. and Gordon, E.W. (1992). *Success Against The Odds.* Washington, DC: Howard University Press.

Brodie, R.D. and Winterbottom, M.R. (1967). Failure in elementary schools as a function of traumata, secrecy and derogation. *Childhood Development* **38**: 701–711.

Buckley, I.G. (1977). *Listen to the Children: A Study of the Impact on the Mental Health of Children of a Parent's Catastrophic Illness.* New York: Cancer Care.

Carver, C.S., Pozo, C., Harris, S.D., Noriega, V., Scheier, M.F., Robinson, D.S., Ketcham, A.S., Moffat, F.L. and Clark, K.C. (1993). How coping mediates the effects of optimism on distress: a study of women with early stage breast cancer. *Journal of Personality and Social Psychology* **65**: 375–391.

Christ, G.H., Siegel, K. and Sperber, D. (1994). Impact of parental terminal cancer on adolescents. *American Journal of Orthopsychiatry* **64**: 604–613.

Compas, B.E., Worsham, N.L., Epping-Jordan, J.E., Grant, K.E., Mireault, G., Howell, D.C. and Malcarne, V.L. (1994). When mom or dad has cancer: markers of psychological distress in cancer patients, spouses, and children. *Heath Psychology* **13**: 507–515.

Compas, B.E., Worsham, N.L., Ey, S. and Howell, D.C. (1996). When mom or dad has cancer II: coping, cognitive appraisals, and psychological distress in children of cancer patients. *Health Psychology* **15**: 167–175.

Haggerty, R.J., Sherrod, L.R., Garmezy, N. and Rutter, M. (Eds) (1994). *Stress, Risk, and Resilience in Children and Adolescents.* New York: Cambridge University Press.

Hoke, L.A. (1996). When a mother has breast cancer: parenting concerns and psychosocial adjustment in young children and adolescents. In K. Hassey Dow (Ed.), *Contemporary Issues in Breast Cancer* (pp. 171–181). Boston, MA: Jones & Bartlett.

Hoke, L.A. (1997). A short-term psychoeducational intervention for families with parental cancer. *Harvard Review of Psychiatry* **5**: 99–103.

Kubler-Ross, E. (1987). *AIDS: The Ultimate Challenge* (p. 3). New York: Collier.

Kupst, M.J. and Schulman, J.L. (1988). Long-term coping with pediatric leukemia: a six-year follow-up study. *Journal of Pediatric Psychology* **7**: 157–174.

Lazarus, R. (1982). Stress and coping as factors in health and illness. In J. Cohen, J. Cullen and R.M. Martin (Eds), *Psychosocial Aspects of Cancer* (pp. 163–190). New York: Raven Press.

Lewis, F.M., Woods N.F., Hough E.E. and Bensley, L.S. (1989). The family's functioning with chronic illness in the mother: the spouse's perspective. *Social Science and Medicine* **9**(11), 1261–1269.

Lewis, F.M. (1990). Strengthening family supports: cancer and the family. *Cancer* **65**: 752–759.

Lewis, F.M. (1996). The impact of breast cancer on the family: lessons learned from the children and adolescents. In L. Baider, C.L. Cooper and A. Kaplan De-Nour (Eds), *Cancer and the Family* (pp. 271–287). Chichester: Wiley.

Lichtman, R.R. (1985). Relations with children after breast cancer: the mother–daughter relationship at risk. *Journal of Psychosocial Oncology* **2**(3) 1–19.

Northouse, L.L. (1991). Psychologic consequences of breast cancer on partner and family. *Seminars in Oncology Nursing*, **7**(3), 216–233.

Rosenfeld, A., Caplan, G., Yaroslavsky, A., Jacobowitz, J., Yuval, Y. and LeBow H. (1983). Adaptation of children of parents suffering from cancer: a preliminary study of a new field for primary prevention research. *Journal of Primary Prevention* **3**: 244–250.

Spiegel, D., Kraemer, H., Bloom, J. and Gottheil, E. (1989). Effect of psychosocial a treatment on survival of patients with metastatic breast cancer. *Lancet* **1**: 888–891.

Waechter, E.H. (1968). Death anxiety in children with fatal illness. Unpublished dissertation, Stanford University.

Weihs, K. and Reiss, D. (1996). In L. Baider, C.L. Cooper and A. Kaplan De-Nour (Eds), *Cancer and the Family* (pp. 3–29). Chichester: Wiley.

Wellisch, D.K., Hoffman, A. and Gritz, E. (1996). Psychological concerns and care of daughters of breast cancer patients. In L. Baider, C.L. Cooper and A. Kaplan De-Nour (Eds). *Cancer and the Family* (pp. 289–305). Chichester: Wiley.

Wellisch, D.K. (1985). Adolescent acting out when a parent has cancer. *International Journal of Family Therapy* **7**: 164–175.

Wellisch, D.K., Gritz, E.R., Schain, W., Wang, H.-J. and Siau, J. (1992). Psychological functioning of daughters of breast cancer patients. Part II: Characterizing the distressed daughter of the breast cancer patient. *Psychosomatics* **33**: 171–179.

Werner, E. and Smith, R. (1982). *Vulnerable but Invincible: A Longitudinal Study of Resilient Children*. New York: Norton.

Wills, T.A., Mariani, J. and Filer, M. (1996). The role of the family and peer relationships in adolescent substance abuse. In G.R. Pierce, B.R. Sarason and I.G. Sarason (Eds), *Handbook of Social Support and the Family* (pp. 521–551). New York: Plenum Press.

Wortman, C. (1984). Social support and the cancer patient: conceptual and methodological issues. *Cancer* **53**(Suppl.): 2239–2360.

Section V
DYNAMIC CHANGES IN FAMILIES WITH A CHILD WITH CANCER

Factors Contributing to the Psychological Adjustment of Parents of Paediatric Cancer Patients

JOSETTE E.H.M. HOEKSTRA-WEEBERS, JAN P.C. JASPERS,
and ED C. KLIP
Department of Medical Psychology, University Hospital Groningen, The Netherlands

WILLEM A. KAMPS
Beatrix Children's Hospital, Division of Pediatric Oncology, University Hospital,
Groningen, The Netherlands

Childhood cancer represents a source of extreme stress for parents. Medical advances in the treatment of different pediatric malignancies have resulted in an overall survival rate of 60% today (Granowetter, 1994), but this means that 40% of the children will still die from the disease. Parents' fear of a possible death is especially strong at initial diagnosis, but continues as parents live with the threat of relapse or death for years (Koocher and O'Malley, 1981). The belief that a child could still die is a strong predictor of post-traumatic stress symptoms of the parents of childhood cancer survivors (Kazak et al., 1998). It is also recognized that multiple stressors during treatment, such as repeated hospital stays, invasive procedures, distressing side effects, disruption of usual family routines, and changes in family roles and responsibilities, coupled with prolonged uncertainty about survival, have implications for both parents and the ill child (Kazak, 1994). While some researchers have found that parents adjust well during the years following the diagnosis (Kupst and Schulman, 1988; Kupst et al., 1995), others have indicated that a substantial amount of distress remains after treatment ends (Kazak et al., 1997). Considerable individual variability in adjustment has been reported for the parents of chronically ill children (Wallander et al., 1998). These findings underline the necessity to identify factors that may facilitate or hinder parental adaptation.

Cancer and the Family, 2nd Edn. Edited by L. Baider, C. L. Cooper and A. Kaplan De-Nour
© 2000 John Wiley & Sons, Ltd

The following model (Figure 15.1) has been used as a framework in our study to help explain the variability in parental psychological functioning by identifying concurrent and prospective predictors of maladjustment. The model is based on the stress–coping–outcome theory of Folkman et al. (1986). Childhood cancer is viewed as an ongoing stressor to which each parent has to adapt. The diagnostic phase is considered an acute traumatic stressor. When the initial treatment phase brings the child into remission, parents enter a phase that can be characterized as a chronic stressor. Stable factors, such as demographic variables and personality character-istics, are distinguished from variables that are likely to change as a function of the course of the disease (coping, social support, marital satisfaction). We have examined the impact of childhood cancer on the psychological functioning of parents; the contribution of different stable and changeable factors to parental psychological adjustment; and the effect of an intervention program.

Eligible for our study were parents of all children newly diagnosed with cancer during a time period of 27 consecutive months. Parents of children who were diagnosed as terminally ill were not included, and neither were those who spoke limited Dutch. Of the 192 eligible parents approached within 14 days of the diagnosis, 164 (=85%) agreed to complete questionnaires (at the hospital) at that time. Six months later (Time2), and 12 months after diagnosis (Time3) 139 and 128 of these parents, respectively, filled in the questionnaires at home. Partners were instructed to do this separately and not to consult one another. Table 15.1 shows the demographic characteristics of the 128 parents who completed the study, and their children. Of the 36 parents who did not complete the study, 19 parents were not asked to continue participation because their child had died, and 17 parents refused. There were no significant differences found between the parents who continued participation and those who dropped out with regard to demographic variables, personality characteristics, coping styles, social support variables, and marital satisfaction. There was only a significant difference found for prognosis ($\chi^2=16.80$, $p<0.001$). Fewer of the parents of children with an estimated chance for survival of $\leqslant 25\%$ completed the study, mainly because their children did not survive the year.

This chapter is divided into the following sections, in which our own results and those of others will be discussed:

1. Parental psychological functioning following cancer diagnosis.
2. The relationship between parental psychological functioning and stable variables: disease-related variables, demographics, life-events, and personality.
3. Associations between parental distress and changeable variables: coping styles, social support, and marital satisfaction.
4. Results of intervention efforts.

We have investigated the concurrent and prospective contributions of different predictor variables. Concurrent analyses have been performed on the data collected on a single measurement (within time analyses). Prospective analyses (across time analyses) involve the contribution of initial predictor variables (measured at diagnosis) to the prediction of future levels of psychological distress (as measured at 12 months post-diagnosis), while controlling for initial distress. We also examined how well change in predictor variables during the year predicted change in psychological distress. In these multiple regression analyses, psychological distress at

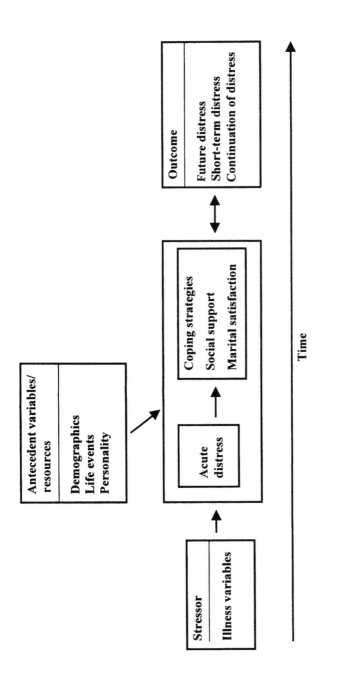

Figure 15.1   Predictive model of factors possibly associated with parental adjustment

Table 15.1 Characteristics of parents and their children

Variable parent		(*n*)	(%)
Gender	Fathers	62	48
	Mothers	66	52
Age	<30	19	15
	30–35	36	28
	35–40	45	35
	>40	28	22
Marital status	Married/cohabiting	127	99
	Widow	1	1
Education	Lower	49	38
	Middle	62	48
	Higher	17	13
Other children	None	9	7
	One	45	36
	Two	59	47
	>Two	13	10
Religious affiliation	Yes	46	36
	No	82	64
Variable children			
Gender	Boy	41	62
	Girl	25	38
Age	<4	25	38
	4–8	10	15
	8–12	18	27
	12–16	13	20
Diagnoses	Leukemias	28	42
	Brain tumors	8	12
	Malignant lymphomas	12	18
	Wilms' tumor	6	9
	Sarcomas—soft tissue	5	8
	Sarcomas—bone	1	2
	Neuroblastoma	2	3
	Germ cell tumor	2	3
	Hepatoblastoma	2	3
Prognosis at diagnosis	>75%	26	39
	25–75%	34	52
	<25%	6	9

12 months was predicted from predictor variables as assessed at 12 months, while controlling for distress level and predictors as measured at diagnosis.

THE EFFECT OF A CHILD'S CANCER ON PARENTAL FUNCTIONING

Parents reported high levels of psychological distress in the acute diagnostic phase as compared to a norm population [assessed using the General Health Questionnaire

(GHQ; Goldberg and Williams 1988)] (Student's t-test: $p < 0.001$). Eighty-five percent of the parents had scores within the clinical range (Hoekstra-Weebers et al., 1996). Comparable results have been reported by others (Manne et al., 1995; Fife et al., 1987). There is mixed evidence on how well parents adjust to the continuing and changing demands made on them during the course of the treatment. Parents were reported to cope well in time and to be able to fulfill their usual daily tasks adequately (Kupst and Schulman, 1988; Kupst et al., 1995; Kazak and Meadows, 1989). Our study showed that, although parental levels of distress decreased during the first year (GHQ: repeated measures analysis of time $F = 62.08$, $p < 0.001$), these levels remained high 1 year after the diagnosis (t-test compared with the norm population $p < 0.001$). This has also been observed by others (Brown et al., 1993). Forty percent of the parents in our study had clinically elevated scores at 1 year after diagnosis, whereas in the norm population only 15% had similarly high scores (Hoekstra-Weebers et al., submitted a). Parents were reported to express continuing concerns about the physical and mental development of their children as well as their future opportunities (Greenberg and Meadows, 1992). Feelings of uncertainty and loneliness persisted long after treatment had ended (Dongen-Melman, et al., 1995).

A factor contributing to the difference in research findings may be found in the difference in instruments used to measure parental adjustment. For example, the Langner Symptom Check List results revealed that parents of pediatric cancer survivors scored within the normal range (Kazak and Meadows, 1989). A later study, in which the Post-traumatic Stress Disorder (PTSD) Reaction Index was used, showed that parents of childhood cancer survivors reported elevated levels of post-traumatic stress symptoms when compared to a control group of parents of healthy children (Barakat et al., 1997). In our own study we found no differences in psychiatric symptomatology between the parents at 1 year after diagnosis and a norm population, using the Symptom Check List (SCL, Derogatis (1977); t-test $p > 0.05$). However, parents reported significantly higher levels of psychological distress at 1 year as compared to a norm publication using the GHQ (t-test $p < 0.001$) (Hoekstra-Weebers et al., 1998a). The SCL gives an absolute value of experienced symptoms, whereas the GHQ evaluates present levels of psychological distress as compared to what one considers usual. So, although parents did not report more psychosomatic complaints, they thought themselves still psychologically out of balance.

We examined the predictive power of initial levels of distress (distress as measured with the GHQ at diagnosis) on future levels of distress (distress reported 12 months later). Initial distress explained 14% of the variance of both parents' future levels of distress (F father $= 19.45$, $p < 0.001$; F mothers $= 21.83$, $p < 0.001$).

PSYCHOLOGICAL ADJUSTMENT AND STABLE VARIABLES

DEMOGRAPHIC VARIABLES

A number of cross-sectional studies investigating the psychological functioning of parents varying from 2 to 6 years after diagnosis concluded that mothers were more at risk for stress than fathers (Speechley and Noh, 1992; Brown et al., 1993; Van Dongen-Melman et al., 1995). In our prospective study, fathers and mothers had similar scores on measures of psychological functioning in the acute diagnostic phase, as well as 6 and 12 months later (paired t-test all $p > 0.05$, Hoekstra-Weebers et al., 1998a). In the general population, women are consistently found to have higher scores than men on measures of psychological distress or psychosomatic complaints (Koeter and Ormel, 1991). It is assumed that women in general are more willing to report distress than men. It may very well be that fathers are more inclined to report their distress in the acute diagnostic phase of a child's cancer and during the first year of intensive treatment. Parents may return to the usual pattern of gender differences as time goes by, as observed in the above-mentioned studies. Therefore, conclusions that mothers are at more risk because of higher scores on measures of psychological distress should be made with care.

Other demographic risk factors of parents mentioned in the literature are: younger age: lower educational and/or occupational level; lower socio-economic status; less income; and no religious affiliation (Barbarin and Chesler, 1986; Van Dongen-Melman et al., 1995; Kupst and Schulman, 1988; Morrow et al., 1984; Sawyer et al., 1993; Speechley and Noh, 1992; Veldhuizen and Last, 1991). Our analyses have shown that age of parent, age and gender of the ill child, level of education, number of other children in the family, and religious affiliation were not significant prospective predictors of parental adjustment at 1 year after diagnosis (multiple regression analyses: all beta values $p > 0.05$, Hoekstra-Weebers et al., 1999).

ILLNESS-RELATED VARIABLES

Objective illness variables, such as the child's estimated chance for survival, type of cancer, response to treatment, length of time in or since treatment, treatment severity, number of days hospitalized and functional impairment were not associated with parental psychological adjustment (Manne et al., 1995; Grootenhuis and Last, 1997; Kazak et al., 1998; Wallander and Varni, 1998; Hoekstra-Weebers et al., 1999). Subjective appraisals of illness and treatment may be more important in explaining parental adjustment (Kazak et al., 1998).

PRIOR AND CONCURRENT LIFE EVENTS

The co-occurrence of other stressing life-events was related to parental maladjustment, according to Kupst and Schulman (1988). We cannot support this conclusion on the basis of our study that examined the predictive power of non-disease-related concurrent life-events (Hoekstra-Weebers et al., 1999). We did find, however, that when parents had experienced more life-events prior to their child's cancer diagnosis, they reported higher distress levels 1 year after diagnosis (multiple regression analysis: $F = 8.23$, $p = 0.0049$, r^2 change $= 0.06$, in addition to initial distress).

PERSONALITY

Very little is known about the contribution of different personality characteristics to the psychological adaptation of parents. One cross-sectional study has shown that intrapersonal characteristics, such as locus of control and social desirability, were unrelated to psychological outcome of parents whose children were diagnosed 2–6 years earlier (Van Dongen-Melman et al., 1995). Our study showed that *trait anxiety*, as assessed at diagnosis (measured with the STAI-t; Spielberger, 1983) is a significant prospective predictor of parents' levels of psychological distress at 12 months post-diagnosis. Trait anxiety explained 18% of fathers' and 7% of mothers' levels of distress, in addition to initial distress. Furthermore, increases in trait anxiety during the year accompanied increases in parental levels of distress (hierarchical multiple regression analysis: fathers, r^2 change=0.20, $p < 0.001$, total r^2=0.52; mothers, r^2 change=0.29, $p < 0.001$, total r^2=0.50). These results correspond with the finding that trait anxiety predicted post-traumatic stress symptoms in parents of childhood cancer survivors (Kazak et al., 1998).

A second personality characteristic that appeared to be of relevance to the adjustment of mothers, but not of fathers, was *assertiveness*. Mothers who used assertive behaviors less frequently with time were more at risk, according to the Scale for Interpersonal Behaviour, a Dutch questionnaire (Arrindell and Ende, 1985). This questionnaire measures how much discomfort a person experiences in a given situation and how often a person enters that situation (Hoekstra-Weebers et al., 1999).

Personality is assumed to be a stable characteristic of a person. However, under the condition of a severe stressor, such as childhood cancer, personality changes may occur that affect adjustment. As such, trait anxiety and assertiveness can be considered appropriate targets for interventions.

PARENTAL ADJUSTMENT AND CHANGEABLE VARIABLES

COPING

It has been suggested that a family's ability to change is associated with their psychological adjustment (Kupst et al., 1988). Others point out the rigidity of some families in handling the changing demands of the illness, even when they cope in a dysfunctional way (Ostroff and Steinglass, 1996). Our prospective study offered the possibility to investigate: whether parents changed their frequency in use of different coping styles; the concurrent and prospective contribution of coping styles on distress; and whether change in coping was associated with change in level of distress. We used the Utrecht Coping List (UCL; Schreurs et al., 1993), a Dutch questionnaire that assesses seven conceptually different coping styles. Parents were asked to respond in connection to their child's illness. Results revealed that both parents used four coping styles significantly less frequently during the year following the diagnosis, namely: active problem focusing; seeking social support; a passive reaction pattern; and comforting cognitions. Fathers also used a palliative reaction pattern and avoidance less frequently with time. Neither parents changed their use of expression or emotions (Hoekstra-Weebers et al., submitted a). These results show that, on the whole, parents decreased their use of different problem-solving and emotion-regulatory strategies with time, as the demands of their child's cancer treatment changed. For example, parents' initial use of problem-focused coping, needed to learn about diagnosis and treatment and find the support they need, may be less useful later when they have come to understand what they can and cannot control about cancer, and when life may have returned to a more stable pattern.

Concurrent analysis of our data revealed that use of the coping styles at diagnosis did not significantly predict fathers' distress at that time (r^2 change=0.18, F change=1.70, controlled for age and education). However, the contribution of the coping styles in predicting mothers' distress was significant (r^2 change=0.28, F change=3.17, $p<0.01$). There was a significant main effect for use of a passive reaction pattern for both parents, meaning that more use of this pattern was related to higher levels of distress. Coping styles as used at 6 months were significant predictors of fathers' distress at that time (r^2 change=0.47, F change=6.55, $p<0.001$) and also of that of the mothers (r^2 change=0.29, F change=3.20, $p<0.01$). A significant main effect was found for a passive reaction pattern for both parents. In addition, more frequent use of a palliative reaction pattern, avoidance, and expression of emotions were uniquely related to higher levels of distress for fathers. Lastly, coping styles as used at 12 months significantly predicted fathers' distress at that time (r^2 change=0.43, F change=5.48, $p<0.001$). This was also found for the mothers (r^2 change=0.44, F change=6.27, $p<0.001$). The parents who used palliative and passive reaction patterns, and avoidance, more frequently reported higher distress levels. In addition, when fathers were more distressed they expressed emotions more frequently.

Prospective analysis showed that use of the seven coping styles at diagnosis had an impact on fathers' distress level 12 months later, although less strongly than their current coping did. Fathers who used avoidance, seeking social support, and expression of emotions more frequently at the time of the diagnosis reported more distress a year later. Mothers' initial use of the coping styles did not have a significant impact on their later levels of distress. However, less use of seeking social support at diagnosis independently predicted higher levels of mothers' distress at 12 months (Hoekstra-Weebers et al., submitted a). These results indicated that whereas fathers' use of the coping styles at diagnosis did not have an effect on their current psychological functioning, it did have longer-lasting effects on their future psychological functioning. The reverse was found for the mothers.

Changes during the year in use of coping were significantly associated with changes in both parents' level of distress. For fathers, increased use of avoidance, a passive reaction pattern and expression of emotions accompanied increased levels of distress. For mothers, increased use of a passive reaction pattern only was associated with higher distress levels (Hoekstra-Weeber et al., submitted a).

In summary, the results underline the assumption that coping should be viewed as a transactional process (Folkman et al., 1986). First of all, parents changed the frequency of use of the coping styles as treatment progressed during the first year after diagnosis. Second, current coping and change in coping had an impact on the psychological functioning at that time. Initial coping did not affect distress 12 months later (mothers), or affected distress at that time less strongly than current coping did (fathers).

We found differences in the effects of coping styles for fathers and mothers. Fathers who sought more social support at diagnosis were more distressed 12 months later. In contrast, mothers who initially sought less support were more distressed later. It has been suggested that a lack of support would be associated with psychological maladjustment (Speechley and Noh, 1992). This seems to be the case for mothers. Our results suggest that fathers, although trying to mobilize support, may not receive the type of support they specifically need. A passive reaction pattern was a consistent risk factor for both parents. A palliative reaction pattern, avoidance, and expression of emotions were additional consistent risk factors for fathers. These coping styles are all emotion-regulatory coping strategies. Active problem focusing was neither an effective nor an ineffective coping style for parents in the specific situation of childhood cancer.

Parents may have more difficulty adjusting when each partner adopts a different coping style of when partners make dissimilar use of a certain coping style (Adams-Greenly, 1986). We found a tendency for couples to use the above-mentioned seven coping styles similarly. However, the more dissimilar a couple's use of palliative and passive reaction patterns, expression of emotions, and comforting cognitions at diagnosis, the more distress the fathers reported at that time. Mothers reported more distress only when there was greater discrepancy in expression of emotions in couples. In contrast, the more dissimilar a couple's use of active problem focusing, palliative and passive reaction patterns, avoidance, and expression of emotions at 12 months after diagnosis, the more distress the mothers reported at that time. Fathers only reported more distress when there was more discrepancy in expression of emotions (Hoekstra-Weebers et al., 1998a). This shift from more distress in fathers at diagnosis to more distress in mothers 12 months later in the case of discrepancies in coping may be explained by traditional role differences between fathers and mothers. When a child is diagnosed with cancer, fathers are seen to spend as much time in the hospital as mothers. Fathers have to give up more of their usual lifestyle of going to their work everyday than mothers who still consider it their responsibility to take care of the family. In addition, fathers have less experience in the nurturing role, which they then have to share with the mothers. Uncertainty about their role may lead to more distress in fathers when there are differences in coping. Twelve months later, life has more or less returned to normal in families with a child that is responding well to treatment. Mothers continue to take care of the child. Coping differences then seem to be related to more distress in mothers. Mothers may feel deserted by the fathers who have picked up their usual everyday life patterns.

SOCIAL SUPPORT

The association between social support and psychological adjustment is well established (Cohen and Wills, 1985). Evidence exists that, among parents of children treated for leukemia social support throughout the cancer treatment was linked to parental adjustment (Kupst and Schulman, 1988). Parents of childhood cancer survivors, and especially fathers, who experience low levels of support were more at risk for psychological distress (Speechley and Noh, 1992). Fewer post-traumatic symptoms were also found in parents of cancer survivors reporting higher levels of perceived support (Kazak et al., 1997). The results of our study (Hoekstra-Weebers et al., submitted b), using the Social Support List–Interactions to measure the amount of support received, and the Social Support List–Discrepancies to assess dissatisfaction with support (Sonderen, 1993), showed that both fathers and mothers received the most support at diagnosis. Parents indicated they received significantly less support during the year. The sharpest decline occurred between the time of diagnosis and 6 months later. Parents who were more distressed at diagnosis received more support. However, parents remained equally satisfied with the amount of support, although the quantity was declining.

Concurrent analysis revealed that these two support variables significantly predicted fathers' levels of distress at diagnosis ($r^2=0.12$), at six months ($r^2=0.16$) and at 12 months ($r^2=0.32$). Mothers' distress at six ($r^2=0.10$) and 12 months ($r^2=0.11$) was significantly predicted by the support variables, but that at diagnosis was not ($r^2=0.00$). Quantity of support had a main effect on fathers' concurrent distress at diagnosis and on mothers' distress at 6 months (more support received was related to more distress). Dissatisfaction with support was independently associated with both fathers' and mothers' level of distress at 6 and 12 months (more dissatisfaction with support was related to more distress).

Prospective analysis showed that a father's level of distress at 12 months was significantly predicted by initial support. This was not found for the mothers. Also in contrast to the mothers, we found that changes during the year in support accompanied changes in fathers' distress level. Notably, the more the fathers were dissatisfied with support at diagnosis and the more dissatisfied fathers grew with time, the more psychological distress they reported a year after diagnosis.

Taken together, these results suggest that social support is a much stronger predictor of fathers' psychological functioning than of that of the mothers. Current support was increasingly important for fathers' distress with time. For mothers, current support at 6 and 12 months just reached significance in predicting their level of distress at that time. Support at diagnosis also affected fathers' distress at 1 year, and changes during the year in support accompanied changes in fathers' level of distress. This was not found for mothers. Dissatisfaction with support was the better predictor of distress. It seems that not so much a lack in *quantity* of support is relevant, but more the dissatisfaction with support.

MARITAL SATISFACTION

Parents may need each other most for support when dealing with the multiple stresses of childhood cancer. The quality of their marriage is therefore of importance. While some found that a higher percentage of parents report marital distress than is normal in the general population (Dahlquist et al., 1993; Fife et al., 1987), others report that marital satisfaction remained unchanged or even increased (Barbarin et al., 1985; Kupst and Schulman, 1988). Our study, using the Maudsley Marital Questionnaire (MMQ; Arrindell et al., 1983), showed that although both fathers and mothers reported significantly more marital dissatisfaction during the year following the diagnosis, their level of dissatisfaction remained comparable with that of a norm population. The level of marital dissatisfaction of the parents was significantly lower than that of a group with recognized marital problems. Our results also showed that while 43% of the parents reported more marital dissatisfaction, 20% indicated more satisfaction (Hoekstra-Weebers et al., 1998c). For some parents, the experience of childhood cancer may have strengthened their relationship, which was also suggested earlier (Barbarin et al., 1985), although a larger subgroup reported the opposite.

Parents each have to cope with the stresses of their child's cancer treatment. This may implicate that not only their own coping strategies but also those of their partner may affect their marital satisfaction. It has been found that use of problem-focused coping was positively associated with marital distress at diagnosis, but not 2 years later (Dahlquist et al., 1996). Our study showed that the marital dissatisfaction of fathers was significantly and positively predicted by their own use of coping styles (unique effects for emotion-focused, but not for problem-focused, coping) but not by that of their partners. In contrast, mothers' marital dissatisfaction was significantly predicted by their partners' coping, rather than by their own (Hoekstra-Weebers et al., 1998c). These results suggest that mothers may be more sensitive or open to the influences of their partners' coping pattern with this life event than fathers are.

It has been suggested that difficulties in a marriage may arise when partners use different coping styles (Koocher and O'Malley, 1981). One study showed that differences in approach or avoidance coping within couples were unrelated to marital distress (Dahlquist et al., 1996). A second study reported that symmetry (equal use) in emotion-focused coping and complementary (differential use) in problem-focused coping was associated with marital quality (Barbarin et al., 1985). Our analyses revealed that discrepancies in coping within couples, and in particular a discrepancy (or asymmetry) in emotion-focused coping, were positively associated with marital distress in both partners (Hoekstra-Weebers et al., 1998c), which partially supports the suggestion of Barbarin et al. (1985).

INTERVENTIONS FOR PARENTS

Only two studies have reported results of the effectiveness of an intervention program for parents of children newly diagnosed with cancer. The first is the study of Kupst and Schulman (1988). They compared parents of children with leukemia who received the usual available care with parents who were offered additional contacts with the pediatric oncology team when initiated by themselves, and with parents who had frequent contacts with a directive therapeutic focus during the period of treatment. While the intervention appeared effective for mothers in the first 6 months following the diagnosis, no effects were found later in time. The second study was undertaken by Hoekstra-Weebers et al. (1998b). Parents of children newly diagnosed with cancer who were receiving the usual standard care and attention from the pediatric oncology team were compared with parents who were offered an additional structured intervention program during the first 6 months following the diagnosis. During eight sessions with individual couples, cognitive–behavioral techniques were used to identify and challenge negative automatic thoughts, to express emotions, to encourage problem-focused coping skills, to train communication and assertiveness skills, to assess the need for support and discuss how to obtain it, and to inform about the possible consequences of the illness and treatment for the entire family. Statistical analyses revealed no beneficial effects of the intervention on psychological functioning, on satisfaction with support received, or on the intensity of negative and positive emotions. However, medium-sized effects were found for both parents on the intensity of negative emotions and for mothers on state anxiety, which means that the intervention did have some clinical relevance. Parents who had received the intervention experienced less negative emotions with time, and mothers were less anxious, than parents who had the usual care. The clinical evaluation of the intervention showed that these parents perceived the sessions as supportive and meaningful. Several suggestions were given to explain the absence of a statistical effect. These included: (a) the use of standardized questionnaires that assess psychological functioning in a general, global way, while more disease-specific questionnaires could have given more insight; (b) the fact that little attention was paid to the changing demands of the treatment, because the intervention was focused on coping with immediate distress resulting from the diagnosis and preparing parents for future potentially stressful events; (c) the timing (immediately after diagnosis) may have been wrong and the intervention time (16 hours in 6 months) may have led to too little continuity; (d) the structured program may not have given enough attention to other possibly more stressful problems.

IMPLICATIONS FOR FUTURE RESEARCH

It is evident from our study as well as from others that many parents, after the initial and devastating shock of the cancer diagnosis, return with time to a level of psychological functioning that is considered normal. However, there remains a substantial subgroup of parents who can be diagnosed as clinically distressed, even though their children are cancer survivors. Efforts should be directed at identifying these vulnerable parents. Therefore, it is necessary to examine risk factors associated with maladjustment.

The model in our prospective study was used to categorize possible risk variables. Demographics and objective illness variables were not related to parental distress. Anxiety intrinsic to personality was a strong predictor for both parents. Coping styles and social support were better predictors for fathers than for mothers. It may well be that mothers' psychological functioning, because they have such a unique care-taking role in the family, is more influenced by variables such as family functioning, mother–child interaction, and perceived parental competence (Kazak et al., 1998; Wallander and Varni, 1998) than by their coping behavior or by social support. The models presented by Wallander and Varni (1998) and Thompson et al., (1994) provide examples in which such variables are included. A second major benefit of their model is that the reciprocal relationship between children's functioning and parents' functioning is addressed.

The results of our study showed how important it is to assess fathers' functioning, which for practical reasons was neglected in many studies (Dolgin and Phipps, 1996). Fathers' level of psychological distress was similar to that of the mothers. However, numerous differences were found between fathers and mothers in variables predicting adjustment. Our study also showed (especially the results on marital functioning) how intertwined the functioning of partners is. Future research should therefore focus on all family members, because individual characteristics and family processes interact in complex and, for the greater part, unknown ways.

Researchers have not given enough attention to the relationship between intrapersonal factors and parental adjustment. Not only was trait anxiety the strongest predictor of future distress, changes in trait anxiety and assertiveness appeared to be associated with changes in distress. This finding is interesting, because personality is often considered to be stable over time. Therefore, longitudinal studies are necessary to replicate or contradict such a finding.

Further longitudinal studies are required because little is known still about the prospective effects of possible predictor variables and the effect of changes in those variables on parental adjustment. The individual parents' adjustment, that of the children and/or that of the whole family system may depend upon changes in such variables as the conditions of the cancer stressor change as a consequence of treatment. A longitudinal design with repeated measures allows for analytical methods to examine the causal direction between various predictor variables and psychological adjustment.

The number of participating parents of childhood cancer patients or survivors in the majority of studies is small, which limits statistical power. Childhood cancer is a rare disease (Miller et al., 1995). Multicentered studies are needed to obtain large enough samples to test multivariate models, using more advanced analytical procedures, such as path analysis, with sufficient power.

The inconsistent findings about parental adjustment can, in part, be attributed to the selection of outcome measure. There is a need for an instrument that, apart from providing information about several dimensions of generic quality of life, is sensitive to areas specifically affected by disease and treatment. For example, Kazak et al. (1998) showed that continuing intrusive memories and flashbacks about cancer were present in parents of childhood cancer survivors, using an instrument assessing post-traumatic stress symptoms.

Parental cognitive processes of appraisals of the stresses of diagnosis and consequent treatment are further relevant concepts. Such event-specific perceptions may influence parental choice for coping behavior, which in turn may affect adjustment (Folkman et al., 1986). Clinical practice indicates that the experience of childhood cancer seems also to profoundly change perceptions of life values (e.g. a choice of time investment in the family over that in the pursuit of a career). These may be healthy, normal responses and represent growth, and parents may report good overall quality of life. However, the opposite may also be true.

Future intervention studies are needed. The studies reviewed have typically offered a relatively similar intervention to all parents. An intervention offered to a subgroup of at-risk parents tailored to their individual and specific needs may be beneficial. This would be clinically relevant and also economical, since there is a serious shortage of both time and money in clinical practice.

ACKNOWLEDGMENTS

This study was funded by the Dutch Cancer Society and the Pediatric Oncology Foundation Groningen.

REFERENCES

Adams-Greenly, M. (1986). Psychological staging of pediatric cancer patients and their families. *Cancer* **58**: 449–453.

Arrindell, W.A., Boelens, W. and Lambert, H. (1983). On the psychometric properties of the Maudsley Marital Questionnaire (MMQ): Evaluation of self-ratings in distressed and 'normal' volunteer couples based on the Dutch version. *Personality and Individual Differences* **4**: 293–306.

Arrindell, W.A. and Ende, J. (1985). Cross-sample invariance of the structure of self-reported distress and difficulty in assertiveness: experiences with the Scale for Interpersonal Behaviour. *Advances in Behaviour Research and Therapy* **7**: 205–243.

Barakat L.P., Kazak, A.E., Meadows, A.T., Casey, R., Meeske, K. and Stuber, M.L. (1997). Families surviving childhood cancer: a comparison of posttraumatic stress symptoms with families of healthy children. *Journal of Pediatric Psychology* **22**: 843–859.

Barbarin, O.A., Hughes, D. and Chesler, M.A. (1985). Stress, coping, and marital functioning among parents of children with cancer. *Journal of Marriage and the Family* **47**: 473–480.

Barbarin, O.A. and Chesler, M.A. (1986). The medical context of parental coping with childhood cancer. *American Journal of Community Psychology* **14**: 221–235.

Brown, R.T., Kaslow, N.J., Madan-Swain, A., Doepke, K.J., Sexson, S.B. and Hill, L.J. (1993). Parental psychopathology and children's adjustment to leukemia. *Journal of the American Academy of Child and Adolescent Psychiatry* **32**: 554–561.

Cohen, S. and Wills, T.A. (1985). Stress, social support, and the buffering hypothesis. *Psychological Bulletin* **98**: 310–357.

Dahlquist, L.M., Czewski, D.I., Copeland, K.G., Jones, C.L., Taub, E. and Vaughan, J.K. (1993). Parents of children newly diagnosed with cancer: anxiety, coping and marital distress. *Journal of Pediatric Psychology* **18**(3): 365–376.

Dahlquist, L.M., Czyzewski, D.I. and Jones, C.L. (1996). Parents of children with cancer: a longitudinal study of emotional distress, coping style, and marital adjustment two and twenty months after diagnosis. *Journal of Pediatric Psychology* **21**(4): 541–554.

Derogatis, L.R. (1997). *SCL-90. Administration, Scoring and Procedures Manual-1 for the Revised Version and Other Instruments of the Psychopathology Rating Scale Series.* Baltimore, MD: Clinical Psychometrics Research Unit, Johns Hopkins University School of Medicine.

Dolgin, M. and Phipps, S. (1996). Reciprocal influences in family adjustment to childhood cancer. In L. Baider, C.L. Cooper and A. Kaplan De-Nour (Eds), *Cancer and the Family* (pp. 73–92). Chichester: Wiley.

Fife, B., Norton, J. and Groom, G. (1987). The family's adaptation to childhood leukemia. *Social Science and Medicine* **24**: 159–168.

Folkman, S., Lazarus, F.S., Dunkel-Schetter C., DeLongis, A. and Gruen, F.J. (1986). Dynamics of a stressful encounter: cognitive appraisal, coping, and encounter outcomes. *Journal of Personality and Social Psychology* **50**: 992–1003.

Goldberg, D.P. and Williams, P. (1988). *A User's Guide to the General Health Questionnaire.* Windsor: NFER–Nelson.

Granowetter, L. (1994). Pediatric oncology: a medical overview. In D.J. Bearson and R.K. Mulhern (Eds), *Pediatric Psychooncology: Psychological Perspectives on Children with Cancer* (pp. 9–34). New York: Oxford University Press.

Greenberg, H.S. and Meadows, A.T. (1992). Psychosocial impact of cancer survival on school-age children and their parents. *Journal of Psychosocial Oncology* **9**: 43–56.

Grootenhuis, M.A. and Last, B.F. (1997). Adjustment and coping by parents of children with cancer: a review of the literature. *Supportive Care in Cancer* **5**: 466–484.

Hoekstra-Weebers, J.E.H.M., Heuvel, F., Boskamp, H.E.P., Kamps, W.A. and Klip, E.C. (1996). Social support and psychological distress of parents of pediatric cancer patients. In L. Baider, C.L. Cooper and A. Kaplan De-Nour (Eds), *Cancer and the Family* (pp. 93–106). Chichester: Wiley.

Hoekstra-Weebers, J.E.H.M., Kamps, W.A. and Klip, E.C. (1998a). Gender differences in psychological adaptation and coping in parents of pediatric cancer patients. *Psycho-Oncology* **7**: 26–36.

Hoekstra-Weebers, J.E.H.M., Jaspers, J.P.C., Kamps, W.A. and Klip, E.C. (1998b). Brief report: an intervention program for parents of pediatric cancer patients: a randomized controlled trial. *Journal of Pediatric Psychology* **23**: 207–214.

Hoekstra-Weebers, J.E.H.M., Jaspers, J.P.C., Kamps, W.A. and Klip, E.C. (1998c). Marital dissatisfaction, psychological distress and the coping of parents of pediatric cancer patients. *Journal of Marriage and the Family* **60**: 1012–1021.

Hoekstra-Weebers, J.E.H.M., Jaspers, J.P.C., Kamps, W.A. and Klip, E.C. (submitted, a). Coping and Psychological Adjustment of Parents of Pediatric Cancer Patients: a longitudinal study.

Hoekstra-Weebers, J.E.H.M., Jaspers, J.P.C., Kamps, W.A. and Klip, E.C. (1999). Risk factors for psychological maladjustment of parents of children with cancer. *Journal of the American Academy of Child and Adolescent Psychiatry* **38**: 1526–1535.

Hoekstra-Weebers, J.E.H.M., Jaspers, J.P.C., Kamps, W.A. & Klip, E.C. (submitted, b). Social support and Psychological Adjustment of Parents of Childhood Cancer Patients.

Kazak, A. and Meadows, A. (1989). Families of young adolescents who have survived cancer: social-emotional adjustment, adaptability and social support. *Journal of Pediatric Psychology* **14**: 175–191.

Kazak, A.E. (1994). Implications of survival: pediatric oncology patients and their families. In D.J. Bearison and R.K. Mulhern (Eds), *Pediatric Psychooncology: Psychological Perspectives on Children with Cancer* (pp. 171–192). New York: Oxford University Press.

Kazak, A.E., Barakat, L.M., Meeske, K., Christakis, D., Meadows, A.T., Casey, R., Penati, B., Stuber, M.L. (1997). Post traumatic stress, family functioning, and social support in survivors of childhood leukemia and their mothers and fathers. *Journal of Consulting and Clinical Psychology* **65**: 120–129.

Kazak, A.E., Stuber, M.L., Barakat, L.P., Meeske, K., Guthrie, D., Meadows, A.T. (1998). Predicting posttraumatic stress symptoms in mothers and fathers of survivors of childhood cancers. *Journal of the American Academy of Child and Adolescent Psychiatry* **37**: 823–831.

Koeter, M.W.J. and Ormel, J. (1991). *General Health Questionnaire* (Dutch manual). Lisse: Swets and Zeitlinger BV.

Koocher, G.P. and O'Malley, J.E. (1981). *The Damocles Syndrome. Psychosocial Consequences of Surviving Childhood Cancer.* New York: McGraw-Hill.

Kupst, M. and Schulman, J. (1988). Long-term coping with pediatric leukemia: a six-year follow-up study. *Journal of Pediatric Psychology* **13**: 7–22.

Kupst, M.J., Natta, M.B., Richardson, C.C., Schulman, J.L., Lavigne, J.V. and Das, L. (1995). Family coping with pediatric leukemia: ten years after treatment. *Journal of Pediatric Psychology* **20**: 601–617.

Manne, S.L., Lesanics, D., Meyers, P., Wollner, N., Steinherz, P. and Redd, W. (1995). Predictors of depressive symptomatology among parents of newly diagnosed children with cancer. *Journal of Pediatric Psychology* **20**: 491–510.

Miller, R.W., Young, J.L. Jr and Novakovic, B. (1995). Childhood cancer. *Cancer* **75**: 395–405.

Morrow, G.R., Carpenter, P.J. and Hoagland, A.C. (1984). The role of social support in parental adjustment to pediatric cancer. *Journal of Pediatric Psychology* **9**: 317–329.

Ostroff, J. and Steinglass, P. (1996). Psychosocial adaptation following treatment: a family systems perspective on childhood cancer survivorship. In L. Baider, C.L. Cooper, A. Kaplan De-Nour (Eds), *Cancer and the Family* (pp. 129–147). Chichester: Wiley.

Sawyer, M.G., Antoniou, G., Toogood, I., Rice, M. and Baghurst, P.A. (1993). A prospective study of the psychological adjustment of parents and families of children with cancer. *Journal of Paediatrics and Child Health* **29**: 352–356.

Schreurs, P.J., Willigen, G. van de, Tellegen, B. and Brosschot, J.F. (1993). *De Utrechtse Coping Lijst: UCL-Handleiding* (The Utrecht Coping List: UCL Manual). Lisse: Swets and Zeitlinger.

Sonderen, E. van. (1993). *The Measurement of Social Support with the SSQ-I and the SSQ-D.* (Dutch manual). Groningen: Noordelijk Centrum voor Gezondheidsvraagstukken.

Speechley, K.N. and Noh, S. (1992). Surviving childhood cancer, social support, and parents' psychological adjustment. *Journal of Pediatric Psychology* **17**: 15–31.

Spielberger, C. (1983). *Manual for the State–Trait Anxiety Inventory.* Palo Alto, CA: Consulting Psychologists' Press.

Thompson, R.J., Gustafson, K.E., George, L.K. and Spock, A. (1994). Change over a 12-month period in the psychological adjustment of children and adolescents with cystic fibrosis. *Journal of Pediatric Psychology* **19**: 189–203.

Van Dongen-Melman, J.E.W.M., Pruyn, J.F.A., DeGroot, A., Koot, H.M., Hählen, K. and Verhulst, F.C. (1995). Late consequences for parents of children who survived cancer. *Journal of Pediatric Psychology* **20**: 567–586.

Veldhuizen, A.M.H. and Last, B.F. (1991). *Children with Cancer. Communication and Emotions*. Amsterdam: Swets and Zeitlinger.

Wallander, J.L. and Varni, J.W. (1998). Effects of pediatric chronic physical disorders on child and family adjustment. *Journal of Child Psychology and Psychiatry* **39**: 29–46.

'My Family and I are in this Together': Children with Cancer Speak Out*

BARBARA M. SOURKES

Montreal Children's Hospital and McGill University, Montreal, Quebec, Canada

RENÉE PROULX

Université du Québec à Montréal, Montreal, Quebec, Canada

My family and I are in this together. We have not been sleeping well lately. . . .

The child-in-the-family is a unit unto itself, with its own distinctive identity, strengths and vulnerabilities. The child's ongoing struggle to withstand and integrate the trauma of cancer unfolds within this framework. His/her ability to cope is greatly influenced by the family—the individual and collective responses of its members. Under optimal circumstances, 'the interior of the family assumes a central role in preserving the patient's psychological integrity' (Rait and Holland, 1986, p. 4). The family affords a refuge in which the child can replenish psychic resources, shielded from the battering assault of the illness (Sourkes, 1995).

From the outset, the child's definition of his/her 'family' (both biological and psychological members) should be elicited. Without such information, the caregiver's assumptions of inclusion or exclusion may be faulty, and valuable sources of support to the child overlooked. The nuclear family of child, siblings and parents is at the core, surrounded by the extended family. In particular, grandparents frequently play a major role in the child's care. Close friends may be indistinguishable from 'family,' especially during crises. The child often names a pet as a family member—a relationship whose importance must not be underestimated. With the changing face of the structure of the family, latitude must be given for alternative and complicated arrangements. These include divorced and reconstituted (blended) families, with their inherent conflictual histories and new alliances; single-parent families; and children of gay parents. Thus, in circumstances that range from the traditional to the extraordinary, the child's definition of 'family' is a significant reality.

*The clinical section of this chapter is adapted from *Armfuls of Time: The Psychological Experience of the Child with a Life-threatening Illness*, by Barbara M. Sourkes, © 1995. Used by permission of the University of Pittsburgh Press.

Cancer and the Family, 2nd Edn. Edited by L. Baider, C. L. Cooper and A. Kaplan De-Nour
© 2000 John Wiley & Sons, Ltd

This chapter will review the literature and address selected clinical issues that pertain to the child who is currently being treated for cancer (not to issues of long-term survivorship).

REVIEW OF THE LITERATURE

THE CHILD'S EXPERIENCE OF THE ILLNESS

For the child with cancer, 'being sick' constitutes a new role that alters relationships—both with others and with self (Schulman 1980; Van Dongen-Melman and Sanders-Woudstra, 1986b; Sourkes, 1998). Although each child lives the illness in a unique way, all children are confronted with universal issues of separation and loss, as well as struggles around competence and control (Brunquell and Hall, 1982; Enskär et al., 1997a; Van Dongen-Melman and Sanders-Woudstra, 1986a,b).

The child's understanding of cancer, as well as his/her concerns, needs, and developmental phase, all influence the lived experience of the illness. Although there is no cognitive comprehension of the illness for the infant and toddler (aged 0–2), the child's sensorimotor functioning means that sensitivity to his/her body and immediate environment is acute (Gibbons, 1988). The repeated experience of invasive medical procedures leads some children to react to any physical contact— even comfort—as threatening and aversive. For the child who does not yet have the ability to conceptualize all that is happening—discomfort, pain, separation from parents—and the level of distress may be profound. Initial research is examining whether the illness and its treatments can have an adverse effect on the early attachment between parents and child. One study of 12 month-olds (Goldberg et al., 1995) found that, as a group, children who were ill (with cystic fibrosis or cardiac problems) differed from healthy children: there were fewer who demonstrated a secure attachment, and more whose attachment was insecure. However, this type of difference was not observed in a study with children with cystic fibrosis aged 12–18 months (Fischer-Fay et al., 1988). Although these studies are only preliminary, they do suggest the importance of understanding the impact of cancer on parent–child attachment when the illness occurs in the early months of life.

The thought processes of the preschooler (3–5 years) are sufficiently mature for the child to begin to seek explanations and to resolve certain problems (Gibbons, 1988), even if he/she cannot yet truly understand the complexity of illness. Given both the egocentric nature of the child's thought, as well as the early development of moral thinking, certain children may interpret the illness and its consequences as a form of punishment for something they have done (Sroufe et al., 1992; Gibbons, 1988). Physical restrictions and the loss of mobility affect the child's newly-emerging sense of competence and control during this stage of development (Brunquell and Hall, 1982).

By about the age of 6, the child has developed a repertoire of cognitive abilities that allow understanding of the illness. His/her initial formulations are closely linked to personal experience (Gibbons, 1988). At first, the child's view of the illness is global and concrete, tied to the immediacy of physiological functions and symptoms. Only gradually does the child understand the illness in a broader context, including concepts of causation and cure as well as psychological aspects (Bibace and Walsh, 1980; Hymovich, 1995). In a study of children with leukemia, aged 5–12 years, the majority of children understood the nature of the illness and the rationale for treatment (Ross, 1989).

The experience of cancer for the school-aged child is marked by the effects of treatment and the isolation from peers, school and other normal activities (Van Dongen-Melman and Sanders-Woudstra, 1986b; Sexson and Madan-Swain,1993; Enskär et al., 1997b). Although the child frequently fears the re-entry process to school, there is evidence that, for children (aged 8–13) newly diagnosed with cancer, the social support provided by schoolmates is the form of support most strongly associated with overall psychosocial adjustment (Varni et al., 1994). Thus, a prompt reintegration into the classroom is crucial (Varni et al., 1994; Sourkes, 1998). Emotional reactions of the school-aged child include fluctuations in mood, feelings of being different, thoughts of death, manifestation of regressive behavior. Pain, fear of pain, and fear of the unknown constitute the most difficult aspects of hospitalization (Enskär et al., 1997b).

As the child approaches adolescence, he/she becomes increasingly capable of thinking about the illness within a broader and more abstract cognitive framework. He/she refers more to the internal experience of living with the illness, and becomes conscious of potentially long-term physical and psychological sequelae (Hymovich, 1995). The child clearly recognizes the repercussions of the illness on his/her life as well as on that of parents and siblings (Enskär et al., 1997a).

The adolescent with cancer, already preoccupied with changes in his or her appearance and with the absence from 'normal life' of peers and school, must also grapple with the intensified dependence on parents at a time when the longing for independence is paramount. The adolescent looks to make sense of all that has happened ('Why me?'). Following diagnosis, adolescents describe a flux of emotions, including disbelief, depression, loneliness, aggressivity. At a time of feeling so powerless, he/she must find some positive belief in the future. The young person seeks support in many arenas: family and friends; teachers and classmates; other young people with cancer; information from professionals or educational associations. The adolescent is particularly sensitive to, and values, a respectful attitude on the part of the professionals involved in his/her care (Enskär et al., 1997a).

The information given to children seems to constitute an important factor in their adjustment (Nannis, Susman et al, 1982). Children differ in their need or desire for information: some want detailed information about their treatment in advance, while others prefer partial information at the time of treatment, or, in some instances, a minimum at any time (Ross, 1989). Proponents of the 'protective' approach believe that certain aspects of the illness, particularly its life-threatening nature, should not be divulged until the child has acquired a mature view of death (Van Dongen-Melman and Sanders-Woudstra, 1986b).

ADJUSTMENT OF THE CHILD WITH CANCER

The stress of cancer is a challenge to any child's resources and vulnerabilities. Studies have shown that children with a chronic physical disorder are at increased risk for psychosocial adjustment problems (Wallander et al., 1988; Lavigne and Faier-Routman,1992; Varni et al., 1994; Wallander and Varni, 1998). Even in children where normal psychological patterns are intact, the illness may cause some to temporarily abandon newly-acquired abilities, to demonstrate regressive behavior, or to develop behavioral problems (Brunquell and Hall, 1982; Van Dongen-Melman and Sanders-Woudstra, 1986b; Hymovich and Roehner, 1989; Brown et al., 1992; Martinson and Bossert, 1994). The most frequently reported problems reported of children on treatment are anxiety and depression (Brown et al., 1992; Varni et al., 1994; Enskär et al., 1997b). In general, these problems are more marked in children within the first year after diagnosis than in those who have finished treatment and are in remission (Brown et al., 1992).

All the reactions demonstrated by children with cancer may be seen as attempts at adaptation within a difficult set of circumstances (Schulman and Kupst, 1980; Van Dongen-Melman and Sanders-Woudstra, 1986b). Children develop new competencies and strategies in problem-solving and emotional regulation as they confront the challenge of the illness (Brown et al., 1992). Many mature quickly and develop a positive attitude toward life (Enskär et al., 1997a,b). Some young people express the wish to 'give something back' and envision, for example, working in the field of health care (Enskär et al., 1997a).

THE CHILD IN THE FAMILY

The adaptation of the child to an illness such as cancer must be seen from an ecological perspective (Wallander et al., 1988; Kazak, 1989, 1993); that is, as an interaction of the child's personal characteristics, the nature and trajectory of the illness, the impact (direct and indirect) of people and life conditions around the child (including sociocultural factors). Without doubt, it is the parents who exert the most influence on the child's adjustment—and it is they who are the most studied.

The exigencies of cancer and its treatment mean that the life of the entire family is governed by the condition of the child (Enskär, 1997c). The parents' personal life plans are upset, their private life as a couple diminished, and relationships with the children change (Enskär, 1997c). 'Special arrangements' multiply as the parents struggle to organize visits to the hospital and clinic, all the while trying to assure the healthy siblings of time and attention (Van Dongen-Melman and Sanders-Woudstra, 1986a).The parents suffer in seeing their child suffer, and feel powerless and incompetent in their role as 'protectors' (Cook, 1984; Van Dongen-Melman and Sanders-Woudstra,1986a; Enskär, 1997c). Many parents report that living with constant uncertainty is the most difficult repercussion of childhood cancer on the family (Sourkes, 1982; Enskär, 1997c). In these stressful circumstances, parents nonetheless struggle to give their ill child the most normal life experience possible (Van Dongen-Melman and Sanders-Woudstra, 1986b; Canam, 1993; Sourkes 1995, 1998). They strive to ensure that the child is neither overprotected nor spoiled (concerns shared by the professional caregivers as well, Davies et al., 1991) during the course of treatment. Parental stress seems to peak about 1 year after diagnosis and then gradually diminishes. In general, however, parents seem to present with good psychosocial adjustment (Brown et al., 1992, 1993). Studies are now demonstrating the reciprocal relationship that exists between child (with cancer)-

parent adjustment, as well as that between parents and the healthy siblings (Dolgin and Phipps, 1996).

Although there has been little research on the immediate impact of the illness on siblings (Shapiro and Brack, 1994), initial findings are that brothers and sisters, like the ill child, are also at increased risk of adjustment problems (Cornam, 1993; Cincotta, 1993; Walker, 1990). Foremost issues in the sibling experience include: loss of parental attention; loneliness; change in family roles, structure, rules and expectations; concerns about the cause of the child's illness; feelings of guilt and anxiety; fear of death; and exacerbated sibling rivalry. Certain siblings express their stress through depression and anxiety; others may develop medical problems (including psychosomatic symptoms) or manifest acting-out behaviors (Koch,1985; Koch-Hattem, 1986; Madan-Swain et al., 1993; Shapiro and Brack, 1994; Sourkes, 1980, 1987; Walker, 1990). In a constructive attempt to regain a sense of control, some siblings invest intensely in their academic work as a means toward mastery (Shapiro and Brack, 1994). Like the ill child, siblings often try to protect their parents from their concerns. Thus, the parents must be particularly attuned to the siblings' expressions of worry, anger and stress.

In conclusion, one cannot talk about the family's adaptation to childhood cancer without naming certain conditions that influence this process. These include: the mental health and preexisting coping styles of the parents; socioeconomic status; structure and functioning of the family; and marital, family and community support (Kupst et al., 1993). Certain life events such as the loss of employment, financial problems or a geographical move can also affect the adaptive process. In the context of the child who is being treated, these concurrent stresses take on a particular impact and can amplify the family distress. When the stresses are closely linked to the illness, they become particularly anxiogenic. The stresses most frequently reported by families are the illness of another family member, medical complications of the ill child, and the death of another child being treated for cancer (Kalnins et al., 1980).

CLINICAL ISSUES

THE IMPACT OF DIAGNOSIS

Cancer is filled with hardship and terror for the child on both a physical and an emotional level. Its ravages are an entity to be reckoned with on an ongoing basis, not a psychic abstraction. From the moment of diagnosis, the illness wends a perilous course; the unknown lies ahead like an uncharted chasm, without boundaries or guides.

> When I heard that I had leukemia, I turned pale with shock. I was scared of blood, needles, of seeing all the doctors, of what was going to happen to me. I was mad about a lot of things: staying in the hospital, taking medicines, bone marrows, spinal taps, IVs, being awakened in the middle of the night. I was sad that I didn't have my toys and that I was missing out on everything. I felt lonely because I was crying about not being at home and not being able to go outside. I also felt hope: for getting better, going home, eating food from home, and seeing my friends.

This 8 year-old child captures the immediacy of the response to the diagnosis of cancer. He articulates the shock; the fear of everything from the concrete medical procedures to the sudden possibility of an altered future ('what was going to happen to me'); the constellation of sadness, grief, and loneliness of separation; and the absence from his normal life. Accompanying all these feelings is a forthright statement of hope.

In another description of the reaction to diagnosis, an 11 year-old child reflected:

> You feel shock—it's like coming to a stop-light, or like being hit by a bolt of lightning. Anger is a very, very dark feeling. You feel scared all the time of what is going to happen to you. Even with people around, you feel alone and very sad. I think of hope as yellow—a sunny color with a lot of light. But you do feel helpless—tiny and scared. Confused . . . you're confused about everything going on and how this could all be happening to you.

Other feelings cited by children include pain, terror, embarrassment, and shame. All these words attest to the overwhelming onslaught of new and frightening experiences that must be quickly assimilated. Such is the 'irreversibly altered reality' (Sourkes, 1982, p. 45) into which the child is catapulted by the diagnosis. Regardless of which aspects of life may appear unchanged, in fact, nothing is the same. The diagnosis thus stands as a dividing line, a marker of 'before and after.' The child, who garners security from predictability, and whose sense of time and timing is not yet well anchored, is thrust into a world of uncertain contingencies. The profundity of the disruption is daunting even to imagine.

Much attention has been devoted to the impact of telling vs. not telling the child the diagnosis and prognosis. The protective stance of the past stated that disclosure to the child would cause increased anxiety and fear. Over the last two decades, however, a shift toward open communication has been evident—toward '*how* to tell' rather than '*whether* to tell'. To shield the child from the truth may only heighten anxiety and cause the child to feel isolated, lonely, and unsure of whom to trust. While the diagnosis is an event in time, 'telling' is a process over time. How to inform the child of the diagnosis should be decided by the parents in consultation with the staff, thereby establishing a crucial alliance from the outset. The parents' design for the disclosure must be carefully heeded: it is they who know the child best, and can gauge his/her resilience in absorbing the news. Furthermore, it is the parents who will see the child through every phase of the illness. The individual child's competence and vulnerability serve as the context for decisions regarding disclosure. Considerations about what, or how much, to tell include: the child's age, cognitive and emotional maturity, family structure and functioning, cultural background, and history of loss. The child's previous experiences with loss bear significantly on his/her reaction to the diagnosis, its meaning and portent. Thus, a child's 'loss history,' and response to it, are crucial to obtain. The history encompasses loss in its broadest sense; for example, illness and death, trauma, change in relationships, especially parental separation/divorce, and geographical moves. Also powerful is the child's past acquaintance with the illness, either personally or through the media. In communication with the life-threatened child at any juncture, 'the truth is not a principle nor a duty nor a rule. The truth is an atmosphere of exchange, of listening, and of respect for the child and his needs. The truth is a state' (Charest and

Douesnard, 1992, p. 473). The precedent for a climate that enables such honest interchange is created from the time of diagnosis.

Anticipatory grief, the experiential process that reflects the anguish of threatened loss, is thrust into being at the time of diagnosis, and ebbs and flows throughout the course of the illness. While the prognosis for many childhood malignancies can now be presented with optimism, the subjective experience of receiving the diagnosis still connotes death. In the following drawings, the child's inward grief for self, and the testimony to the family's grief, are illustrated and articulated.

- *A nine-year-old boy* portrayed his older brother as a rock singer, his mother cooking, another brother, his father, and his pet hamster (Figure 16.1). When asked what had changed after his diagnosis, he added tears to each person. With regard to the omission of himself he explained: 'I didn't include myself, because at the time I was in the hospital, and didn't think I'd be back in the picture.' The little hamster imprisoned in the cage may well be his symbolic self-representation. Thus, the boy graphically conveyed anticipatory grief: the threat of his own absence from his family.

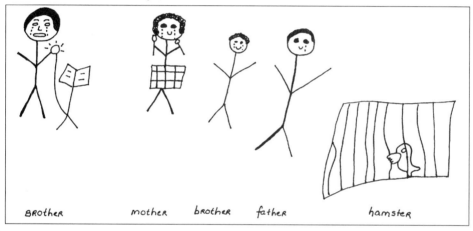

Figure 16.1

- *An 8 year-old boy* hastily drew stick figures to illustrate the members of his family. (Figure 16.2) One brother was playing baseball, another playing hockey, and the patient himself was bald, had no mouth, and was not doing anything. Neither were the parents engaged in any activity. When asked what changed in his family after he became ill, the boy immediately scrawled: 'They all cry.' This is a striking portrait of the child's awareness of anticipatory grief within the family system.

- *A 10 year-old boy*, who had been diagnosed at the age of 6, drew an active and engaging family portrait. When asked what had changed after he got sick, he added slashes of rain to the sky. He then crossed out his little brother, with the commentary: 'my little brother wasn't alive then.' His choice of words—'wasn't alive then', rather than 'wasn't born yet'—attests to the valence of the life–death dichotomy of the diagnosis. He added tears to his mother and showed his father thinking, 'poor kid.' He erased himself playing ball and re-portrayed himself as he was then—in a wheelchair. (Figures 16.3, 16.4).

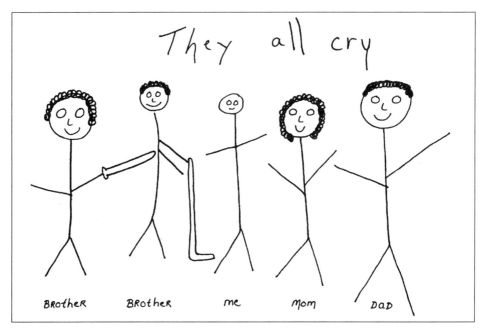

They all cry

BROtheR   BROtheR   me   Mom   DaD

Figure 16.2

FAMILY FUNCTIONING WHEN A CHILD HAS CANCER

The myth that a child's cancer either unites or destroys a family reduces complexity to oversimplification. In fact, resilience or vulnerability to the stress of the illness depends upon a myriad of factors. A family's experience and means of coping with adversity in the past will, to some extent, predict its response in the present. Salient dimensions of family functioning, which must be viewed through a sociocultural as well as a psychological lens, include: open/closed style of communication (both informational and affective); close/distant emotional involvement; flexible/rigid roles; organized/chaotic overall structure. How power and control are defined and delegated within the family, as well as how children are viewed (in terms of their individualism and competence), must be understood. The availability of support from extended family, friends and community is also an important consideration. Inextricably linked with all these variables are the nature and course of the disease itself. Certain factors severely compromise a family's capacity to adapt to the exigencies of a child's illness. For example, a history of psychiatric disturbance, marital conflict, addiction, abuse, and financial problems put a family at elevated risk.

Within a systems view, stress in one part of the family affects all the other members. Bowen (1976), a founder of family therapy, referred to the 'emotional shock wave' phenomenon:

> . . . a network of underground 'aftershocks' of serious life events that can occur anywhere in the extended family system in the months or years following serious

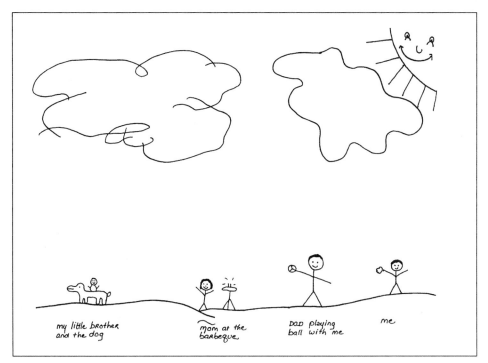

Figure 16.3

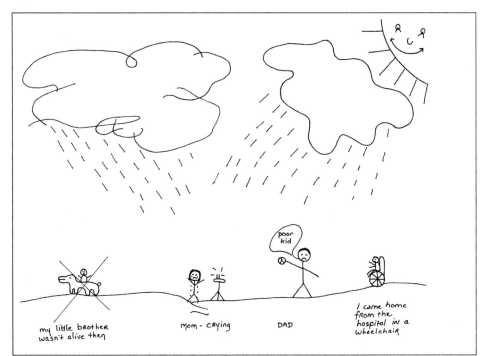

Figure 16.4

emotional events in a family. It occurs most often after the death or the *threatened death* [italics added] of a significant family member (1976, p. 339).

The child witnesses these reverberations, and instinctively locates his/her illness as the cause. Guilt is a common response, even in the rational light of knowing that he/she did not ask for the illness to happen.

- *An 11 year-old girl* reflected sadly: 'My mother and father had a hard life. It's not that I think that it's my fault. There was nothing I could do about being sick. But it was like I was the last straw.'

- *A 4 year-old 'only' child* asked his parents: 'Are you not having a new baby because you don't want another sick kid?'

- *A 9 year-old boy* had barely sat down before he began to speak: 'I think that my illness causes problems for everybody. They all have to worry a lot. Last night when I'd already gone to bed, I heard my parents arguing about money. *They'd have enough money if I were dead.*' He burst into tears.

- *A 10 year-old girl* listed each family member's reaction to her illness (excluding herself): 'Mother—cried [sadness and anticipatory grief]; father—got thinner, but gained it back when I got better [psychosomatic expression]; brother—got uptight easily [chronic tension]; sister—got a boyfriend [peer support—or flight from pain in family].' The girl's cryptic descriptions portray the manifestations of stress in her family.

In many instances, the child denies that the illness has caused problems for the family. He/she may report positive changes, but is reluctant or unable to think of difficulties. It is as if the child cannot afford to acknowledge any stress because of the guilt associated with being its 'cause.'

- In response to what had changed in her family, *a 12 year-old girl* stated: 'To me, I couldn't see a change, although my family may have had to adjust themselves.' She thus began with denial, and then vaguely conceded that perhaps there was some impact.

Changes in Pre-existent Roles and Relationships

The presence of cancer, while linked most obviously to the ill child, creates changes in all the pre-existent roles and relationships within the family. Most common is the intensification of the relationship between the child and the parents (especially the mother), and the exclusion of the healthy siblings. The centrality of attention accorded to the child is understandable, and even necessary, during critical periods. However, when this focus becomes the norm over time, a complicated tangle of dysfunction can result. The child wields too much power, the marital dyad is disrupted, and the siblings lose their visibility in the family. While the child often observes and worries about the imbalances incurred by the illness, his/her state of vulnerability and need overshadows these concerns. Furthermore, it is not the child's responsibility to redress the balance of the family constellation.

- *A 6 year-old 'only' child* constantly tried to prevent his parents from going out on their own. He would predict terrible thunderstorms prior to their departure, or have a temper tantrum when the babysitter arrived. When the therapist addressed the fact that parents need to spend time together, without kids, the boy responded: 'See that window? I'm going to throw you out of it, and I'm going to handcuff my parents' hands together to a piece of furniture in here.'

- *A 9 year-old girl* explained: 'I think that my brother and sister are really mad at me, because I get all the presents and a lot of attention. They think I'm spoiled. I'd be mad at me if I were them. But they don't have to go for treatments like I do.'

If the child has functioned in some pivotal way in the family, his/her role may be dramatically affected by the onset of the illness.

- A mother referred to her *9 year-old daughter* as 'our own family therapist.' When the girl became sick, and thus unavailable for her usual role, her parents recognized how much they had relied on her to carry out their mandate.

'Protection'

The issue of 'protection' within the family may emerge in various guises throughout the course of the illness. The child's anger that the parents were not able to keep him/her out of harm's way reflects a profoundly shaken sense of safety. Each time the child encounters a new crisis, or undergoes a painful procedure, the loss of protection is evoked anew. He/she learns early that parents are neither omnipotent nor invulnerable, and that threatening forces operate beyond even their control. In witnessing the child's agony, the parents face their own helplessness.

In another facet of protection, the child tries to spare the parents the intensity of his/her fear and sadness. This stance is matched by the parents' attempts to shield the child from any further hardship, especially from witnessing *their* distress. Eventually a cycle is set in motion. This cycle isolates the child and parents from one another at exactly those times that mutual disclosure would create a comforting bridge.

SIBLING RELATIONSHIPS

Sibling relationships are a crucial axis in the family, a subsystem of their own (Sourkes, 1980,1987). The predominant themes that emerge between the child with cancer and the well siblings are mutual anger/resentment and mutual protectiveness/caring.

Siblings may resent the extra attention and privileges accorded the patient, while simultaneously feeling guilty about being healthy. The patient, angry to be sick, voices the injustice ('it's not fair that *I* got sick. . . .'). However, these protests bring only short-lived relief, followed by remorse and guilt at his/her 'monopoly' on the parents' time and energy.

- *A seven-year-old girl* cheerfully announced that she had finished her family picture, after having methodically drawn her parents and younger brother. When the therapist casually asked: 'And what about you?' she responded, startled: 'Oh! I forgot!' Only then did the girl put herself into the picture—solidly on top of her

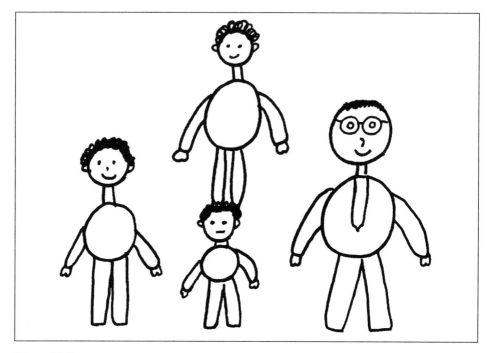

Figure 16.5

brother's head. This triumphant placement reflected the resentment that she had been expressing to her mother in recent weeks: 'Why is he always so healthy and I'm so sick all the time?' (Figure 16.5).

Most children with cancer demonstrate an impressive capacity for concern about the siblings.

● *A child with cancer* said to the therapist: 'Please could you go and talk to my sister *alone*. She needs someone to talk to. Please do it as a favor to me.'

It is not unusual for a child to declare that a brother or sister has been a 'best friend' through the hardship. He/she discovers a new appreciation for the sibling's abiding presence and companionship. To ignore or undervalue the positive caring between the patient and siblings is to neglect an invaluable resource for the children's coping.

*   *   *

CONCLUSION

I have a closer relationship with my family than most other kids because I've needed them more these last years.

This simple and direct statement attests to the inextricable bond between the child with cancer and his/her family. It also reinforces that fact that in terms of psychological care, the 'patient' is the entire family, not only the child who is ill.

With the intrusion of the illness, the relationship between child and family organizes around the pivot of potential loss. Thus, if a child is seen in individual psychotherapy, it is critical that the therapist not intercede as a divisive wedge between them. From the outset, an ongoing alliance between the child's therapist and the parents diminishes this threat and optimizes the outcome of the work. Such collaboration is a *sine qua non* of the process.

Family therapy can play a pivotal role in sustaining, strengthening, and repairing family resources. The profound and enduring impact of the child's illness on the family is addressed within this context. In no way does family therapy preclude or contradict the individual psychotherapy with the child. Rather, it affirms the family unit as a whole, and provides a framework for its healing.

REFERENCES

Bibace, R. and Walsh, M.E. (1980).   Development of children concepts of illness. *Pediatrics* **66**: 912–917.

Bowen, M. (1976).   Family reaction to death. In P.J. Guerin (Ed.), *Family Therapy*. New York: Gardner.

Brown, R.T., Kaslow, N.J., Hazzard, A.P., Madan-Swain, A., Sexson, S.B., Lambert, R., and Baldwin, K. (1992).   Psychiatric and family functioning in children with leukemia and their parents. *Journal of the American Academy of Child and Adolescent Psychiatry* **31**(3): 495–502.

Brown, R.T., Doepke, K.G. and Kaslow, N.J. (1993).   Risk-Resistance Adaptation Model for Pediatric Chronic Illness: Sickle Cell Syndrome as an example. *Clinical Psychology Review* **13**: 133–167.

Brunnquell, D. and Hall, M.D. (1982).   Issues in the psychological care of pediatric oncology patients. *American Journal of Orthopsychiatry* **52**(1): 32–44.

Canam, C. (1993).   Common adaptive tasks facing parents of chidren with chronic conditions. *Journal of Advanced Nursing* **18**: 46–53.

Charest, M.C. and Douesnard, S. (1992).   La vérité sort de la bouche des enfants. *Psychiatrie Recherche et Intervention en Santé Mentale de l'enfant* **2**: 471–480.

Cincotta, N. (1993).   Psychosocial issues in the world of children with cancer. *Cancer* **71**(10): 3251–3260.

Cook, J.A. (1984).   Influence of gender on the problems of parents of fatally ill children. *Journal of Psychosocial Oncology* **2**(1): 71–91.

Cornam, J. (1993).   Childhood cancer: Differential effects on the family members. *Oncology Nursing Forum* **20**: 1559–1566.

Davies, W.H., Noll, R.B., DeStefano, L, Bukowski, W.M. and Kulkarni, R. (1991).   Differences in the child-rearing practices of parents of children with cancer and controls: The perspectives of parents and professionals. *Journal of Pediatric Psychology* **16**(3): 295–306.

Dolgin, M.J. and Phipps, S. (1996).   Reciprocal influences in family adjustment to childhood cancer. In L. Baider, C.L. Cooper and A. Kaplan De-Nour (Eds), *Cancer and the Family*. Chichester: Wiley.

Enskär, K., Carlsson, M., Golsäter, M. and Hamrin, E. (1997a).   Symptom distress and life situation in adolescents with cancer. *Cancer Nursing* **20**(1): 23–33.

Enskär, K., Carlsson, M., Golsäter, M., Hamrin, E., and Kreuger, A. (1997b).   Life situation and problems as reported by children with cancer and their parents. *Journal of Pediatric Oncology Nursing* **14**(1): 18–26.

Enskär, K., Carlsson, M., Golsäter, M., Hamrin, E. and Kreuger, A. (1997c).   Parental reports of changes and challenges that result from parenting a child with cancer. *Journal of Pediatric Oncology Nursing* **14**(3): 156–163.

Fischer-Fay, A., Goldberg, S., Simmons, R. and Levison, H. (1988). Chronic illness and infant–mother attachement: Cystic fibrosis. *Developmental and Behavioral Pediatrics* **9**(5): 266–270.

Gibbons, M.B. (1988). Coping with childhood cancer: a family perspective. In P.W. Power, A.E. Dell Orto and M.B. Gibbons (Eds), *Family Interventions Throughout Chronic Illness and Disability*. New York: Springer.

Goldberg, S., Gotowiec, A. and Simmons, R.J. (1995). Infant–mother attachment and behavior problems in healthy and chronically ill preschoolers. *Development and Psychopathology* **7**: 267–282.

Hymovich, D. and Roehner, J. (1989). Psychosocial consequences of childhood cancer. *Seminars in Oncology Nursing* **5**: 56–62.

Hymovich, D.P. (1995). The meaning of cancer to children. *Seminars in Oncology Nursing* **11**(1): 51–58

Kalnins, I.V., Churchill, M.P. and Terry, G.E. (1980). Concurrent stresses in families with a leukemic child. *Journal of Pediatric Psychology* **5**(1): 81–92.

Kazak, A. E. (1993). Editorial: psychological research in pediatric oncology. *Journal of Pediatric Psychology* **18**(3): 313–318.

Kazak, A.E. (1989). Families of chronically ill children: a systems and social-ecological model of adaptation and challenge. *Journal of Consulting and Clinical Psychology* **57**(1): 25–30.

Koch, A. (1985). 'If only it could be me': the families of pediatric cancer patients. *Family Relations* **34**: 63–70.

Koch-Hattem, A. (1986). Siblings' experience of pediatric cancer: interviews with children. *Health and Social Work* **11**(2): 107–117.

Kupst, M.J. (1993). Family coping: supportive and obstructive factors. *Cancer* **71**(10): 3337–3341.

Lavigne, J.V. and Faier-Routman, J. (1992). Psychological adjustment to pediatric physical disorders: a meta-analytic review. *Journal of Pediatric Psychology* **17**(2): 133–157.

Madan-Swain, A., Sexson, S.B., Brown, R. T. and Ragab, A. (1993). Family adaptation and coping among siblings of cancer patients, their brothers and sisters, and non-clinical controls. *American Journal of Family Therapy* **21**(1): 60–70.

Martinson, I. and Bossert, E. (1994). The psychological status of children with cancer. *Journal of Child and Adolescent Psychiatry Nursing* **7**: 16–23.

Nannis, E.D., Susman, E.J., Strope, B.E., Woodruff, P.J., Hersh, S.P., Levine, A.S. and Pizzo, P.A. (1982). Correlates of control in pediatric cancer patients and their families. *Journal of Pediatric Psychology* **7**(1): 75–84.

Rait, D.S. and Holland, J. (1986). Pediatric cancer: psychosocial issues and approaches. *Mediguide to Oncology* **6**: 1–5.

Ross, S.A. (1989). Childhood leukemia: the child's view. *Journal of Psychosocial Oncology* **7**(4): 75–90.

Schulman, J.L. (1980). Psychosocial Aspects of Childhood Cancer: A Bibliography. In J.L. Schulman and N.J. Kupst (Eds.), *The Child with Cancer*. Charles C. Thomas: Springfield, Illinois, p. 86–105.

Sexson, S.B. and Madan-Swain, A. (1993). School re-entry for the child with chronic illness. *Journal of Learning Disabilities* **26**(2): 115–125.

Shapiro, M. and Brack, G. (1994). Psychosocial aspects of siblings' experiences of pediatric cancer. *Elementary School Guidance and Counseling* **28**: 264–273.

Sourkes, B.M. (1980). Siblings of the pediatric cancer patient. In J. Kellerman (Ed.), *Psychological Aspects of Childhood Cancer*. Springfield: Charles C. Thomas.

Sourkes, B. (1982). The Deepening Shade: *Psychological Aspects of Life-threatening Illness*. Pittsburgh: University of Pittsburgh Press.

Sourkes, B.M. (1987). Siblings of the child with a life-threatening illness. *Journal of Children in Contemporary Society* **19**: 159–184.

Sourkes, B.M. (1995). *Armfuls of Time. The Psychological Experience of the Child with a Life-threatening Illness*. Pittsburgh: University of Pittsburgh Press.

Sourkes, B.M. (1998). Psychologic aspects of leukemia and other hematologic disorders. In D.J. Nathan and S.H. Orkin (Eds), *Hematology of Infancy and Childhood*, 5th Edn. Philadelphia, PA: W.B. Saunders.

Sroufe, L.A., Cooper, R.G. and DeHart, G.B. (1992). *Child Development. Its Nature and Course*, 2nd Edn. New York: McGraw-Hill.

Van Dongen-Melman, J.E.W.M. and Sanders-Woudstra, J.A.R. (1986a). The chronically ill child and his family. In R. Michels and J.O. Cavenar (Eds), *Psychiatry*. Philadelphia, PA: J.B. Lippincott.

Van Dongen-Melman, J.E.W.M. and Sanders-Woudstra, J.A.R. (1986b). Psychosocial aspects of childhood cancer: A review of the literature. *Journal of Child Psychology and Psychiatry* **27**(2), 145–180.

Varni, J.W., Katz, E.R., Colegrove, R. Jr. and Dolgin, M. (1994). Perceived social support and adjustment of children newly diagnosed cancer. *Developmental and Behavioral Pediatrics* **15**(1): 20–26.

Walker, C.L. (1990). Siblings of children with cancer. *Oncology Nursing Forum* **17**(3): 355–360.

Wallander, J.L. and Varni, J.W. (1998). Effects of pediatric chronic physical disorders on child and family adjustment. *Journal of Child Psychology and Psychiatry and Allied Disciplines* **39**(1): 29–46.

Wallander, J.L., Varni, J.W., Babani, L., Banis, H.T. and Wilcox, K.T. (1988). Family resources as resistance factors for psychological maladjustment in chronically ill and handicapped children. *Journal of Pediatric Psychology* **14**(2): 157–173.

Maternal Problem-solving Training in Childhood Cancer

MICHAEL J. DOLGIN

Israel Institute for the Treatment and Study of Stress, Haifa, Israel

SEAN PHIPPS

St. Jude Children's Research Hospital, Memphis, Tennessee, USA

PSYCHOSOCIAL ADJUSTMENT TO CHILDHOOD CANCER (PACC) RESEARCH CONSORTIUM*

Research on the adjustment of children with cancer has long recognized the importance of family factors in determining outcome, as well as the systemic and interactional nature of the individual adjustment of patients, parents and siblings within families (Chesler and Barbarin, 1987; Dolgin and Phipps, 1996; Horowitz and Kazak, 1990; Kupst et al., 1982). Thus, the adjustment of the child-patient or sibling to the diagnosis of childhood cancer will be both directly and indirectly related to the adjustment of the parents. The Psychosocial Adjustment to Childhood Cancer (PACC) research consortium, which began with a focus on the determinants of adjustment in siblings of children with cancer (Sahler et al., 1994), recognized that the primary factors that were common to both sibling and patient adjustment reflected the role of parental and, in particular, maternal behavior and psychological functioning. This led to the current PACC research focus, which aims to capitalize on the systemic nature of adjustment in families by intervening with mothers of children newly diagnosed with cancer in order to promote optimal adjustment in all family members. The intervention utilizes 'Problem-solving Skills Training' (PSST), an approach that has been effective in many populations, including adult cancer patients (D'Zurilla and Nezu, 1999; Nezu et al., 1999a,b), but has not previously been applied to parents of children with cancer.

This chapter reviews the research leading to the current PACC focus on PSST as a treatment approach in the childhood cancer setting. First, the research literature on

---

*This chapter reviews work by the investigators of the Psychosocial Adjustment to Childhood Cancer Research Consortium (PACC): Olle Jane Sahler, University of Rochester (Principal Investigator); Robert W. Butler, Oregon Health Sciences University: Donna R. Copeland, University of Texas, MD Anderson Cancer Center; Ernest R. Katz, Children's Hospital of Los Angeles; Raymond K. Mulhern, St. Jude Children's Research Hospital; Robert B. Noll, Children's Hospital and Medical Center, Cincinnati; and James W. Varni, Children's Hospital, San Diego.

---

patient, sibling, and family adjustment to childhood cancer is reviewed, pointing naturally towards a focus on mothers as a primary target of intervention. Next, an overview of PSST as a clinical technique is presented, focusing on its relevance, application, and potential benefits, through maternally focused problem-solving training, as an intervention for childhood cancer. Finally, the work of the PACC group on Maternal Problem-solving Skills Training (MPSST) is described, along with the conceptual model underlying this work and preliminary findings from a randomized outcome study evaluating MPSST in this population.

FAMILY ADJUSTMENT TO CHILDHOOD CANCER

The rationale for developing a PSST intervention for mothers is based on the intersection of three lines of research: (a) the adaptation of children with cancer and other chronic illnesses, and its relationship to family factors and parental (particularly maternal) adjustment; (b) the adaptation of healthy siblings to having an ill or disabled brother or sister, and its relationship to family factors and parental adjustment; and (c) the impact of childhood cancer on parental (maternal) adjustment, and the role of maternal adjustment/psychological functioning in determining the level of adaptation of both ill and healthy children in the family.

ADAPTATION OF CHILDREN WITH CANCER

The earliest investigations regarding the adjustment of children with chronic illness or disability revealed that the proportion of maladjustment among these children was about twice that of the physically healthy population (Pless and Roughmann, 1971). Studies conducted subsequently have found less of a difference between ill children and controls, and have suggested that chronically ill or disabled children display, on the average, more behavioral and social problems than would be expected when compared to a normative sample, but less than children who are typically referred for clinical treatment (Drotar et al., 1981; Gayton et al., 1977; Wallander et al., 1988). Thus, it has become common to characterize these children as 'at-risk' for psychosocial maladjustment, i.e., they tend to display more behavioral problems as a sign of their distress, but these problems do not generally reach the threshold of psychopathology.

Certainly, children with cancer who undergo lengthy and intensive treatment regimens, as well as their families, fit the category of an at-risk population (Mott, 1990; Van Dongen-Melman and Sanders-Woudstra, 1986). Yet it is important to emphasize that considerable variability has been noted in how individual children adapt to their physical disability, leading investigators to search for those intrinsic or extrinsic factors which facilitate or impede successful coping. A primary source of factors determining the adequacy of the patient's coping comes from within the family system.

The relationship of family factors to child adjustment begins with sociodemographic variables. For example, children with cancer from single-parent families, those from families where the parents had less formal education, and those who had young mothers are at greatest risk for social and behavioral problems (Mulhern et al., 1989, 1993). Beyond sociodemographic variables, research has shown a consistent relationship between the measures of the family environment and adjustment in the child with cancer. Higher levels of family adaptability have been associated with higher scores on measures of child social and academic functioning, self-esteem, and overall mental health (Kazak and Meadows, 1989; Raitt et al., 1992). Likewise, higher levels of family cohesion and organization, and lower levels of family conflict, have been associated with better child outcomes (Phipps and Mulhern, 1995; Raitt et al., 1992; Wallander et al., 1989; Varni et al., 1998). Phipps and Mulhern (1995) demonstrated that both family cohesion and expressiveness serve as protective factors in the adjustment of children undergoing bone marrow transplantation. The adjustment of children with cancer has been shown to relate directly to parental functioning, i.e., high levels of parental distress or the presence of parental psychopathology are consistently associated with greater adjustment difficulties (Brown et al., 1993; Fritz et al., 1988; Kupst, 1993; Kupst and Schulman, 1988). A consistent finding is the strength of the relationship between parental adjustment and the child-patient's adjustment to illness (Kupst, 1993). In summary, available studies indicate that the family environment is a source of potential targets for intervention to improve the adaptation of the pediatric patient.

ADAPTATION OF HEALTHY SIBLINGS

Although much research has been conducted on how healthy siblings cope with the stress of a life-threatening chronic disease in the family, the reported findings, much like those for their ill brother or sister, have been inconsistent. Indeed, findings have ranged from evidence for considerable maladjustment, to little or no effect, to indications of a positive influence on psychological development (Breslau et al., 1981; Cadman et al., 1988; Dyson, 1989; Ferrari 1984; Lavigne and Ryan, 1979).

Specifically with regard to the siblings of children with cancer, it appears that this population is at risk for adjustment problems, such as poor academic achievement and impaired social interactions, as well as more undesirable behaviors, such as guilt, aggressiveness, withdrawal, anxiety, fearfulness, and jealousy (Cairnes et al., 1979; Carr-Gregg and White, 1979; Tritt, 1988). In addition, Cairnes and colleagues (1979) found that siblings have difficulties with body image and excessive anxiety that are similar to that of their ill brother or sister. They are also more likely to perceive themselves as socially isolated and to view their parents as being overindulgent with the ill child. In the initial PACC study of sibling adaptation, Sahler et al. (1994) reported that the prevalence of emotional/behavioral problems among healthy siblings of children with cancer was similar to that of the general population prior to the diagnosis of cancer, but the prevalence of such problems after diagnosis more than doubled. However, similar to the adjustment outcomes in the cancer patient, there is wide variability in how well siblings adapt. Again, it appears that the impact of a serious illness in a sibling is best viewed as a risk factor that is mediated by other personal characteristics (e.g., temperament), environmental variables, and, perhaps most importantly, by family resources that can positively or negatively affect adaptation.

As was found in studies with the child-patient, adjustment of siblings is related to family adaptability (Horowitz and Kazak, 1990), family cohesion (Gogan and Slavin, 1981; Dolgin et al., 1997), and family support and expressiveness (Dolgin et al., 1997). In a study noteworthy for its cross-cultural findings, Dolgin et al. (1997) found similar significant correlations between sibling behavioral adjustment and measures of family support, expressiveness, and conflict in both US and Israeli samples. Results also indicated that maternal coping through utilization of interpersonal support resources was significantly related to better behavioral adjustment among siblings.

FAMILY FACTORS, MATERNAL ADJUSTMENT, AND CHILD ADAPTATION

Early research findings regarding the adjustment of parents of children with cancer and other chronic disease suggested that some caregivers have long-term difficulties with excessive anxiety and depression (Fife et al., 1987; Hughes and Lieberman, 1990; Overholsin and Fritz, 1990). Mothers, in particular, experience post-traumatic stress symptoms, with an incidence as high as 40% (Hall and Baum, 1995; Pelcovitz et al., 1996; Stuber et al., 1994, 1996). These findings are, however, not universal. Kupst and co-workers, for example, report results on numerous measures of parental psychological functioning that were within normal limits as early as 6 months after diagnosis of cancer in their child (Kupst and Schulman, 1988). More importantly, several studies have found significant relationships between individual parental, especially maternal, reports of their own mental and physical health and measures of adaptation to stressful life events among their children (Hetherington and Martin, 1986; Daniels et al., 1987; Jessop et al., 1988). That is, on an individual basis, the level of functioning of a specific parent appears to have a direct effect on the level of functioning of the child, whether that child is ill/disabled or a healthy sibling.

Another important factor influencing psychological and functional outcome of children appears to be the degree to which their respective parents, especially mothers, identify family and extended social systems as supportive (Morrow et al., 1981; Speechly and Noh, 1992; Thompson et al., 1992), which may serve to moderate and protect the parent from the impact of stress. In turn, the parent may then serve to buffer the impact of stressful experiences on his/her own children. For example, Mulhern et al. (1992) evaluated 99 sets of pediatric cancer patients and their mothers and found maternal self-reported depression to be the single best predictor of child depression, whether measured by child self-report or by maternal report. Furthermore, reduced social support and increased medical symptoms of the child were significantly associated with increased maternal depression. In a report from the PACC sibling study, Zeltzer et al. (1996) found that sibling reports of somatic symptoms and use of health care services were directly related to maternal utilization and mothers' subjective sense of well-being. In addition, sibling somatic complaints, by both parent- and self-report, were significantly related to parental somatization and maternal health status. Indeed, these parent variables emerged among the strongest predictors of sibling health/somatic outcomes. Thus, mothers who felt emotionally and physically better, and who found the resources and support systems on which they relied to be helpful, have children who adapt more favorably.

In another report from the PACC sibling study, Sahler et al. (1997) found that, when healthy siblings were categorized according to level of adaptation (dysfunctional to resilient), the mothers' general well-being and resource utilization were correlated with their children's level of adaptation. Interestingly, the mothers with children who were dysfunctional accessed more support resources but their satisfaction was lower. Whether this relationship was due to accessing the wrong resources, to their inability to articulate their needs sufficiently to obtain appropriate help, or to their inability to effectively apply whatever advice or guidance was offered, is unknown.

In instances where maternal support systems and resource utilizations are ineffective, it may be that the mother has incomplete understanding or poorly processed information specific to a condition or situation related to the child's cancer. Thus, a systematic method for providing skills the mother can use to, among other things, access essential information, so that she can acquire greater and more useful knowledge, could have a direct and beneficial effect on her ability to find and use appropriate resources. Another desirable effect would be a reduction in her frustration and anxiety (thus increasing her general level of well-being), which would, indirectly, serve to enhance the patient's and siblings' levels of adaptation.

Although there is overall agreement that a mother's depression is a definite risk factor for her child in general (Green, 1993), as well as in the particular context of pediatric cancer (Cohen et al., 1994), the exact etiology of negative affectivity in parents of children with cancer is unclear. It may be the result of a major stressor, such as the diagnosis of the cancer itself, and/or it may arise as the result of the accumulation of the many microstressors associated with tasks of daily living that are made more difficult by having a child with cancer. Regardless of the etiology, women, in general, are particularly reactive to negative events within the family (Conger et al., 1993). Unlike fathers, who are more likely to respond to stressors such as childhood cancer by turning to substance abuse or other forms of antisocial behavior, mothers tend to develop depression, anxiety, and somatization disorders (Culbertson, 1997).

These findings led us to believe that an intervention which decreased such reactions in mothers would improve maternal functioning and have a beneficial spillover effect on her children's (both patient and sibling) coping. This is a particularly appealing model because skills training that is targeted at the pivotal primary caregiver (most often, the mother) also has the potential to enhance spousal relationships and family and community relationships, as well as to strengthen parent–child relationships adversely affected by the stress experienced by the mother. Research suggests that skills training aimed at the wife/mother would be a key intervention for maintaining the integrity of the family. For example, 74% of men reported that they talk primarily to their spouse when upset (Antonucci and Akiyama, 1987). Further, men typically depend on their spouse to maintain contact with friends, family, and the community. Thus, targeting the mother/wife as the pivotal caretaker has the potential to enhance parent–child, spousal, family, and community relationships and to provide particularly helpful support to families in which mothers are the sole caregiver.

PROBLEM-SOLVING SKILLS TRAINING

Social problem solving refers to a process whereby the individual is able to identify effective means for coping with stressful events. It has been suggested that a deficit in problem-solving skills may serve as an important risk factor for ineffective coping with either a major stress or smaller but continuous stressors, and that learning new problem-solving skills can improve the individual's ability to manage daily challenges that were previously associated with distress. PSST had been shown to be an effective treatment in decreasing negative affectivity and enhancing functioning in depressed adults (D'Zurilla and Chang, 1995; Nezu 1986, 1987; Nezu and Perri, 1989). Studies have demonstrated the relationships between problem-solving skills and psychological stress, depression, anxiety, positive affectivity, negative affectivity, optimism, pessimism, and knowledge acquisition (Chang and D'Zurilla, 1996; D'Zurilla and Chang, 1995; D'Zurilla and Nezu, 1990; D'Zurilla and Sheedy, 1991). In addition, social problem solving has been applied successfully with newly diagnosed pediatric cancer patients for targeted problems such as reintegrating into their school, community, and peer group (Katz and Varni, 1993; Varni et al., 1994).

D'Zurilla and Goldfried (1971) first conceptualized problem-solving theory and research as a five-stage process:

1. *Problem orientation—the cognitive and motivational set with which the individual approaches problems in general.*
2. *Problem definition and formulation—*delineation of a problem into concrete and specific terms and the identification of specific goals.
3. *Generation of alternatives—*production of an exhaustive listing of possible solutions.
4. *Decision making—*systematic evaluation of the range of alternative solutions with regard to their consequences and the selection of optimal choices.
5. *Solution implementation and verification—*monitoring and evaluating the chosen solution outcome after its implementation.

D'Zurilla (1986) had translated these steps into specific techniques for application in stress management and prevention.

1. *Problem orientation—*this step involves the notion that individuals may confront multiple problems, challenges and decisions which, while extremely stressful and personally taxing, may be normal and common, and that many of these can be resolved through a systematic problem-solving approach. During this step, a distinction is drawn between those stressors that are clearly beyond one's control and those that may be modifiable. The principal purpose of PSST, therefore, is to identify and target those aspects of situational stress that are within one's control. The mutual influence of thoughts (cognitions) and feelings (emotions) is emphasized, as is the importance of specificity, creativity, and activity in problem solving and stress reduction.
2. *Problem definition and formulation—*the accurate and precise definition of a problem, conflict or decision to be made is an essential step toward resolving the challenge. A clearly operationalized and articulated problem will greatly facilitate the subsequent generation of possible solutions, their evaluation, and outcome assessment. The objective of this step is to clearly define the problem.
3. *Generation of alternative solutions—*the primary function of this step is to produce, through brainstorming, a number of high-quality potential solutions

to the problem situation. A non-critical posture is recommended during this step in order to facilitate the search for the best or most effective strategies.

4. *Decision making*—during this step, a careful cost–benefit analysis is made regarding the list of alternative solutions generated. As a result, a 'best choice (or choices)' solution with the highest probability of positive outcome is arrived at for subsequent implementation.

5. *Solution implementation and verification*—here, an action plan for implementing the 'best' solution is carried out. Within this step, any anticipated obstacles are addressed. Unanticipated obstacles are managed by referring back to the earlier PSST steps, including redefinition of the problem, attempting an alternative solution, generating additional solutions, etc. Self-monitoring and self-evaluation are taught in order to assess solution outcome, and self-reinforcement is encouraged for accomplishing problem resolution and achieving a desirable outcome.

Throughout the PSST process, specific strategies for relapse prevention, i.e. a return to pre-PSST methods of functioning, are emphasized. These often include: (a) bibliotherapy, in the form of detailed hand-outs for ongoing and future reference; (b) identifying high-risk situations to which the individual has previously been vulnerable; (c) identifying the signs of emotional distress to serve as 'red flags' indicating that problem solving techniques are called for; and (d) emphasizing the importance of a positive problem orientation and cautioning against the hazards of complacency.

BRIGHT IDEAS: MATERNAL PSST IN CHILDHOOD CANCER

CONCEPTUAL MODEL

The conceptual model adopted by the PACC study group in its research on PSST views a crisis situation as having the potential for negative outcomes. Given a crisis of childhood cancer in the family, our model postulates that: (a) in response to a given stressor/crisis, the PSST intervention may alter the course of negative outcomes; (b) the primary desired outcome of the intervention is an increase in problem-solving skills; (c) higher levels of problem-solving skills will decrease negative affectivity and improve adjustment (secondary outcome); and (d) individual moderating factors may influence how successfully problem-solving skills are mastered and implemented. Figure 17.1 depicts the hypothesized pathways for the effects of the PSST intervention as these have guided the PACC research in this area.

PROGRAM FORMAT AND GUIDELINES

To make the overall philosophy and steps of the PSST program more easily understood and remembered, we developed the acronym "**Bright IDEAS**" and the logo of a lighted bulb. "**Bright**" signifies the sense of optimism and positive problem orientation about solving problems that is essential for successful implementation. The letters **I** (Identify the problem), **D** (Determine the options), **E** (Evaluate options and choose the best), **A** (Act), and **S** (See if it worked) signify the five essential steps of problem solving, as articulated by D'Zurilla and Nezu and reinterpreted by us

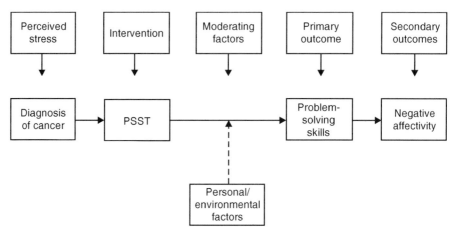

Figure 17.1 Conceptual model

(Varni et al., 1998) (Figure 17.2). Instructional materials developed to guide the PSST include a treatment manual, summary brochure, problem-solving worksheets, and trigger cartoons.

The PSST protocol consisted of six to eight individual treatment sessions conducted by a trained psychosocial professional (minimum of MA in psychology or social work with at least 2 years of work experience) who had undergone a specialized training seminar in PSST for the purposes of this study, and who continued to receive ongoing supervision at each of the eight PACC study sites—all major pediatric cancer centers in the USA and in Israel—by each site's principal investigator. The initial treatment sessions focused on imparting the essential steps in the problem-solving process, modeling and illustration of the problem-solving process via specific and highly relevant training vignettes, and identification of the specific problems encountered by individual mothers. Subsequent sessions guided mothers through the application of the PSST steps to their own particular stressors and circumstances. A Problems Checklist, especially developed for the purpose and listing a range of common stressors among mothers of children with cancer, provided additional stimulation of individually relevant situations to focus on in the PSST sessions. Ongoing reference to the 'Bright IDEAS' problem-solving model guided the entire course of PSST intervention, aided by the worksheets and other materials. Throughout, the emphasis was on imparting a generic coping skill that could be applied as needed to the specific, relevant stressors experienced over time by each individual mother, thereby promoting skills generalization and relapse prevention.

The PSST program we have designed for mothers has been conducted to date in individual sessions. Although a group format is possible, we have found that it is typically more convenient for the mother to schedule the instructional sessions during regularly scheduled clinic appointments for medical treatment or during her child's extended hospitalizations. The variability in scheduling, combined with unforeseen events of a medical or family nature, make it very difficult to consistently bring together a small group. Since the instructional sessions are individualized, the

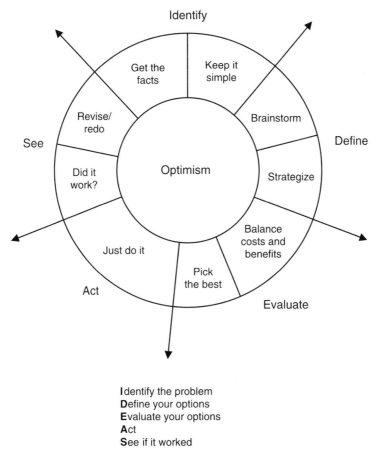

Identify the problem
Define your options
Evaluate your options
Act
See if it worked

Figure 17.2   The Bright IDEAS model for Problem Solving

entire intervention program is typically conducted in six 1–1.5 hour instructional sessions over a 6–8 week period. The format for the PSST session is standardized, and is outlined in Table 17.1.

TREATMENT CONSIDERATIONS AND PROCESS ISSUES

Establishing the parent–therapist partnership is the essential first step in conducting PSST. Warmth, empathy, trust, and genuineness set the stage for the parent's receptivity to learn the specific problem-solving strategies. Further, emphasizing the collaborative nature of the PSST as a skills training approach, as opposed to a psychotherapeutic endeavor aimed at reducing parental psychopathology, enhances the parent's perception that the therapist is treating the patient as an individual, and that the therapist depends on the parent's active cooperation to make PSST relevant and effective in addressing the parent's needs. This mutual collaboration fosters a sense of teamwork, where the therapist contributes general strategies and the treatment approach to problems and the parent brings all the information and

Table 17.1 PSST Format

Session 1
1. Introduction to problem-solving steps
2. Discuss problem orientation philosophy (**Bright IDEAS**)
3. Discuss problem definition/formulation (**I**dentify the problem)
4. Discuss generation of alternative solutions (**D**etermine the options)
5. Discuss decision-making process (**E**valuate options)
6. Discuss solution implementation (**A**ct and check the best)
7. Discuss solution verification (**S**ee if it worked)
8. Apply PSST steps to selected training vignettes
9. Review current problems to facilitate problem identification
10. Discuss worksheets
11. Begin PSST process with selected problem
12. Designate homework assignment
13. Overview of subsequent session

Sessions 2–5
1. Review previous session
2. Review homework assignments
3. Apply PSST steps to selected problem
4. Steps 3–12 (without 8) for unresolved or new problem

Session 6
1. Review homework assignments
2. Discuss relapse prevention strategies

---

details unique to her experiences. The sense of collaboration and the expectation that the parent is facing solvable problems is heightened by recognizing that problem solving is an integral part of everyday life, which the parent handled quite adequately until faced with the catastrophic event of childhood cancer, which interferes with and strains usual coping mechanisms and support networks.

In order to promote this sense of collaboration, as well as to increase the overall effectiveness of the intervention, several intervention principles and process are adhered to:

1. *Define the rationale behind problem-solving training*—at the initial stage of instruction, the parent needs to be given the rationale for learning the targeted skills. The parent is provided with information about the usefulness and inherent advantages of each step in the Bright IDEAS strategy in order to be a successful problem-solver. The parent needs to be provided with information about the value of problem-solving skills, based on the potential positive consequences and benefits of having these skills in her repertoire as they apply to coping with childhood cancer.

2. *Define the skills to be taught*—in addition to describing the reasons why the problem-solving skills are valuable, the therapist also presents in detail the specific cognitive–behavioral components of each skill. Verbal and written instructions are provided to specify in concrete terms exactly what cognitions and behaviors are required and how they need to be performed in order to accomplish problem resolution. We achieve this by distributing written

handouts defining the PSST steps along with vignette examples illustrating the successful application of PSST. Verbal and written instructions help break down the overall skill into separate cognitive and behavioral components that can be identified and learned.

3. *Modeling*—modeling by the therapist provides direct examples of the problem-solving components and elucidates the problem-solving strategies for the parent. A combination of modeling by the instructor, along with detailed instructional handouts and parent *in vivo* practice, provides the integrated learning experience needed to acquire the subtleties of skill performance. Instructor modeling affords flexibility in illustrating or highlighting particular aspects of the problem-solving skills process. Further, modeling depicts in vivid detail the cognitive and behavioral processes intrinsic to particular problem-solving that verbal and written instructions alone cannot convey.

4. *Behavioral rehearsal*—behavioral rehearsal is a form of structured role playing that enables the parent to act out and practice the problem-solving process just modeled. After the parent observes the therapist model the cognitive self-instructions and behavioral components intrinsic to the particular problem-solving skill, the instructor then sets up an illustrative problematic situation in which the parent is given the opportunity to rehearse or practice the specific and behavioral components of the problem-solving process during the session.

5. *Performance feedback*—performance feedback is defined as providing the parent with detailed information on how well she has enacted the specific cognitive and behavioral components during behavioral rehearsal. After the parent rehearses the designated problem-solving skills, performance feedback is provided immediately.

6. *Generalization and maintenance*—generalization, or transfer of learning, is an essential component of the PSST program. It ensures that the newly acquired problem-solving skills are applied in appropriate situations in the parent's everyday environment. Rather than the 'train and hope' approach, where transfer of learning is not specifically planned but is passively hoped for as a function of simply teaching the new skill, generalization must be a planned component of each skills training session. Thus, specific programming needs to be built into the skills training intervention to facilitate the generalization of the skills to different settings and different people over time. For newly learned skills to transfer from the training setting to the natural environment, carefully planned structured homework and practice assignments must be incorporated into each training session. In addition to programming generalization across situations and people, the instructor reinforces and encourages the parent's utilization of the newly learned problem-solving skills in the natural environment. Finally, teaching the parent specific self-reinforcement and positive cognitive self-instructional procedures further optimizes generalization and maintenance.

The initial step in the PSST process—establishing a positive problem orientation—is of special importance, especially in dealing with a population under extreme or catastrophic circumstances. This step involves the cognitive appraisal that having to cope with numerous problems, decisions, and challenges associated with the diagnosis and treatment of childhood cancer is common and normal for this extraordinary life event, and that many of these challenges can be surmounted and resolved through the systematic problem-solving approach. It is essential to emphasize that while the diagnosis of childhood cancer is not within their control, there are a myriad of potentially solvable problems that accompany the diagnosis and treatment of childhood cancer. The primary focus, therefore, of the problem-solving intervention is to identify and target those aspects of the diagnosis and treatment process that are within the control of parents.

From this perspective, parents need to be reassured that, while the emotional distress associated with the diagnosis of childhood cancer will most likely always be present, the intensity of their distress will lessen as they overcome multiple problems and challenges that are within their control to resolve. Parents need to be instructed that feelings of depression, anxiety, and anger may in part be explained by all the everyday problems and decision-making challenges they must confront, and that these emotions should serve as cues that they may be feeling frustrated by unresolved conflicts and problems. Emphasis is on those characteristics of the diagnosis and treatment process which are modifiable, or if not directly modifiable, are at least reduced in impact by modifying the cognitive processes that elicit the emotions associated with unresolvable problems. Since there will be aspects of the disease and treatment which are not completely under the parents' control, helping them to alter their cognitive appraisal of certain problematic situations may ameliorate some of the emotional distress they may be experiencing.

Steps 2 (problem definition and formulation), 3 (generation of alternative solutions) and 4 (decision-making) in the PSST process, as described earlier, set the stage for the crucial step (5) of solution implementation and verification. The actual implementation of the 'best' solution alternative selected in the previous steps is essential in achieving the desired outcome. Four component aims are involved in this process:

1. *Solution performance*—the parent is instructed to implement the 'best' solution arrived at via the earliest PSST steps. If unanticipated obstacles arise in the actual implementation of the parent's solution plan (e.g., skill deficit, elevated emotional distress, lack of cooperation from others), the parent is instructed to: (a) cycle back to previous problem-solving steps and consider choosing a different solution from the previously developed solution alternatives list or generate a new alternative solution plan; or (b) reformulate the overall problem and include steps to overcome the obstacles to effective solution performance.

2. *Self-monitoring*—in order to measure solution implementation and outcome through accurate and objective assessment of solution performance, parents are helped to develop a checklist or rating system to monitor their implementation of the chosen solution.

3. *Self-evaluation*—If the match between the observed and desired outcomes is satisfactory, the parent moves on to self-reinforcement. If the parent is not satisfied with the match between expected and obtained outcome, then the parent is instructed to troubleshoot the mismatch by attempting to determine whether the source of the difficulty lies with the previous problem-solving steps

(e.g., skill deficits, obstacles). At this point, the parent may choose to cycle back and reformulate, or may decide that more information or expert help is needed.

4. *Self-reinforcement*—parents are encouraged to reward themselves for accomplishing problem resolution or the expected outcome. This may entail verbal self-statements or praise, or actually arranging for a tangible pleasurable activity to reinforce effort and success. It is at this step of accomplishment that the cognitive attribution of 'learned optimism' should be strongly encouraged— that, to help parents recognize that they can control aspects of the process involved with the diagnosis and medical treatment of their child's cancer.

In our application of PSST with mothers, specific strategies are aimed at minimizing relapse prevention. 'Relapse' implies a return to strategies utilized prior to PSST. Apart from periodic booster sessions after the treatment intervention has been completed, other primary relapse prevention strategies include:

1. providing parents with clear, detailed handouts of material taught during the treatment intervention. This material can be referred to after the PSST intervention has been completed to remind the parents what they have been taught, to elicit positive self-statements, and to maintain a positive problem orientation.

2. identifying high-risk situations, i.e., problematic situations where the parent has typically responded in an impulsive manner, 'not stopping and thinking' prior to acting. Thus, we encourage discussion of effective coping with high-risk situations in the future.

3. using emotional distress as a 'red flag' or cue that the problem-solving techniques taught during the intervention need to be rigorously utilized to address these feelings.

4. emphasizing to parents the importance of not becoming complacent, i.e., gradually lapsing into old ways of coping over time.

5. enthusiastically emphasizing the concepts of self-efficacy and learned optimism, i.e., that the problem-solving strategies work, and that the parent can solve problems successfully by adhering to the principles taught during PSST.

CASE STUDY

Susan was the 29 year-old mother of 6 year-old David, diagnosed with leukemia 6 weeks prior to beginning PSST. She had been spending a great deal of time with her son in the hospital due to his recurrent infections and fever. She was a bright and pleasant woman, but was clearly worn and depressed by the extended hospital stays. Susan's anger at the professional staff soon began to surface, with the recurring complaint that she was not being kept adequately informed and that the communication between her and her son's primary physician was poor.

After establishing a positive problem orientation—that her sense of helplessness could be relieved by adopting a systematic approach to problem-solving—her therapist introduced Susan to the initial step of problem identification, explaining that just about any problem, no matter how major it may look at first, is solvable if broken down into small parts. Beginning with the broad problem of 'poor communication', Susan was encouraged to explore and define exactly what that meant. After some discussion, she was able to identify three specific communication problems that caused her the greatest frustration: (a) the fact that her son's doctor did not speak with her each day when her son was in the hospital; (b) the fact that the doctor used medical terms she did not understand; (c) the fact that the doctor did not inform her of test results following her son's outpatient visits.

Addressing the next step, defining options for problem resolution, Susan chose to focus on the most distressing issue for her at the time—the fact that the doctor did not speak with her each day when her child was in hospital. She and her therapist explored why this situation may have come about. Susan reported that the doctor often visited her child before she got to the hospital in the morning and after she left in the afternoon. She complained that the doctor had so many patients to see and that his visits to her son's room were often very brief and rushed. Finally, she claimed that the doctor frequently conveyed information through the nursing staff, while she wanted direct communication with him. Based on this, she arrived at three potential options for gaining more direct communication with her son's doctor: (a) she could come to the hospital earlier or leave later; (b) she could ask the doctor when it would be convenient to meet at another time of the day and where; (c) she could ask the doctor when it would be convenient to talk by telephone about her child's care.

Susan was led through the next step—decision making—based on a cost–benefit analysis of the options she had generated. She began with her first option—Come earlier/go later. She explained that she had two other children who were in school and that she could not leave the house until 8.30 a.m. (doctor rounds were at 7.30 a.m.). She also had to be home to supervise at 3 p.m. (afternoon rounds were at 4 p.m.). Furthermore, her husband left for work at 7.30 a.m. and returned home at 5 p.m. He had no vacation or sick time left and a baby-sitter in the afternoon would introduce a difficult financial burden. Also, Susan wanted very much to be home for her other children. Assessing a second option, Susan offered that she could make herself available between 9 a.m. and 2.30 p.m. Because she knew the doctor sometimes had emergencies or other duties, she could offer to be in her child's room between 11.30 a.m. and 1 p.m. each day. This would mean eating lunch early or late and not being able to leave the hospital room until after the doctor's visit. As a third option, she considered the possibility of making herself available during those same hours, but that the doctor could call rather than come to her child's room. The barriers to this option would be the same as those listed above, but, in addition, she would not see the doctor face-to-face, which she felt was important to her.

Of the three options, Susan decided that the second would be best. Adjusting her lunchtime was not a problem, she would not pay for a sitter, she could be home with her two other children before and after school, and she would be able to actually meet with the doctor. She also decided to keep a small notepad in her purse so she could write down questions she, her husband, or other family members had, so that she could make the most of the 10–15 minutes with the doctor.

Susan began the next day and for two days the plan worked well. On the third day the doctor had an emergency and she got word from the nurses that the meeting had to be cancelled. Evaluating whether the plan was working well or whether she needed to make some changes, she concluded that: (a) 2 days out of 3 was an improvement and she could save her questions; (b) it would be all right for the doctor to call if a visit was impossible; (c) she could go to the clinic rather than wait at her child's bedside; (d) someone else (e.g., the nurse) could talk with her. Susan decided that daily contact with the doctor was essential. She and the doctor discussed calling as an alternative when meeting was not possible. Both agreed that talking on the telephone was preferable to either skipping a meeting, going to the clinic (which was busy and not very private), or having someone else answer her questions. Over the next week she was satisfied with seeing the doctor almost every day and talking on the phone occasionally to meet her needs for information and communication.

EVALUATION OF PSST IN MOTHERS OF CHILDREN WITH CANCER

The PACC study group conducted an initial pilot study of PSST in mothers of newly diagnosed patients. This study was carried out at six major pediatric cancer facilities in the USA and Israel and set for itself two primary objectives: first, to develop, field test, and evaluate a novel PSST curriculum package for mothers of children with cancer; second, to collect preliminary data from a randomized trial of the efficacy of PSST in enhancing problem-solving skills (primary effect) and decreasing negative affectivity (secondary effects). Following beta testing with 12 mothers (two per site) and materials refinement, a randomized trial was conducted in which 36 mothers of children with newly diagnosed cancer (2–16 weeks post-diagnosis) received PSST and were compared to a control group of 36 mothers who received only the standard psychosocial services offered at their institution. In order to evaluate PSST impact, three assessment points were selected: T1 (baseline, pre-treatment), T2 (immediately post-treatment), and T3 (3 month follow-up). Assessment of primary treatment effects—improvements in problem-solving abilities—was obtained by administering the Social Problem Solving Index–Revised (SPSI-R). Secondary effects, reductions in negative affectivity, were measured by the Profile of Mood States (POMS) and the Beck Depression Inventory (BDI),

Preliminary analyses from this cohort indicate significant changes in the desired direction as a result of intervention from T1 to T2. Specifically, SPSI-R and POMS scores show significant positive changes from pre-treatment levels to immediate post-treatment levels in the intervention group as compared to the control group. This is the case when examining absolute change scores from T1 to T2 in subjects and controls, and when comparing T2 scores between subjects and controls within an analysis of covariance model using T1 scores as the covariate. Gains in problem-solving scores among recipients of PSST persisted at significantly higher levels when compared to controls at T3, 3 months after training. In addition, anecdotal reports and subjective ratings of both subjects and trainers suggest the PSST curriculum to be a potent, well-received, and highly relevant treatment approach in this population. The PACC study group is currently conducting a large-scale investigation of PSST in mothers of newly diagnosed patients, as well as the development, application, and evaluation of technology-based PSST methods using computer-assisted multimedia programs.

CONCLUSION

Mothers of children with cancer are an important target population, not only in terms of the distress they experience as a result of their child's illness, but also due to their pivotal role in functioning and adaptation of the child-patient and other family members. PSST is a treatment approach that lends itself to persons in crisis situations—those in which pre-existing coping methods may be impaired. PSST has demonstrated benefits for a wide range of clinical populations, and has been recently empirically validated in mothers of children with cancer. Clearly there exists a need for specific intervention methods, of which PSST may be only one, for applications in pediatric oncology. To date, only a minute proportion of the vast literature on psychosocial pediatric oncology describes applied intervention methods and, of those, few have been subjected to the test of empirical validation. Randomized, controlled intervention research is needed. Directions for future research include parents, both mothers and fathers, as well as other caregivers (e.g., medical staff), and, of course, children. The simplicity and considerable face validity of PSST render it a generic and highly applicable approach in persons coping with the myriad of challenges inherent in the cancer experience.

REFERENCES

Antonnucci, T.C. and Akiyama, H. (1987). An examination of sex differences in social support among older men and women. *Sex Roles* **17**: 737–749.

Breslau, N., Weitzman, M. and Messenger, K. (1981). Psychologic functioning of siblings of disabled children. *Pediatrics* **67**: 344–353.

Brown, R.T., Kaslow, N.J., Madan-Swain, A., Doepke, K.J., Sexson, S.B. and Hill, L.J. (1993). Parental psychopathology and children's adjustment to leukemia. *Journal of the American Academy of Child and Adolescent Psychiatry* **32**: 554–561.

Cadman, D., Boyle, M. and Afford, D.R. (1988). The Ontario Child Health Study: social adjustment and mental health of siblings of children with chronic health problems. *Journal of Developmental and Behavioral Pediatrics* **9**: 117–121.

Cairnes, N.U., Clark, G.M., Smith, S.D. and Lansky, S.B. (1979). Adaptation of siblings to childhood malignancy. *Journal of Pediatrics* **95**: 484–487.

Carr-Gregg, M. and White, L. (1987). Siblings of paediatric cancer patients: a population at risk. *Medical and Pediatric Oncology* **15**: 62–68.

Chang, E.C. and D'Zurilla, T.J. (1996). Relations between problem orientation and optimism, pessimism, and trait affectivity: a construct validation study. *Behaviour Reseach and Therapy* **34**: 185–194.

Chesler, M.A. and Barbarin, O.A. (1987). *Childhood Cancer and the Family*. New York: Brunner-Mazel.

Cohen, D.S., Friedrich, W.N., Jaworski, T.M., Copeland, D.R. and Pendergrass, T. (1994). Pediatric cancer: predicting sibling adjustment. *Journal of Clinical Psychology* **50**: 303–319.

Conger, R.D., Lorenz, F.O., Elder, G.H., Simmons, R.L. and Ge, X. (1993). Husband and wife differences in response to undesirable life events. *Health and Social Behavior* **34**: 71–88.

Culbertson, F.M. (1977). Depression and gender: an international review. *American Psychologist* **52**: 25–31.

D'Zurilla, T.J. (1986). *Problem-solving Therapy: A Social Competence Approach to Clinical Intervention*. New York: Springer.

D'Zurilla, T.J. and Chang, E.C. (1995). The relations between social problem solving and coping. *Cognitive Therapy and Research* **19**: 547–562.

D'Zurilla, T.J. and Goldfried, M. (1971). Problem-solving and behavior modification. *Journal of Abnormal Psychology* **78**: 104–126.

D'Zurilla, T.J. and Nezu, A.M. (1990). Development and preliminary evaluation of the Social Problem-Solving Inventory (SPSI). *Psychological Assessment* **2**: 156–163.

D'Zurilla, T.J. and Nezu, A.M. (1999). *Problem-Solving Therapy: A Social Competence Approach to Clinical Intervention*, 2nd Edn. New York: Springer.

D'Zurilla, T.J. and Sheedy, C.F. (1991).   The relation between social problem-solving ability and subsequent level of psychological stress in college students. *Cognitive Therapy and Research* **16**: 589–599.

Daniels, D., Moos, R.H., Billings, A.G. and Miller, J.J. III (1987).   Psychological risk and resistance factors among children with chronic illness, healthy siblings, and healthy controls. *Journal of Clinical Child Psychology* **15**: 295–308.

Dolgin, M.J., Blumensohn, R., Mulhern, R.K., Orbach, J., Sahler, O.J.Z., Roghmann, K.J., Carpenter, P.J., Barbarin, O.A., Sargent, J.R., Zeltzer, L.K. and Copeland, D.R. (1997).   Sibling adaptation to childhood cancer collaborative study: cross-cultural aspects. *Journal of Psychosocial Oncology* **15**: 1–15.

Dolgin, M.J. and Phipps, S. (1996).   Reciprocal influences in family adjustment to childhood cancer. In L. Baider, C.L. Cooper and A.K. Kaplan De-Nour (eds), *Cancer and the Family* (pp. 73–92). New York: Wiley.

Drotar, D., Doershuk, C.F., Stern, R.C., Boat, C.F., Boyer, W. and Matthews, L. (1981).   Psychosocial functioning of children with cystic fibrosis. *Pediatrics* **67**: 338–343.

Dyson, L.L. (1989).   Adjustment of siblings of handicapped children: a comparison. *Journal of Pediatric Psychology* **14**: 125–229.

Ferrari, M. (1984). Chronic illness: psychosocial effects on siblings. I. Chronically ill boys. *Journal of Child Psychology and Psychiatry* **25**: 459–476.

Fife, B., Norton, J. and Groom, G. (1987).   The family's adaptation to childhood leukemia. *Journal of Social Science in Medicine* **24**: 159–168.

Fritz, G.K., Williams J.R. and Amylon, M.D. (1988).   After treatment ends: psychosocial sequelae in pediatric cancer survivors. *American Journal of Orthopsychiatry* **58**: 552–561.

Gayton, W.F., Friedman, S.B., Tavormina, J.F. and Tucker, F. (1977).   Children with cystic fibrosis. I. Psychological testing findings of patients, siblings and parents. *Pediatrics* **5**: 888–894.

Gogan, J.L. and Slavin, L.A. (1981).   Intervening with brothers and sisters. In G.P. Koocher and J.P. O'Malley (Eds), *The Damocles Syndrome* (pp.101–111). New York: McGraw-Hill.

Green, M. (1993). Maternal depression: bad for children's health. *Contemporary Pediatrics* **10**: 28–36.

Hall, M. and Baum, A. (1995).   Intrusive thoughts as determinants of distress in parents of children with cancer. *Applied Social Psychology* **25**: 1215–1230.

Hetherington, E.M. and Martin, B. (1986).   Family factors and psychopathology in children. In H.C. Quay and J.S. Werry (Eds), *Psychopathological Disorders of Childhood* (pp. 332–389). New York: Wiley.

Horowitz, W.A. and Kazak, A.E. (1990).   Family adaptation to childhood cancer: siblings and family system variables. *Journal of Consulting and Clinical Psychology* **19**: 221–228.

Hughes, P.M. and Lieberman, S. (1990).   Troubled parents: vulnerability and stress in childhood cancer. *British Journal of Medical Psychology* **63**: 53–64.

Jessop, DJ., Riessman, C.K. and Stein, R.E.K. (1988).   Chronic childhood illness and maternal mental health. *Journal of Developmental and Behavioral Pediatrics* **9**: 147–156.

Kazak, A.E. and Meadows, A.T. (1989).   Families of young adolescents who have survived cancer: social-emotional adjustment, adaptability, and social support. *Journal of Pediatric Psychology* **14**: 175–191.

Katz, E.R. and Varni, J.W. (1993).   Social skills training for newly diagnosed children with cancer. *Cancer* **71**: 334–339.

Kupst, M.J., Schulman, J.L., Honig, G., Maurer, H., Morgan, E. and Fochtman, D. (1982).   Family coping with childhood leukemia: one year after diagnosis. *Journal of Pediatric Psychology* **73**: 157–174.

Kupst, M.J. and Schulman, J.L. (1988).   Long-term coping with pediatric leukemia. A six-year follow-up study. *Journal of Pediatric Psychology* **13**: 7–22.

Kupst, M.J. (1993). Family coping: supportive and obstructive factors. *Cancer* **71**: 3337–3341.

Lavigne, J.V. and Ryan, M. (1979).   Psychologic adjustment of siblings of children with chronic illness. *Pediatrics* **63**: 616–627.

Morrow, G.R., Hoagland, A. and Varnrike, C.L.M. (1981). Social support and parental adjustment to pediatric cancer. *Journal of Consulting and Clinical Psychology* **49**: 763–765.

Mott, M.G. (1990). A family in crisis: a child with cancer. *British Medical Journal* **301**: 133–134.

Mulhern, R.K., Carpentieri, S., Shema, S., Stone, P. and Fairclough, D. (1993). Factors associated with social and behavioral problems among children recently diagnosed with brain tumor. *Journal of Pediatric Psychology* **18**: 339–350.

Mulhern, R.K., Fairclough, D.L., Smith, B. and Douglass, S.M. (1992). Maternal depression assessment methods, and physical symptoms affect estimates of depressive symptomatology among children with cancer. *Journal of Pediatric Psychology* **17**: 313–326.

Mulhern, R.K., Wasserman, A.L., Friedman, A.G. and Fairclough, D. (1989) Social competence and behavioral adjustment of children who are long-term survivors of cancer. *Pediatrics* **83**: 18–25.

Nezu, A.M. (1986). Cognitive appraisal of problem-solving effectiveness: relation to depression and depressive symptoms. *Journal of Clinical Psychology* **42**: 847–852.

Nezu, A.M. (1987). A problem-solving formulation of depression: a literature review and proposal of a pluralistic model. *Clinical Psychology Review* **7**: 121–144.

Nezu, A.M. and Perri, M.G. (1989). Problem-solving therapy for unipolar depression: an initial dismantling study. *Journal of Consulting and Clinical Psychology* **57**: 408–413.

Nezu, A.M., Nezu, C.M., Houts, P., Faddis, S., Friedman S. (1999a). *Helping Cancer Patients Cope: A Problem-solving Approach.* Washington, DC: American Psychological Association.

Nezu, A.M., Nezu, C.M., Houts, P., Friedman, S. and Faddis, S. (1999b). Relevance of problem-solving therapy to psychosocial oncology. *Journal of Psychosocial Oncology* **16**: 5–26.

Overholsin, J.C. and Fritz, G.K. (1990). The impact of childhood cancer on the family. *Journal of Psychosocial Oncology* **8**: 71–85.

Pelcovitz, D., Goldenberg, B., Kaplan, S., Weinblatt, M., Mandel, F., Meyers, B. and Vinciguerra, V. (1996). Post-traumatic stress disorder in mothers of pediatric cancer survivors. *Psychosomatics* **37**: 116–126.

Phipps, S. and Mulhern, R.K. (1995). Family cohesion and expressiveness promote resilience to the stress of pediatric bone marrow transplant: a preliminary report. *Journal of Developmental and Behavioral Pediatrics* **16**: 257–263.

Pless, I.B. and Roghmann, K.J. (1971). Chronic illness and its consequences: observations based on three epidemiologic surveys. *Journal of Pediatrics* **79**: 357–359.

Raitt, D.S., Ostroff, J.S., Smith, K., Cella, D.F., Tan, C. and Lesko, L.M. (1992). Lives in a balance: perceived family functioning and the psychosocial adjustment of adolescent cancer survivors. *Family Process* **31**: 383–397.

Sahler, O.J.Z., Roghmann K.J., Carpenter, P.J., Mulhern, R.K., Dolgin, M.J., Sargent, J.R., Barbarin, O.A. Copeland, D.R. and Zeltzer, L.K. (1994). Sibling adaptation to childhood cancer collaborative study: prevalence of sibling distress and definition of adaptation levels. *Journal of Developmental and Behavioral Pediatrics* **15**: 353–366.

Sahler, O.J.Z., Roghmann, K.J., Mulhern, R.K., Carpenter, P.J., Sargent, J.R., Copeland, D.R., Barbarin, O.A., Zeltzer, L.K. and Dolgin, M.J. (1997). Sibling adaptation to childhood cancer collaborative study: the association of sibling adaptation with maternal well being, physical health, and resource use. *Journal of Developmental and Behavioral Pediatrics* **18**: 233–243.

Speechley, K.N. and Noh, S. (1992). Surviving childhood cancer, social support, and parents' psychological adjustment. *Journal of Pediatric Psychology* **17**:15–33.

Stuber, M.L., Christakis, D.A., Houskamp, B. and Kazak, A.E. (1996). Post-traumatic symptoms in childhood leukemia survivors and their parents. *Psychosomatics* **37**: 254–261.

Stuber, M.L., Gonzales, S., Meeske, K., Guthrie, D., Houskamp, B.M., Pynoos, R. and Kazak, A. (1994). Post-traumatic stress after childhood cancer. II. A family model. *Psycho-Oncology* **3**: 313–319.

Thompson, R.J., Gustafson, K.E., Hamlett, K.W. and Spock A. (1992). Stress, coping and family functioning in the psychological adjustment of mothers of children and adolescents with cystic fibrosis. *Journal of Pediatric Psychology* **17**: 573–585.

Tritt, S.G. and Esses, L.M. (1988). Psychosocial adaptation of siblings of children with chronic medical illnesses. *American Journal of Orthopsychiatry* **58**: 211–220.

Van Dongen-Melman, J.E.W.M. and Sanders-Woudstra, J.A.R. (1986). Psychosocial aspects of childhood cancer: a review of the literature. *Journal of Child Psychology and Psychiatry* **27**: 145–180.

Varni, J.W., Katz, E.R., Colegrove, R. and Dolgin, M. (1994). The impact of social skills training on the adjustment of children with newly diagnosed cancer. *Journal of Pediatric Psychology* **18**: 751–767.

Varni, J.W., Sahler, O.J., Katz, E.R., Mulhern, R.K., Copeland D.R., Noll, R.B., Phipps, S., Dolgin, M.J. and Roghmann, K. (1998). Maternal problem solving therapy in pediatric cancer. *Journal of Psychosocial Oncology* **16**: 41–72.

Wallander, J.L., Varni, J.W., Babani, L.V., Banis, H.T. and Wilcox, K.T. (1988). Children with chronic physical disorders: maternal reports of their psychological adjustments. *Journal of Pediatric Psychology* **13**: 197–212.

Wallander, J.L., Varni, J.W., Balbani, L., Banis, H.T. and Wilcox, K.T. (1989). Family resources as resistant factors for maladjustment in chronically ill and handicapped children. *Journal of Pediatric Psychology* **14**: 157–173.

Zeltzer, L.K., Dolgin, M.J., Sahler, O.J.Z., Roghmann, K.J., Barbarin, O.A., Carpenter, P.J., Copeland, D.R., Mulhern, R.K. and Sargent, J.R. (1996). Sibling adaptation to childhood cancer collaborative study: health outcomes of siblings of children with cancer. *Medical and Pediatric Oncology* **27**: 98–107.

Section VI
SEXUALITY: PERCEPTION
OF SELF

Sexual Self-concept for the Woman with Cancer

BARBARA L. ANDERSEN and DEANNA M. GOLDEN-KREUTZ

Department of Psychology, Ohio State University, Columbus, OH, USA

Cancer patients often experience sexual difficulties following treatment. In fact, it is the one area which is most likely to undergo disruption, more so than other major life areas, such as interpersonal relations and employment (Welch-McCaffrey et al., 1989). Review of disease site data suggests that disease and treatment factors, in part, account for much of the sexual dysfunction which occurs, as the majority of adult cancer patients with solid tumors (approximately 85% of all adult patients) are vulnerable to sexual dysfunction. Contemporary reviews highlight the importance of sexuality for cancer survivors, in general, as Gotay and Muraoka (1998) note:

> The aspects of QoL (quality of life) that pose the most difficulty for survivors are likely to vary by cancer site, but this literature strongly implies that sexual functioning and/or satisfaction is a common issue for many survivors, regardless of diagnosis or treatment.

There are several examples of the ways in which cancer treatments can impact a woman's sexuality. For example, there are gynecologic changes (e.g., vaginal discharge) associated with long-term adjuvant tamoxifen therapy for breast cancer (Wolf and Jordan, 1992), or what has been termed 'female androgen deficiency syndrome' from cytotoxic agents and/or bilateral salpingo-oophorectomies (Kaplan and Owett, 1993). Additionally, data suggests that if sexual problems develop, they do so as soon as intercourse resumes, and, if untreated, they are unlikely to resolve (Andersen et al., 1989). Thus, a significant number of female cancer survivors will experience sexual problems of either an acute or a chronic nature, and this may be one of the primary factors leading to problems with depression and their seeking of alternative therapies (e.g. herbal medicine, massage; Burstein et al., 1999).

We review the central findings regarding sexuality in women with cancer (see companion chapter by Schover et al., this volume, for review of sexuality in men). Three sections are included. First, we identify the common malignancies for women and provide a site-specific discussion of sexual morbidity. Predicting which women are at risk for sexual dysfunctions is an important need and is the focus of the second section. We provide our model for identifying which women will be at risk for mild,

Cancer and the Family, 2nd Edn. Edited by L. Baider, C. L. Cooper and A. Kaplan De-Nour
© 2000 John Wiley & Sons, Ltd

moderate, or severe sexual difficulty. Third, we discuss the individual difference variable, sexual self-schema, that can predict sexual outcomes for women with cancer. Moreover, we elaborate how cancer stress can provide the diathesis for the development of sexual dysfunction for women with a negative sexual self-schema. The third and final section presents a conceptual model for understanding the processes of sexual problem development and discusses various options currently available for the treatment of sexual dysfunctions in cancer patients.

COMMON MALIGNANCIES AND ASSOCIATED SEXUAL MORBIDITY

For women, cancer is a leading cause of death, usually ranking either first or second across age groups. Table 18.1 displays data from the USA on the incidence and death rates in women by site (Landis et al., 1999), and Table 18.2 provides incidence and death rate data from selected world areas (Parkin et al., 1999). Cancers vary in their prevalence and mortality—notice the geographic differences as displayed in Table 18.2 (e.g., overall death rates of 117.7 in the USA compared to 77.1 in China). Nonetheless, in examining the death rates worldwide, the top killers of women include breast, colon and rectum, stomach, lung, and gynecologic cancers (Parkin et al., 1999). We will focus on these four sites, as they account for the majority of all female cancer cases.

BREAST

Surgery is the initial treatment for virtually all women, and minimally involves axillary nodal biopsy or sampling and removal of the tumor (lumpectomy or breast-conserving therapy, BCT) or, more typically, axillary nodal dissection and the removal of the entire breast (modified radical mastectomy, MRM). Not all women receiving a modified radical mastectomy are eligible for breast reconstruction [e.g.,

Table 18.1   Cancer incidence and deaths in women by site—1999 US estimates

Incidence (total est. 598 000)			Deaths (total est. 272 000)		
Site	Number	(%)	Site	Number	(%)
Breast	175 000	(29)	Lung/bronchus	68 000	(25)
Lung/bronchus	77 600	(13)	Breast	43 000	(16)
Colon/rectum	67 000	(11)	Colon/rectum	28 000	(11)
Uterine corpus	37 400	(6)	Pancreas	14 500	(5)
Ovary	25 000	(4)	Ovary	14 500	(5)
Non-Hodgkin's lymphoma	24 200	(4)	Non-Hodgkin's lymphoma	12 300	(5)
Melanoma of skin	18 400	(3)	Leukemia	9700	(4)
Urinary bladder	15 100	(3)	Urinary corpus	6400	(2)
Pancreas	14 600	(2)	Brain/nervous system	5600	(2)
All other sites	130 000	(23)	Multiple myeloma	5600	(2)
			All other sites	57 200	(21)

Adapted from Landis et al. (1999).

Table 18.2   Age-standardized incidence and death rates for all sites in adult females per 100 000 for selected world areas

World area	Incidence	Deaths
Northern Africa	145.3	81.3
North America	277.5	117.7
South America (tropical)	185.0	111.0
Eastern Asia: China	105.3	77.1
Eastern Asia: Japan	166.8	79.9
Eastern Europe	172.8	102.9
Northern Europe	234.5	125.4
Western Europe	210.4	106.5
Australia/New Zealand	254.0	109.2
Developed countries	208.9	105.4
Developing countries	122.0	78.0

Adapted from Parkin et al. (1999).

tissue expander with implant, autologous tissue transfer from the abdomen or gluteal area, or permanent implant under a rotated latissimus dorsi (abdominal) flap], but those that are may elect to receive it at the time of mastectomy. Still other women may elect to have a bilateral mastectomy (removal of the breast with the tumor as well as removal of the other, disease-free, breast). Even though this is rare, women who request such extended surgery are typically those women with a strong familial history (i.e., a first-degree relative, a mother or sister who died of the disease at a young age), who are young when diagnosed (e.g., 45 years), and who actively want to reduce their risk of recurrence, as the remaining breast is the most common site for disease progression (Harris et al., 1993). Since breast cancer often spreads to the surrounding nodal areas, radiation, chemotherapy and/or hormonal therapy, and/or bone marrow transplant are the current adjuvant treatment options following surgical recovery.

The stage of disease/extent of initial surgical treatment are influential variables in determining sexual outcome for women with breast cancer. A meta-analysis of psychosocial outcomes of breast cancer surgery reported consistent psychologic advantages for lumpectomy (i.e., breast-conserving surgery) in contrast to mastectomy for body image and, to a lesser but still significant effect, for marital/sexual adjustment (Moyer, 1997). In fact, Moyer (1997) concluded: 'The largest and most robust effect size, showing benefits for breast-conserving surgery for body/self-image, is already a firmly established finding (p. 290).' For those women who receive mastectomy, by choice or necessity, reconstructive surgery may be included. Since reconstruction at the time of mastectomy incurs added cost and surgical morbidity (e.g., slower wound healing, extra days in hospital, added blood loss and anesthesia), research is needed to determine the benefit added. A certain motivation for reconstruction is for 'better' quality of life outcomes than with MRM alone.

We studied 190 women with Stage II or III breast cancer (Yurek et al., in press). Results indicated that during the immediate post-surgery period, women receiving breast reconstruction (MRMw/R) experienced disrupted sexual behavior and sexual responses, significantly more so than women receiving lumpectomy or mastectomy without reconstruction. Moreover, our data suggested that the reconstruction achieves no reduction in stress about the body changes, at least when assessed during the early post-surgery period, as the reconstruction group reported levels of stress equivalent to those of the women receiving mastectomy without reconstruction, and both mastectomy groups reported body change stress significantly higher (in some cases twice as high) as the responses of the women receiving lumpectomy. Descriptive data on the few women who requested bilateral mastectomy suggested that more radical surgical therapy does, indeed, result in greater psychological and behavioral morbidity.

COLON AND RECTUM

There is limited data on the sexual functioning of women after receiving treatment for colorectal cancer. In a review of the available literature after radical surgical treatment of rectal cancer (nine studies), van Driel et al. (1993) found that 20–78% of women experience loss of sexual desire postoperatively, with 38–65% discontinuing intercourse. Severe dyspareunia was found to be common. These rates are significantly higher than those found for individuals receiving related surgical treatments for benign conditions, such as ulcerative colitis treated with ileostomy (Kuchenoff et al., 1981). In particular, several factors were found to be related to sexual dysfunction after surgery in female rectal cancer patients, including type of surgery and reconstruction, and increased age (van Driel et al., 1993).

LUNG

Currently, no available data exists on sexual functioning in female lung cancer patients and/or their partners. However, we do know that there has been a striking increase in lung cancer incidence among women. Smoking is considered to be the major etiologic agent as the increase is directly related to women's changed smoking patterns in the 1940s, 1950s, and 1960s. Since 1987 in the USA, for example, more women have annually died of lung than breast cancer (Landis et al., 1999), a trend which is expected to continue for at least the next 15–20 years (Holleb, 1985). Untreated, 95% of lung cancer patients will die within 1 year. Even with treatment, the 5 year survival rate (e.g., the number of diagnosed patients who are still alive 5 years following treatment) is approximately 10% (American Cancer Society, 1999).

GYNECOLOGIC TUMORS

Cervix, Endometrial, and Ovary

There are three major sites for gynecologic cancer: the cervix (accounting for 9.8 of all new cases worldwide in women), the ovary (4.4 of new cases) and the endometrium (accounting for 3.7 of all new cases; Parkin et al., 1999). Vulvar cancer, accounting for the majority of remaining gynecologic cases, will be discussed below.

Cervix cancer is the seventh most common (third in mortality) malignant disease. It has had a world-wide decline in incidence, especially in developed countries. Potential risk factors include: early age at first intercourse; number of different sexual partners at an early age, along with intercourse with 'high-risk' males (i.e., males who have had contact with multiple partners); and being diagnosed with human papillomavirus (HPV). Symptoms often include abnormal bleeding or vaginal discharge; pain is often associated with advanced disease. Treatment strategies for cervical cancer include surgery, radiation, or a combination. For those with recurrent disease or extensive disease at diagnosis, the scenario is much more difficult and may include radical pelvic surgery, pelvic exenteration. This is a strategy for cure, but it incurs considerable behavioral, psychological, and sexual morbidity. The operation usually involves removal of the uterus, tubes, ovaries, bladder and/or rectum, and vagina, as well as part of the vulva for some women. The result is dramatic body alteration—one if not two abdominal stomas for urinary or fecal diversion, and necessary vaginal reconstruction, if it is possible and the woman desires it.

Risk factors for ovary disease include age, nulliparity, and familial history of breast or ovarian cancer. Only one-quarter are diagnosed with limited disease, compared to 50–80% of women with other types of gynecologic cancer. Treatment usually consists of debulking surgery (e.g., removal of the uterus, tubes, ovaries, lymphadenectomy, and all other visible signs of tumor), and lengthy, cytotoxic chemotherapy, usually with multiple agents.

Endometrial cancer rates show a sharp increase in the perimenopausal years, with a peak occurrence at ages 55–66. Risk factors include early age at menarche, late age of menopause, infertility, and obesity. Treatment for endometrial cancer usually consists of surgery (e.g., total abdominal hysterectomy and bilateral salpingo-oophorectomy) and, possibly, radiation, hormone therapy, and/or chemotherapy.

Sexual Disruption before Diagnosis Clinical studies have noted that postcoital bleeding or pelvic pain, for example, may alert a woman to the need for medical care. For instance, Andersen et al. (1986) found that prior to the onset of cancer signs/symptoms, gynecologic cancer patients reported similar patterns of sexual activity and responsiveness as healthy women, but with the appearance of disease signs/symptoms (e.g., fatigue, postcoital bleeding, vaginal discharge, pain), the women experienced significant sexual difficulties. In fact, women have reported that they have initiated changes in intercourse frequency because of bleeding (or fear of), pain, and anxiety (Harris et al., 1982). Thus, it appears that women who experience a substantial change in sexual functioning tend to negatively interpret this disruption and seek medical attention.

Surgery, Radiation, and/or Chemotherapy   The three primary treatments for localized or regional pelvic disease for cervix, endometrial, and ovarian cancer have potentially different effects on sexuality. Considering radical hysterectomy and related surgeries (e.g., total abdominal hysterectomy), controlled prospective longitudinal data confirm that even simple hysterectomy for benign disease produces significant sexual disruption (Andersen et al., 1989; Weijmar Schultz et al., 1991). Thus, the vaginal shortening with radical hysterectomy (approximately one-third of the upper vagina is removed) can contribute to subjective feelings for the woman that the vagina is 'too short' for intercourse. Nerve and vascular disruption to the pelvis (as may occur with lymphadenectomy) may also result in loss of sensitivity and orgasmic disruption. Premature menopause, with the direct effects of atrophic vaginitis from estrogen deprivation, can also result in sexual difficulties (e.g., vaginal narrowing or closing).

Radiation therapy destroys ovarian functioning and, thus, induces menopausal symptomatology for premenopausal women and causes vaginal atrophy and stenosis for all women. These outcomes are most severe for women treated with vaginal irradiation (intracavitary radium/cesium implants; see Andersen et al., 1984, for a discussion of the psychological aspects of this difficult treatment) when it is used alone or in combination with external beam irradiation (Karlsson and Andersen, 1986). Estrogen therapy following treatment can control such symptoms as 'hot flushes' and aid in the healing of the vaginal epithelium (Walling et al., 1990), and use of vaginal dilators can reduce or eliminate fibrosis (e.g., the vaginal walls 'sticking' together; Krumm and Lamberti, 1993). However, due to the magnitude of the vaginal changes, dyspareunia may still occur.

Chemotherapy is used in the treatment of advanced disease and/or when residual tumor is left after surgery and/or radiotherapy. In addition to the general side-effects of chemotherapy (e.g., nausea/vomiting, bladder/kidney toxicity, and bone marrow suppression), it can induce and/or increase menopausal symptoms which result in sexual dysfunctions.

Radical Surgery (Pelvic Exenteration)   As noted, this radical surgery is used for extensive but resectable disease at diagnosis, for some women with centrally recurrent disease, and, more recently, to lengthen survival time in patients with recurrent disease. Clinical reports, not surprisingly, have reported the cessation of sexual activity for many women (e.g., 15%, according to Corney et al., 1993; 80–90% according to Andersen and Hacker, 1983a). For the majority of women and couples, the prospect of ending their sexual life (as most couples cease all sexual activity when intercourse becomes impossible) is distressing and may be a source of continuing marital discord.

Vaginal reconstruction (e.g., with a loop of bowel or portions of inner thigh muscle) is a possibility for some and enables a woman to maintain sexual activity that includes intercourse. However, many sexual difficulties often remain, including problems with the physical characteristics of the new vagina (e.g., the cavity is too large, too narrow), arousal and/or orgasm, or dyspareunia and/or bleeding with intercourse. Regardless of whether or not women with pelvic exenteration undergo vaginal reconstruction, these women face the greatest disruption to their sexual body and functioning of any female cancer group.

Combined Therapies   Patients treated with combination therapy usually receive a lower total dose of radiation than those treated with radiotherapy only. In addition, depending on the surgical procedure, the apex of the vagina, which is exposed to the largest dose of radiation when intracavitary treatment is included, is removed during surgery. Thus, the remaining portion of the vagina is less affected and, perhaps, less vulnerable to problems of dyspareunia. These patients would be expected to be at greater risk for sexual morbidity because of the combination therapy.

In general, the rates of sexual behavior disruption and dysfunction are comparable between surgery and radiation treatments (see Andersen and van der Does, 1994, for a review). Following cancer treatment, women have reported awareness of fewer signs of sexual excitement and lower arousability for sexual activities with their partner (Andersen et al., 1989), especially women who have received radiation (Cull et al., 1993). The most likely reason for the arousal deficits is the co-occurrence of significant disruptors (e.g., dyspareunia, due in part to radiation effects and/or induced menopause). Data consistent with these results have been reported by others (e.g., Cull et al., 1993; Krumm and Laberti, 1993; Weijmar Schultz et al., 1991). Additionally, Krumm and Laberti (1993) have noted that poor compliance with treatment may lead to sexual avoidance and ultimately to sexual difficulties (e.g., older women who do not feel comfortable using vaginal dilators). As it has been estimated that radiation-induced tissue changes continue for upwards of 5 years following the completion of therapy, the need to adhere to treatment recommendations is critical.

Vulva

This cancer is rare and occurs most commonly among older/elderly women. When a woman seeks treatment, vulvar itching is often a long-standing complaint, although a mass or growth is most common. Ignorance or misinterpretation of the symptoms is common for patients and physicians alike, such that delay is a major problem. Surgery is the primary treatment modality, and can vary from a wide local excision of the lesion to a modified radical vulvectomy, which removes all labial tissue and often the clitoris and usually the lymph nodes in the groin and/or pelvis. Radiation therapy can accompany surgery.

Treatment can produce extreme genital disfigurement and many women have difficulty adjusting to the body changes (Andersen and Hacker, 1983b). Even though the population of women diagnosed with vulvar cancer is older than the 'average' patient with cervical or ovary disease, there is no data to suggest that they will be less distressed by changes to their sexuality. Not surprisingly, the reports of women who are treated with vulvectomy vs. wide local excision are dramatically different, with the former patients becoming non-orgasmic and the latter patients maintaining orgasm and other sexual responses (DiSaia et al., 1979).

Andersen and colleagues have also provided data on the sexual outcomes for women treated with wide local excision and related treatments for *in situ* disease. Overall, it appears that *in situ* patients as a group are more likely to be sexually inactive at follow-up, whether or not they have available sexual partners, than age-matched healthy counterparts. Additionally, the outcomes for women with *in situ* disease contrast markedly with those for women with invasive disease, many of whom are treated with vulvectomy, with or without groin dissection. The general trend is consistent: at least 30–50% of patients become sexually inactive, and of the women remaining active, 60–70% have multiple sexual dysfunctions. For the women who become sexually inactive, many factors may be contributory, including negative feelings (by the woman or her partner) about the physical changes to the body, and severe dyspareunia related to narrowed introitus. However, despite poorer sexual responding (Weijmar Schultz et al., 1990), the majority of women would have preferred to remain sexually active rather than to have all intimacy end (e.g., Andersen and Hacker, 1983b).

PREDICTING RISK FOR SEXUAL MORBIDITY

Sufficient psychosocial research has been conducted in the last two decades on sexual outcomes to begin to develop models to predict which women will be at risk for psychological or behavioral morbidity. Earlier, Schag et al. (1993) noted the importance of identifying characteristics of women at risk for psychosocial distress. In a test of predictors for women with breast cancer, women who were at moderate to high risk for problem development at diagnosis had concerns, such as continuing psychological distress, difficult communication with marital partners, negative body image, and disrupted sexuality at the 12 month follow-up. In this section we provide a model and identify variables, both medical and psychological, which predict sexual difficulties following cancer in women. The majority of the variables identified are ones that are known at the times of diagnosis and early recovery.

MEDICAL CONTRIBUTORS

The previous review clarifies the significant role of medical factors, such as the extent of disease and magnitude of treatment, in negatively influencing sexual outcomes. We have formulated a model of disease and treatment pathways which can yield differential levels of risk for sexual morbidity (see Figure 18.1; see also Andersen, 1993). Variables are introduced according to a disease time line, from cancer appearance to the immediate post-treatment recovery period, as disease-relevant events provide a meaningful framework for understanding psychological adjustment to cancer.

Turning to the model (Figure 18.1), at the onset of cancer we consider the occurrence of disruptive signs/symptoms. When the disease is detected and produces sexual disruption, this is the first point of psychological/behavioral morbidity. It is clear that such early disruption occurs for women eventually diagnosed with gynecologic cancer (Andersen et al., 1986). With the appearance of disease indicants (e.g., fatigue, postcoital bleeding, vaginal discharge, pain), women reported a dramatic change in sexual functioning which can include loss of desire, lowered excitement, and dyspareunia. We found a four- to five-fold increase in the frequency of sexual dysfunctions from pre- to post-appearance of cancer signs/symptoms. This early change is included because of its role in increasing a woman's emotional distress and alerting her to the potential for subsequent life changes.

The model indicates that the extent of disease and treatment are major determinants of risk. As indicated, the disease and treatment status is summarized

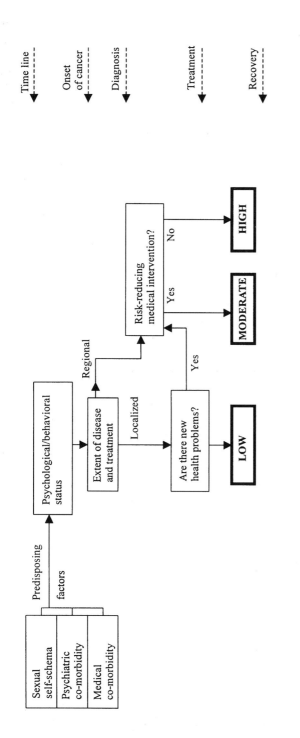

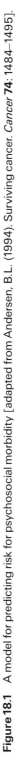

Figure 18.1 A model for predicting risk for psychosocial morbidity [adapted from Andersen, B.L. (1994). Surviving cancer. *Cancer* **74**: 1484–1495].

into routes of 'limited' vs. 'extensive;' these alternatives should have supporting medical endpoint data, as well as stage and magnitude of treatment information. The limited/extensive distinction is based in part on the classification of disease stage—localized vs. regional or metastatic—and its direct relationship to survival for most disease sites. The model goes one step further and suggests that the extent of disease be considered in the context of the magnitude of treatment received. For example, women with localized or regional breast cancer receive the same surgical treatment—modified radical mastectomy—and might only differ in the provision of adjuvant chemotherapy. Thus, even though the women differ in the extent of the disease, they can receive the same (or closely related) cancer therapies.

For those women whose therapy can not be modified, the model next considers the availability of risk-reducing medical interventions. For those with extensive disease/treatment, the availability of such interventions may potentially reduce the level of risk from 'high' to 'moderate.' Examples of rehabilitative medical efforts include vaginal reconstruction for pelvic exenteration patients, labia preservation for vulva cancer patients, or breast reconstruction for women treated with a modified radical mastectomy. For women who have had such interventions, psychological, behavioral, and sexual outcomes may be better, although the interventions are not panaceas (e.g., Andersen and Hacker, 1983a,b; Yurek et al., in press, for data).

For those with limited disease/treatment, the availability of medical interventions could potentially reduce their risk from 'low' to approximate that of healthy individuals (i.e., the base rate). For example, some women experiencing a surgical menopause following treatment for localized cervical cancer can be treated with hormonal replacement therapy, just as are healthy women who experience a natural menopause with its attendant difficulties (Matthews et al., 1990).

The final contributor to risk is new health problems (e.g., hormonal changes and/or continuing stressors from the disease/treatment). Consideration of hormonal changes includes two issues: induced menopause and infertility. As discussed, many women undergo premature menopause because of their treatment. Menopausal changes produce significant sexual effects (see Walling et al., 1990, for a review). Also, ovary removal/sterilization ends child bearing—a potential stressor for some, particularly young, women. Continuing stressors can be heterogeneous. Examples include chronic fatigue (Meyerowitz et al., 1983) or late morbidities from treatments (e.g., a bowel fistula following pelvic irradiation). Should such problems arise, the model considers the availability of effective treatments.

In sum, multiple pathways can lead to high or moderate morbidity risk, but only those individuals who have limited disease/treatment and who have no new or continuing problems are hypothesized to have the lowest risk.

SEXUAL SCHEMA AND OTHER PSYCHOLOGICAL CONTRIBUTORS

While the factors noted above may contribute to morbidity, psychological/behavioral variables may be important as well. Moreover, psychological variables have the potential to be influenced (i.e. changed) and so are positioned to be the most important in predicting, as well as reducing, sexual morbidity. The model in Figure 18.1 begins with 'baseline' psychological/behavioral factors—age, sexual status (active/inactive), and prior frequency of important sexual activities (such as intercourse). These factors have emerged as important predictors of sexual activity in the earliest research on sexuality (e.g., Kinsey et al., 1953), as well as contemporary variants (e.g., Newcomb, 1986; Wyatt et al., 1988a,b). These variables are important predictors in studies of healthy individuals, but their predictive utility is also found in studies of individuals with chronic conditions and illnesses (e.g., Curry et al., 1993; Keil et al., 1992). Thus, we note these variables in preface to the discussion below.

In identifying a psychological variable relevant to sexual or body change outcomes, many investigators proposed body image (e.g., Derogatis, 1980). While this undoubtedly occurred because of its intuitive appeal, body image was also a variable seen as relevant to sexuality for healthy women (Cash, 1991). There have been descriptive findings of poor body concept among cancer patients, particularly in early studies of women with breast cancer (de Haes and Welvaart, 1985). However, in the majority of these studies the measures of the body image construct are not validated. In fact, psychometric studies have found weak theoretical notions of the construct and poor operationalizations (e.g., measures of poor reliability/validity; Andersen and LeGrand, 1991). In our empirical tests, we found that body image measures could not predict outcome either among breast cancer patients (Andersen and Jochimsen, 1985) or in multiple samples of women with gynecologic cancer (Andersen and LeGrand, 1991).

Rather than examining a view of the body *per se* we have proposed a more central perspective—a woman's view of herself as a sexual person or her sexual self-schema—as a predictor of sexual morbidity. *Sexual self-schema (or sexual self-concept)* is a cognitive view about sexual aspects of oneself; it is derived from past experience, manifest in current experience, and it guides the processing of domain-relevant social information (Andersen and Cyranowski, 1994; Andersen et al., 1999).

With this conceptual formulation, extensive psychometric work was done to operationalize the construct and develop a measure of sexual schema for women (Andersen and Cyranowski, 1994) and men (Andersen et al., 1999). Using the trait adjective methodology, the brief scale assesses a cognitive self-view of sexuality. For women, the scale includes two positive aspects—an inclination to experience romantic/passionate emotions and a behavioral openness to sexual experiences and/or relationships—and a negative aspect—embarrassment and/or conservatism—which appears to be a deterrent to sexual expression. For men, the scale includes three positive aspects—an inclination to experience romantic/passionate emotions; stereotypical characteristics of men, such as aggressive and independent attributes; and a behavioral openness to sexual experiences and/or relationships.

Sexual self-schemas represent basic or core beliefs regarding sexual aspects of the self. We contend that individual differences in sexual self-view represent an important cognitive diathesis for predicting sexual difficulty or dysfunction. The Sexual Self-Schema Scales provide brief, easy-to-administer, reliable, and stable assessments of both males' and females' views of the sexual self. Moreover, the subtle and unobtrusive nature of this cognitive assessment approach represents an important advance over alternative, sexually-explicit measures that may be hampered by respondent discomfort, social desirability, or other response biases (see Catania et al., 1990; Weinhardt et al., 1998). Such measurement characteristics make this self-report scale a practical assessment tool for use in both clinical and research settings.

The specificity of the sexual self-schema construct, the relationship of sexual schemas to relevant sexual outcomes, and the potential interaction of sexual schemas with sexually-relevant stressors, all contribute to considering that sexual schemas may represent a significant vulnerability factor or diathesis. Our research suggests that positive, sexual self-views may facilitate sexual functioning. However, when sexual self-schemas are extremely negative, conflicted, or weak, they may diathesize for the occurrence of subsequent sexual dysfunction. Stressful events or assaults to the sexual system—such as certain medical or psychological stressors—may interact with negative (or, for males, weak) sexual self-schema to create deficits in sexual functioning.

As an initial test of this diathesis-stress model of sexual dysfunction, we have tested the construct in the context of risk for sexual morbidity following gynecologic cancer (Woods et al., 1997) and breast cancer (Yurek et al., in press). Consistent with our definition of the construct, we anticipated that women 'low' in sexual self-concept, in contrast to women with a 'high' sexual self-concept, would be at greatest risk for sexual difficulty. Low-sexual-schema women would be expected to have more difficulties because they are, in general, less romantic/passionate in their emotions, less open to sexual experiences, and more likely to have negative feelings about their sexuality. Thus, in the context of cancer—with disease or treatment factors causing direct changes to the sexual body or sexual responses—we find that women with 'low' sexual self-schemas are at greater risk. Women with negative self-views of their sexuality find that their sexual arousability is lower, they are less apt to try new sexual activities as a way to cope with their sexual difficulties, and they have more negative cognitions or feelings, such as embarrassment, about any body changes. Indeed, they are more vulnerable to traumatic stress reactions from changes to their sexual body, such as outcomes with breast cancer surgeries (Yurek et al., in press). This research indicated that sexual self-schema scores accounted for a full 28% of the variance in women's post-treatment sexual responsiveness, over and above such variables as previous sexual frequency, extent of disease-treatment, and menopausal status.

We propose that interventions to prevent sexual morbidity or provide rehabilitation when difficulties arise will be important for the woman with a negative sexual self-concept. Interventions can provide specific strategies for managing sexual difficulties, but interventions could challenge the women's typical—i.e. negative—sexual self-view. Interventions can provide strategies for enhancing sexual self-schema, such as strategies for becoming aroused during sexual activity, open to sexual experiences, and less inhibited, embarrassed, or nervous. In the next section, we provide a process model of sexual activity and sexual response cycle problem development among women with cancer (Andersen and Elliot, 1993). It details the differences between 'dysfunctional' and 'non-dysfunctional' response patterns. The 'dysfunctional' pattern is based on our empirical findings (e.g., Andersen et al., 1989), but it is characterized by low arousal, behavioral inhibition, and negativity—a constellation of responses which mirror the responses of women with more negative sexual self-schemas.

INTERVENTIONS FOR SEXUAL MORBIDITY

Psychological interventions can reduce distress, hasten resumption of routine activities, and improve social outcomes for groups at high risk for psychological or behavioral morbidity, such as those with disseminated or recurrent disease, as well as those at low or moderate risk (see Andersen, 1992, for a review). When controlled studies have been reviewed, effective therapy components have included: an emotionally supportive context to address fears and anxieties about the disease (e.g., Cain et al., 1986; Capone et al., 1980; Maguire et al., 1983), information about the disease and treatment (e.g., Cain et al., 1986; Fawzy et al., 1990), behavioral coping strategies (e.g., role playing difficult discussions with family or the medical staff; Fawzy et al., 1990), cognitive coping strategies (Cain et al., 1986; Telch and Telch, 1986), and relaxation training to lower 'arousal' and/or enhance one's sense of control (Fawzy, et al., 1990). There are insufficient data to choose among components, but the literature would suggest an emphasis on relaxation, coping, social support, and disease-specific components (Andersen, 1992).

A CLINICAL PROCESS MODEL OF SEXUAL DYSFUNCTION FOLLOWING TREATMENT

The clinical formulation described here provides a conceptual basis for the formulation of interventions for sexual difficulties (see Table 18.3). In brief, this is a process model of the development of significant sexual dysfunction. We contrast specific 'dysfunctional' behaviors and responses with 'functional' ones. The model begins with an explicit initiation for sexual activity, as couples attempt to return to their prior 'routines' for sex. Longitudinal data indicate that from the beginning couples make few changes to accommodate the fact that the woman has had cancer (Andersen et al., 1989). The only accommodation that is usually made is 'waiting' to resume intercourse. We include the interactions of behavioral, cognitive, affective, and physiologic processes.

We focus first on sexual behavior—the frequency and context for sexual activity. It is typical that the frequency of intercourse declines significantly during the early post-treatment recovery period and remains at a lowered level during the first year of recovery. This general effect of reduction in intercourse frequency has been replicated across gynecologic and breast patients, although the reductions are more extreme (intercourse occurs rarely or never) for women receiving the most radical genital surgeries (e.g., Andersen and Hacker, 1983a,b). We also know that global behavioral disruption does not usually occur; that is, when couples engage in intercourse, albeit less often, they continue the same pattern of sexual behaviors that had occurred prior to cancer diagnosis. This suggests that no 'prompting' of the sexual behavior repertoire is needed, but it also shows that couples do not spontaneously vary their sexual behavior. Indeed, couples continue to engage, perhaps unadvisedly, in the same range and type of sexual activities, even when the result is significant sexual disruption or even intercourse pain for the woman.

Regarding sexual desire, many data suggest that upwards of 50% of women will be diagnosed with a sexual desire disorder during the early post-treatment period (Andersen and van der Does, 1994). One half of these cases will resolve during the first post-treatment year; however, there will be a comparable number of new, late cases by 1 year post-treatment. The higher rate of desire problems early in the post-treatment year may be due in part to the emotional crisis surrounding diagnosis and

Table 18.3 Model of the psychological processes of sexual dysfunction following cancer and comparison with the functional pattern of healthy women. Explicit initiation of sexual activity (e.g. an interested partner and "usual" contexts for sexual interactions)

	Functional pattern	Dysfunctional pattern
Change in the contexts for sexual activity	None usually occurs, although the woman is adaptive and may even initiate minor alterations	Changes in the timing of sexual activity (e.g. a change in a "routine" from intercourse in the evening hours to the morning) or the contexts (e.g. coital position) may require explicit planning and communication with the sexual partner which may be beyond the woman's repertoire or require known but unfamiliar strategies. The absence or failure of efforts can result in continued timing/contextual difficulties
Frequency of sexual activity	Frequency pattern is established which is flexible to acute and time limited stressors	Intercourse may have been halted due to medical treatment and other sexual interactions or intimacy are significantly reduced or absent
Sexual desire	Sexual thoughts/fantasies occur, affect is neutral to positive regarding sexual activity, and the individual initiates and/or responds to partner's initiations for sexual activity	The woman may not feel "sexual" or have sexual thoughts/fantasies. General affect may be labile and/or negative due to the recent diagnosis, disease, and/or treatment. There are few, if any, initiations for sexual activity and there is lowered interest in responding to her partner's initiations
Sexual excitement (arousal): Cognitive, affective, and behavioral responses	Sexual cognitions occur with positive affect and expectancies. Psychological arousal facilitates efficient focus on erotic cues and further increases in arousal	Lack of information or uncertainty about "changed" sexual responses and anatomy predominates sexual cognitions and leads to a "spectatoring" for signs/symptoms of pre-diagnosis sexual response. The ability to focus on erotic cues is significantly impaired and alternative foci of visible sexual body changes (e.g. mastectomy scar) and/or new disruptors from disease/treatment (e.g. dyspareunia) lowers erotic focus further. The affective experience is neutral to negative, and behavioral strategies to enhance arousal may not be known or, if known, are plagued by confirmed fears of disrupted sexual responses

Sexual excitement: Physiologic responses	The individual experiences the signs of sexual arousal (e.g. lubrication, bodily warmth). If difficulties occur, only minor changes (e.g. changing the focus of stimulation, fantasizing) are required and the strategies have a high rate of success	Any change from pre-disease/treatment response (e.g. absence of vaginal lubrication) confirms fears and anxiety of changed sexuality. Psychological efforts (e.g. fantasizing) to facilitate physiological arousal may have limited success if the changes are permanent. If the latter is not the case, the psychological/behavioral efforts may require an unfamiliar or expanded behavioral repertoire for the woman and perhaps her partner (e.g. masturbation with intercourse; alternative intercourse positions; body touching without the expectation for intercourse)
Orgasm	Orgasm may occur with positive anticipation and accrued sexual arousal. Signs of the response are felt (e.g. rhythmic contractions) with the accompanying psychologic sensations of release and pleasure	Lowered arousal or inhibitors/distractors predominate such that orgasm does not occur. If it does occur, it may be experienced as "different" (e.g. subjectively not as intense) or may be accompanied by interfering sensations (e.g. pain). Any orgasm disruption reinforces the negative cognition of changed sexuality and negative affective responses of fear and frustration.
Resolution	The woman views her sexual responses as functional and her sexual activities as positive. Psychological contentment and satisfaction and physiologic relaxation accompany the positive cognitions	The woman views her responses as impaired and their performance as dysfunctional. For those who experienced some arousal without orgasm, there may be residual sexual tension or residual discomfort if sexual activity was accompanied with pain. Doubts about sexuality have been confirmed and compensatory strategies may have been absent, or if attempted, may have failed. Affect is globally negative with the possibility of specific reactions of depressed, anxious, or angry mood
Responses to subsequent sexual opportunities	The individual continues to approach sexual encounters. There are neutral to positive cognitive and affective responses and effective physiologic responses	The individual avoids or, if engages, seeks an early termination of a sexual episode, as there are negative cognitions and affects with disrupted or permanently impaired physiologic responses. The individual may engage only out of "duty" to the partner with a further lowering of their own erotic focus

treatment. This suggests that interventions to reduce affective distress would be important and that lowered distress might enhance sexual desire.

Of all the phases of the sexual response cycle, sexual excitement—including cognitive, affective, behavioral, and physiologic responses—undergoes the greatest disruption with cancer treatment. This disruption takes the form of women viewing themselves as dysfunctional, reporting lowered arousability and reduced awareness of physiologic signs of arousal (e.g., body/pelvic warmth, lubrication). The lowered arousability is specific to foreplay and intercourse (Andersen et al., 1989), suggesting that women's ability to focus on erotic cues is significantly impaired. Some women, particularly those treated for pelvic tumors (e.g., cervix, ovary, colon) may also have dyspareunia (the most significant and distracting sensation to sexual arousal). In addition, women also report negative cognitions about their bodies, with a narrowing of negative thoughts and evaluations for the body part that has undergone change (e.g., the breast, the pelvis, the genitals; Andersen and LeGrand, 1991).

In view of these difficulties, it is not surprising that orgasm can be impaired. For example, there is a four-fold increase (e.g., 7–25%) in the frequency of orgasmic dysfunction from pre- to post-treatment (Andersen et al., 1989) among women treated for gynecologic cancer. Orgasmic difficulty for women produces moderate distress and provides a salient indicator to women that their sexual responses are significantly impaired. For some, the high levels of dyspareunia during intercourse is a probable contributor to orgasmic dysfunction.

Finally, the resolution phase is also disrupted for many women. There may be residual pain following intercourse. In addition, women may view their sexual life as significantly changed. Again, our data indicate that their evaluation worsens with the 'magnitude' of disease/treatment; for women with cervix, endometrial, ovary, or breast cancer these evaluations are 'below average' (e.g., Andersen et al, 1989), for women with vulvar disease the evaluation is 'inadequate' (Andersen and Hacker, 1983b), and for women treated with pelvic exenteration, the evaluation is 'poor' (Andersen and Hacker, 1983a).

Data suggest that the problems described above are most severe in the earliest post-treatment months and they begin as soon as intercourse is resumed. Further, the development of sexual problems for the male partner (e.g., delayed ejaculation in particular) may be sequelae to the women's problems. For couples that abandoned sexual activity, our longitudinal data indicated that the typical scenario was that a couple would resume intercourse in the early months, experience significant sexual problems, and then not make future attempts. Thus, for both the woman and her partner, the sexual interaction is initially problematic, it can become more difficult, and the situation may worsen with the lack of knowledge or failed efforts to change. Thus, we hypothesize that the response to subsequent sexual opportunities may be avoidance after these initial, difficult times. The avoidance mechanism then results in a further reduction in the frequency of sexual activity, resulting in a negative feedback loop.

INTERVENTION STRATEGIES

In addition to focusing on sexual functioning, many therapists might wish to offer sexual therapy within the context of a broad-based stress and coping framework.

Such interventions might be designed, for example, to reduce stress, enhance coping and effective problem solving, provide information regarding the effects of the disease and treatment, enhance social adjustment, and address gynecologic specific sexual concerns—sexual self-concept, sexual behavior, and sexual functioning.

Three intervention studies have included sexuality components as part of a multicomponent effort. Two studies included women at low morbidity risk. Capone et al. (1980) provided a brief, crisis-oriented intervention. For sexually active women, a sexual therapy component included sexual information and methods to cope and reduce anxiety when resuming intercourse. Fifty-six newly diagnosed women (88% were Stage I–III) with gynecologic cancer were included. A non-equivalent control group was obtained by recruiting previously treated women. Analyses indicated no differences between groups or within the intervention group on the measures of emotional distress, but substantial differences were found between the groups in the resumption and frequency of intercourse across all post-treatment assessments (e.g., 16% of the intervention vs. 57% of the control women reported less or no sexual activity at 12 months post-treatment). The second quasi-experimental investigation was reported by Houts et al. (1986) and used a peer counseling model. Interventions were delivered in telephone contacts and booklet descriptions of the coping strategies. Thirty-two women, 14 intervention and 18 control, participated. Analyses indicated no differences between groups at any point in time.

The only study with moderate-risk women is that of Cain et al. (1986) comparing individual and group therapy formats. The intervention included discussion of the causes of cancer at diagnosis, impact of the treatment(s) on body image and sexuality, relaxation training, and setting goals for the future to cope with uncertainty and fears of recurrence, delivered in 8 sessions. Seventy-two women with gynecologic cancer (21 individual intervention, 22 group intervention, and 29 no-treatment control) completed the study. Analyses indicated that there were no differences between the intervention formats, but both intervention groups reported less depression and anxiety, better psychosocial adjustment (including health perspectives and use of leisure time) and sexual functioning than the no-treatment control group. In summary, these quasi-experimental designs suggest that even broad-based interventions in which sexuality occupies a relatively minor focus can produce significant improvements in sexual functioning.

Selection of specific therapeutic techniques and content for a sexuality intervention can be guided by the literature in psychosocial intervention research with cancer patients (for review, see Andersen, 1992), behavioral sex therapy techniques, and clinical experience treating women during health crises or for sexual dysfunction. For the sexuality portions, one can rely on many of the same sexual therapy principles and techniques that have documented effectiveness with healthy individuals (Masters and Johnson, 1970; Rosen and Beck, 1988), as many of the sexual problems described above are common ones (e.g., anticipatory concerns about resuming sexual activity following abstinence, arousal deficits, orgasmic dysfunction). However, other problems are unique (e.g., dyspareunia due to radiation-induced vaginal atrophy or stenosis), more severe (e.g., orgasmic dysfunction due to nerve and/or vascular disruption/removal, rather than a skills deficit), or more distressing or difficult to overcome (e.g., body disfigurement, which is permanent). Thus, development of some new techniques may be necessary, although the basic principles of social learning interventions (e.g. graduated assignments; development of a non-demanding performance environment) will be important. Finally, an oft-preferred strategy for conducting a sexual intervention is with couples when both individuals are available and interested in participating. However, it is clear that significant gains can be achieved by treating the individual, whether the woman has cancer or is healthy (Andersen, 1981).

Stress Reduction

There are three central components that many therapists find useful. First is providing the woman with a way to conceptualize or think about the cancer stressor experience. For example, one model is that of Gatchel et al.'s (1989) model of stress as a psychophysiological process. Second, teaching a woman adaptive coping strategies (e.g., seeking information, positive appraisal) can be offered as skills that can be learned and applied generically. Third, some strategy to reduce overall tension and anxiety, such as guided imagery or progressive muscle relaxation (e.g., Bernstein and Borkovec, 1973), is useful. It can be used as a method for lowering overall body tension and women can be provided with audiotapes for home use.

Disease and Treatment Information

Didactic materials on general disease/treatment can be developed, but in most countries the federal or national agencies often publish patient education materials that can be used.

Cognitive Restructuring and Problem Solving

There are two components that may be useful. Cognitive restructuring can be used to identify current manifestations of the cancer stressor (e.g., low mood, low energy/fatigue, disrupted relationship with spouse). The A (Activity/event)–B (Beliefs/automatic thoughts)–C (Consequences/feelings and behaviors) model can be offered as a conceptual framework, and then specific examples from the woman's experience would be important. Problem solving can follow the same cognitive principles. The procedure typically consists of five stages: (a) overview of the principles; (b) how to define and formulate target problems; (c) generation of problem solutions; (d) decision making; and (e) verification of solutions. To learn the principles, women could be provided with 'hands-on' experience by working on solutions for one or two common problems confronting women with cancer, such as fatigue and time management.

Enhancing Social Adjustment and Support

There are typically three components to such interventions. First, the intervention effort *per se* can be used to direct social comparisons among women. This is done most easily if treatment is offered in a group format, as members then learn that many of their reactions to the cancer are normal and shared by others (e.g., Shelley Taylor's conceptualization of adjustment to threatening events; Taylor et al., 1984).

Second, a useful technique is to help a woman identify her social network so that she may more clearly assess and access social support. One simple way is to use a concentric circle model (with the patient at the center). One can then systematically cover other levels of social relationships (e.g., close friends and family—parents/in laws, siblings; children of all ages; spouse/spouse equivalent) and identify sources of satisfaction and clarify areas of difficulty. This is especially important, as it is not uncommon for family members' distress to approach that of the patient's (Cassileth et al., 1985; Given et al., 1993). In fact, higher distress levels in patients are correlated with distress levels in spouses (Baider and Kaplan De-Nour, 1984, 1988; Cassileth et al., 1985; Northouse and Swain, 1987; Oberst and James, 1985). Finally, the teaching of assertive communication skills, modeled after the work of Jakubowski and Lange (1978), can assist women in expressing their thoughts, feelings, and needs in a manner which facilitates support from, and communication with, members of their social networks. Four techniques are often used: (a) specifying and clarifying of one's message; (b) direct communication; (c) 'owning' one's message (use of 'I,' 'my', etc., in statements); and (d) asking for feedback. These skills can be practiced across the levels of social relationships identified above. This is especially important as disruption in the family exacerbated by the patient's cancer diagnosis and treatment can evolve into a chronic problem if not addressed (Northouse, 1988).

Sexuality

There are six components we find helpful:

1. Coping with cancer and the potential impact on one's body can include didactic information on the specific disease, treatment modality, and changes anticipated/received for body parts and functions. Therapy sessions can include dialogue regarding the woman's feelings about the didactic information, problem solving for immediate concerns (e.g., recuperation from surgery, coping with menopausal symptoms, fear of recurrence), and role play of communication skills for facilitating problem solving and soliciting the support/assistance of others.

2. It is useful to consider the context for physical and sexual (body) changes and attempt to enhance sexual self-esteem. Didactic components can review the bodily changes brought by treatment, with an emphasis on female sexual anatomy and physiology (coverage of the sexual response cycle and expected changes), sexual activity as a natural function, identifying and relabeling pain/ discomfort or other difficult-to-control symptoms that may occur following treatment, and learning about one's body through touch. Homework components are often necessary and will need to be individualized depending on the disease site and treatment. Regardless of the site, however, assignments often include self-exploration of the body in bath/shower, with or without including the breasts/genitals, a clinical look at the genitals/breasts, and Kegel (vaginal) exercises, for example.

3. Broadening the contexts for sexual activity, and facilitating and enhancing sexual communication is important. Didactic/therapy sessions can include: consideration of optimal timing for sexual activity, given current health status;

consideration of broadening the behavioral repertoire (e.g., sexual activities in lieu of intercourse, alternative intercourse positions); sexual desire as an 'appetite;' and strategies to facilitate desire (e.g., fantasy, erotic materials). Role plays of negotiating with a partner for changes in sexual routines and sharing information with a partner about anticipated changes (e.g., diminished lubrication, intercourse pain, difficulty with orgasm) are useful for women. Homework sessions might include body explorations with erotic focus, making choices about the contexts and types of sexual activities, and information sharing with partner.

4. Efforts must be taken to manage dyspareunia (or other symptom/sign distractors during sexuality). Didactic information can include discussion of the causes (specific and general) of the sexually disruptive symptoms/signs with regard to the woman's disease/treatment. For vaginal pain, a multimodal strategy is often useful, combining behavioral strategies (e.g., use of vaginal dilators to gauge pain and decide about advisability of intercourse), the use of aids such as artificial lubricants, and relaxation procedures. For women with severe vaginal atrophy/stenosis, a regimen of dilator usage may be necessary. Homework sessions can include the use of dialators and use of the above treatments/aids with the continuation of vaginal Kegel exercises. In all cases, however, it is important to assess the advisability of sexual activity in the context of pain, vaginal or otherwise.

5. Discovering the partner's sexuality concerns and communicating one's own sexual concerns and needs is important. Didactic sessions can include discussion of male anatomy/physiology and anticipated partner reactions to the woman's illness, body changes, and sexual changes. Therapy may also include discussion of the woman's concerns about her partner's reaction to disease, illness, and changes in health and sexuality. Role playing a discussion with her partner on topics of concern to the woman can be helpful to clarify the woman's feelings and begin to understand the possible reactions her partner may be having. For women without partners, one can discuss strategies for sharing information about one's cancer and treatments to a prospective partner, if the woman wishes. Homework, if appropriate, could be specific discussions with partner.

6. Specific efforts to enhancing arousal and orgasm may be needed. Strategies to facilitate orgasm, if it has been disrupted with treatment, can be suggested, such as including additional manual stimulation. Therapeutic efforts need to encourage a woman's experimentation with alternative sexual activities as well as engaging in activities to maintain interpersonal intimacy.

SUMMARY

For approximately half of the women diagnosed, cancer is a survivable disease. Available data suggests cautious optimism that psychological and sexual outcomes can be improved through general psychological interventions, but it is likely that even greater gains could be achieved if sexuality-specific interventions were a central part of a therapeutic effort. We offer a strategy, shown in Figure 18.1, for considering the medical factors which may contribute to risk for sexual morbidity. This model is empirically supported with our survivor data, as well as conceptual replications by other investigators studying other cancer groups (see Gordon et al., 1980). Moreover, a foundation of clinical research in cancer and basic research in sexuality has led to the proposal of the individual difference variable, sexual self-schema, that can be used to predict which women will be at risk for significant sexual morbidity. Assessing sexual self-schema and applying the morbidity risk model would be an important step forward in the identification of women at risk for sexual difficulties. Longitudinal data have highlighted the early trajectory of sexual problem development. The concluding section offers a clinical model for the design of interventions for sexual rehabilitation and suggests specific intervention strategies which are based on the difficulties of women with non-positive sexual self-concepts.

REFERENCES

American Cancer Society. (1999). *Cancer Facts and Figures—1999*. New York: American Cancer Society.

Andersen, B.L. (1981). A comparison of systematic desensitization and directed masturbation in the treatment of primary orgasmic dysfunction in females. *Journal of Consulting and Clinical Psychology* **49**: 568–570.

Andersen, B.L. (1992). Psychological interventions for cancer patients to enhance the quality of life. *Journal of Consulting and Clinical Psychology* **60**: 552–568.

Andersen, B.L. (1993). Predicting sexual and psychological morbidity and improving quality of life for women with gynecologic cancer. *Cancer* **71**: 1678–1690.

Andersen, B.L., Anderson, B. and deProsse, C. (1989). Controlled prospective longitudinal study of women with cancer: I. Sexual functioning outcomes. *Journal of Consulting and Clinical Psychology* **57**: 683–691.

Andersen, B.L. and Cyranowski, J.C. (1994). Women's sexual self schema. *Journal of Personality and Social Psychology* **67**: 1079–1100.

Andersen, B.L., Cyranowski, J. M. and Espindle, D. (1999). Men's sexual self-schema. *Journal of Personality and Social Psychology* **76**: 645–661.

Andersen, B.L., and Elliott, M.L. (1993). Sexuality for women with cancer: assessment, theory, and treatment. *Sexuality and Disability* **11**: 7–37.

Andersen, B.L. and Hacker, N.F. (1983a). Psychosexual adjustment following pelvic exenteration. *Obstetrics and Gynecology* **61**: 331–338.

Andersen, B.L. and Hacker, N.F. (1983b). Psychosexual adjustment after vulvar surgery. *Obstetrics and Gynecology* **62**: 457–462.

Andersen, B.L. and Jochimsen, P.R. (1985). Sexual adjustment among breast cancer, gynecologic cancer, and healthy women. *Journal of Consulting and Clinical Psychology* **53**: 25–32.

Andersen, B.L., Karlsson, J.A., Anderson, B. and Tewfik, H.H. (1984). Anxiety and cancer treatment: response to stressful radiotherapy. *Health Psychology* **3**: 535–551.

Andersen, B.L., Lachenbruch, P.A., Anderson, B. and deProsse, C. (1986). Sexual dysfunction and signs of gynecologic cancer. *Cancer* **57**: 1880–1886.

Andersen, B.L. and LeGrand, J. (1991). Body image for women: conceptualization, assessment, and a test of its importance to sexual dysfunction and medical illness. *Journal of Sex Research* **28**: 457–477.

Andersen, B.L. and van der Does, J. (1994). Surviving gynecologic cancer and coping with sexual morbidity: an international problem. *International Journal of Gynecologic Cancer* **4**: 225–240.

Baider, L. and Kaplan De-Nour, A. (1984). Couples' reaction and adjustment to mastectomy. *International Journal of Psychiatry in Medicine* **14**: 265–276.

Baider, L. and Kaplan De-Nour, A. (1988). Adjustment to cancer: who is the patient—the husband or the wife? *Israel Journal of Medical Sciences* **24**: 631–636.

Bard, M. and Sutherland, A.M. (1955). Psychological impact of cancer and its treatment: IV. Adaptation to radical mastectomy. *Cancer* **4**: 656–672.

Bernstein, D.A. and Borkovek, T.D. (1973). *Progressive Muscle Relaxation Training*. Champaign, IL: Research Press.

Burstein, H.J., Gelber, S., Guadagnoli, E. and Weeks, J.C. (1999). Use of alternative medicine by women with early-stage breast cancer. *New England Journal of Medicine* **340**: 1733–1739.

Cain, E.N., Kohorn, E.I., Quinlan, D.M., Latimer, K. and Schwartz, P.E. (1986). Psychosocial benefits of a cancer support group. *Cancer* **57**: 183–189.

Cash, T.F. (1991). *Body Image Therapy: A Program for Self-directed Change*. New York: Guilford.

Cassileth, B.R., Lusk, E.J., Strouse, T.B., Miller, D.S., Brown, L.L. and Cross, P.A. (1985). A psychological analysis of cancer patients and their next-of-kin. *Cancer* **55**: 72–76.

Capone, M.A., Good, R.S., Westie, K.S. and Jacobson, A.F. (1980). Psychosocial rehabilitation of gynecologic oncology patients. *Archives of Physical Medicine and Rehabilitation* **61**: 128–132.

Catania, J. A., Gibson, D. R., Chitwood, D. D. and Coates, T. J. (1990). Methodological problems in AIDS behavioral research: influences on measurement error and participation bias in studies of sexual behavior. *Psychological Bulletin* **108**: 339–362.

Corney, R.H., Crowther, M.E., Everett, H., Howells, A. and Shepherd, J.H. (1993). Psychosexual dysfunction in women with gynecological cancer following radical pelvic surgery. *British Journal of Obstetrics and Gynaecology* **100**: 73–78.

Cull, A., Cowie, V.J., Farquharson, D.I.M., Livingstone, J.R.B., Smart, G.E. and Elton, R.A. (1993). Early stage cervical cancer: psychosocial and sexual outcomes of treatment. *British Journal of Cancer* **68**: 1216–1220.

Curry, S.L., Levine, S.B., Jones, P.K. and Kurit, D.M. (1993). Medical and psychosocial predictors of sexual outcome among women with systemic lupus erythematosus. *Arthritis Care and Research* **6**: 23–30.

de Haes, J.C. and Welvaart, K. (1985). Quality of life after breast cancer surgery. *Journal of Surgical Oncology* **28**: 123–125.

Derogatis, L. (1980). Breast and gynecologic cancers: their unique impact on body image and sexual identity in women. In J.M. Vaeth (Ed.), *Frontiers of Radiation Therapy and Oncology*, Vol. 14 (pp. 1–11). Basel: Karger.

DiSaia, P.J., Creasman, W.T. and Rich, W.M. (1979). An alternate approach to early cancer of the vulva. *American Journal of Obstetrics and Gynecology* **33**: 825.

Fawzy, F.I., Cousins, N., Fawzy, N., Kemeny, M.E., Elashoff, R. and Morton, D. (1990). A structured psychiatric intervention for cancer patients: I. Changes over time in methods of coping and affective disturbance. *Archives of General Psychiatry* **47**: 720–725.

Gatchel, R.J., Baum, A. and Krantz, D.S. (1989). *An Introduction to Health Psychology*, 2nd Edn. New York: Random House.

Given, C.W., Stommel, M., Given, B., Osuch, J., Kurtz, M.E. and Kurtz, J.C. (1993). The influence of cancer patients' symptoms and functional states on patients' depression and family caregivers' reaction and depression. *Health Psychology* **12**: 277–285.

Gotay, C.C. and Muraoka, M.Y. (1998). Quality of life in long-term survivors of adult-onset cancers. *Journal of the National Cancer Institute* **90**: 656–667.

Harris, J. R., Morrow, M. and Bonadonna, G. (1993). Cancer of the breast. In V. T. DeVita, S. Hellman and S. A. Rosenberg (Eds), *Cancer: Principles and Practice of Oncology*, 4th Edition (pp. 1264-1332). Philadelphia: J. B. Lippincott Company.

Harris, R., Good, R.S., & Pollack, L. (1982). Sexual behavior of gynecologic cancer patients. *Archives of Sexual Behavior* **11**: 503–510.

Holleb, A.I. (1985). Lung cancer: a feminist issue. *CA—A Cancer Journal for Clinicians* **35**: 125–126.

Houts, D., Whitney, C., Mortel, R. and Bartholomew, M. (1986). Former cancer patients as counselors of newly diagnosed cancer patients. *Journal of the National Cancer Institute*, **76**: 793–796.

Jakubowski, P. and Lange, A. (1978). *The assertive option: Your rights and responsibilities.* Champaign, IL: Research Press Co.

Kaplan, H.S. and Owett, T. (1993). The female androgen deficiency syndrome. *Journal of Sex and Marital Therapy* **19**: 3–24.

Karlsson, J.A. and Andersen, B.L. (1986). Radiation therapy and psychological distress: outcomes and recommendations for enhancing adjustment. *Journal of Psychosomatic Obstetrics and Gynecology* **5**: 283–294.

Keil, J.E., Sutherland, S.E., Knapp, R.G., Waid, L.R. and Gazes, P.C. (1992). Self-reported sexual functioning in elderly blacks and whites: the Charleston Heart Study experience. *Journal of Aging and Health* **4**: 112–125.

Kinsey, A.C., Pomeroy, W.B., Martin, C.E. and Gebhard, P.H. (1953). *Sexual Behavior in the Human Female.* Philadelphia, PA: W.B. Saunders.

Krumm, S. and Lamberti, J. (1993). Changes in sexual behavior following radiation therapy for cervical cancer. *Journal of Psychosomatic Obstetrics and Gynecology* **14**: 51–63.

Kuchenoff, J., Wirsching, M. and Druner, H.V. (1981). Coping with a stoma: a comparative study of patients with rectal carcinoma or inflammatory bowel disease. *Psychotherapy and Psychosomatics* **36**: 98–104.

Landis, S.H., Murray, T., Bolden, S. and Wingo, P.A. (1999). Cancer statistics, 1999. *CA—A Cancer Journal for Clinicians* **49**(1): 8–31.

Maguire, P., Brooke, M., Tait, A., Thomas, C. and Sellwood, R. (1983). The effect of counselling on physical disability and social recovery after mastectomy. *Clinical Oncology* **9**: 319–324.

Masters, W.H. and Johnson, V.E. (1970). *Human Sexual Inadequacy.* Boston, NA: Little, Brown.

Matthews, K.A., Wing, R.R., Kuller, L.H., Meilahn, E.N., Kelsey, S.F., Costello, E.J. et al. (1990). Influences of natural menopause on psychological characteristics and symptoms of middle-aged healthy women. *Journal of Consulting and Clinical Psychological* **58**: 345–351.

Meyerowitz, B.E., Watkins, I.K. and Sparks, F.C. (1983). Psychosocial implications of adjuvant chemotherapy: a two-year follow-up. *Cancer* **52**: 1541–1545.

Moyer, A. (1997). Psychosocial outcomes of breast-conserving surgery versus mastectomy: a meta-analytic review. *Health Psychology* **16**(3): 284–298.

Newcomb, M.E. (1986). Notches on the bedpost: generational effects of sexual experience. *Psychology, A Quarterly Journal of Human Behavior* **23**: 37–46.

Northouse, L. (1988). Social support in patients' and husbands' adjustment to breast cancer. *Nursing Research* **37**: 91–95.

Northouse, L. and Swain, M.A. (1987). Adjustment of patients and husbands to the initial impact of breast cancer. *Nursing Research* **36**: 221–225.

Oberst, M.T. and James, R.H. (1985). Going home: patient and spouse adjustment following cancer surgery. *Topics in Clinical Nursing*: 46–57.

Parkin, D.M., Pisani, P. and Ferlay, J. (1999). Global cancer statistics. *CA—A Cancer Journal for Clinicians* **49**(1): 33–64.

Renneker, R. and Cutler, M. (1952). Psychological problems of adjustment to cancer of the breast. *Journal of the American Medical Association* **148**(10): 833–838.

Rosen, R.C. and Beck, J.G. (1988). *Patterns of Sexual Arousal.* New York: Guilford.

Schag, C.A.C., Ganz, P.A., Polinsky, M.L., Fred, C., Hirji, K. and Petersen, L. (1993). Characteristics of women at risk for psychosocial distress in the year after breast cancer. *Journal of Clinical Oncology* **11**: 783–793.

Taylor, S.E., Lichtman, R.R. and Wood, J.V. (1984). Attributions, beliefs about control, and adjustment to breast cancer. *Journal of Personality and Social Psychology* **46**: 489–502.

Telch, C.F. and Telch, M.J. (1986). Group coping skills instruction and supportive group therapy for cancer patients: A comparison of strategies. *Journal of Consulting and Clinical Psychology* **54**: 802–808.

van Driel, M.F., Weymar Schultz, W.C.M., van de Wiel, H.B.M., Hahn, D.E.E. and Mensink, H.J.A. (1993). Female sexual functioning after radical surgical treatment of rectal and bladder cancer. *European Journal of Surgical Oncology* **19**: 183–187.

Walling, M.K., Andersen, B.L. and Johnson, S.R. (1990). Hormonal replacement therapy for postmenopausal women: sexual outcomes and related gynecologic effects. *Archives of Sexual Behavior* **119**: 119–137.

Weijmar Schultz, W.C.M., Van de Wiel, H.B.M. and Bouma, J. (1991). Psychosexual functioning after treatment for cancer of the cervix: a comparative and longitudinal study. *International Journal of Gynecologic Cancer* **1**: 37–46.

Weijmar Schultz, W.C.M., van de Wiel, H.B.M., Bouma, J., Janssens, J. and Littlewood, J. (1990). Psychosexual functioning after treatment for cancer of the vulva: a longitudinal study. *Cancer* **66**: 402–407.

Weinhardt, L.S., Forsyth, A.D., Carey, M.P., Jaworski, B.C. and Durant, L.E. (1998). Reliability and validity of self-report measures of HIV-related sexual behavior: progress since 1990 and recommendations for research and practice. *Archives of Sexual Behavior* **27**: 155–180.

Welch-McCaffrey, D., Hoffman, B., Leigh, S.A., Loescher, L.J. and Meyskens, F.L. (1989). Surviving adult cancers. Part 2: Psychosocial implications. *Annals of Internal Medicine* **111**: 517–524.

Wolf, D.M. and Jordan, V.C. (1992). Gynecologic complications associated with long-term adjuvant tamoxifen therapy for breast cancer. *Gynecologic Oncology* **45**: 118–128.

Woods, X.A., Copeland, L.J. and Andersen, B.L. (1997). Sexual self-schema and sexual morbidity among gynecologic cancer survivors. *Journal of Consulting and Clinical Psychology* **65**: 221–229.

Wyatt, G.E., Peters, S.D. and Guthrie, D. (1988a). Kinsey revisited, Part I: comparisons of the sexual socialization and sexual behavior of white women over 33 years. *Archives of Sexual Behavior* **17**: 201–239.

Wyatt, G.E., Peters, S.D. and Guthrie, D. (1988b). Kinsey revisited, Part II: comparisons of the sexual socialization and sexual behavior of black women over 33 years. *Archives of Sexual Behavior* **17**: 289–331.

Yurek, D., Farrar, W.B. and Andersen, B.L. (in press). Breast cancer surgery: comparing surgical groups and determining individual differences in post-operative sexuality and body change stress. *Journal of Consulting and Clinical Psychology*.

19

Deciding to Have Children after Cancer

LESLIE R. SCHOVER

University of Texas M. D. Anderson Cancer Center, TX, USA

Although the definition of 'family' varies across human cultures, it is fairly universal that a family includes, at the least, a parent and children. Thus, an important family issue for younger cancer survivors is whether their experience of illness changes their likelihood of becoming parents or their experience of parenthood.

Although the majority of survivors of cancer have had children before their diagnosis, those whose malignancies occurred during childhood, adolescence, or young adulthood, before family-building was complete, must decide whether to have children after cancer. They may face infertility, so that their only options for parenthood are to adopt a child or participate in some form of third-party reproduction, such as using donated sperm or oocytes, or having a surrogate mother carry their embryos. Women who are able to conceive and carry a pregnancy after cancer treatment may worry about whether pregnancy would trigger a cancer recurrence. If their treatment included chemotherapy, or radiation therapy to the pelvis or abdomen, women may be at risk for pregnancy complications (Critchley et al., 1992). Both men and women who are thinking of having children after cancer may worry about the health of their potential offspring. Could a parent's cancer treatment cause a birth defect in a child conceived afterwards? Would this second generation of children be more likely to experience cancer themselves? Recent publicity about inherited cancer syndromes may increase survivors' perceptions of risk for their children.

Resolving these concerns and making a decision to have a child after cancer thus involves not only examining one's thoughts and feelings about parenthood, but also comprehending complex medical information that even oncology health care providers do not fully understand or communicate (Schover, 1997).

DOES THE CANCER EXPERIENCE DECREASE THE WISH TO HAVE CHILDREN?

One possible outcome of these concerns about having children is that survivors would have less desire to become parents. Mental health professionals have observed

Cancer and the Family, 2nd Edn. Edited by L. Baider, C. L. Cooper and A. Kaplan De-Nour

that many aspects of the lives of survivors of childhood or adolescent cancer are affected by the perceived threat of recurrence. The 'Damocles syndrome', as this anxiety has been termed (Koocher and O'Malley, 1981), may prevent survivors from investing energy in their futures. As new information accumulates about the long-term risk of second malignancies or other medical late effects of cancer treatment, such as cardiac or lung disease (Kalapurakal and Thomas, 1997; Parsons and Brown, 1998), survivors of pediatric cancer may feel uneasy about their ability to see their potential children through to adulthood.

Indeed, research has found that some pediatric cancer survivors are as likely as their peers to engage in risky health behaviors, such as smoking (Tyc et al., 1997). Survivors have also been observed, compared to their siblings, to have poorer educational (Evans and Radford, 1995) or occupational attainment (Zeltzer et al., 1997). Survivors might forego parenthood if their illness limited their occupational or financial achievements, and they felt unable to care adequately for a child. Another factor that could deter cancer survivors from becoming parents would be trouble finding a mate because of their cancer history and its physical sequelae. Two studies of pediatric cancer survivors did find lower rates of marriage than expected (Byrne et al., 1989; Green, et al., 1991), although divorce rates were no different between a large group of survivors and their sibling controls (Byrne et al., 1989). A recent study of breast cancer survivors also confirmed that cancer diagnosed in adulthood does not precipitate any unusual rates of divorce (Dorval et al., 1999).

We recently investigated some of these issues, surveying a sample of cancer survivors from our tumor registry who had been diagnosed before age 35, and were currently at least age 18 and free of known disease (Schover et al., 1999). Our response rate was 47%, and the only significant demographic bias was that women were more likely than men to return the questionnaire. The average age at cancer diagnosis of our respondents was 26, so that we had primarily a sample treated in young adulthood. They were currently a mean of 5.5 years post-diagnosis.

Even within this group that contained few survivors of pediatric cancer, 54% remained childless at the time of the survey. Within the childless group, 76% still would like to have a child in the future, and only 6% felt that having cancer decreased their wish for children. However, survivors who had already been parents at the time of their cancer diagnosis were less likely to want additional children; only 31% wanted another child and 29% felt that having cancer decreased their wish for further children. Thus, the impact of cancer on the desire for parenthood is quite different for those who have not yet had children at diagnosis, compared to those who were already parents.

We asked about specific barriers to parenthood after cancer. Ninety-four percent of our sample viewed themselves as healthy enough to be good parents. Only 15% felt that cancer had limited their financial ability to take good care of a child, and 12% believed that cancer had limited their chance of attracting the right mate with whom to start a family. Only 18% would not want to be a parent if they were to die at a prematurely young age, although 58% agreed with a statement that they would not want to leave their partner with young children to raise alone as a single parent.

As one woman, diagnosed with rectal carcinoma at age 30, wrote on her questionnaire:

God has been with me through my cancer and life, and I trust him to guide my path. I feel so blessed to have two beautiful children. If I die young from cancer or anything, I trust God's plan and know my children will be okay. No-one knows the time of their death—I could die young with cancer or in a car accident, etc. . . . You can't put your life on hold for what might be.

Thus, at least for this group of survivors, primarily of malignancies in young adulthood, most feel ready and able to be parents.

DOES THE CANCER EXPERIENCE MAKE SURVIVORS BETTER PARENTS?

Although books have given cancer patients advice about how to communicate with children during their treatment (Harpham, 1997), neither researchers nor clinicians have given much thought to the idea that cancer survivors may be better parents because of their experience of illness. Survivors often comment that coping with cancer reduces their reactivity to the hassles of daily life and gives them a greater appreciation of the moment. These are valuable skills for parenting. Those able to have a child after cancer may view their offspring as especially valued and cherished, much like children born after parents endure treatment for non-cancer-related infertility (Golombok et al., 1995). Couples who were committed to each other before the cancer diagnosis also often report feeling closer because of their experience during the illness, gaining a new appreciation of each other, more open communication about emotions, and increased flexibility in exchanging roles in the family (Schover et al., 1987). Enhancements of a couple's relationship could also have a positive impact on their parenting.

Our survey found that 78% of survivors agreed with the statement: 'My experience of cancer has made or will make me a better parent.' This is an aspect of cancer survivorship that should be studied, using both self-report scales on parenting and behavioral observation of the family.

THE PAIN OF INFERTILITY AFTER CANCER

Having established in our survey that the great majority of childless cancer survivors did want children, it was not surprising that infertility was a significant concern for many of them. Of respondents who were childless at the time of the survey, 44% viewed themselves as less fertile than others of similar age and gender, and 26% had worried at least a fair amount about infertility. Men and women did not differ significantly on these variables. Although 18% of this group had tried for a pregnancy for over a year without success, only 6% of childless survivors had sought medical treatment for infertility. This is quite a bit lower than statistics that suggest that about 44% of couples with infertility in the USA eventually seek help (Stephen and Chandra, 1998). Our sample was relatively young, and some may not yet have felt ready to pursue trying to conceive. It also may be especially threatening for a young cancer survivor to contemplate infertility treatment, with its frequent medical visits, unpleasant and invasive tests, and uncertain outcome. One of our respondents, diagnosed with Hodgkin's disease as a teenager and now aged 30, wrote:

> My husband and I will be married 10 years this year and are expecting our first child! Last year we began doing some searching for a doctor to discuss infertility. In the past I was told that it was not necessary to do any testing until we were consistently trying to get pregnant. I was fearful of the test results because a diagnosis of 'infertile' seemed too permanent. I believe that is why I put off seeing a specialist for so long.

Our survey also highlighted the problem that information about infertility after cancer may not be adequately discussed by oncology health care providers. Of our respondents, only 65% of those who received a cancer treatment with potential to damage fertility recalled the topic being brought up, in about half of these cases by the physician who had treated their cancer. Others had discussed their fertility with a specialist (25%), a nurse (8%), or a family doctor (6%).

Some educational materials are available for patients about cancer-related infertility. The American Society of Reproductive Medicine publishes a pamphlet, *Fertility after Cancer Treatment: A Guide for Patients* (American Society of Reproductive Medicine, 1995), and the present author has written a comprehensive self-help book that explains the causes and treatments for infertility after cancer (Schover, 1997).

Cancer survivors may need more than just medical information, however, to feel ready to confront the emotional roller coaster of infertility treatment. One issue in readiness to start treatment is whether infertility was a surprise or not. Some survivors of childhood cancer may never have been informed that infertility is a possible long-term consequence of their chemotherapy or radiotherapy, whereas others may have been prepared emotionally by their families, years ahead of time, for that eventuality. I would speculate, however, that the survivors most distressed about fertility would be those treated during adolescence, when cancer treatment can interfere with puberty and the development of a healthy feeling of attractiveness and self-worth. The influence of age at diagnosis on coping with cancer-related infertility is thus another topic worthy of research.

MAKING CHOICES ABOUT FERTILITY AT THE TIME OF DIAGNOSIS

Young adults or even teenagers who are diagnosed with cancer may have to make choices about preserving their fertility at the time they are to begin treatment, when the life-and-death concerns of the illness are still paramount. Men, who may undergo combination chemotherapy or localized radiation therapy that could damage the testes, have the option of banking sperm before cancer treatment (Schover et al., 1998). Sperm banking used to be impractical for most men newly diagnosed with cancer, since they often have poor semen quality. Another barrier was that, under the traditional schedules for sperm banking, it might take as long as two weeks to collect enough semen samples to provide a basis for successful infertility treatment at a later date.

Not only has research shown that adequate semen samples can be collected on a tighter schedule, but also the advent of a new technique of *in vitro* fertilization (IVF), called intracytoplasmic sperm injection (ICSI), has made it worthwhile to bank even very small quantities of semen, regardless of quality. With ICSI, one sperm cell is injected into each oocyte retrieved from the female partner in a couple undergoing

IVF. Even though the freezing and thawing process destroys many sperm cells, ICSI only requires that a very few remain living at the time of IVF. Once the semen is frozen, it can be stored for many years without further damage until it is thawed for use.

Sperm banking remains underutilized by men having cancer treatment. In our recent survey (Schover et al., 1999), only 24% of childless male cancer survivors had banked sperm before their treatment. Many of the men who did not bank sperm did not recall being informed of the option, although we provide a full-service sperm bank within our hospital and have educational brochures available. Physicians, especially those practicing outside of major cancer centers, may not be well-educated about advances in sperm-banking, or may not know where to refer their patients. Financial issues also may be a deterrent. Although some insurers cover sperm banking, patients could have up to $2000 in out-of-pocket costs for the procedure and several years of storage (Schover et al., 1998).

Addressing the topic of sperm banking takes patience and expertise. The health care provider must be able to explain why sperm banking is helpful, including educating the patient about IVF and other infertility treatments. Young men who are unmarried often are accompanied by family members at the time of cancer diagnosis. It is probably best in most cases to bring up the idea of sperm banking with a young man alone, since it involves the sensitive subject of using masturbation to collect semen samples, as well as his desire for children in the future. On the other hand, parents may be helpful in helping young men make a decision. Adolescents, in particular, often disregard health risks. They may believe that they will never become infertile in spite of the statistics about their cancer treatment's side effects, or may discount the distress they would feel if they could not become a father in the future. Another very delicate subject that should be raised is creating an advance directive about the disposition of the frozen semen in the event of the patient's death.

If the young man is under age 18, the parents will need to be involved in the informed consent process. It would even be advisable to ask the parents' permission before educating their son about the option of banking sperm. Parents may also need to be informed if the collection room has erotic materials in it, such as magazines or videos.

Although sperm banking brings some complex emotional challenges, it is technically simple and successful. Unfortunately, there is not an option to preserve female fertility that begins to approach the ease of sperm banking. Women who are about to undergo chemotherapy that may permanently damage their ovaries, or who will have their ovaries removed surgically or exposed to radiation, have limited choices. A few women delay their cancer treatment until they can undergo a cycle of IVF, taking hormones for several weeks to stimulate their ovaries to ripen multiple eggs, having the oocytes 'harvested' under anesthesia via an ultrasound-guided needle through the upper vagina, and having the eggs fertilized with sperm cells from the woman's husband or committed partner—or, if she is single, perhaps from an anonymous semen donor. Any embryos that result from successful fertilization are frozen and stored until the woman has finished her cancer treatment and is ready to try to become pregnant. Then some embryos can be thawed and transferred to her uterus.

Not only is IVF very expensive, time-consuming, and limited in its success, but women with hormone-sensitive tumors, breast cancer in particular, may be taking a risk using fertility drugs. Some women with breast cancer have chosen to try 'natural cycle' IVF before beginning chemotherapy. Their spontaneous ovulation is monitored using ultrasound studies and hormone tests. When the one oocyte (or perhaps two) is almost ready for ovulation, it is harvested instead, and fertilized using the ICSI procedure. If an embryo develops, it can be frozen for later transfer. Unfortunately, the pregnancy rates from natural cycle IVF are very low, less than 10% per cycle (Daya et al., 1995; Surbone and Petrek, 1997).

Recently, advances have been made in freezing either ovarian tissue or unfertilized eggs. When these techniques are perfected, a true equivalent to sperm banking will be available for women (Moomjy and Rosenwaks, 1998). Two technical problems must be overcome, however. The first is that even fully mature oocytes do not have a high rate of survival when frozen and thawed before fertilization takes place. They may also be more vulnerable than embryos to genetic damage during the freezing process. Nevertheless, the first pregnancies using a frozen and thawed egg have recently been reported. The next problem is that most oocytes that can be easily collected from the ovary are in the immature state. Getting them to mature successfully in the laboratory is the most difficult part of the process. We need to be able to freeze eggs in the immature state, ripen them in the laboratory, and then successfully fertilize them before egg banking will be viable.

In animals, an alternative line of research involves removing and freezing a strip of ovarian tissue containing hundreds of immature oocytes. After thawing, the tissue can be transplanted back into the female, where it grows a new blood supply so that it can produce hormones and mature oocytes. At least one lamb has been born from this process, but it has not yet been demonstrated to be successful in humans.

Around the USA, a number of centers are offering to freeze women's ovarian tissue now, before cancer treatment. The hope is that by the time the women want to have babies, some means of using the immature, frozen oocytes will be available. This is obviously a gamble. When the cost of the procedures to remove and store the ovarian tissue is paid by a research grant, and the woman is well-informed about the speculative nature of the whole process, there seems minimal ethical concern. Some women, however, are paying several thousand dollars to store their own tissue. Even with informed consent, I find it worrisome to offer an unproved method to women desperate to preserve their fertility at a time when they are already emotionally overwhelmed. It reminds me of the companies that offer to freeze corpses, in the hopes that humans of the next millennium will have the knowledge to resurrect them and cure their fatal illnesses.

WOMEN'S WORRIES ABOUT THE SAFETY OF PREGNANCY

For those women still able to conceive a pregnancy after cancer, the decision to become pregnant may be anxiety-provoking. Oncologists typically counsel women to wait at least 2 years after cancer treatment to become pregnant since, for most malignancies, this is the period of greatest risk for a recurrence. Women may misinterpret this advice, however, and worry that pregnancy itself could promote a cancer recurrence.

For women who have had breast cancer, a specific concern is the high levels of circulating estrogen in the bloodstream during pregnancy (Surbone and Petrek,

1997). If cancer cells remained, it is possible that estrogen could promote their growth. However, recent epidemiologic studies have been reassuring that women who survive breast cancer and subsequently become pregnant do not have any poorer health outcomes (Kroman et al., 1997; Surbone and Petrek, 1998; van Schoultz et al., 1995). For women with other types of cancer, even melanoma, in which pregnancy was formerly thought to be dangerous (Grin et al., 1998), there is little reason to suppose that pregnancy would promote a recurrence.

Women are often not well-informed about the safety of pregnancy after cancer, however. In our survey, only one-third of women recalled a health care provider discussing pregnancy after cancer with them. Not surprisingly, 17% of the women we surveyed had worried at least a fair amount that pregnancy would cause their cancer to return—with essentially no difference in the degree of concern between women who had had breast cancer and those with other malignancies.

A more realistic concern is that some women may be at risk for pregnancy complications as a result of having had treatment for cancer. Women appear to be far less worried about these risks than they are about the possible link between pregnancy and cancer recurrence. This lack of anxiety probably reflects a lack of knowledge. In our survey, only 14% of the women who wanted children in the future planned to consult a high-risk obstetrician about pregnancy. Yet, women who have had chemotherapy that impairs their heart or lung capacity could develop serious pulmonary or cardiac complications during a pregnancy (Brierley et al., 1998). Women whose uterus received a dose of radiation therapy in childhood or later on are at increased risk of having miscarriage, premature birth, or low-birthweight infants (Critchley et al., 1992). Women who are cancer survivors need to be given full and accurate information about carrying a pregnancy successfully. Those who potentially are at risk for pregnancy complications should be counseled to consult a high-risk obstetrician before attempting to conceive.

CONCERNS ABOUT THE HEALTH OF CHILDREN BORN AFTER CANCER

How worried are cancer survivors about having children with genetic abnormalities or other health problems triggered by a parent's exposure to chemotherapy or radiation? Our survey suggested that those who had children worried more about the issue (30% worrying at least a fair amount vs. 9% of childless survivors). Again, only about one-third of those with children recalled ever discussing this topic with a health professional, and even fewer (12%) of childless survivors received information about health risks to potential children. This lack of communication is discouraging, given that a fairly large number of children born after a parent's cancer treatment have been followed, without any unusual rates of birth defects or other health problems being observed (Byrne et al., 1998). A recent follow-up of 24 babies exposed to chemotherapy for breast cancer during the second or third trimesters of pregnancy also found no clear damage to health (Berry et al.,1999). It is very sad to think that some couples may forego having children because of exaggerated fears for their offsprings' health, and that others are worrying needlessly about the children they already have.

CONCERNS ABOUT CHILDREN'S RISK FOR CANCER

Perhaps the most frightening thought for a survivor who is trying to decide whether to become a parent is that his/her children are doomed to have cancer as well. As one of our respondents wrote:

> In my opinion, if I had the opportunity to know *for certain* that I would pass on cancer through my children, *I would not have children.* However, if there was only a *small risk,* I probably would take the risk. Some things in life are worth it. Of course, involved in this decision is the opinion of my doctors.

Again, however, only 22% of childless survivors in our study had discussed their children's risk of inheriting cancer with a health professional, compared to 53% of those who had at least one child (which is still a disappointingly low percentage). This difference suggests that when a parent is diagnosed with cancer, he/she often fears for existing children and seeks out information about their cancer risk. Perhaps because of recent publicity about inherited cancer syndromes, about 40% of our respondents believed that their children would have a higher than normal risk of getting cancer in their lifetimes. About 26% of the sample thought they might pursue genetic counseling to determine their own familial cancer risk and to aid them in deciding whether to have children.

These fears also have little basis in reality. Currently, inherited genetic mutations are thought to account for only 5–10% of all malignancies. Even though parents and children also share environmental risk factors, the parent with cancer has already experienced many years of a non-shared environment before his/her children are born. It is not surprising that recent epidemiologic studies find that the only increased risk of malignancy in the offspring of survivors of pediatric cancer is in the rare families with a truly inherited cancer syndrome, such as some forms of retinoblastoma (Sankila et al., 1998).

MAKING CHOICES ABOUT CHILDREN
IN INHERITED SYNDROME FAMILIES

The few men or women who do belong to families in which an inherited cancer syndrome has been identified have to sort out extremely complex issues when making decisions about having children. Most of the known genetic syndromes are inherited in an *autosomal dominant* fashion, which means that the person who carries a mutated gene increasing his/her cancer risk has a 50% chance of passing that gene on to each child. The technology is already available, if a couple want to use genetic testing, to see if a fetus carries one of these gene mutations (Wagner and Ahner, 1998). In my clinical experience with women considering genetic testing for mutations in the BRCA1 or BRCA2 genes that increase risk for breast cancer (Burke et al., 1997a), most would not consider having prenatal testing in order to terminate a healthy pregnancy. These gene mutations do not confer a 100% lifetime risk of breast cancer. A female baby carrying the mutation would have perhaps a 40–80% lifetime risk of breast cancer in adulthood, depending on the mutation and the environment. A typical comment made by women seeking genetic testing for themselves was that by the time a daughter grew up, they believed there would be a cure for breast cancer. The issues for carriers of the mutations that increase risk for hereditary non-polyposis colon cancer would be similar, except that the gender of the fetus would not be an issue in decision-making (Burke et al., 1997b).

An additional reason to avoid prenatal genetic testing for these late-onset disorders is that it would undoubtedly lead to situations in which a couple decided to go ahead with a pregnancy *despite* knowing that the fetus carried the relevant gene mutation. This outcome would violate ethical guidelines, which prevent genetic testing in children for adult-onset disorders. This prohibition was developed because of the risk that families would stigmatize a child at future risk for cancer, or inadvertently would communicate to that child a sense of doom, or at least of limited life possibilities (Wertz et al., 1994). Ethical oversight committees also fear that widespread use of prenatal testing and pregnancy termination might lead to insurers refusing to pay for the medical care of children 'allowed' to be born with a genetic disorder, i.e. whose parents had refused genetic testing or chose not to terminate an affected fetus.

Although there are powerful arguments to forbid prenatal genetic testing for late-onset disorders, most women I have interviewed feel that society should leave the choice up to the couple. In families that have lost several young people to inherited breast, ovarian, or colon cancer, the suffering is intense. Young adults who know they carry the familial mutation may wish to have a child who will not face the same risks. Parents may have an even stronger desire to consider prenatal testing when genetic cancer syndromes potentially affect children or adolescents, such as inherited retinoblastoma, the Li–Fraumeni syndrome that can include childhood leukemia or sarcoma, or familial adenomatous polyposis (FAP).

FAP is an autosomal dominant disorder in which mutation carriers begin to develop colon polyps in childhood (Petersen and Brensinger, 1996). If left untreated, virtually all carriers will develop colon cancer as young adults. When a parent is known to have FAP, children begin screening by colonoscopy at around age 10. Children of this age are considered eligible to have genetic testing, because of the benefit that those who do not carry the mutation can escape this unpleasant surveillance regime. Mutation carriers are recommended to have prophylactic removal of the colon, and often also the rectum, as teenagers or very young adults. Even with the threat of colon cancer removed, many people with FAP die prematurely of gastric cancer or complications of benign tumors called desmoids. A survey in the UK of 62 adults who themselves had FAP revealed that 64% would use prenatal testing if available, although only 24% would consider terminating an affected fetus (Whitelaw et al., 1996). Almost all (93%) believed that prenatal testing should be made available to families carrying the mutation for FAP.

Another option to prevent the birth of children at risk for inherited cancer syndromes is the use of preimplantation genetic diagnosis (PGD). When a gene mutation has been identified in a parent, the wife in the couple can undergo a cycle of IVF in order to create multiple embryos. While the embryos are growing in the laboratory, one or several cells can be safely removed for a genetic 'biopsy.' Only embryos that do not carry the feared mutation would be replaced into the mother's uterus for attempted pregnancy. Affected embryos would be discarded. Although the idea of destroying an embryo is much more palatable to many couples than is pregnancy termination, PGD is very expensive, and typically none of the costs are covered by private insurers. The woman also has to undergo the medical risks of IVF, even though she usually is of normal fertility. The pregnancy rate after PGD is limited, not only by the success rates of IVF itself, but by the potential exclusion of many of the embryos that are created. Nevertheless, the first attempt to use PGD for FAP was recently reported (Asangla et al., 1998).

Women who carry BRCA1 or BRCA2 mutations have the most difficult choices of all since, for them, the risks that pregnancy could promote a malignancy are still unknown (Burke et al., 1997a). Today, most women undergoing genetic testing for these mutations have already been diagnosed with breast or ovarian cancer and are concerned for the children they already have (Lerman et al., 1996). As younger women learn that they could be at risk, however, and as estimates of the lifetime risk of breast cancer decrease for these syndromes, women are faced with agonizing choices. Should they forego childbearing entirely, out of concern that it would trigger breast cancer? Is it worthwhile considering prophylactic mastectomy, perhaps even before getting pregnant, or will breast-feeding prove protective against cancer for these women, as it has for women who do not carry an inherited mutation? In families with known ovarian cancer risk, should a woman have her children as early in life as possible and then have prophylactic oophorectomy? Using oral contraceptives appears protective against ovarian cancer, even for women who carry mutations (Narod et al., 1998). Will having a child also prove to have preventive value, as it does for most women? It is impossible yet to sort out these competing possibilities.

ADOPTION AS AN OPTION FOR FAMILY BUILDING

In our society, couples with infertility are often encouraged to adopt. Couples who choose this option are perceived as giving a loving home to a child who otherwise might be neglected, whereas those who pursue high-technology infertility treatment are sometimes stigmatized as wasting money in a desperately selfish effort to perpetuate their own genes. Yet, the realities of adoption are not so rosy in the USA and most countries of Western Europe. As contraception became increasingly available, abortion on demand became legalized in many countries, and raising a child outside of marriage lost its stigma, the number of children available for adoption decreased radically (Bachrach et al., 1992; Chippindale-Bakker and Foster, 1996). In the USA, couples who want to adopt a healthy infant face waiting lists years long from public agencies or extremely high costs for independent domestic adoptions or international adoptions. Caucasian infants are in the highest demand.

If one parent has a history of cancer, even if a physician is willing to attest to their excellent prognosis, it is unclear how much the barrier to adoption may rise. Public agencies are reluctant to specify their evaluation criteria for adoptive parents. Private adoptions increasingly involve appealing directly to birth mothers through networking or advertising on the Internet. An individual birth mother may be scared away just by the mention of cancer in a potential adoptive couple, particularly if she has many families vying for her baby.

Although it is easier to adopt older children with health problems or histories of abuse or neglect, raising a special needs child calls for stamina, excellent health insurance, and willingness to deal with the medical system—resources that may not be available to some cancer survivors.

In our survey, 62% of respondents said they would at least hypothetically consider adoption if they were infertile because of cancer treatment. Having a child did not impact on these largely favorable attitudes to adoption. Yet, I could not find even one empirical study of the success of cancer survivors in adopting compared to individuals or couples who attempt adoption after infertility unrelated to a life-threatening disorder. Clearly, such a study would be valuable in guiding men and women who would like to adopt after cancer.

THIRD-PARTY REPRODUCTION AFTER CANCER

A non-traditional way to have children after cancer interferes with fertility is to enlist the help of a third person, either to donate a sperm or egg, or to carry a pregnancy for a woman who cannot do so successfully herself. In some *surrogate pregnancies*, the woman who agrees to carry the baby also supplies the oocyte. Other women are *gestational carriers*, who become pregnant with transferred embryos created from the oocyte of the mother in the recipient couple and the sperm of the father.

Using a *gamete donor* is undoubtedly the most common type of third-party reproduction among cancer survivors. Yet, it still remains less accepted than adoption. In our survey, only about a quarter of respondents would consider using a donated sperm or egg to have a child if cancer caused infertility. Still, the attitudes of this group of survivors are more favorable than those of the general population (Braverman and Corson, 1995). Research suggests that people who have experienced infertility develop more openness to the idea of gamete donation than those who have never had trouble having a child. Our own research also demonstrated, however, that when medical factors allow couples a choice between using a donated gamete and pursuing IVF with their own mutual genetic material, the great majority prefer to have their genetic offspring (Schover et al., 1996).

For some cancer survivors, third-party reproduction is the only medical alternative to adoption. Given the costs and difficulty of adoption, using simple office insemination with donor sperm is a far less expensive and complex alternative (Vercollone et al., 1997). Modern sperm banks can assure that donors are free of sexually-transmitted diseases and common genetic disorders. Becoming pregnant via embryos from donated oocytes is also relatively simple and easy for the woman who is a survivor of cancer with non-functional ovaries but an intact uterus. She does not have to take the fertility drugs that would raise her own estrogen levels to abnormal heights, although she will undergo the normal hormonal changes of pregnancy. Finding an oocyte donor is often difficult, however, unless a good friend or family member is willing and available. Since the donor must undergo a cycle of IVF, with all the discomfort and medical risks involved, volunteer donors are typically paid at least $3000 currently in the USA. The recipient couple must also pay for the IVF cycle. The costs are usually less than those for an independent or international adoption, but even with very high success rates, there is no guarantee of a living baby.

Couples who have a child using third-party reproduction face dilemmas about telling the child or others about this unconventional conception. Most mental health professionals advocate always telling the child about his/her true genetic origins to avoid the potential damaging influence of such a family secret on parent–child relationships. Yet, the great majority of couples have not told their offspring about the gamete donation (Schover and Thomas, 1999). Some worry that their children would be stigmatized by the extended family or community, especially if the family is part of a religious group that does not condone gamete donation or has a strong element of ethnic pride. Others fear that the child would want to know more about the donor's heritage and would be frustrated by the very limited amount of information available about anonymous gamete donors. Those who had a family member or friend serve as a donor may worry that the child would develop a competing parental attachment to their genetic father or mother. Many couples express the fear that knowing about third party reproduction would simply cause pain to their child without enriching the child's life in any way. On the other hand, when one parent has a history of cancer, especially as part of an inherited cancer syndrome, it may be a relief to a child to know that he/she does not share that same genetic potential.

Although couples who pay a woman to carry a pregnancy often plan at first to keep in contact with the surrogate mother and to have some future contact between her and the child, it is unclear how often such intentions are carried through (Ragone, 1994). Researchers have not yet studied any differences in how much contact couples and children have with traditional surrogates who are the genetic mother of the baby vs. gestational carriers who carry a fetus unrelated to them biologically. Since surrogates often have a large role in choosing the couples with whom they work, it would also be important to know how often women in this group would refuse, out of anxiety or lack of knowledge about cancer, to enter into partnership with a couple in which one spouse had a cancer history.

CONCLUSIONS

For those whose lives were interrupted by cancer before they had created their ideal family, there are an increasing number of options to become parents. Yet, researchers have only begun to examine the attitudes and experiences of cancer survivors about having and raising children. It is time to go beyond simply documenting the medical impact of cancer treatment on fertility, the safety of pregnancy, and the health of the next generation of children. Researchers in behavioral oncology must examine the ways in which having cancer influences men's and women's decisions about having children; develop and evaluate new educational programs to increase survivors' knowledge about the medical aspects of cancer and reproduction; compare cancer survivors to others who experience infertility in terms of barriers to having medical infertility treatment, being able to adopt, or to utilize third party reproduction; and examine the impact of the cancer experience on survivors' parenting skills and attitudes towards their children.

REFERENCES

American Society for Reproductive Medicine (1995). *Fertility after Cancer Treatment: A Guide for Patients*. Birmingham, AL: American Society for Reproductive Medicine.

Asangla, A.O., Wells, D., Handyside, A.H., Winston, R.M. and Delhanty, J.D. (1998). Pre-implantation genetic diagnosis of inherited cancer: familial adenomatous polyposis coli. *Journal of Assisted Reproduction and Genetics* **15**: 140–144.

Bachrach, C.A., Stolley, K.S. and London, K.A. (1992). Relinquishment of premarital births: evidence from national survey data. *Family Planning Perspectives* **24**: 27–32, 48.

Berry, D.L., Theriault, R.L., Holmes, F.A., Parisi, V.M., Booser, D.J., Singletary, S.E., Buzdar, A.U. and Hortobagyi, G.N. (1999). Management of breast cancer during pregnancy using a standardized protocol. *Journal of Clinical Oncology* **17**: 855–861.

Braverman, A.M. and Corson, S. L. (1995). Factors related to preferences in gamete donor sources. *Fertility and Sterility* **63**: 543–549.

Brierley, J.D., Rathmell, A.J., Gospodarowicz, M.K., Sutcliffe, S.B., Munro, A., Tsang, R. and Pintilie, M. (1998). Late effects of treatment for early-stage Hodgkin's disease. *British Journal of Cancer* **77**: 1300–1310.

Burke, W., Daly, M., Garber, J., Botkin, J., Ellis Kahn, M.J., Lynch, P., McTiernan, A., Offit, K., Perlman, J., Petersen, G., Thomson, E. and Varricchio, C., for the Cancer Genetics Studies Consortium (1997a). Recommendations for follow-up care of individuals with an inherited predisposition to cancer. II. BRCA1 and BRCA2. *Journal of the American Medical Association* **277**: 997–1003.

Burke, W., Petersen, G., Lynch, P., Botkin, J., Daly, M., Garber, J., Ellis Kahn, M.J., McTiernan, A., Offit, K., Thomson, E. and Varricchio, C., for the Cancer Genetics Studies Consortium (1997b). Recommendations for follow-up care of individuals with an inherited predisposition to cancer; I. Hereditary non-polyposis colon cancer. *Journal of the American Medical Association* **277**: 915–919.

Byrne, J., Fears, T.R., Steinhorn, S.C., Mulvihill, J.J., Connelly, R., Austin, D.F., Holmes, G.F., Holmes, F.F., Latourette, H.B. and Teta, M.J. (1989). Marriage and divorce after childhood and adolescent cancer. *Journal of the American Medical Association* **262**: 2693–2699.

Byrne, J. Rasmussen, S.A., Steinhorn, S.C., Connelly, R.R., Myers, M.H., Lynch, C.F., Flannery, J., Austin, D.F., Holmes, F.F., Holmes, G.E., Strong, L.C. and Mulvihill, J.J. (1998). Genetic disease in offspring of long-term survivors of childhood and adolescent cancer. *American Journal of Human Genetics* **62**: 45–52.

Chippindale-Bakker, V. and Foster, L. (1996). Adoption in the 1990s: sociodemographic determinants of biological parents choosing adoption. *Child Welfare* **74**: 337–355.

Critchley, H.O., Wallace, W.H., Shalet, S.M., Mamtora, H., Higginson, J. and Anderson, D.C. (1992). Abdominal irradiation in childhood: the potential for pregnancy. *British Journal of Obstetrics and Gynaecology* **99**: 392–394.

Daya, S., Gunby, J., Hughes, E.G., Collins, J.A., Sagle, M.A. and Young Lai, E.V. (1995). Natural cycles for *in vitro* fertilization: cost-effectiveness analysis and factors influencing outcome. *Human Reproduction* **10**: 1719–1724.

Dorval, M., Maunsell, E., Taylor-Brown, J. and Kilpatrick, M. (1999). Marital stability after breast cancer. *Journal of the National Cancer Institute* **91**: 54–59.

Evans, S.E. and Radford, M. (1995). Current lifestyle of young adults treated for cancer in childhood. *Archives of Disease in Childhood* **72**: 423–426.

Golombok, S., Cook, R., Bish, A. and Murray, C. (1995). Families created by the new reproductive technologies: quality of parenting and social and emotional development of the children. *Child Development* **66**: 285–298.

Green, D.M., Zevon, M.A. and Hall, B. (1991). Achievement of life goals by adult survivors of modern treatment for childhood cancer. *Cancer* **67**: 206–213.

Grin, C.M., Driscoll, M.S. and Grant-Kels, J.M. (1998). The relationship of pregnancy, hormones, and melanoma. *Seminars in Cutaneous Medicine and Surgery* **17**: 167–171.

Harpham, W.S. (1997). *When A Parent Has Cancer: A Guide to Caring for Your Children.* New York: Harper Collins.

Kalapurakal, J.A. and Thomas, P.R. (1997). Pediatric radiotherapy. An overview. *Radiologic Clinics of North America* **35**: 1265–1280.

Koocher, G.P. and O'Malley, J.E. (Eds) (1981). *The Damocles Syndrome.* New York: McGraw-Hill.

Kroman, N., Jensen, M.B., Melbye, M., Wohlfahrt, J. and Mouridsen, H.T. (1997). Should women be advised against pregnancy after breast cancer treatment? *Lancet* **350**(9074): 319–322.

Lerman, C., Narod, S., Schulman, K., Highes, C., Gomez-Caminero, A., Bonney, G., Gold, K., Trock, B., Main, D., Lynch, J., Fulmore, C., Snyder, C., Lemon, S.J., Conway, T., Tonin, P., Lenoir, G. and Lynch, H. (1996). BRCA1 testing in families with hereditary breast–ovarian cancer: a prospective study of patient decision making and outcomes. *Journal of the American Medical Association* **275**: 1885–1892.

Moomjy, M. and Rosenwaks, Z. (1998). Ovarian tissue cryopreservation: the time is now. Transplantation or *in vitro* maturation: the time awaits. *Fertility and Sterility* **69**: 999–1000.

Narod, S.A., Risch, H., Moslehi, R., Dorum, A., Neuhausen, S., Olsson, H., Provencher, D., Radice, P., Evans, G., Bishop, S., Brunet, J.S. and Ponder, B.A. (1998). Oral contraceptives and the risk of hereditary ovarian cancer: Hereditary Ovarian Cancer Clinical Study Group. *New England Journal of Medicine* **339**: 424–428.

Parsons, S.K. and Brown, A.P. (1998). Evaluation of quality of life of childhood cancer survivors: a methodological conundrum. *Medical and Pediatric Oncology* **1** (Suppl): 46–53.

Petersen, G.M. and Brensinger, J.D. (1996). Genetic testing and counseling in familial adenomatous polyposis. *Oncology* **10**: 89–94.

Ragone, H. (1994). *Surrogate Motherhood: Conception in the Heart* (pp. 133–135). Boulder, CO: Westview.

Sankila, R., Olsen, J.H., Anderson, H., Garwicz, S., Glattre, E. and Hertz, H. (1998). Risk of cancer among offspring of childhood cancer survivors. Association of the Nordic Cancer Registries and the Nordic Society of Paediatric Haematology and Oncology. *New England Journal of Medicine* **338**: 1339–1344.

Schover, L.R. (1997). *Sexuality and Fertility after Cancer.* New York: Wiley.

Schover, L.R., Agarwal, A. and Thomas, A.J. (1998). Cryopreservation of gametes in young patients with cancer. *Journal of Pediatric Hematology and Oncology* **20**: 426–428.

Schover, L.R., Evans, R.B. and von Eschenbach, A.C. (1987). Sexual rehabilitation in a cancer center: diagnosis and outcome in 384 consultations. *Archives of Sexual Behavior* **16**: 445–461.

Schover, L.R., Rybicki, L.A., Martin, B.A. and Bringelsen K.A. (1999). Having children after cancer: a pilot survey of survivors' attitudes and experiences. *Cancer* **86**: 697–709.

Schover, L.R. and Thomas, A.J. (2000). *Overcoming Male Infertility: Understanding Its Causes and Treatments.* New York: Wiley.

Schover, L.R., Thomas, A.J., Miller, K.F., Falcone, T., Attaran, M. and Goldberg J. (1996). Preferences for intracytoplasmic sperm injection (ICSI) vs. donor insemination (DI) in severe male factor infertility: a preliminary report. *Human Reproduction* **11**: 101–104.

Stephen, E.H. and Chandra, A. (1998). Updated projections of infertility in the United States: 1995–2025. *Fertility and Sterility* **70**: 30–34.

Surbone, A. and Petrek, J.A. (1997). Childbearing issues in breast carcinoma survivors. *Cancer* **79**: 1271–1278.

Surbone, A. and Petrek, J.A. (1998). Pregnancy after breast cancer. The relationship of pregnancy to breast cancer development and progression. *Critical Reviews in Oncology–Hematology* **27**: 169–178.

Tyc, V.L., Hudson, M.M., Hinds, P., Elliott, V. and Kibby, M.Y. (1997). Tobacco use among pediatric cancer patients: recommendations for developing clinical smoking interventions. *Journal of Clinical Oncology* **15**: 219–2204.

van Schoultz, E., Johansson, H., Wilking, N. and Rutqvist, L. E. (1995). Influence of prior and subsequent pregnancy on breast cancer prognosis. *Journal of Clinical Oncology* **13**: 430–434.

Vercollone, C.F., Moss, H. and Moss, R. (1997). *Helping the Stork: The Choices and Challenges of Donor Insemination.* New York: Macmillan.

Wagner, T. and Ahner, R. (1998). Prenatal testing for late-onset diseases such as mutations in the breast cancer gene 1 (BRCA1). Just a choice or a step in the wrong direction? *Human Reproduction* **13**: 1125–1126.

Wertz, D.C., Fanos, J.H. and Reilly, P.R. (1994). Genetic testing for children and adolescents: who decides? *Journal of the American Medical Association* **272**: 875–881.

Whitelaw, S., Northover, J.M. and Hodgson, S.V. (1996). Attitudes to predictive DNA testing in familial adenomatous polyposis. *Journal of Medical Genetics* **33**: 540–544.

Zeltzer, L.K., Chen, E., Weiss, R., Buo, M.D., Robison, L.L., Meadows, A.T., Mills, J.L., Nicholson, H.S. and Byrne, J. (1997). Comparison of psychologic outcome in adult survivors of childhood acute lymphoblastic leukemia versus sibling controls: a Cooperative Children's Cancer Group and National Institutes of Health study. *Journal of Clinical Oncology* **15**: 547–556.

Section VII
GENETICS: FAMILIAL RISK

20

Communication of Individualized Cancer Risk Information within the Family Context

JOAN L. BOTTORFF, PAMELA A. RATNER and JOY L. JOHNSON
School of Nursing, University of British Columbia, Vancouver, BC, Canada

MARY K. McCULLUM
Hereditary Cancer Program, British Columbia Cancer Agency, Vancouver, BC, Canada

Scientists' ability to determine personal risk information is changing our understanding of health and illness. Over the past 25 years the 'at-risk health status' has joined those of acute and chronic illness as legitimate health states. Kenen (1996) argued that this status is often accompanied by a diagnostic invitation, in which individuals are encouraged to learn more about their at-risk status. The increased attention that has been directed toward cancer risk and the legitimization of the at-risk status has prompted a public demand for personal risk and diagnostic information.

Many factors place an individual at risk for cancer, including behavioral, environmental, and hereditary factors. One of the strongest risk factors is that of heredity, which is currently believed to account for approximately 5–10% of all malignancies (Claus et al., 1991; Lynch and Lynch, 1991). Recent genetic research has made it possible to offer individuals within identified 'cancer families' more specific information about their cancer risk. This development has created a growing demand for individualized risk information fueled by media reports that laud the benefits of genetic testing (Lynch and Lynch, 1999) and heightened by the public's concern. Advances made in genetic testing for cancer have raised the legitimacy of the at-risk status and have introduced complexities into the communication of risk information, particularly within the family context. For this reason, much of this chapter on communication of cancer risk focuses on hereditary risk.

In this chapter we provide a summary of emerging issues and challenges in communicating individualized cancer risk information with a focus on the family. The chapter begins with a description of the context in which the sharing of risk

Cancer and the Family, 2nd Edn. Edited by L. Baider, C. L. Cooper and A. Kaplan De-Nour
© 2000 John Wiley & Sons, Ltd

information takes place. A case study exemplifies issues that arise when sharing cancer risk information. This is followed by a discussion of how risk perceptions are formed. The chapter concludes with a consideration of potential psychological and behavioural sequelae that arise when individualized cancer risk information is shared.

THE CONTEXT OF SHARING CANCER RISK INFORMATION

Procedures for sharing cancer risk information can be summarized in the following three steps: (a) provide accurate information; (b) formulate appropriate recommendations; and (c) offer emotional and psychological support (Mahon, 1998). While these steps may appear straightforward, they are complicated by several factors, most important of which is the context in which this risk information is provided and received. Context can be thought of as the circumstances relevant to an event. Communication, by necessity, involves at least two people. In the communication of cancer risk information, the contexts of the individual and of the health professional(s) inform the communication process, influencing what is said and what is heard. In addition, this communication takes place in a larger societal context in which messages about cancer inform risk perceptions. Each of these three contexts is considered in turn.

THE INDIVIDUAL CONTEXT

The health education and counseling literature has tended to conceptualize risk counseling as a process that focuses on an individual. In this process, individuals are counseled about how factors in their lives place them at risk for cancer. The problem with this individualized focus is that it does not acknowledge that at-risk individuals are members of families. While this point is true for all health-care communication, situating cancer risk communication within the family context is particularly important. Families may provide support and encouragement to those who are undergoing risk counseling, yet, because family history is a significant risk factor for cancer, family members and their cancer histories also constitute a risk factor. In other words, the individuals who, by virtue of their histories, place a person at risk for cancer, are often the same people the person is connected with and cares about (Wellisch and Hoffman, 1998). This paradox is further confused by the fact that the information that is obtained about an individual's risk, particularly genetic risk, may also have a great bearing on his/her family members' individual risk perceptions.

The term 'family' is used to recognize those who are connected by blood, those who share the same household, or those who have close kinship ties. Kin and household members often hold similar values and practices, and accordingly the behaviors that may put them at risk for cancer are often shared, such as smoking, sun exposure, and diet. Consequently, informing individuals that their behavior places them at risk for cancer also has implications for their household and kinship networks. Individuals may be reluctant to consider modifying their risk behaviors if they are closely tied to family 'ways.' Accordingly, practitioners need to move beyond an individualized approach to risk communication and find ways to address this larger family context. Empirical studies suggest that families who are at higher risk for cancer are amenable to considering lifestyle changes that will moderate their cancer risk (Kristeller et al., 1996).

A second sense of family is the sense of 'blood ties.' It is this sense that is particularly important when discussing family history and genetics in relation to cancer risk. While individuals may want to know their 'individual risk' of cancer, risk assessments necessitate knowing a great deal about the family. The very act of seeking this information may quickly turn an individual matter into a family matter. Individuals do not experience their families as 'neat biological links', but rather as variable social relationships. These relationships are marked sometimes by conflict, and consequently information may be unavailable or inaccessible (Armstrong et al., 1998).

The need to expand individual risk counseling into a family context is perhaps most apparent in the area of genetics. To conduct linkage testing, DNA specimens are required from members who have the cancer and from those who do not. Obviously, the information obtained from these samples can profoundly affect more than the individual seeking genetic risk information. In addition to providing information about the cancer risk, the process of conducting these linkage studies has been known to uncover issues of paternity, for example. Thus, an individual's request for cancer risk information can lead to profound implications for the entire family.

It is noteworthy that family members often do not make distinctions between blood ties and other family ties. In the context of risk assessment, the practitioner's need to distinguish between these forms of ties can be confusing for families. The way a person comes to consider his/her risk is rarely based on an understanding of Mendelian genetics (Richards, 1996b). Family life varies widely, and inevitably an understanding of being at risk for cancer depends, in part, on this context. It is this understanding that informs the communication process between clients and health professionals.

THE CONTEXT OF THE HEALTH CARE PROFESSIONAL

Risk communication is a part of clinical risk management, yet many health professionals are reluctant to share risk information with their clients. This reluctance stems from a perceived lack of skill about how to communicate risk information, a perceived lack of information about what places people at risk, and a concern that individuals may be unduly stressed by risk information. There is an emerging recognition among professionals that providing risk information requires skill. 'We need some sort of training in the communication of risk in everyday terms' (Edwards et al., 1998, p. 296). Communicating risk is particularly challenging because the way that the message is framed can affect the way it is heard, and the action that is likely to arise (Sarfati et al., 1998). In addition, the use of medical terminology can create barriers to understanding (Chapple et al., 1997).

Another challenge in communicating risk information arises from the perception that the facts about cancer risk are not readily available and are constantly changing. Information about cancer risk is rapidly emerging and practitioners are challenged to sift through information and to understand what constitutes risk. As one nurse commented, 'I feel the main problem is when experts keep moving the goal posts' (Edwards et al., 1998, p. 299).

Risk information cannot be thought of as a single set of neutral facts; these 'facts' can be interpreted differently by practitioners. A survey of clinical geneticists revealed that even when experts were provided the same information about families, their interpretations about risk and their suggestions about risk management varied widely (Rosser et al., 1996). Physicians have been found to hold widely varying ideas about what constitutes breast cancer risk factors. At times these ideas are based on mere opinion and lead to erroneous conclusions, such as 'promiscuity causes breast cancer' (McMullin et al., 1996). The ways that practitioners understand risk depends on the type of information that is allowed to enter their explanatory models. In addition to understanding what places a person at risk, practitioners have considerable discretion about which risks to emphasize in their encounters with clients. These choices are influenced by factors such as the professional's own values and assumptions (Buetow et al., 1998).

Some professionals are concerned that patients are incapable of coping with or understanding risk information. Confronted with the ambiguity of risk information, and wanting to offer clear information, they are reluctant to convey the limitations of cancer risk knowledge, fearing it could be misconstrued. As a general practitioner commented, '[Patients] are bound to perceive that a risk is perhaps greater if they are getting equivocal advice' (Edwards et al., 1998, p. 299). Other practitioners are concerned that risk information will cause their patients stress and anxiety (Buetow et al., 1998). Health professionals have reportedly argued that personalized risk information will increase anxiety and fear and that 'people don't learn from fear' (Bottorff et al., 1997). The concern underlying this sentiment is that individuals may become so frightened by the prospect of cancer that they might not engage in screening activities that could assist with early detection (Royak-Schaler et al., 1996). This concern is not unfounded; psychological distress associated with breast cancer risk has been found to reduce adherence to mammography screening recommendations (Lerman et al., 1995).

THE SOCIETAL CONTEXT

Communication between a client and health professional about cancer risk does not take place in a vacuum; it is shaped by the larger societal context, including social attitudes and public perceptions about the nature of risk and responsibility (Reagan, 1997). To address the emerging demand, information sources about cancer risk have flourished. As a result, the discourse about health risk in general and cancer risk in particular is no longer the sole domain of the clinician. Today, many sources of public information on cancer risk are available via print media, radio, television, and the Internet. While this information is addressing a need, these materials have been noted to contain contrary and often confusing information (Marino et al., 1999).

Despite the tremendous amount of information available about cancer risk, the public remains confused. Inaccuracies and ambiguities present in the media further complicate risk communication between a client and practitioner. Patients often believe they must educate their practitioners, while in turn practitioners believe they must combat the knowledge their clients obtain via the media. One physician stated,

'If something is there in black and white in a newspaper, if that is slightly inaccurate, even if you have an excellent relationship with your patients, they tend to believe the inaccurate report rather than yourself and it's a big task then changing their views' (Edwards et al., 1998, p. 296).

Because of the demand for risk information, professionals find themselves in the position of explaining to individuals that perceive themselves to be at high risk for cancer why they are not eligible for genetic testing (Bottorff et al., in press). A challenge that lies ahead for health professionals is to meet this demand by developing effective strategies to help the public determine whether they are at particular risk, and what type of risk counseling they require (Bottorff et al., 1998).

Professionals involved in providing cancer risk information are cautioned to remain cognizant of the contexts that inform their communication with clients. Communication of cancer risk information must move beyond an exclusive focus on the individual. In the next section, a case study is presented to exemplify how these contexts inform the decision to seek and receive individualized cancer risk information. While the 'facts' described in the case study represent actual family experiences, a composite of several families has been used to preserve confidentiality. A genogram is provided to assist the reader (see Figure 20.1).

THE TYLER FAMILY: A CASE STUDY

Jane's mother Barb was diagnosed with breast cancer when Jane was 13 and died 3 years later. Over the course of her illness, Barb and her husband talked openly with Jane and her siblings about the cancer and its treatment, encouraging them to ask questions and to express their concerns. They were a close family that became even closer in the last months of Barb's life. Two of Barb's younger sisters were frequent visitors and sources of support, juggling the care of their own children to be with Barb's family. Her other sister and brother were not involved, and Jane remembers their infrequent visits as uncomfortable.

After watching a television program about families who had undergone genetic testing for breast and ovarian cancer, Jane, now 25 years of age, decided to investigate whether this might be possible for her family. Her family doctor, who admitted knowing little about the subject, reluctantly referred her to a cancer genetics program, where she was asked to provide details about her family's history. Jane's maternal grandmother died of ovarian cancer in her mid-50s, and a maternal great-aunt also died of ovarian cancer. Barb had often remarked that ovarian cancer was her fear; she had not worried about breast cancer because she was so young.

Jane requested that her grandfather and three aunts provide further details of the family history. Anita and Cheryl were very interested and asked to be involved in future appointments with the genetic counselor. Nancy made it clear that she had no interest in participating. She stated, 'I've already done what I needed to do and cancer has no place in my life now.' When Jane asked for clarification, Nancy reluctantly shared that 2 years earlier she had undergone bilateral prophylactic mastectomy and oophorectomy, 'to be sure that I never have to go through what my

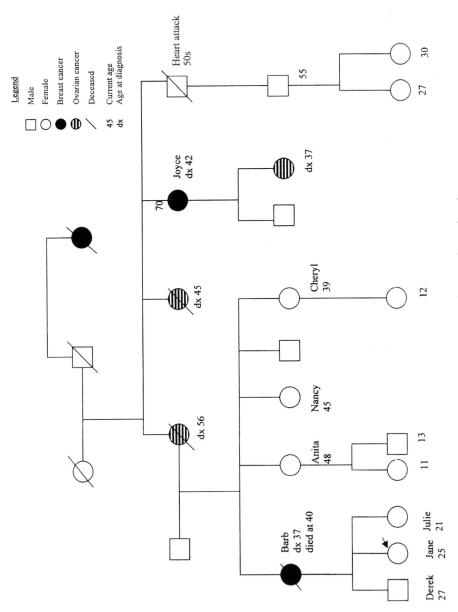

Figure 20.1   Tyler family genogram at initial genetics consultation, the arrow denotes the proband

mother and Barb went through.' She had decided not to tell her sisters or nieces because she believed they would think she had over-reacted.

Her grandfather put Jane in touch with Joyce, her grandmother's only surviving sibling. Jane had never met the woman and was apprehensive about contacting her, especially to ask about the family history of cancer. She was surprised when Joyce promptly returned her call. Jane was more surprised to learn that Joyce had had breast cancer at the age of 42 and that her 37 year-old daughter was completing chemotherapy for ovarian cancer. Joyce provided information about her brother and his family, and indicated that she believed her father's sister had died of breast cancer. She described her own breast cancer experience and was not enthusiastic about genetic testing. 'Helping my daughter through her chemotherapy takes all my energy right now.'

Accompanied by Anita, Cheryl, and Julie, Jane took the family history information to an appointment with a genetic counselor. Their 2 hour appointment included telling their stories as members of a 'cancer family' and being provided with information about genes, mutations, inheritance, cancer risk, and the possibility of genetic testing. The counselor explained that their family history was certainly suggestive of a hereditary cancer syndrome, with six closely related women in three generations being diagnosed either with breast cancer at a young age or with ovarian cancer. She described the possibility that an inherited mutation in the BRCA1 or BRCA2 genes might explain their situation, and that it could be important information for both the men and the women in the family.

Jane immediately wanted to know when they could have their blood tested. The counselor explained that for genetic testing to provide a useful result, the first person to have her blood tested should be someone who had had breast or ovarian cancer. If a mutation was found, then interested family members could choose to find out whether they had inherited the specific gene mutation. The four women were distressed at this news, because it meant that Joyce or her daughter would need to participate, which was unlikely. The counselor reminded them that the decision to have testing required careful consideration by each person. She gave them an information booklet to send to their relatives, indicating that any member of the family was welcome to contact her.

Several events over the next year caused the family to book another appointment with the genetic counselor. Anita discovered a lump in her right breast, confirmed by mammography and biopsy to be a very small breast cancer. Cheryl and she met with the genetic counselor and Anita gave a blood sample for testing. It seemed ironic to them that it took another cancer diagnosis in the family to make testing possible. A short time later, Joyce informed Jane that her daughter's ovarian cancer had not responded to chemotherapy and she was not expected to live. Joyce indicated that her daughter's imminent death had changed her mind about genetic testing, and she arranged to meet with a genetic counselor in a city nearby. She expressed the hope that she and her daughter could have their blood tested to find an explanation for the 'toll that cancer was taking in their family.' Arrangements were made for blood samples from Joyce and her daughter to be tested and they talked about how valuable Joyce's assistance would be in informing the extended family when a result became available.

While the family waited for the test results, Jane booked an appointment with the counselor to discuss her own situation. She was considering marriage and was struggling with how to tell her partner that she could have a very high risk of cancer. He knew that her mother had died of breast cancer but they had discussed neither the cancer history in her family, nor her own risk. As Jane described, 'I didn't want to tell him too soon and scare him off, but I can't plan a future with him if he doesn't know this important piece of information about me.'

Eventually Anita was advised that her testing was complete. Accompanied by her husband and sister Cheryl, she learned that a BRCA1 gene mutation had been identified and that the same mutation had been found in her aunt's and cousin's blood samples. This was taken as good news by Anita and Cheryl, who finally felt they had an explanation. Now, the rest of the family could be tested, and perhaps some would even learn that they did not carry the mutation. Anita's husband sat quietly, with tears in his eyes. He shared that he did not see this as good news; he could only focus on the significant chance that Anita might develop another cancer, and that their children might also inherit this predisposition.

Cheryl shared the news with Jane and Julie, knowing that they had a good understanding of what it meant, and suggested that the three of them go together to have their blood taken. Jane was ready to go that afternoon, but Julie was not so sure. She stated, 'I look so much like mom that I don't really need to have the test. I already know that I have it.' Their brother Derek thought it was all very interesting and that he 'might as well find out,' although he did not think it would make much difference to him.

Anita contacted Nancy and they had a difficult conversation. because testing had not previously been possible, and Nancy had already had prophylactic surgery, the sisters had not told her about their initial genetic counseling appointment, neither had they informed their brother. Now Anita was disclosing her recent breast cancer diagnosis, and the fact that there was a 'defective' gene in their family. Nancy stated that she still thought it was a bad idea and had no interest in having such testing. She also wanted to try to convince Jane and Julie not to ruin their lives by having the test done.

When Jane called Joyce to discuss how to advise the rest of the family, she found that Joyce had already contacted her brother's adult granddaughters and they were very interested in learning more. They had no direct experience with cancer, but expressed the opinion that it was good to have as much information as possible, even if that included learning you had a high risk of cancer. They did not think that their father would want to get involved, so wanted to get the testing done and tell him of the results later. This story could continue with details of the decisions made by each of the members of this family and the impact on their lives.

This case study highlights many issues including: considerations of when individuals should seek risk information, misconceptions about heredity and risk, family dynamics, the impact of genetic information on future plans and reconciliation of past decisions, and, most important, the recognition that these actions are not solely those of any one individual—they hold serious implications for the entire family. In the remainder of the chapter we focus on factors underlying the formation of risk perception and the implications of communicating risk information for individuals and their families.

FORMULATION OF RISK PERCEPTION

The following section addresses how individuals within families in which a cancer diagnosis has been made form perceptions of their own risk or susceptibility to cancer. Scientists have made great advances in identifying individuals who are at high risk for cancer based either on risk factors or, more recently, on the basis of genetic mutations. The lay public may have some knowledge of this science, but, for the most part, come to assess their own risk of cancer based on their subjective experience, and cognitive and emotional factors.

Typically, individuals with family histories of cancer hold a pessimistic bias regarding cancer risk; they have a tendency to overestimate their risk for cancer. This phenomenon may occur across cancers, although little empirical work is available in areas other than breast cancer risk perception. Accordingly, much of what follows arises from the psychosocial literature related to women's perceptions of their breast cancer risk.

The prevalent phenomenon that individuals tend to estimate their risk of acquiring a particular disease as less than the chances of similar others (termed 'unrealistic optimism' by Weinstein, 1982, 1984), does not appear to occur in those who define themselves as members of 'cancer families,' particularly those who believe in hereditary causation (Richardson et al., 1994). Weinstein's (1987, 1989) work suggests that unrealistic optimism, or optimistic bias, most likely occurs when diseases are considered preventable or controllable by individual action. Those who have experienced cancer within the family may conceptualize the disease as uncontrollable and consequently adopt fatalistic notions of their own susceptibility or risk. For example, Hallowell et al. (1998) interviewed a woman with a family history of cancer who had been advised that her lifetime risk of ovarian and breast cancer was 32%:

> I think if there's cancer in your family, I mean we've got no one in our family that's ever died of a heart attack, nobody. They've all died of cancer, one way or another. I mean my father had lung cancer, which is totally different. But it still puts the fear of God into you really . . . and I just think, well, I'm obviously the next one on the cards (p. 357).

The pessimistic bias observed in individuals with family histories of cancer may result from their personal experience with the disease (i.e., having a family history). For example, McCaul and O'Donnell (1998) found that women with a family history of breast cancer made higher estimates of their risk than did women without a family history. Women with a first-degree relative with breast cancer (e.g., mother or sister) estimated their risk, on average, at 50%, while women with a second- or third-degree relative with breast cancer (e.g., grandmother or great-aunt) estimated their risk to be as high as 43%. It is still unclear how pervasive this thinking is. Richardson et al. (1994) reported that 55% of women who were twin sisters of women with breast cancer diagnoses perceived their lifetime chance of breast cancer as higher or almost inevitable, compared to other women. What we do not know is what the women, particularly those that believed their risk to be the same or less than other women (45%), believed the average women's risk to be; it may have been overestimated. In another study of women with family histories of breast or ovarian cancer, 76%

perceived themselves to be at higher risk than women in general and 20% regarded a diagnosis of cancer as inevitable (Hallowell et al., 1998).

At first blush, the association between perceived risk and family history of cancer might be patently obvious. After all, positive family history is a risk factor. However, a Dutch study found that, among women with family histories of breast cancer, only 46% knew that women who have a first-degree relative with breast cancer are at increased risk (Drossaert et al., 1996). These women believed they were susceptible to breast cancer, and more likely to think so than those with negative family histories. Those who knew that family history was a risk factor achieved the highest susceptibility scores. This might suggest that it is not knowledge of risk factors alone that heightens this population's sense of susceptibility, but rather the experience of breast cancer in the immediate environment. For example, in the Richardson et al. (1994) study, 75% of the women who were twins of women with breast cancer reported that their twin sister's diagnosis made them feel more susceptible to cancer. Yet, when asked about the causes of cancer in their twin sisters, 70% responded that it was caused by stress. 58% responded that inherited make up or heredity was the cause, and three-quarters of these respondents also cited stress. Over half (52%) cited poor eating habits, and lesser-mentioned factors included being physically 'run down,' environmental chemicals, natural hormone levels, smoking, alcohol consumption, viruses, hormone medications, childbearing, injuries to the breast, and sexual history or activity.

What other factors influence the formation of individuals' risk estimates, particularly among those with a positive family history? In many instances, individuals point to genetics, even though they may not have particular information about a genetic mutation, may be describing unrelated cancers, or may have a family history that is not suggestive of a genetic mutation (e.g., one distant relative who was diagnosed with a cancer late in life). In McCaul and O'Donnell's (1998) study of women's perceived breast cancer risk, 90% of those with a family history of cancer cited genetics, heredity, and family history (including cancers other than breast cancer) as the reason behind their risk estimate. It is likely that many individuals conflate notions of genetic predisposition (inherited susceptibility) with familial risk (common risk factors). Quotations from the respondents interviewed in the study of Hallowell et al. (1998) illustrate this sense of heightened susceptibility:

> Because obviously I lost my mum, and it wasn't very nice because in the end she died of a brain tumor and I had to watch her die in a hospice and I wouldn't wish that on anybody. . . . And then my sister started, obviously I thought, Oh my God! I am next!
> I am expecting to get it [ovarian cancer] to be honest. Going by my family's history so far, just about every female on my mother's side has had some sort of cancer . . . I am expecting to have cancer sort of in my forties and fifties (p. 353).

Similarities observed between affected relatives and the self may contribute to heightened susceptibility. For example, an individual's age is often contrasted with an affected relative's age at the time of diagnosis:

> It was sort of in the 40s where I realized I better start taking a look. I am getting older now. My mom died at 46 . . . that breast cancer thing is coming into focus now (Chalmers and Thomson, 1996, p. 271).

Chalmers and Thomson (1996) also noted that comparisons are made between an individual's personality, lifestyle and physical characteristics (e.g., response to stress, diet, and breast size) and those of an affected relative.

When an individual believes that he/she is at risk for cancer by virtue of being a member of a 'cancer family,' a complex cognitive schema emerges with an intertwining of objective and subjective risk information. The individual's perception of his/her risk is unavoidably complicated by personal values and biases, and is often subject to error (Bottorff et al., 1998).

There are dissimilar ideas about the meaning of risk that vary across health professionals and between professionals and the lay public. Hansson (1989) suggested that professionals look upon the term as a unidimensional, technical concept that relates to a specific, known probability. The public, however, assigns various meanings to the word. A noteworthy outcome of this discrepancy is that there can be significant differences between the estimated magnitude of different risks and individuals' perceptions and interpretations of those risks. For example, after being counseled that her lifetime risk of breast risk was 40%, a woman in the Hallowell et al. (1998) study stated:

> Cancer's not a thing, it's not like a cold, you've got a chance of getting it or you won't. It's either there or it's not. Now, if it don't come up in the breast and there's nowhere for it to come up, it will come up somewhere else and it won't be as easy to find (p. 355).

This woman's statement also points to a common cognitive bias that informed her understanding of numeric data.

Parsons and Atkinson (1992) found that when individuals are provided with estimates of their risk stated in percentages, they often restate those values in categorical terms. Such unsophisticated readings (e.g., 'high,' 'low,' or 'fifty–fifty') may be more decipherable, but the intrinsically probabilistic quality of risk information is transformed into definitive pronouncements and 'the probabilistic . . . [is] expressed as a matter of certainty' (Parsons and Atkinson, 1992, p. 454). Lippman-Hand and Fraser (1979) found that recipients of risk information often reduce the information to a dichotomous interpretation (i.e., either it will or will not happen).

The interpretation of risk information is delimited by personal beliefs and assumptions that may be discordant with scientific and epidemiologic knowledge. Individuals that are generally pessimistic are likely to magnify the seriousness of a given risk value (Moran, 1970). Pearn (1973) suggested that, even in the presence of low risk, such individuals believe that their 'bad luck' increases their risk, almost in a 'metaphysical way' (p. 132).

Even the most sophisticated individuals tend to have difficulty understanding the nature of risk and probability and frequently rely on heuristic devices to comprehend probabilistic problems. In the end, the individual must come to understand the information in ways that make it meaningful. Reassurances that adverse outcomes occur rarely, such as in less than 10% of a population, hold little comfort for those who may believe that they are destined to be that one person in 10. No matter what the probability of risk may be, to the individual, it is an all-or-none phenomenon; they will be affected or they will not be (Bogardus et al., 1999). This phenomenon arises because, in addition to cognitive biases that influence one's understanding, there are social biases, particularly those arising from one's family history (Frankenberg, 1993). It is evident that individuals that consider their risk to be high because of their family history do not view risk as hypothetical. The meaning they attribute to risk is informed by social and familial meanings, and any risk information encountered must conform to a well-established causal schema (Tversky and Kahneman, 1982). When faced with contrary information suggesting that their risk is lower than perceived, these individuals may be averse to amending expansive and coherent schemas. For example, a woman with a family history of breast cancer who was advised that her lifetime risk was 20%, and lower than what she perceived, insisted:

> I know I'm going to get it, it's just when I'm going to get it. So there was no thought that I wasn't at any less risk . . . I wanted to hear that [that her risk was lower than perceived], but I still thought, well, I'm still going to get it . . . I've said straight from the start, it's too close to me for me to just brush it off . . . I didn't for once think that they were going to say, you're not at any risk, and even if they'd said it I wouldn't have believed it, because I know I am, so anything that would have been said any different wouldn't have changed my view at all (Hallowell et al., 1998, p. 357).

Watson et al. (1999) found that 61% of women with a family history of breast cancer, who overestimated their risk, continued to do so following genetic counseling. Despite corrective information related to their lifetime risk, these women remained 'fixed' in their understanding.

The basis upon which individuals that identify as members of 'cancer families' form estimates of their own susceptibility is complex and not easily modified. This pessimistic bias is likely to hold many implications for the psychological well-being of this population, in addition to their preventive behaviour and response to health education and counseling. As genetic testing continues to attract media attention, and as the lay public is exposed to information about genetic susceptibility, there is a pressing need to understand better how this information is incorporated into the complex understandings that individuals possess relative to their personal risk, how new information is processed, how health professionals can assist in promoting accurate risk estimation, and how individuals' perceived risk influences their psychological health and preventive (screening) behaviour.

THE IMPACT OF RISK INFORMATION

Although relatively few individuals receive confirmation of their genetic risk for cancer, many are identified to be at high risk based on their family history and other risk factors. The impact of risk information for individuals that are confirmed or potential genetic mutation carriers and their families is not well understood. Despite acknowledgement of the role of relatives and family relationships in discussions of the impact of genetic disease, most researchers have focused on individual, rather than family, experiences of the receipt of cancer risk information.

The receipt of cancer risk information can be conceptualized as a 'new traumatic situation' (Alby, 1998) that shapes an 'at-risk identity' (Hallowell, 2000). The consequences of receiving a risk estimate are likely to be very different from those associated with a cancer diagnosis. Developments in genetic testing approaches no longer require sampling of whole families. Consequently, individuals can obtain risk information despite family disagreements about the value of knowing one's risk. Information about the risk status of any one individual, however, can heighten concerns of unaffected relatives, both for themselves and their children. From a few research studies and clinical experience with genetic testing for cancer risk, two important areas of impact are apparent: (a) psychological sequelae for individuals and their families; and (b) influences on health behaviour.

PSYCHOLOGICAL SEQUELAE FOR INDIVIDUALS AND THEIR FAMILIES

Although information about risk can be important in motivating individuals to engage in cancer screening, it has been associated with a range of psychological consequences that vary with the strength of the family history, experiences with cancer, and expectations related to risk status. Responses to results that indicate high risk have included acceptance when expectations are confirmed and relief from anxiety when uncertainty is reduced (Lynch et al., 1999). For others, emotional reactions to test results may be so strong that they compromise one's quality of life and subsequent screening practices. Even with the pre- and post-test counseling, women tested for BRCA1 gene mutations have exhibited relatively high levels of distress (Croyle et al., 1997), especially those with information-seeking coping styles (Lerman et al., 1994, 1996).

Individuals who are found to be negative for a genetic mutation also experience a range of emotions, including relief, disbelief, or 'survivor's guilt.' In some instances, emotional reactions associated with risk information may begin shortly after application for testing and may persist for some time, indicating a need for ongoing psychological and educational interventions (Grosfeld et al., 1996). For example, individuals that initially feel a sense of disbelief upon receiving cancer risk information may require time to fully understand their results (Mahon and Casperson, 1995).

Individual reactions to testing are often linked with family concerns. In a qualitative study of 13 individuals with hereditary cancer syndrome, participants attributed high levels of anxiety to concerns for their children rather than themselves (Mahon and Casperson, 1995). Ambivalent feelings about favourable test outcomes are common when individuals are worried about the test results of other relatives (Grosfeld et al., 1996). Non-carriers often feel isolated because of a sense of disconnection from family members that are carriers.

Family responses to the communication of cancer risk information are not well understood; most empirical literature concerning the impact of testing addresses the affected individual (Croyle and Lerman, 1995). Nevertheless, clinical experience suggests that the receipt of risk information may profoundly affect families (Macdonald et al., 1995). This may be intensified if difficulties are encountered when at-risk individuals openly discuss cancer and explain test results (Grosfeld et al., 1996), and by pre-existing family dysfunction (Engelking, 1995). Discussions of cancer risk information with children present unique challenges that vary with age and sometimes gender.

Interviews with women at risk for breast and ovarian cancer who sought genetic counseling provide insights into family communication patterns and issues raised as a consequence of seeking cancer risk information (Daly et al., 1999; Green et al., 1997). Although most of the women in these studies reported that they could talk openly about cancer with a majority of their relatives, the quality and pattern of communication varied with the nature of family relationships. Green et al. (1997) reported that taboos related to talking about cancer and reproductive parts of the female body influence communication patterns. Further, women found it difficult to seek information from some family members (e.g., if the person was old or ill), not wanting to upset individuals with painful memories, and occasionally withheld information to avoid alarming or burdening relatives by 'opening up' the cancer experience. Often relatives may not support or understand an individual's need to seek risk information. We know little about individuals' experiences in asking relatives to provide necessary blood samples or family members' responses to such requests.

Patterns of disclosing results of testing to family members are beginning to be described. Once informed of their risk status for breast and ovarian cancer, women often feel duty-bound to inform family members, although they approach this cautiously to avoid upsetting others.

> I think it would be better if it was spoken rather than a letter, because a letter is frightening, because you think—if I thought those girls [nieces] weren't doing anything [i.e., having screening] and I was told that they are really at a high risk, I think in conversation I would say to them, do you have these checks that are available, you know? They are really a good idea. That what—I think I would bring it up in a light way with them (Green et al., 1997, p. 55).

Others have observed that men are often excluded from family conversations about breast cancer and in some instances report actively avoiding such discussions (McAllister et al., 1998). Although relatively little is known about how families discuss cancer risk and make use of risk information, there are important consequences for families when inadequate communication occurs. Grosfeld et al. (1996) described one family's experience related to genetic testing for medullary thyroid carcinoma, which is associated with several hereditary cancer syndromes. One woman, who was very worried about her children's risk, successfully pressured her husband to participate in testing. Because he refused to discuss the matter any further, she had to cope with her despair over the possible test results on her own and conflicts arose. This family's experience illustrates the difficulties that families are often prepared to undergo when obtaining risk information. In another example, Lynch et al. (1999) reported that a woman with breast cancer was said to blame her father (a BRCA1 carrier) and his family for passing the genetic mutation to her. Although the blame may have been perceived rather than real, it resulted in intense guilt for the father.

In other families, at-risk individuals are able to discuss the experience with some, if not all, relatives. One woman explained:

> I have a daughter of 24. We can talk quite openly about the family history and my risks and hers too. Initially, she said that she wouldn't want to know if she carried the gene but is now able to consider the advantages of knowing. . . . My husband has never found it easy to talk about the issue. I think he would rather not think about the possibilities and he has never initiated discussion on the topic with me. I have no other blood

relatives that I keep in regular contact with to share the situation, and my parents-in-law do not feel comfortable talking about cancer at all (Richards, 1996a, p. 38).

The receipt of risk information has been noted to change relationships within families. Improved contact and closer bonds between carriers of genetic mutations within nuclear and extended families have been observed, although sometimes at the cost of reducing contact with family members not at-risk (Grosfeld et al., 1996). Stigmatization and coercion can also occur within family networks.

These examples illustrate how family dynamics can influence the process of adjusting to risk information and cause strain within some families. Further research is required to identify and describe effective family communication patterns and strategies that are sensitive to the issues related to disclosure of cancer risk information. Individuals who have participated in genetic counseling for hereditary cancer have expressed dissatisfaction with the provision of information about how to discuss hereditary cancer with their children and other relatives (Bleiker et al., 1997). The sequelae of risk communication for individuals and families require more attention by researchers. There may be other important psychological outcomes related to receiving cancer risk information that should be explored. For example, there is some evidence that the concept of perceived personal control may be helpful in understanding the success with which individuals cope following genetic counseling (Berkenstadt et al., 1999).

INFLUENCES ON HEALTH BEHAVIOR

Risk assessment provides a basis for decision making about a variety of health behaviours, including preventive action and surveillance. These decisions, however, are not always straightforward. For example, women at high risk for breast and ovarian cancer can choose among several options, none of which is guaranteed, including rigorous screening, chemoprevention such as tamoxifen, and prophylactic surgery (Lerner, 1999). Furthermore, these risk management strategies carry potential adversities, including false reassurance, changes in body image, anxiety, and other health risks.

Factors influencing risk-management decisions include individual factors, such as coping style, anxiety, and expectations of risk status. A qualitative study of responses to genetic testing for familial adenomatous polyposis (FAP) revealed that, even when testing indicated an extremely low risk of developing disease, a desire to continue regular bowel screening persisted, despite it being extremely aversive (Michie et al., 1996). Several explanations are offered by Michie et al., including the need to maintain a sense of risk to make sense of past efforts, a lack of skill to deal with the removal of the threat, and the immutability of critical aspects of the perceived risk. Similar results have been found among women who received low risk results after genetic testing for breast and ovarian cancer (Lynch et al., 1993). Seven of nine women indicated that they would proceed with intensive surveillance, and two wished to proceed with prophylactic mastectomy despite their low-risk status. It remains unclear whether these responses to risk information are modifiable.

The family also appears to have an influence on risk management decisions. Women at risk for familial breast and ovarian cancer have been observed to frame their decisions in the context of family relationships, considering the consequences for their children, partners, and other family members (Hallowell, 1998). A strong motivator to consider prophylactic surgery is a sense of obligation to one's family to manage risk and to optimize survival (Hallowell, 1998, 2000).

Few studies have examined the health behaviour of family members of individuals who have received risk information. Ayme et al. (1993) found that changes to health behavior among family members are limited, because genetic information is not transmitted to all relatives or does not make clear the necessity for further information or action. This is further complicated when an affected individual does not wish information to be disclosed to anyone else, or when family members do not wish to be informed of the results of testing. Evidence suggests that simply being a member of a cancer family appears to have an important influence on health behavior. One study of women with a family history of breast cancer provides some evidence that women construct their own personal meaning of the benefits and limitations of breast self-examination, and make decisions to use this surveillance strategy along with prioritizing a 'risk-reducing' lifestyle to gain control over their feelings of threat (Chalmers and Luker, 1996). Whether the receipt of individualized cancer risk information by one or more members of a family modifies relatives' health behaviour remains unknown.

Efficacious interventions are required to enhance psychological adjustment and adoption of recommended health practices and to prevent or ameliorate the negative sequelae of risk information. Recommendations have been extrapolated from interventions to promote cancer screening and psychosocial interventions for coping with cancer. Drawing on the latter, Kash and Lerman (1998) recommended a variety of behavioural interventions (e.g., support groups, individual psychotherapy, psycho-educational interventions), coping skills training and decision counseling. These interventions, however, are often focused on at-risk individuals rather than their families. Innovative interventions are needed to address family issues associated with cancer risk information. Assessments of openness to discuss cancer may help identify families with a potential to encounter difficulties (Mesters et al., 1997).

CONCLUSION

Attributions and discussions of cancer risk inevitably involve a focus not only on the individual but also on family systems. Despite developments in risk assessment, our knowledge about how to communicate risk estimates effectively within the family context is underdeveloped. There are no clear directives about how to ensure that the probabilistic nature of risk estimates is accurately communicated and understood. While there is a clear need to move beyond the individual to the family context, the sequelae of providing cancer risk information to individuals and their families are only beginning to be understood.

New discoveries about genetic links in cancer are increasingly shared with the public and many, including those with cancer, question their genetic risk. Given the rapid developments in genetic testing, a new challenge is emerging in cancer care, necessitating that health professionals address issues related to the communication of risk information. Increasingly, health professionals will be called on to provide cancer risk information in ways that support or augment services available through familial cancer genetics programs.

REFERENCES

Alby, N. (1998). Comment on 'The psychological impact of genetic testing for breast cancer'. *European Journal of Cancer* **34**: 1986.

Armstrong, D., Michie, S. and Marteau, T.M. (1998). Revealed identity: a study of the process of genetic counselling. *Social Science and Medicine* **47**: 1653–1658.

Ayme, S., MacQuart-Moulin, G., Julian-Reynier, C., Chabal, F. and Giraud, F. (1993). Diffusion of information about genetic risk within families. *Neuromuscular Disorders* **3**: 571–574.

Berkenstadt, M., Shiloh, S., Barkai, G., Katznelson, M.B.-M. and Goldman, B. (1999). Perceived personal control (PPC): a new concept in measuring outcome of genetic counseling. *American Journal of Medical Genetics* **82**: 53–59.

Bleiker, E.M.A., Aaronson, N.K., Menko, F.H., Hahn, D.E.E., van Asperen, C.J., Rutgers, E.J.T., ten Kate, L.P. and Leschot, N.J. (1997). Genetic counseling for hereditary cancer: a pilot study on experiences of patients and family members. *Patient Education and Counseling* **32**: 107–116.

Bogardus, S.T., Holmboe, E. and Jekel, J.F. (1999). Perils, pitfalls and possibilities in talking about medical risk. *Journal of the American Medical Association* **281**: 1037–1041.

Bottorff, J.L., Balneaves, L.G., Buxton, J., Ratner, P.A., McCullum, M., Chalmers, K. and Hack, T. (in press). Falling through the cracks: women's experiences of ineligibility for genetic testing for breast cancer risk. *Canadian Family Physician*.

Bottorff, J.L., Johnson, J.L., Ratner, P.A., Joab, A. and Olson, K. (1997). *The provision of personal breast cancer risk information: Service or disservice?* Poster presented at the National Workshop on Organized Breast Cancer Screening Programs, Ottawa, ON, Canada, April.

Bottorff, J.L., Ratner, P.A., Johnson, J.L., Lovato, C.Y. and Joab, S.A. (1998). Communicating cancer risk information: the challenges of uncertainty. *Patient Education and Counseling* **33**: 67–81.

Buetow, S., Cantrill, J. and Sibbald, B. (1998). Risk communication in the patient–health professional relationship. *Health Care Analysis* **6**: 261–268.

Chalmers, K. and Thomson, K. (1996). Coming to terms with the risk of breast cancer: perceptions of women with primary relatives with breast cancer. *Qualitative Health Research* **6**: 256–282.

Chalmers, K.I. and Luker, K.A. (1996). Breast self-care practices in women with primary relatives with breast cancer. *Journal of Advanced Nursing* **23**: 1212–1220.

Chapple, A., Campion, P. and May, C. (1997). Clinical terminology: anxiety and confusion amongst families undergoing genetic counseling. *Patient Education and Counseling* **32**: 81–91.

Claus, E.B., Risch, N. and Thompson, W.D. (1991). Genetic analysis of breast cancer in the cancer and steroid hormone study. *American Journal of Human Genetics* **48**: 232–242.

Croyle, R.T. and Lerman, C. (1995). Psychological impact of genetic testing. In R.T. Croyle (Ed.), *Psychological Effects of Screening for Disease Prevention and Detection* (pp. 11–38). New York: Oxford University Press.

Croyle, R.T., Smith, K.R., Botkin, J.R., Baty, B. and Nash, J. (1997). Psychological responses to BRCA1 mutation testing: preliminary findings. *Health Psychology* **16**: 63–72.

Daly, M., Farmer, J., Harrop-Stein, C., Montgomery, S., Itzen, M., Costalas, J.W., Rogatko, A., Miller, S., Balshem, A. and Gillespie, D. (1999). Exploring family relationships in cancer risk counseling using the genogram. *Cancer Epidemiology, Biomarkers and Prevention* **8**: 393–398.

Drossaert, C.C., Boer, H. and Seydel, E.R. (1996). Perceived risk, anxiety, mammogram uptake, and breast self-examination of women with a family history of breast cancer: the role of knowing to be at increased risk. *Cancer Detection and Prevention* **20**: 76–85.

Edwards, A., Matthews, E., Pill, R. and Bloor, M. (1998). Communication about risk: diversity among primary care professionals. *Family Practice* **15**: 296–300.

Engelking, C. (1995). Genetics in cancer care: confronting a Pandora's Box of dilemmas. *Oncology Nursing Forum* **22** (2 Suppl.): 27–34.

Frankenberg, R. (1993). Risk anthropological and epidemiological narratives of prevention. In S. Lindenbaum and M. Lock (Eds), *Knowledge, Power and Practice: The Anthropology of Medicine and Everyday Life* (pp. 219–242). Los Angeles, CA: University of California Press.

Green, J., Richards, M., Murton, F., Statham, H. and Hallowell, N. (1997). Family communication and genetic counseling: the case of hereditary breast and ovarian cancer. *Journal of Genetic Counseling* **6**: 45–60.

Grosfeld, F.J.M., Lips, C.J.M., Ten Kroode, H.F.J., Beemer, F.A. and Van Spijker, H.G. (1996). Psychological consequences of DNA analysis for MEN type 2. *Oncology* **10**: 141–146.

Hallowell, N. (1998). 'You don't *want* to lose your ovaries because you think "I might become a man".' Women's perceptions of prophylactic surgery as a cancer risk management option. *Psycho-Oncology* **7**: 263–275.

Hallowell, N. (2000). Reconstructing the body or reconstructing the woman? Perceptions of prophylactic mastectomy for hereditary breast cancer risk. In L.K. Potts (Ed.), *Ideologies of Breast Cancer: Feminist Perspectives* (pp. 153–180). London: Macmillan/St. Martin's Press.

Hallowell, N., Statham, H. and Murton, F. (1998). Women's understanding of their risk of developing breast/ovarian cancer before and after genetic counseling. *Journal of Genetic Counseling* **7**: 345–354.

Hansson, S.O. (1989). Dimensions of risk. *Risk Analysis* **9**: 107–112.

Kash, K.M. and Lerman, C. (1998). Psychological, social, and ethical issues in genetic testing. In J.C. Holland (Ed.), *Psycho-oncology* (pp. 196–207). New York: Oxford University Press.

Kenen, R.H. (1996). The at-risk health status and technology: a diagnostic invitation and the 'gift' of knowing. *Social Science and Medicine* **42**: 1545–1553.

Kristeller, J.L., Hebert, J., Edmiston, K., Liepman, M., Wertheimer, M., Ward, A. and Luippold, R. (1996). Attitudes toward risk factor behavior of relatives of cancer patients. *Preventive Medicine* **25**: 162–169.

Lerman, C., Daly, M., Masny, A. and Balshem, A. (1994). Attitudes about genetic testing for breast-ovarian cancer susceptibility. *Journal of Clinical Oncology* **12**: 843–850.

Lerman, C., Lustbader, E., Rimer, B., Daly, M., Miller, S., Sands, C. and Balshem, A. (1995). Effects of individualized breast cancer risk counseling: a randomized trial. *Journal of the National Cancer Institute* **87**: 286–292.

Lerman, C., Schwartz, M.D., Miller, S.M., Daly, M., Sands, C. and Rimer, B.K. (1996). A randomized trial of breast cancer risk counseling: interacting effects of counseling, educational level, and coping style. *Health Psychology* **15**: 75–83.

Lerner, B.H. (1999). Great expectations: historical perspectives on genetic breast cancer testing. *American Journal of Public Health* **89**: 938–944.

Lippman-Hand, A. and Fraser, F.C. (1979). Genetic counseling—the postcounseling period: I. Parents' perceptions of uncertainty. *American Journal of Medical Genetics* **4**: 51–71.

Lynch, H.T. and Lynch, J.F. (1991). Familial factors and genetic predisposition to cancer: population studies. *Cancer Detection and Prevention* **15**: 49–57.

Lynch, H.T. and Lynch, J.F. (1999). Pros and cons of genetic screening for breast cancer. *American Family Physician* **59**: 43–45.

Lynch, H.T., Watson, P., Conway, T.A., Lynch, J.F., Slominski-Caster, S.M., Narod, S.A., Feunteun, J. and Lenoir, G. (1993). DNA screening for breast/ovarian cancer susceptibility based on linked markers. A family study. *Archives of Internal Medicine* **153**: 1979–1987.

Lynch, H.T., Watson, P., Tinley, S., Snyder, C., Durham, C., Lynch, J., Kirnarsky, Y., Serova, O., Lenoir, G., Lerman, C. and Narod, S.A. (1999). An update on DNA-based

BRCA1/BRCA2 genetic counseling in hereditary breast cancer. *Cancer Genetics Cytogenetics* **109**: 91–98.

Macdonald, K.G., Doan, B., Kelner, M. and Taylor, K.M. (1995). Genetic vulnerability: the unwanted inheritance. Sociobehavioural implications of cancer risk. In K.M. Taylor and D. DePetrillo (Eds), *Critical Choices: Ethical, Legal and Sociobehavioural Implications of Heritable Breast, Ovarian and Colon Cancer* (pp. 19–60). Toronto: International Research and Policy Symposium.

Mahon, S.M. (1998). Cancer risk assessment: conceptual considerations for clinical practice. *Oncology Nursing Forum* **25**: 1535–1547.

Mahon, S.M. and Casperson, D.S. (1995). Hereditary cancer syndrome: part 2. Psychosocial issues, concerns, and screening—results of a qualitative study. *Oncology Nursing Forum* **22**: 775–782.

Marino, C. and Gerlach, K.K. (1999). An analysis of breast cancer coverage in selected women's magazines, 1987–1995. *American Journal of Health Promotion* **13**: 163–170.

McAllister, M.F., Evans, D.G.R., Ormiston, W. and Daly, P. (1998). Men in breast cancer families: a preliminary qualitative study of awareness and experience. *Journal of Medical Genetics* **35**: 739–744.

McCaul, K.D. and O'Donnell, S.M. (1998). Naive beliefs about breast cancer risk. *Women's Health* **4**: 93–101.

McMullin, J.M., Chavez, L.R. and Hubbell, F.A. (1996). Knowledge, power and experience: variation in physicians' perceptions of breast cancer risk factors. *Medical Anthropology* **16**: 295–317.

Mesters, I., van den Borne, H., McCormick, L., Pruyn, J., De Boer, M. and Imbos, T. (1997). Openness to discuss cancer in the nuclear family: scale, development, and validation. *Psychosomatic Medicine* **59**: 269–279.

Michie, S., McDonald, V. and Marteau, T. (1996). Understanding responses to predictive genetic testing: a grounded theory approach. *Psychology and Health* **11**: 455–470.

Moran, E. (1970). Clinical and social aspects of risk-taking. *Proceedings of the Royal Society of Medicine* **63**: 1273–1277.

Parsons, E. and Atkinson, P. (1992). Lay constructions of genetic risk. *Sociology of Health and Illness* **14**: 437–455.

Pearn, J.H. (1973). Patients' subjective interpretation of risks offered in genetic counselling. *Journal of Medical Genetics* **10**: 129–134.

Reagan, L.J. (1997). Engendering the dread disease: women, men, and cancer. *American Journal of Public Health* **87**: 1779–1787.

Richards, M. (1996a). Daily life and the new genetics: some personal stories. In T. Marteau and M. Richards (Eds), *The Troubled Helix: Social and Psychological Implications of the New Genetics* (pp. 3–59). Cambridge: Cambridge University Press.

Richards, M. (1996b). Families, kinship and genetics. In T. Marteau and M. Richards (Eds), *The Troubled Helix: Social and Psychological Implications of the New Human Genetics* (pp. 249–273). Cambridge: Cambridge University Press.

Richardson, J.L., Mondrus, G.T., Deapen, D. and Mack, T.M. (1994). Future challenges in secondary prevention of breast cancer for women at high risk. *Cancer* **74** (Suppl. 4): 1474–1481.

Rosser, E.M., Hurst, J.A. and Chapman, C.J. (1996). Cancer families: what risks are they given and do the risks affect management? *Journal of Medical Genetics* **33**: 977–980.

Royak-Schaler, R., Cheuvront, B., Wilson, K.R. and Williams, C.M. (1996). Addressing women's breast cancer risk and perceptions of control in medical settings. *Journal of Clinical Psychology in Medical Settings* **3**: 185–199.

Sarfati, D., Howden-Chapman, P., Woodward, A. and Salmond, C. (1998). Does the frame affect the picture? A study into how attitudes to screening for cancer are affected by the way benefits are expressed. *Journal of Medical Screening* **5**: 137–140.

Tversky, A. and Kahneman, D. (1982). Causal schemas in judgements under uncertainty. In D. Kahneman, P. Slovic and A. Tversky (Eds), *Judgement under Uncertainty: Heuristics and Biases* (pp. 117–128). Cambridge: Cambridge University Press.

Watson, M., Lloyd, S., Meyer, L., Eeles, R., Ebbs, S. and Murday, V. (1999). The impact of genetic counselling on risk perception and mental health in women with a family history of breast cancer. *British Journal of Cancer* **79**: 868–874.

Weinstein, N.D. (1982). Unrealistic optimism about susceptibility to health problems. *Journal of Behavioral Medicine* **5**: 441–460.

Weinstein, N.D. (1984). Why it won't happen to me: perceptions of risk factors and susceptibility. *Health Psychology* **3**: 431–457.

Weinstein, N.D. (1987). Unrealistic optimism about susceptibility to health problems: conclusions from a community-wide sample. *Journal of Behavioral Medicine* **10**: 481–500.

Weinstein, N.D. (1989). Optimistic biases about personal risks. *Science* **246**: 1232–1233.

Wellisch, D.K. and Hoffman, A. (1998). Daughters of breast cancer patients: genetic legacies and traumas. In Y. Danieli (Ed.), *International Handbook of Multigenerational Legacies of Human Trauma* (pp. 603–619). New York: Plenum.

21

Genetic Counseling for Cancer: A Family Issue

EVELINE M.A. BLEIKER and NEIL K. AARONSON

Department of Psychosocial Research and Epidemiology,
The Netherlands Cancer Institute, Amsterdam, The Netherlands

Over the past ten years, genes responsible for the familial occurrence of breast/ovarian cancer, colorectal cancer, and some less frequently occurring cancer syndromes have been identified. In particular, the cloning of two major breast cancer susceptibility genes (BRCA1 and BRCA2) has boosted public awareness of these novel developments. These findings have stimulated the use of genetic counseling programs for familial forms of cancer. The primary goal of genetic counseling for cancer susceptibility is to educate individuals about cancer risk and cancer prevention, which may eventually lead to a reduction in morbidity and mortality from cancer. At the same time, provision of risk information may also impact on the psychosocial health of the counseled individuals and their family members.

In this chapter, psychosocial issues in genetic counseling encountered by patients and their family members are reviewed. What becomes clear is that the psychosocial, behavioral, and practical implications of the genetic counseling reach beyond the individual counselee to the immediate and extended family. Additionally, a case study is presented which illustrates the type of psychosocial issues surrounding genetic counseling for cancer. Finally, recommendations are given for translating research findings into effective psychosocial services, and for directions for future research efforts.

GENETIC COUNSELING AND CANCER: WHERE ARE WE NOW?

It has long been suspected that the familial occurrence of certain types of cancer may be due to a familial predisposition (Claus et al., 1991). Well-known families in which familial clustering of cancer was observed included those of Napoleon Bonaparte, afflicted by gastric cancer (Ewing, 1922), and the wife of the French surgeon Broca, diagnosed with breast cancer. Broca (1866) published one of the first

Cancer and the Family, 2nd Edn. Edited by L. Baider, C. L. Cooper and A. Kaplan De-Nour

well-documented medical reports on a family pedigree as it relates to hereditary cancer.

However, it was not until recently that genes were identified and diagnostic tests became available that allow genetic testing for several types of cancer. Diagnostic tests are now available for familial cancer syndromes such as breast and/or ovarian cancer, colorectal cancer and some rare cancer syndromes, such as MEN2 (multiple endocrine neoplasia type 2) (Gardner et al., 1993), and Li–Fraumeni syndrome (characterized by a frequent occurrence of sarcoma, breast cancer, brain tumors, leukemia, or adrenocortical carcinoma in the family) (Malkin et al., 1990). These diagnostic tests can, in some families, indicate who is a carrier of a specific germ-line mutation. Germ-line mutations are associated with significantly increased risk of developing cancer, even up to 100% in some cancer syndromes. In this chapter we will focus on family issues in the most common hereditary cancer syndromes: hereditary breast and ovarian cancer (HBOC) and hereditary non-polyposis colorectal cancer (HNPCC).

HEREDITARY BREAST AND OVARIAN CANCER (HBOC)

During the past decade, two genes—BRCA1 and BRCA2—have been identified which, when exhibiting mutations, increase significantly the risk of developing breast and/or ovarian cancer (Wooster et al., 1995; Miki et al., 1994). The existence of other dominantly inherited predisposing genes has been suggested. Between 5% and 10% of breast and ovarian cancers are thought to be attributable to the inheritance of a gene conferring a high risk (King et al., 1993). Women with a BRCA1/2 mutation are estimated to have a strong increased risk of developing cancer before the age of 70 years. These estimates vary from 56% to 85% for breast cancer, and 16% to 60% for ovarian cancer, depending on the population studied (Easton et al., 1995; Struewing et al., 1997). In contrast to sporadic breast cancer, hereditary breast cancer is characterized by an early age of onset and an increased incidence of bilateral breast cancer (Verhoog et al., 1998).

Current preventive health recommendations for female carriers of BRCA1/2 mutations include: yearly mammography, semi-annual physical examinations, monthly breast self-examination, or preventive mastectomy (with or without a breast reconstruction) (van Geel et al., 1997). Women at risk of developing ovarian cancer can choose between yearly screening of the ovaries, and prophylactic oophorectomy. Preventive surgery is expected to reduce the risk of developing cancer at that specific site (van Geel et al., 1997; Schrag et al., 1997), but a small risk of developing cancer near that specific site still exists.

COLORECTAL CANCER

In Western and industrialized countries, colorectal cancer (CRC) continues to be one of the major forms of neoplastic morbidity and mortality (Allum et al., 1994). It is estimated that approximately 5% of all CRC cases represent one well-delineated genetic syndrome: hereditary non-polyposis colorectal cancer (HNPCC, or Lynch syndrome) (Lynch and Lynch,1996). This condition, like BRCA1 and BRCA2, has an autosomal dominant pattern of inheritance. Children of carriers have a 50%

likelihood of inheriting the deleterious gene. Furthermore, it is characterized by early onset (age 44 years), as compared with sporadic colorectal cancer (Lynch et al., 1993). Until recently, the basic genetic defect of HNPCC was unknown. In 1993 and 1994, genes associated with HNPCC were identified, rendering possible pre-symptomatic DNA-based diagnosis (Bronner et al., 1994; Papadopoulos et al., 1994; Fishel et al., 1994; Leach et al., 1993). The lifetime risk of CRC is approximately 80% in gene carriers (Vasen et al., 1996). Additionally, the increased lifetime risk for endometrial cancer in female HNPCC mutation carriers may be as high as 42% (Dunlop et al., 1997). Individuals at risk for HNPCC are now being referred for genetic counseling and genetic testing (Heouaine et al., 1996).

Mutations in mismatch repair genes are responsible for HNPCC. The underlying mutation can be detected in approximately 50% of HNPCC families (Holtzman, 1996; Nystrom-Lahti et al., 1995). In the remaining 50% of families, DNA studies are 'non-informative', i.e., the causative mutation cannot be detected with current diagnostic methods. These latter families, with an inconclusive DNA test result, receive a risk estimate and a screening advice based on the family data.

HNPCC mutation carriers are advised to undergo either colonoscopy or sigmoidoscopy every 2–3 years. Individuals with a strong family history who receive an inconclusive genetic test result are advised to undergo colon screening every 3–5 years (Vasen, 1996; Vasen et al., 1996).

WHO ATTENDS A FAMILY CANCER CLINIC?

The majority of clinic attendees are currently women seeking counseling for the familial occurrence of breast/ovarian cancer (Bleiker et al., 1999; Richards et al., 1995). Some counselees come alone. Others are accompanied by their sister(s), brother(s), partner, parents, children, or other family members. A recent study conducted at the family cancer clinic of The Netherlands Cancer Institute showed that half of the counselees who visited the clinic during May 1995 and June 1996 had been treated for cancer in the past (Bleiker et al., submitted). The average age of the clinic attendees was 45 years (SD = 12). In the majority of cases, individuals were referred by their medical specialist. Approximately 20% were self-referred, some-times triggered by a television program or an article in the popular press. Only a few (2%) were referred by their general practitioner. In a study by Richards et al. (1995), it was found that, in many cases, clinic visits were prompted by the diagnosis of cancer or death of a close relative from cancer, or because the counselee was approaching the age at which a relative (most often the mother) developed the disease.

The most important reasons for which individuals seek genetic counseling and testing for cancer is to obtain a greater degree of certainty about personal risk, to be able to take preventive actions and to estimate the risk of cancer for their children (Bleiker et al., 1997). Other reasons include marriage and family planning, to 'take better care of oneself', and to contribute to research (Lerman et al., 1995; Kash, 1995). Studies conducted to date (primarily among women at risk of breast and/or ovarian cancer), suggest that those who seek genetic counseling often overestimate their risk of developing cancer (Kash et al., 1995; Gagnon et al., 1996; Evans et al., 1993; Lerman et al., 1994b). A number of studies have reported that those women with a familial risk of breast cancer who seek genetic counseling often exhibit heightened levels of psychological distress and cancer-related worry as compared to women at normal risk (Lloyd and Watson, 1996; Gagnon et al., 1996; Lerman et al., 1994a; Valdimarsdottir et al., 1995). In contrast, in a recent study, a curvilinear relationship was found between cancer-specific distress and the decision to undergo genetic testing: women with moderate levels of cancer-specific distress were more likely to undergo genetic testing than women with either high or low levels of such distress (Valdimarsdottir et al., 1999).

THE PROCEDURE OF GENETIC COUNSELING: A FAMILY ISSUE

The primary goal of genetic counseling for cancer susceptibility is to educate individuals about cancer risk and cancer prevention, which may eventually lead to a reduction in morbidity and mortality from cancer. Individuals who request genetic counseling for themselves are typically asked to provide detailed information about cancer in first-, second-, and third-degree relatives: who had cancer, what type of cancer, and when was it diagnosed? In some cases, permission is requested to verify this information by contacting the hospitals where family members were treated for cancer. Sometimes informed consent from primary relatives is needed for verification via tumor material or blood samples of deceased family members. In some families, the cooperation of family members with cancer is preferred, because blood (i.e., DNA) from affected individuals may be more informative (i.e., the likelihood of identifying a mutation in affected family members is increased). Therefore, in most cases where individuals seek individual counseling, involvement of family members is highly desirable. For the counselee who has to contact family members and inform them about the aim of the genetic counseling, obtaining this information is not always an easy task. Not infrequently, counselees describe family communication as limited, either because there are long-standing conflicts between family members, or because they have lost contact with more distant branches of the family following the death of a family member (Richards et al., 1995). This may lead some individuals to withdraw from the genetic counseling process, due to concerns about the additional family stresses that it may cause.

After obtaining all necessary information from the family, a range of issues is typically discussed during the genetic counseling, including the family history of cancer, possibility of DNA testing, motivation for undergoing and potential benefits and limitations of such testing, and possible consequences of counseling and testing for the counselee and his/her family members. If possible, DNA testing is offered. In an American study among members of HBOC families, 58% requested their BRCA1 test results, whereas 42% preferred not to be informed of their genetic status (Lerman et al., 1997). Cancer-specific distress was significantly and positively related to requests for test results. In a small study in the UK, the uptake of BRCA1 testing in high-risk families was 41% (Watson et al., 1996). It should be noted that both of these studies included special research cohorts, which may not be representative of the larger population that presents for genetic counseling.

The analysis and reporting of DNA results takes between 2–6 months, depending on the facilities available and whether a mutation has already been identified in a family. At the time of disclosure of the test results, the possible psychosocial impact on the counselee and his/her family is discussed and screening and prophylactic treatment options are considered (Wigbout, 1997; Bleiker et al., 1997). Studies indicate that 17–45% of women with an increased risk of developing breast/ovarian cancer *consider* undergoing prophylactic mastectomy, and 33–76% prophylactic oophorectomy (Hallowell, 1998; Lynch et al., 1997; Lerman et al., 1996). However, there are as yet no accurate estimates available on the percentage of women who actually opt for preventive surgery.

At the family cancer clinic of The Netherlands Cancer Institute our experience is that it is preferable to counsel family members separately. This holds particularly for the release of the genetic test results (Wigbout, 1997). This separation of family members is important, so that every individual is taken seriously and personal doubts and questions can be discussed freely, without the possible pressure or strong opinions of other family members.

THE PSYCHOSOCIAL IMPACT OF GENETIC COUNSELING

The provision of genetic risk information may impact on the psychosocial health of the counseled individual (Botkin et al., 1996). Psychosocial health includes such issues as psychological distress, family functioning, feelings of worry and guilt related to cancer risk assessment, and practical problems associated with health and life insurance, work, and family planning.

GENERAL AND SPECIFIC PSYCHOLOGICAL DISTRESS

In a retrospective study of women with a family history of breast cancer who attended genetic counseling, levels of generalized psychological distress (as measured by the Brief Symptom Inventory) were found to be similar to those of age-matched controls without a family history of breast cancer. However, breast cancer-specific distress (as assessed by the Impact of Events Scale (IES)) was significantly higher among the former group (Lloyd and Watson, 1996). Comparable results were obtained in a prospective study on the psychological impact of genetic testing for BRCA1 (Croyle et al., 1997). It was reported that gene mutation carriers manifested significantly higher levels of genetic test-related psychological distress (IES), as compared with non-carriers. The highest levels of test-related distress were observed among mutation carriers without a history of cancer or cancer-related surgery. Generalized distress (state anxiety as measured by the Spielberger State–Trait Anxiety Inventory) declined after DNA testing (Croyle et al., 1997). Importantly, heightened levels of psychological distress have also been observed among individuals who have been informed that they are not carriers of a gene mutation (Huggins et al., 1992; Hayden, 1991), and those who withdraw from DNA testing or receive equivocal results (Lerman et al., 1998; Wiggins et al., 1992).

FAMILY INVOLVEMENT

Illness of any kind may cause changes in relationships within families. However, genetically-linked health conditions, because of their hereditary nature, may have specific and far-reaching consequences for family dynamics and relationships. Drawing a family tree (i.e., establishing the pedigree) is a standard, early step in the process of genetic counseling. The process of generating the pedigree can have profound effects on family relationships, quite independently of the genetic risk profiles that may follow (Richards, 1996). Usually, clinic attendees are forewarned that they will need to provide health-related information about their relatives. This may require their re-establishing contact with 'lost' relatives, or it may revive memories of severed relationships and family rifts. Individuals may become upset as they recount details of the illness and death of their relatives. Not uncommonly, relatives will have to be approached to provide relevant health-related information. This is an important and often difficult task for the initial clinic attendee. The role of 'messenger' informing relatives of the hereditary character of cancer in the family can be a very stressful one (Dudok de Wit et al., 1997).

Even before a family tree is drawn, other psychological processes may be set in motion as a result of concern about the risk of hereditary illness. The best known of these had been termed *preselection* (Kessler and Bloch, 1989; Kessler, 1988). This is a family process whereby a family member is singled out, *a priori*, as the one most likely to develop the disease in question. In studies of families with Huntington's disease (Tibben et al., 1990; Bloch et al., 1989; Kessler, 1988) and families with MEN-2A (Grosfeld et al., 1996), it was found that some families had very explicit ideas about who would and who would not be a carrier. If a preselected individual is tested and found not to carry the gene mutation, there are likely to be significant family repercussions. It is our experience that similar family dynamics are also present in some hereditary breast and ovarian cancer families.

FEELINGS OF WORRY AND GUILT

In a study by Lerman et al. (1994b), one-third of the women at increased risk for developing breast cancer reported having worries and concerns of a sufficient magnitude to impair their daily functioning. In a study by Kash et al. (1995), feelings of guilt were found to be pervasive among women at high risk of developing breast cancer. In some cases, this guilt was related to feelings of inadequacy in helping other relatives who had had cancer. Other women felt guilty because they may have passed a gene on to their offspring. Many women felt guilty about their 'preoccupation' with the possibility of developing breast cancer in the future, given that they were currently healthy. In some cases, women experienced so-called 'survivor guilt', i.e., feelings of guilt that they had not (yet) developed breast cancer, while other relatives had. Similar findings were reported in a study of relatives of ovarian cancer patients (Lerman et al., 1994a): 25% of the women indicated that they would feel guilty if they were to test negative for a hereditary breast–ovarian cancer susceptibility gene. In a particularly striking case, we observed a male carrier of a BRCA1 gene who had passed the gene on to his two daughters. One daughter developed breast cancer at an early age, and the other underwent preventive mastectomy. The healthy father felt that he was responsible for this misfortune in his daughters and reported intense feelings of guilt and depression.

PRACTICAL IMPLICATIONS

Genetic counseling may have significant consequences in the areas of insurance, work, and family planning (Bassford and Hauck, 1993). Most concerns about discrimination against carriers of genetic conditions revolve around insurance coverage (Marteau and Anionwu, 1996). A common concern is that genetic counseling may be made mandatory for some insurance schemes (Billings et al., 1992), and that this may result in limited coverage or outright denial of insurance. A small US survey of individuals who had undergone DNA testing for a range of genetic conditions has provided some evidence of such discriminatory practices, including denial of health insurance, exclusion from company plans, and denial of life insurance (Natowicz et al., 1992). To our knowledge, such discriminatory practices have not yet been documented in other countries, but may be expected in the future.

With regard to work discrimination, Billings and his colleagues (1992) have reported a range of problems experienced by individuals with a variety of genetic health conditions, including difficulty in obtaining employment, early termination, being passed over for promotion, and mandatory job transfer. Finally, in the area of family planning, Kash and her colleagues (1995) have reported that many women counseled in a familial cancer clinic in New York, who had been found to be at increased risk of developing breast cancer, postponed marriage and/or decided not to have children. These women reported that they felt certain that they would eventually develop breast cancer, and would die of their disease, and thus chose to avoid the long-term commitments associated with marriage and child-bearing.

A CASE STUDY

The complex family dynamics that individuals may encounter when undergoing genetic counseling for cancer can perhaps best be illustrated with a case study. The experiences of Miss A and her family shed light on the procedure of genetic counseling, the possible dilemmas encountered in the counseling process, and the decisions that need to be made.

Miss A (see pedigree, Figure 21.1, III: 4) attended the family cancer clinic for genetic counseling for breast cancer. She is a 39 year-old healthy woman. Her sister (III: 3), aged 43, was diagnosed with breast cancer at the age of 40. This sister had breast-conserving surgery with adjuvant radiotherapy. The mother of Miss A had died of breast cancer when Miss A was 16 years of age. The experience of the mother's disease and death had had a great impact on the lives of Miss A and her sister, who were adolescents at that time. In addition, an aunt (mother's sister, II: 1) had died of breast cancer at the relatively young age of 45 years. Grandmother (I: 2) had died at the age of 55, possibly of breast cancer (unconfirmed).

Because of the frequent occurrence of breast cancer in the family, Miss A had undergone periodic breast screening since the age of 35. At the last breast screening, her doctor had recommended that Miss A and her sister undergo genetic counseling. After some hesitation ['Do I really want to know whether I have a high risk of developing (a recurrence of) breast cancer?'], Miss A and her sister decided to undergo counseling. At the clinic, a genetic nurse explained the genetic counseling process (see Bleiker et al., 1997) and completed the family pedigree (Figure 21.1). Subsequently, a first meeting was held with the clinical geneticist (a physician) who explained in detail the possibilities and limitations of DNA testing.

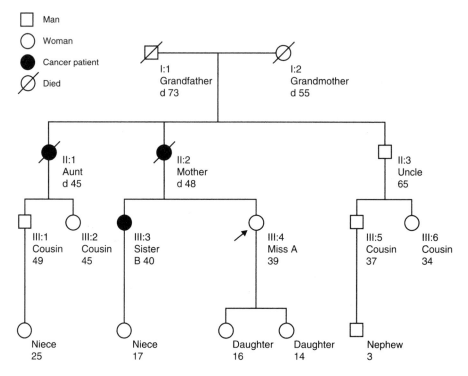

Figure 21.1 Pedigree (or genogram) of the family of Miss A

Miss A and her sister decided to undergo DNA testing, and provided a blood sample. Since tumor material of the deceased mother could be of help in determining the genetic risk, Miss A's father was asked to give his consent to analyze his deceased wife's body tissue, which had been preserved at the hospital after her surgery. Although this was somewhat confusing and distressing for the father, who was now aged 72, he eventually agreed. The results of the DNA testing of family A were available about 6 months later. Miss A and her partner, and Miss A's sister and her partner, were seen separately by the clinical geneticist.

A BRCA1 mutation was found in the family of Miss A. Miss A was found not to be a carrier of this mutation and thus she could discontinue breast screening until the age of 50, at which time she would be invited to participate in the population-based breast cancer screening in The Netherlands. Miss A expressed relief for herself, but more importantly for her two daughters. At the same time, Miss A was very concerned for her sister, who was found to be a carrier of a BRCA1 mutation (the same mutation was found in the tissue of her mother). Her sister was neither shocked nor terribly upset. She had expected this result because she had already been treated for breast cancer. Nevertheless she was concerned, especially for her daughter of 17 years, who had a 50% chance of being a carrier of this BRCA1 mutation. Should she be tested? At what age? What should she be told? What would be the consequences for her if she were to be found to be a carrier? Would her health insurance premium be raised? Would she have difficulty finding employment? What is the best policy regarding the use of oral contraceptives? Miss A's sister also became concerned about whether her breast-conserving treatment had been sufficient, as well as about the most appropriate preventive action for her remaining breast (screening or preventive mastectomy). She was informed that she also had an increased risk of developing ovarian cancer—something she did not expect, since there was no ovarian cancer in her family. Should she go for periodic screening of the ovaries, which is not completely reliable, or should she opt for preventive oophorectomy? Miss A's sister discussed her concerns with a psychosocial worker who helped her to put the pros and the cons of the various options in perspective. She also discussed the possibilities and limitations of a surgical intervention with a surgeon.

Miss A and her sister were also aware (see Figure 21.1) that their aunt (II: 1) and uncle (II: 3) might be carriers of the same BRCA1 mutation. Since their mother had died, the contact with their uncle (II: 3) had been infrequent. However, if he was a carrier, the uncle's daughter (III: 6) could also be at increased risk. Should Miss A contact her uncle and her cousin? She would have to convey bad news to someone she had not been in contact with for years. What about their right 'not to know?'. Even more difficult was the relationship with the family of the older sister of their mother (II: 1). This aunt (II: 1) had died many years earlier, and her partner had subsequently remarried. Due to family conflicts, contact with this branch of the family had broken down many years ago. Should Miss A make contact with this part of her family? On the one hand, she felt a moral obligation to tell them about the breast cancer mutation in the family, and the possible increased risk of breast cancer for her cousin and niece. On the other hand, Miss A was hesitant to contact them, expecting an escalation of the family conflict. Finally, Miss A decided not to contact this branch of the family, although she did not feel perfectly comfortable with this decision.

This case illustrates the complex family dynamics and decision-making process involved in genetic counseling for cancer. For every family member, the benefits and limitations of genetic counseling should be considered before further steps are taken. Professional psychosocial support can be of real help for these families, especially since their natural support system is typically composed of close family members, each of whom may have his/her own anxieties and worries.

IMPLICATIONS FOR PSYCHOSOCIAL SERVICES

As illustrated above, genetic counseling for cancer is a family issue. It is important that, during the initial session at the family cancer clinic, the possible impact of the genetic counseling for the counselee, and also for his/her relatives, is discussed. Additionally, consideration needs to be given to the provision of professional psychosocial support as well as standard genetic counseling. This raises the important question of which individuals are at increased risk for psychosocial problems as a result of genetic counseling, and what types of support should be available?

Support services should be provided for counselees who have problems in communicating with their family members. Recognition and support of the counselee who is the 'messenger' and who is the 'first utilizer' of predictive testing in the family is important, especially when the counselee has the feeling that he/she has to provide a good example for the rest of the family (Dudok de Wit et al., 1997).

From earlier studies of patients with (breast) cancer, we have learned that those individuals who have experienced high levels of psychological distress before the diagnosis are at risk of poor adjustment to their disease and treatment (Bleiker et al., in press; Tjemsland et al., 1998). This has also been reported for couples: early difficulties and distress in couples facing breast cancer predicted later problems (Northouse et al., 1998). Similarly, distress or depressive symptoms experienced before genetic counseling and testing is predictive of levels of distress during and after the counseling process (Bleiker et al., 1999; DudokdeWit et al., 1998).

Results of a study of the daughters of breast cancer patients suggest that the experience of cancer within the family, especially during adolescence (11–20 years), may have a significant impact on levels of cancer-related distress (Wellisch et al., 1992). At greatest risk for distress were the adolescent daughters of mothers with a poor prognosis or mothers who died of breast cancer.

Another vulnerable group is formed by those counselees who have recently lost a close relative to cancer. In fact, it may be appropriate to delay the genetic counseling in order to provide time to cope with the loss and grief. The recent occurrence of metastases in a relative with cancer may result in identification with the patient and increased death-anxiety among identified gene carriers and individuals at high risk. This may lead to the wish to hasten the predictive testing procedure (Dudok de Wit et al., 1994). For these counselees it is important to allow sufficient time for an informed decision to be made with regard to genetic testing and/or preventive actions.

First results of a study conducted at The Netherlands Cancer Institute indicated that the *perceived need* for psychosocial support does not depend on the genetic test results: a similar percentage of the counselees with a positive test, a negative test, and a non-informative test result reported the need for additional psychosocial support (Bleiker, submitted). In line with this result, Dudok de Wit et al. (1998) reported that the genetic test result, as such, did not determine the degree of distress experienced after testing.

In contrast, levels of depressive symptoms and cancer-related distress have been reported to decrease after testing for non-carriers, and to remain stable in carriers. Higher levels of test-related distress have been observed in the subgroup of carriers without a personal history of cancer. Therefore, special attention might be given to healthy individuals who are found to be carriers (pre-symptomatic testing) (Croyle et al., 1997).

However, psychosocial support should be available not only for those who are found to be carriers of a mutation, but also for the non-carriers. They can harbor feelings of guilt for not being a carrier (when their loved ones are). Feelings of confusion are often reported: relief for themselves, and especially for their own children, but concern and worry about the persistent increased risk among their close family members.

Attention should also be paid to those counselees who come for genetic testing but who later decline to receive the test results. These individuals may be at increased risk for depression (Lerman et al., 1998).

Finally, attention should be paid to those families in which clear expectations exist about (non)carriership. Grosfeld et al. (1996) found that, if the test outcome differs from what is anticipated, families have more difficulty adapting. Such expectations are often based on perceived similarities, either with regard to physical appearance or personality, with affected individuals; factors which in reality have no bearing on an individual's chance of being a carrier (Davison, 1996).

DIRECTIONS FOR FUTURE RESEARCH

While a number of studies have been performed on the psychosocial impact of genetic testing in cancer, there is still a paucity of information about the impact of such testing on family functioning. A contributing factor to this state of affairs may be that 'family functioning' is difficult to assess. To our knowledge, no valid and reliable questionnaires are available that assess the impact on family relationships of an event such as cancer. Extant questionnaires focus on the nuclear family (father, mother and children), and do not cover the relationships of adults with their siblings, aunts, uncles, cousins, or grandchildren. Furthermore, because families differ widely in their size, composition, and dynamics, it is difficult to employ standardized questionnaires. The use of semi-structured interviews may be a more appropriate means of data collection in this research setting.

An important topic of investigation in genetic counseling for cancer is the various roles adopted by family members (Dudok de Wit et al., 1997). In addition, future studies should take into account the developmental stage of a family (Northouse, 1994). It is likely that the psychosocial impact of genetic counseling and testing may vary significantly between families without children, families with school-aged vs. adult children, etc. (Gualthérie van Weezel, 1995).

As described in this chapter, the experience of cancer within the family, especially during adolescence (11–20 years), may have a significant impact on the levels of cancer-related distress later in life (Wellisch et al., 1992). Similarly, previous experiences with cancer in the family (i.e., age at which a close relative developed cancer, involvement in the treatment, and whether or not this relative survived/died) may have a significant impact on the way in which the genetic counseling process is experienced.

Future studies should preferably use a prospective, longitudinal design with assessments before, as well as at several time points during and after, the counseling and testing. Additionally, we know little about the impact of genetic counseling and testing in the long term (several years after disclosure of genetic test results). Therefore, studies with a long-term follow-up are needed.

To assess distress in family members with hereditary cancer syndromes, we recommend using specific questionnaires, such as the IES (Horowitz et al., 1979), or the Cancer Worries Scale of Lerman et al. (1994a). While more general distress measures, such as the State–Trait Anxiety Inventory (Spielberger, 1983) and the Center for Epidemiologic Studies–Depression Scale (Bouma et al., 1995), may provide an accurate estimate of the prevalence of non-specific anxiety and depression, prior research suggests that the levels of these more generalized forms of distress are not typically affected by genetic counseling and testing.

Little is known about the psychosocial consequences of receiving inconclusive DNA test results. This represents a relatively large and potentially vulnerable segment of the counseled population worthy of additional study.

Risk perception, cancer worries, screening behavior, and the impact of genetic counseling on family relationships may vary as a function of culture. Cross-cultural studies in this field would be welcomed.

Finally, there is a need for developing and rigorously testing (psychosocial) counseling models in which family systems and dynamics play a central role. Preferably, this should take the form of randomized controlled studies whose central goal is to identify the most effective form of counseling for both the individual and the family unit.

REFERENCES

Allum, W.H., Slaney, G., McConkey, C.C. and Powell, J. (1994). Cancer of the colon and rectum in the West Midlands, 1957–1981. *British Journal of Surgery* **81**: 1060–1063.

Bassford, T.L. and Hauck, L. (1993). Human genome project and cancer: the ethical implications for clinical practice. *Seminars in Oncology Nursing* **9**: 134–138.

Billings, P.R., Kohn, M.A., de Cuevas, M., Beckwith, J., Alper, J.S. and Natowicz, M.R. (1992). Discrimination as a consequence of genetic testing. *American Journal of Human Genetics* **50**: 476–482.

Bleiker, E.M.A., Aaronson, N.K., Menko, F.H., Hahn, D.E., van Asperen, C.J., Rutgers, E.J., et al. (1997). Genetic counseling for hereditary cancer: a pilot study on experiences of patients and family members. *Patient Education and Counseling* **32**: 107–116.

Bleiker, E.M.A., Aaronson, N.K., Menko, F.H. et al. Health-related quality of life prior to and following genetic counseling for cancer (submitted).

Bleiker, E.M.A., Pouwer, F., van der Ploeg, H.M., Leer, J.-W.H. and Ader, H.J. (in press). Psychological distress two years after diagnosis of breast cancer: frequency and prediction. *Patient Education and Counseling*.

Bloch, M., Fahy, M., Fox, S. and Hayden, M.R. (1989). Predictive testing for Huntington disease: II. Demographic characteristics, life-style patterns, attitudes, and psychosocial assessments of the first fifty-one test candidates. *American Journal of Medical Genetics* **32**: 217–224.

Botkin, J.R., Croyle, R.T., Smith, K.R., Baty, B.J., Lerman, C., Goldgar, D.E. et al. (1996). A model protocol for evaluating the behavioral and psychosocial effects of BRCA1 testing. *Journal of the National Cancer Institute* **88**: 872–882.

Bouma, J., Ranchor, A.V., Sanderman, R. and van Sonderen, E. (1995). Het meten van symptomen van depressie met de CES-D. Een handleiding. Noordelijk Centrum voor gezonheidsvraagstukken, Rijksuniversiteit Groningen.

Broca, P. (1866). *Traite de tumeurs*. Paris: Asselin.

Bronner, C.E., Baker, S.M., Morrison, P.T., Warren, G., Smith, L.G., Lescoe, M.K. et al. (1994). Mutation in the DNA mismatch repair gene homologue hMLH1 is associated with hereditary non-polyposis colon cancer. *Nature* **368**: 258–261.

Claus, E.B., Risch, N. and Thompson, W.D. (1991). Genetic analysis of breast cancer in the cancer and steroid hormone study. *American Journal of Human Genetics* **48**: 232–242.

Croyle, R.T., Smith, K.R., Botkin, J.R., Baty, B. and Nash, J. (1997). Psychological responses to brca1 mutation testing: preliminary findings. *Health Psychology* **16**: 63–72.

Davison, C. (1996). Predicitive genetics: the cultural implications of supplying probable futures. In T. Marteau and M. Richards (Eds), *The Troubled Helix. Social and Psychological Implications of the New Human Genetics*. Cambridge: Cambridge University Press.

Dudok de Wit, C., Meijers-Heijboer, E.J., Tibben, A., Frets, P.G., Klijn, J.G.M., Devilee, P. et al. (1994). Effect on a Dutch family of predictive DNA-testing for hereditary breast and ovarian cancer. *Lancet* **344**: 197.

Dudok de Wit, A.C., Tibben, A., Duivenvoorden, H.J., Niermeijer, M.F. and Passchier, J. (1998). Predicting adaptation to presymptomatic DNA testing for late onset disorders:

who will experience distress? Rotterdam Leiden Genetics Workgroup. *Journal of Medical Genetics* **35**: 745–754.

Dudok de Wit, A.C., Tibben, A., Frets, P.G., Meijers-Heijboer, E.J., Devilee, P., Klijn, J.G. et al. (1997). BRCA1 in the family: a case description of the psychological implications. *American Journal of Medical Genetics* **71**: 63–71.

Dunlop, M.G., Farrington, S.M., Carothers, A.D., Wyllie, A.H., Sharp, L., Burn, J. et al. (1997). Cancer risk associated with germline DNA mismatch repair gene mutations. *Human Molecular Genetics* **6**: 105–110.

Easton, D.F., Ford, D. and Bishop, D.T. (1995). Breast and ovarian cancer incidence in BRCA1-mutation carriers. Breast Cancer Linkage Consortium. *American Journal of Human Genetics* **56**: 265–271.

Evans, D.G., Burnell, L.D., Hopwood, P. and Howell, A. (1993). Perception of risk in women with a family history of breast cancer. *British Journal of Cancer* **67**: 612–614.

Ewing, J. (1922). *Neoplastic Diseases: A Treatise on Tumors*. Philadelphia, PA: Saunders.

Fishel, R., Lescoe, M.K., Rao, M.R., Copeland, N.G., Jenkins, N.A., Garber, J. et al. (1994). The human mutator gene homolog MSH2 and its association with hereditary non-polyposis colon cancer. *Cell* **77**: 167.

Gagnon, P., Massie, M.J., Kash, K.M., Gronert, M., Heerdt, A.S., Brown, K. et al. (1996). Perception of breast cancer risk and psychological distress in women attending a surveillance program. *Psycho-Oncology* **5**: 259–269.

Gardner, E., Papi, L., Easton, D.F., Cummings, T., Jackson, C.E., Kaplan, M. et al. (1993). Genetic linkage studies map the multiple endocrine neoplasia type 2 loci to a small interval on chromosome 10q11.2. *Human Molecular Genetics* **2**: 241–246.

Grosfeld, F.J., Lips, C.J., Ten Kroode, H.F., Beemer, F.A., Van Spijker, H.G. and Brouwers-Smalbraak, G.J. (1996). Psychosocial consequences of dna analysis for men type 2. *Oncology (Huntington)* **10**: 141–146.

Gualthérie van Weezel, L.M. (1995). Leven in de verlenging; kanker in het gezin. *Systeemtherapie* **7**: 23–33.

Hallowell, N. (1998). 'You don't want to lose your ovaries because you think "I might become a man".' Women's perceptions of prophylactic surgery as a cancer risk management option. *Psycho-Oncology* **7**: 263–275.

Hayden, M.R. (1991). Predictive testing for Huntington disease: are we ready for widespread community implementation? [Editorial]. *American Journal of Medical Genetics* **40**: 515–517.

Heouaine, A., Mareni, C., Varesco, L., Genuardi, M. and Neri, G. (1996). Genetic counseling in hereditary non-polyposis colorectal cancer. *Tumori* **82**: 136–142.

Holtzman, N.A. (1996) Are we ready to screen for inherited susceptibility to cancer? *Oncology (Huntington)* **10**: 57–64.

Horowitz, M., Wilner, N. and Alvarez, W. (1979). Impact of Event Scale: a measure of subjective stress. *Psychosomatic Medicine* **41**: 209–218.

Huggins, M., Bloch, M., Wiggins, S., Adam, S., Suchowersky, O., Trew, M. et al. (1992). Predictive testing for huntington's disease in Canada: adverse effects and unexpected results in those receiving a decreased risk. *American Journal of Medical Genetics* **42**: 508–515.

Kash, K.M. (1995). Psychosocial and ethical implications of defining genetic risk for cancers. *Annals of the New York Academy of Science* **768**: 41–52.

Kash, K.M., Holland, J.C., Osborne, M.P. and Miller, D.G. (1995). Psychological counseling strategies for women at risk of breast cancer. *Monographs of the National Cancer Institute* **17**: 73–79.

Kessler, S. (1988). Invited essay on the psychological aspects of genetic counseling. V. Preselection: a family coping strategy in Huntington's disease. *American Journal of Medical Genetics* **31**: 617–621.

Kessler, S. and Bloch, M. (1989). Social system responses to Huntington's disease. *Family Processes* **28**: 59–68.

King, M., Rowell, S. and Love, S.M. (1993). Inherited breast and ovarian cancer: what are the risks? What are the choices? *Psycho-Oncology* **5**: 33–38.

Leach, F.S., Nicolaides, N.C., Papadopoulos, N., Liu, B., Jen, J., Parsons, R. et al. (1993). Mutations of a mutS homolog in hereditary non-polyposis colorectal cancer. *Cell* **75**: 1215–1225.

Lerman, C., Daly, M., Masny, A. and Balshem, A. (1994a). Attitudes about genetic testing for breast–ovarian cancer susceptibility. *Journal of Clinical Oncology* **12**: 843–850.

Lerman, C., Kash, K. and Stefanek, M. (1994b). Younger women at increased risk for breast cancer: perceived risk, psychological well-being, and surveillance behavior. *Monographs of the National Cancer Institute* **16**: 171–176.

Lerman, C., Hughes, C., Lemon, S.J., Main, D., Snyder, C., Durham, C. et al. (1998). What you don't know can hurt you: adverse psychologic effects in members of BRCA1-linked and BRCA2-linked families who decline genetic testing. *Journal of Clinical Oncology* **16**: 1650–1654.

Lerman, C., Narod, S., Schulman, K., Hughes, C., Gomez-Caminero, A., Bonney, G. et al. (1996). BRCA1 testing in families with hereditary breast–ovarian cancer: a prospective study of patient decision making and outcomes. *Journal of the American Medical Association* **275**: 1885–1892.

Lerman, C., Schwartz, M.D., Lin, T.H., Hughes, C., Narod, S. and Lynch, H.T. (1997). The influence of psychological distress on use of genetic testing for cancer risk. *Journal of Consulting and Clinical Psychology* **65**: 414–420.

Lerman, C., Seay, J., Balshem, A. and Audrain, J. (1995). Interest in genetic testing among first-degree relatives of breast cancer patients. *American Journal of Medical Genetics* **57**: 385–392.

Lloyd, S. and Watson, M. (1996). Risk perception, mental health and health behaviours in women with a family history of breast cancer presenting for genetic counselling. (Abstract). *Psycho-Oncology* **5**: 355–356.

Lynch, H.T., Lemon, S.J., Durham, C., Tinley, S.T., Lynch, J.F., Surdam, J. et al. (1997). A descriptive study of BRCA1 testing and reactions to disclosure of test results. *Cancer* **79**: 2219–2228.

Lynch, H.T. and Lynch, J. (1996). Genetic counseling for hereditary cancer. *Oncology (Huntington)* **10**: 27–34.

Lynch, H.T., Smyrk, T.C., Watson, P., Lanspa, S.J., Lynch, J.F., Lynch, P.M. et al. (1993). Genetics, natural history, tumor spectrum, and pathology of hereditary non-polyposis colorectal cancer: an updated review. *Gastroenterology* **104**: 1535–1549.

Malkin, D., Li, F.P., Strong, L.C., Fraumeni, J.F. Jr, Nelson, C.E., Kim, D.H. et al. (1990). Germ line p53 mutations in a familial syndrome of breast cancer, sarcomas, and other neoplasms. *Science* **250**: 1233–1238.

Marteau, T.M., Anionwu, W. (1996). Evaluating carrier testing: objectives and outcomes. In T. Marteau and M. Richards (Eds), *The Troubled Helix. Social and Psychological Implications of the New Human Genetics*. Cambridge: Cambridge University Press.

Miki, Y., Swensen, J., Shattuck-Eidens, D., Futreal, P.A., Harshman, K., Tavtigian, S. et al. (1994). A strong candidate for the breast and ovarian cancer susceptibility gene BRCA1. *Science* **266**: 66–71.

Natowicz, M.R., Alper, J.K. and Alper, J.S. (1992). Genetic discrimination and the law. *American Journal of Human Genetics* **50**: 465–475.

Northouse, L.L. (1994). Breast cancer in younger women: effects on interpersonal and family relations. *Monographs of the National Cancer Institute* **16**: 183–190.

Northouse, L.L., Templin, T., Mood, D. and Oberst, M. (1998). Couples' adjustment to breast cancer and benign breast disease: a longitudinal analysis. *Psycho-Oncology* **7**: 37–48.

Nystrom-Lahti, M., Kristo, P., Nicolaides, N.C., Chang, S.Y., Aaltonen, L.A., Moisio, A.L. et al. (1995). Founding mutations and alu-mediated recombination in hereditary colon cancer. *Nature Medicine* **1**: 1203–1206.

Papadopoulos, N., Nicolaides, N.C., Wei, Y.F., Ruben, S.M., Carter, K.C., Rosen, C.A. et al. (1994). Mutation of a mutL homolog in hereditary colon cancer. *Science* **263**: 1625–1629.

Richards, M. (1996). Families, kinship and genetics. In T. Marteau and M. Richards (Eds), *The Troubled Helix. Social and Psychological Implications of the New Human Genetics* Cambridge: Cambridge University Press.

Richards, M.P.M., Hallowell, N., Green, J.M., Murton, F. and Statham, H. (1995). Counseling families with hereditary breast and ovarian cancer: a psychosocial perspective. *Journal of Genetic Counseling* **4**: 219–233.

Schrag, D., Kuntz, K.M., Garber, J.E. and Weeks, J.C. (1997). Decision analysis—effects of prophylactic mastectomy and oophorectomy on life expectancy among women with BRCA1 or BRCA2 mutations. *New England Journal of Medicine* **336**: 1465–1471.

Spielberger, C.D. (1983). *Manual for the State–Trait Anxiety Inventory STAI-Form Y.* Palo Alto, CA: Consulting Psychologists' Press.

Struewing, J.P., Hartge, P., Wacholder, S., Baker, S.M., Berlin, M., McAdams, M. et al. (1997). The risk of cancer associated with specific mutations of BRCA1 and BRCA2 among Ashkenazi Jews. *New England Journal of Medicine* **336**: 1401–1408.

Tibben, A., Vegter, V.D., Vlis, M., Niermeijer, M.F., Kamp, J.J., Roos, R.A., Rooijmans, H.G., et al. (1990). Testing for Huntington's disease with support for all parties (letter). *Lancet* **335**: 553.

Tjemsland, L., Soreide, J.A. and Malt, U.F. (1998). Post-traumatic distress symptoms in operable breast cancer III: status one year after surgery. *Breast Cancer Resesearch and Treatment* **47**: 141–151.

Valdimarsdottir, H.B., Bovbjerg, D.H., Brown, K., Jacobsen, P., Schwartz, M.D., Bleiker, E. et al. (1999). Cancer-specific distress is related to women's decisions to undergo BCRA1-testing. *Cancer Research and Therapeutic Control* **8**: 61–68.

Valdimarsdottir, H.B., Bovbjerg, D.H., Kash, K.M., Holland, J.C., Osborne, M.P. and Miller, D.G. (1995). Psychological distress in women with a familial risk of breast cancer. *Psycho-Oncology* **4**: 133–141.

Van Geel, A.N., Rutgers, E.J., Vos-Deckers, G.C., de Vries, J. and Wobbes, T. (1997). (Women with hereditary risk of breast cancer: consensus of surgical representatives of study groups for hereditary tumors regarding intensive monitoring, diagnosis and preventive resection). (in Dutch). *Nederlands Tijdschrift voor Geneeskunde* **141**: 874–877.

Vasen, H.F., Wijnen, J.T., Menko, F.H., Kleibeuker, J.H., Taal, B.G., Griffioen, G. et al. (1996). Cancer risk in families with hereditary non-polyposis colorectal cancer diagnosed by mutation analysis. *Gastroenterology* **110**: 1020–1027.

Vasen, H.F.A. (1996). Erfelijk en familiair colorectaal carcinoom: richtlijnen voor beleid. *Patient Care* 28–34.

Verhoog, L.C., Brekelmans, C.T.M., Seynaeve, C., van den Bosch, L.M.C., Dahmen, G., van Geel, A.N. et al. (1998). Survival and tumour characteristics of breast-cancer patients with germline mutations of BRCA1. *Lancet* **351**: 316–321.

Watson, M., Lloyd, S.M., Eeles, R., Ponder, B., Easton, D., Seal, S. et al. (1996). Psychosocial impact of testing (by linkage) for the BRCA1 breast cancer gene: an investigation of two families in the research setting. *Psycho-Oncology* **5**: 233–239.

Wellisch, D.K., Gritz, E.R., Schain, W., Wang, H.J. and Siau, J. (1992). Psychological functioning of daughters of breast cancer patients. Part ii: Characterizing the distressed daughter of the breast cancer patient. *Psychosomatics* **33**: 171–179.

Wigbout, G. (1997). Poliklinisch advies over erfelijke kanker. *Kanker* **21**: 30–31.

Wiggins, S., Whyte, P., Huggins, M., Adam, S., Theilmann, J., Bloch, M. et al. (1992). The psychological consequences of predictive testing for Huntington's disease. Canadian collaborative study of predictive testing. *New England Journal of Medicine* **327**: 1401–1405.

Wooster, R., Bignell, G., Lancaster, J., Swift, S., Seal, S., Mangion, J. et al. (1995). Identification of the breast cancer susceptibility gene BRCA2. *Nature* **378**: 789–792.

Familial Cancer and Genetics: Psychosocial and Ethical Aspects

KATHRYN M. KASH and MARY KAY DABNEY
Beth Israel Cancer Center, New York, USA

JIMMIE C. HOLLAND
Memorial Sloan–Kettering Cancer Center, New York, USA

MICHAEL P. OSBORNE and DANIEL G. MILLER
Strang Cancer Prevention Center, New York, USA

In the past 5 years there has been a plethora of research involving cancer susceptibility genes. Several major cancer susceptibility genes have been cloned and sequenced, including the APC gene for familial adenomatous polyposis (FAP) (Leppert et al., 1990), the BRCA1 and BRCA2 genes for hereditary breast and/or ovarian cancer (HBOC) (Miki et al., 1994; Wooster et al., 1995), and the MLH1, MSH2, MSH6, PMS1, and PMS2 genes for hereditary non-polyposis colon cancer (HNPCC) (Nicolaides et al., 1994; Peltomäki et al., 1993). These scientific advances offer new opportunities for members of families with several relatives with various cancers to discover whether or not they carry a mutation in a cancer susceptibility gene and subsequently have an increased risk to develop cancer. Approximately 186 000 new cases of breast cancer will be diagnosed this year in the USA, with an estimated 44 000 women dying of the disease (American Cancer Society, 1999). Although only 5–10% of all breast cancers are thought to be inherited (Miki et al., 1994; Wooster et al., 1995), women with family histories of the disease are being targeted for genetic testing research. Given the high breast cancer rate and the preponderance of media attention to breast and ovarian cancer susceptibility genes, many women want to have genetic testing without understanding the full ramifications of the process.

Before genetic testing was available for cancer susceptibility genes, there were studies done looking at the interest in genetic testing and the emotional distress of individuals at risk for Huntington's disease (HD). A study of predictive testing for HD showed that the presence of intrusive symptoms at baseline increased the likelihood of poor adjustment after revealing the test results (Tibben et al., 1993).

Cancer and the Family, 2nd Edn. Edited by L. Baider, C. L. Cooper and A. Kaplan De-Nour
© 2000 John Wiley & Sons, Ltd

The HD data from Wiggins and colleagues (1992) showed that those who did not receive their test results were most distressed and those who did receive their results (positive or negative) were less distressed at 1 year post-test. In one of the first outcome studies of BRCA1 testing, Croyle et al. (1997) reported on the short-term (1–2 week) impact of testing on general distress and breast cancer-specific distress in high-risk women. Although BRCA1 carriers did not demonstrate increases in general distress, they did report significantly higher post-test levels of intrusive thoughts. Recently, Lerman and colleagues (1996) reported interim data from a prospective cohort study of members of several HBOC families. At baseline and 1 month follow-up, all carriers, non-carriers, and decliners of BRCA1 testing scored in the normal ranges on these measures. However, non-carriers exhibited significant decreases in depressive symptoms and role impairment and marginally significant decreases in sexual impairment, as compared to carriers and decliners.

For the past several years, we have been conducting research on genetic testing for cancer susceptibility genes, as well as individual mutations in cancer genetic counseling in the clinical and research setting. In our first study we wanted to identify the psychological and behavioral factors related to genetic testing issues. The second study was done to determine whether there were differences in knowledge of, attitudes towards, and willingness to undergo genetic testing in women at average risk for breast cancer and women at increased risk, due to their family histories of the disease. What is reported and discussed in this chapter is the psychological sequelae of being at risk for breast and other cancers, as well as the ethical issues involved in testing for BRCA1 and BRCA2 and APC gene mutations.

RESEARCH STUDY

The study presented here examined differences in knowledge of, attitudes towards, and willingness to undergo genetic testing for breast cancer in women at average risk (one in eight; 12%) and increased risk (13–50%) for the disease, based on their family histories of breast cancer. In addition, we sought to identify the psychological and behavioral factors that were related to genetic testing. This project was based on the transtheoretical model of behavior change and decisional balance (Prochaska et al., 1992), the Health Belief Model (Rosenstock et al., 1988), and how patients make decisions (Redelmeier et al., 1993). We anticipated that women who perceived their risk to be higher, who saw more positive aspects of genetic testing, who had greater knowledge of breast cancer and genetic testing, and who reported greater breast cancer anxiety, would be the most willing to undergo genetic testing when it becomes available on a clinical basis.

This study was conducted as part of a larger study investigating attitudes towards, and willingness to undergo, genetic testing in women at increased risk for breast cancer. Currently there are 14 785 women across the USA enrolled in the Strang Cancer Prevention Center's National High Risk Registry. This Registry was begun in 1990 as a research program to identify women with personal and family histories of breast and ovarian cancers and to provide them with basic information regarding their risk (Claus et al., 1992) for developing breast cancer, and appropriate breast cancer screening recommendations. Potential participants at increased risk were randomly selected from the 1000 women who participated in the larger study and who provided us with the name, address, and phone number of a friend (who had no first-degree relative with breast cancer and was within 5 years of their own age) who would be willing to complete a questionnaire. The participants were 391 women at increased risk for breast cancer, who were part of Strang's National High Risk Registry. We compared them with 382 women who were at average (population-based) risk for breast cancer, who had no first-degree relative with breast cancer, and who were age- and geographically-matched controls. None of the women had a personal history of cancer.

The following information was obtained on all participants: (a) sociodemographic information, such as age, race/ethnicity, marital status, education, employment status, occupation, religion, income, and town size; (b) knowledge of genetic testing; (c) knowledge of breast cancer; (d) knowledge of risk factors for breast cancer; (e) willingness to undergo genetic testing; (f) attitudes toward genetic testing; (g) breast cancer anxiety; (h) family history of breast cancer; and (i) perception of risk of developing breast cancer and being a gene mutation carrier.

RESULTS

The demographic characteristics of the total sample of 773 women were divided into risk levels according to the Claus et al. (1992) model: 12% (average risk), $n = 382$; 13–20% = 132; 20–35%, $n = 125$; and 35–50%, $n = 134$. The mean age was 44, with a range from 20 to 76. Sixty-eight percent of the women lived in rural areas (population under 20 000) or small cities (population from 20 000 to 150 000. The majority were Caucasian (97%), married (78%), had children (74%), and were college-educated (59%). There were no significant differences between women at average risk and women at increased risk on any demographic variables. All of the women ($n = 391$) at increased risk had one first-degree relative with breast cancer under the age of 50; 85 (22%) had two first-degree relatives with breast cancer and nine had three first-degree relatives with breast cancer.

Within the group of 391 women at increased risk for breast cancer (13–50%), 73% overestimated their risk, 3% underestimated their risk and 24% accurately reported their risk for breast cancer. Within the cohort of 382 women at average risk (10–12%) for breast cancer, 79% overestimated their risk and 21% accurately reported their risk for breast cancer. There was a significant difference in perception of risk between women at average risk and women at increased risk, $t(768) = 3.09$, $p < 0.002$. All groups overestimated their risk for breast cancer, with women at average risk having a mean of 30.66% (SD = 18.28) and the women at high risk with a mean of 54.73% (SD = 21.26). Women at average risk were significantly less likely ($p < 0.0001$) to perceive their risk of being a mutation carrier than women at increased risk. Only 1.3% of average-risk women thought it was very to extremely likely that they were gene mutation carriers as compared with 31.5% of women at increased risk.

Women at average risk had the lowest scores on breast cancer specific anxiety (mean = 8.44; SD = 7.57) and women at high risk had the highest scores (mean = 21.85; SD = 10.72). There was a significant difference between women at average risk and women at increased risk ($p < 0.0001$), but no difference within the three groups of women at increased risk. There were no differences on any other measure of psychological distress (e.g., depression, general anxiety, intrusive or avoidant thoughts).

GENETIC TESTING ISSUES

The major reasons women would undergo genetic testing were: (a) plan on doing breast self-examination regularly; (b) have certainty about their gene mutation status; (c) plan on going for mammograms and clinical breast examinations on a regular basis; and (d) their mutation status would help family members decide about testing. The most important negative aspects of genetic testing were: (a) knowing that their mutation status would not predict when breast cancer would occur; (b) knowing that their mutation status would cause concern for their children; (c) they would worry about their siblings; (d) they would live with the uncertainty; and (e) worry about health insurance coverage.

Only 36% of the women at average risk and 65% of the women at increased risk had heard about genetic testing for breast cancer. Despite this lack of information, 43% of average-risk women and 72% of high-risk women reported that they would have their blood taken for genetic testing and get their results immediately. There were several predictors of a woman's willingness to undergo genetic testing. Women who reported fewer negative aspects of testing ($p < 0.0001$) and more positive aspects of testing ($p < 0.0001$) were most likely to undergo genetic testing. Greater anxiety about breast cancer influenced a woman's decision to undergo genetic testing ($p < 0.0005$). The greater the perception of risk, the more willing to undergo genetic testing ($p < 0.0001$). The less formal education and the less knowledge of genetic testing, the more willing women were to undergo genetic testing ($p < 0.01$).

CONCLUSIONS FROM STUDY

The finding that greater breast cancer anxiety motivates the use of genetic testing is worrisome, because is suggests that the individuals most likely to request testing may be more psychologically vulnerable. Distressed individuals may be more vulnerable to adverse psychological consequences upon learning their positive (or negative) genetic status. In the study by Croyle et al. (1997) mentioned above, the highest levels of distress were found in carriers who had had no prior cancer diagnosis or preventive surgery. This group is most similar to our women at increased risk for breast cancer because of their family histories.

While the potential uptake for high-risk women is similar to those approached for HD, it is perplexing that almost half of women at average risk would consider genetic testing for breast and ovarian cancers. However, previous studies of HD have shown that intention to have a hypothetical genetic test often do not correspond to subsequent test utilization (Craufurd et al., 1989). It is clear from our data that the more knowledge women have, the less likely they are to undergo genetic testing. All women need to be educated regarding the benefits, risks, and limitations of genetic testing.

While the two initial reports (Croyle et al., 1997; Lerman et al., 1996) do not provide evidence for significant or pervasive adverse psychological effects of BRCA1 testing, caution is warranted in generalizing these findings to other populations and settings. Participants in those studies were members of high-risk families in hereditary cancer registries, many of whom were involved in prior cancer genetics studies. Those families had been included in the registries because of their unusually high prevalence of cancer. As a consequence of witnessing cancer in many close family members, the emotional responses of study participants may have been blunted. In our current work we are looking at emotional distress in women undergoing genetic testing. We found that the most distressed individuals are women who least expect to be gene mutation carriers and have positive test results. Women who expect to be positive and have a positive test result have certainty in what they have always believed to be true. In some cases, worrying about the possibility of being a mutation carrier may be no less distressing than having that belief confirmed.

ETHICAL PRINCIPLES OF GENETIC TESTING

A multitude of ethical and legal issues surrounding genetic counseling is compounded by the uncertainty of the outcome of genetic testing. The current ethical principles guiding risk notification and genetic testing were derived from the Canadian collaborative study of predictive testing for Huntington's disease (Huggins et al., 1990) and expanded by the Institute of Medicine (Andrews et al., 1994). The Canadian group was the first to look at the impact of testing for a genetic disease. While there are major differences between hereditary susceptibility for Huntington's disease and for cancers, both areas involve genetic counseling and testing, and both have similar ethical and psychological implications (Andrews et al., 1994).

When one applies these principles to genetic testing, several principles are important. The first is respect for autonomy. This refers to the rights of those approached for testing to be fully informed as to the profound effects and implications testing may have on their lives, so that they can exercise autonomy in making a decision. An individual should only agree to testing if he/she wants the information for his/her own purposes, not to accommodate relatives, health care providers, or anyone else. For FAP families, the parents are the ones who make the decision regarding genetic testing of their children, authorize the test, and are present at the results disclosure session. With regards to BRCA1/2 testing, children do not generally undergo genetic testing because breast and ovarian cancers are adult-onset diseases.

The principle of beneficence has application in genetic testing. 'First, do no harm' is a salient concept for those providing genetic counseling, whose role requires attention to possible adverse effects of improper counseling methods. In genetic counseling for cancer susceptibility, counselors ought to consider whether or not the test results will do 'more harm than good' rather than 'more good than harm'.

In terms of confidentiality or privacy, it is important that test results not be disclosed to third parties or other family members without discussing such a move with the person tested and getting his/her approval for what will be revealed, and to whom the information may be disseminated. Confidentiality of data is also crucial in terms of employment and insurance as many patients are concerned that they may lose or be denied health and life insurance or not be hired or promoted by employers due to their positive gene mutation status (Billings et al., 1992; Ostrer et al., 1993).

In terms of the principle of equity or justice, there should be equal access for all to genetic counseling and genetic testing. One question that needs to be addressed is who will pay for genetic counseling and genetic testing individuals whose family histories are congruent with hereditary susceptibility but cannot pay. Will testing be offered to those who can pay but are at the lowest risk for susceptibility? Genetic counseling and testing should be obtainable for appropriate family members regardless of ethnicity, geographical location, or ability to pay. In this sense, 'justice' refers to fairness for all.

CASE STUDIES

In the following section we will describe five cases involving FAP and HBOC families, in which there were many psychological and ethical issues. Each case demonstrates different issues that arise in the genetic counseling and testing process. The problems identified are: (a) a change in familial relationships as a result of genetic testing; (b) the distress associated with learning mutation status; (c) the ethical dilemma of confidentiality; (d) pressure from other family members to undergo genetic counseling and testing; and (e) genetic testing of children for an adult-onset disease.

The first case involves a FAP family (Figure 22.1). Mr AD is a 46 year-old man who was clinically diagnosed with FAP at age 30. FAP is a genetic condition in which polyps are inherited. Individuals with FAP can develop hundreds to thousands of polyps in the colon as teenagers and young adults. Polyps are a concern because they can develop into cancer. This condition is inherited and can be passed from generation to generation via mutations in the APC (adenomatous polyposis coli) gene on chromosome 5. At age 30, Mr AD had his colon removed and had an ileorectal anastomosis. As can be seen from the pedigree, Mr AD has a family history of FAP. He underwent genetic testing so that his children could learn their APC gene mutation status. He was found to have a mutation in the APC gene. Mr AD's son has not undergone genetic testing and was clinically diagnosed with FAP at age 17. To date, he has refused surgery. However, Mr AD's two daughters did undergo genetic testing. The 18 year-old did not inherit the APC gene mutation from her father, while the 15 year-old did inherit the APC gene. After the disclosure session, the 18 year-old stated that she felt very guilty once she realized that her younger sister had inherited the APC gene mutation. This is called 'survivor guilt', which can occur when one person tests negative while other family members are positive for the gene mutation. The relationship between Mr AD and his wife was not strong prior to the genetic testing of his daughters. Additionally, the father was always close to the 18 year-old, while the mother was always close to the 15 year-old. However, after the 15 year-old tested positive, the father began to bond with her. The mother's relationship with the 15 year-old became strained and she even told her daughter not to have children. Within a year, Mr AD developed rectal cancer, his son still refused surgery, the 15 year-old was devastated regarding her father's diagnosis of cancer, and Mr AD and his wife separated.

The second case (Figure 22.2) is one in which a woman had been diagnosed with breast cancer at age 44 and her sister had been diagnosed with both breast and ovarian cancers in her 40s. This family history is consistent with HBOC, and a

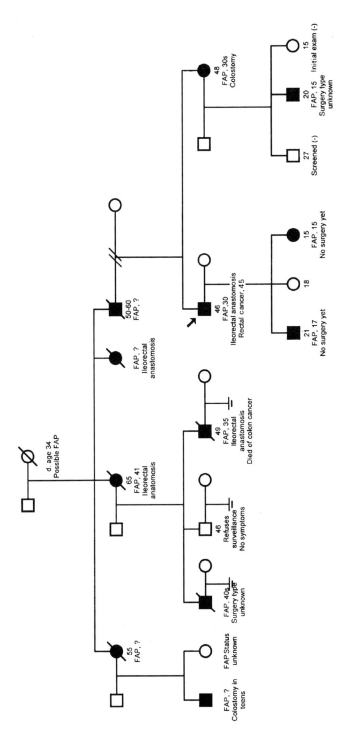

Figure 22.1 Pedigree of an FAP family. Arrow indicates Mr AD. Squares=males; circles=females; dark shading=FAP; oblique line=deceased

mutation in the breast and ovarian cancer predisposition gene, BRCA1, on chromosome 17 was suspected. In 1992, Ms TL participated in a research protocol in which she provided a blood sample to help clone the BRCA1 gene and characterize its mutations. The informed consent stipulated that results would be released to study participants or a specified family member. In 1995, the researchers learned that Ms TL had tested positive for a mutation in the BRCA1 gene. However, Ms TL died of breast cancer before her results could be disclosed. Ultimately her husband and three daughters, aged 30, 29 and 27, were given the information and offered genetic counseling and testing. All three received genetic counseling and decided to undergo genetic testing. All three women inherited the BRCA1 gene mutation from their mother. One of the daughters had believed that her chances of being a gene mutation carrier were very slim, and thus she became quite distressed upon learning that she was positive. Another sister decided to begin a family immediately and delayed surveillance procedures for breast and ovarian cancer. The third sister began surveillance procedures immediately. In the disclosure session, all three sisters agreed that at least none of them would feel 'survivor guilt'.

The third case (Figure 22.3) involves a young woman, Ms SB, who developed breast cancer at age 30. Since she believed her paternal aunt had died of breast cancer around her age, she was very worried about developing a recurrence. Consequently, she sought psychological help related to her distress about breast cancer and in decision-making regarding prophylactic surgery and genetic testing. In a phone conversation, Ms SB's mother informed Ms SB's therapist that the man Ms SB believed to be her father was not. Since Ms SB's father was unable to produce children, the family doctor had obtained sperm from the same donor for each of her four children. None of the children were aware of this, as the parents always felt it was not necessary because the sperm donor could not be identified. The family is of Ashkenazi Jewish ancestry and the sperm donor was also Jewish. Ms SB's mother feels they are a close family and that her husband is a wonderful 'father' to their children. The problem here is that the therapist was unable to reveal this information to Ms SB because it would be a breach of confidentiality. Ms SB, however, is basing some of her decision making regarding prophylactic surgery and genetic testing on the death of a paternal aunt, who is not biologically related to her. Unbeknown to Ms SB, her younger sister underwent genetic counseling and testing. She tested positive for a BRCA2 gene mutation and was going to have prophylactic mastectomies and prophylactic oophorectomies. Consequently, Ms SB underwent genetic testing and was found to have a BRCA1 gene mutation and now is at increased risk to develop a contralateral ovarian cancer. Ms SB was very distressed about having an increased risk to develop ovarian cancer and had prophylactic mastectomies and prophylactic oophorectomies. In addition, there has been some interest shown from the institution where the sisters had their genetic testing, to have the parents tested. Since two mutations in one family or even in one person is rare, the institution wanted to determine the parent of origin for each mutation. The father tested positive for a BRCA1 mutation and the mother tested positive for a BRCA2 mutation.

The fourth case (Figure 22.4) involves Ms KM, who is currently 51 years old. Her identical twin sister was diagnosed with breast cancer at age 44 and underwent a lumpectomy with radiation therapy and chemotherapy. Ms KM has adhered to the

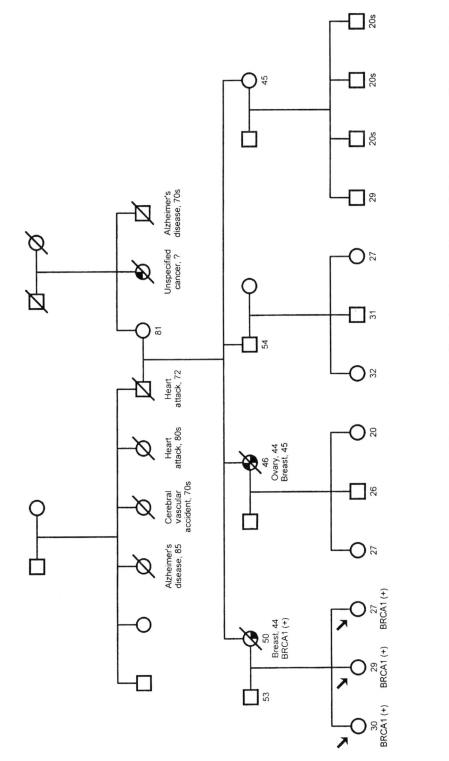
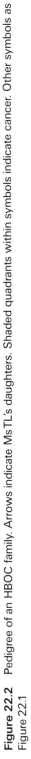

Figure 22.2 Pedigree of an HBOC family. Arrows indicate MsTL's daughters. Shaded quadrants within symbols indicate cancer. Other symbols as Figure 22.1

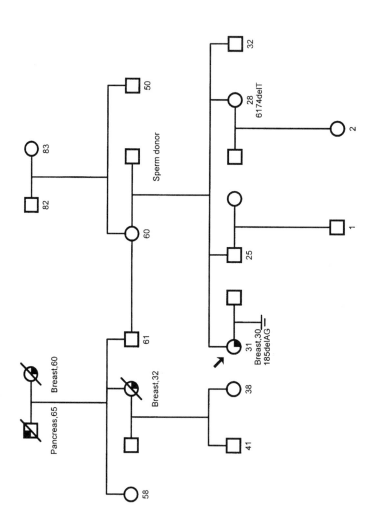

Figure 22.3   Pedigree of Ms SB's family. Arrow indicates Ms SB. Shaded quadrants within symbols indicate cancer. Other symbols as in Figure 22.1

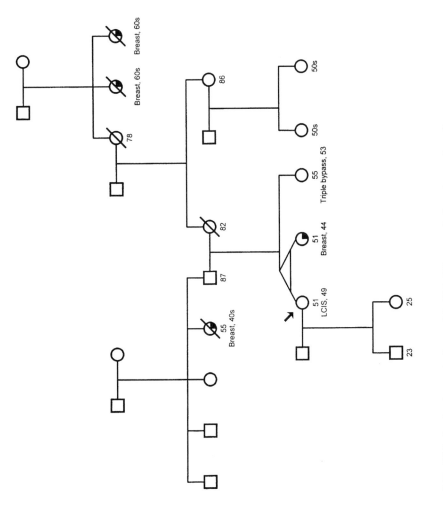

Figure 22.4 Pedigree of Ms KM's family. Arrow indicates Ms KM. Other symbols as in previous figures

recommended screening guidelines for breast cancer since her sister was diagnosed, and keeps up with the current literature regarding screening for breast cancer and the genetics of breast cancer. Two years ago Ms KM was diagnosed with lobular carcinoma *in situ* (LCIS), which is considered a marker of increased risk for invasive breast cancer. At this time, Ms KM prefers to participate in a breast cancer surveillance program, rather than undergo genetic testing or prophylactic surgery. However, Ms KM's 25 year-old daughter feels that her mother is a gene mutation carrier and wants her to undergo genetic testing as soon as possible. While Ms KM is making a fully informed decision not to have genetic testing, a family member is attempting to coerce her.

The fifth case (Figure 22.5) involves a 37 year-old man with a strong family history of breast cancer. In fact, four of his sisters with breast and/or ovarian cancer have tested positive for a mutation in the BRCA1 gene. Mr BR is very ambivalent about genetic testing and does not want to undertake it at this time. Mrs BR is angry with her husband, as she wants to know his gene mutation status in order to decide about genetic testing for her three small daughters, aged 7, 5, and 2½. In view of Mr BR's reluctance to discuss his ambivalence with his wife or undergo genetic testing, Mrs BR is now requesting testing for all three daughters. While it has been explained to Mrs BR that it is inappropriate to test children for an adult-onset disease, she is insistent and vows to find someone who will do it for her. There are many psychological problems that could arise with her daughters as a result of genetic testing. For example, Mrs BR may treat a daughter who is a gene mutation carrier differently from a daughter who is negative for a gene mutation. The subsequent psychological sequelae may be quite deleterious for both daughters. To date, no one has been willing to do genetic testing for her daughters.

SUMMARY

Perhaps the most serious limitation of genetic testing is that state-of-the-art diagnostics and therapies do not match test information. To receive positive test results when there is no adequate treatment can be tragic. It is important to remember that the genetic counselor should provide fully informed consent regarding the risks, benefits, and limitations of genetic testing and to be aware of the potential problems of testing. The genetic counselor should also recommend screening guidelines regardless of testing results. The psychologist's role is to make sure that the individual is psychologically equipped to deal with the emotional distress regarding testing and to help individuals cope with the results of testing. We need to target specific populations (e.g., women at average risk, women at increased risk) and tailor messages for each group in a randomized intervention trial. In this manner, we will be able to learn the most effective ways of communicating risk and decreasing the negative psychological sequelae of genetic testing. A multitude of ethical and legal issues surrounding genetic counseling is compounded by the uncertainty of genetic testing. The case studies illustrate the familial problems with both FAP and breast/ovarian cancer, as well as ethical questions regarding genetic testing. These questions revolve around the autonomy of individuals, genetic testing of children, confidentiality of information, stigmatization of gene mutation carriers, and complex family issues surrounding genetic testing.

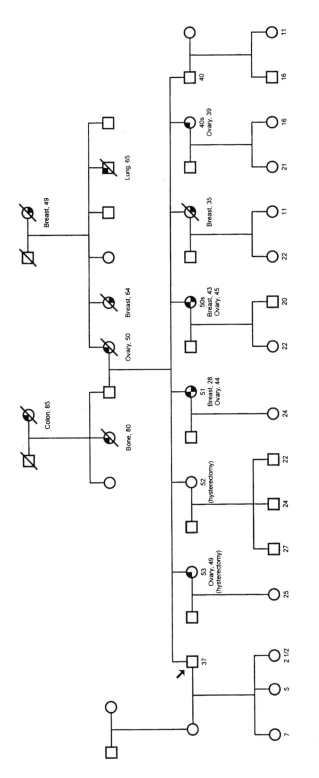

Figure 22.5 Pedigree of Mr BR's family. Arrow indicates Mr BR. Other symbols as in previous figures

REFERENCES

American Cancer Society (1999). *Cancer Facts and Figures: 1999*. New York: American Cancer Society.

Andrews, L.B., Fullarton, J.E., Holtzman, N.A., Motulsky, A.G. (Eds) (1994). Assessing genetic risks: implications for health and social policy. Committee on Assessing Genetic Risks, Division of Health Sciences Policy, Institute of Medicine. Washington, DC: National Academy Press.

Billings, P.R., Kohn, M.A., de Cuevas, M. et al. (1992). Discrimination as a consequence of genetic testing. *American Journal of Human Genetics* **50**: 476–482.

Claus, E.B., Risch, N. and Thompson, W.D. (1992). Age of onset as an indicator of familial risk of breast cancer. *American Journal of Epidemiology* **131**: 961–972.

Craufurd, D., Dodge, A., Kerzin-Storrar, L. and Harris, R. (1989). Uptake of presymptomatic predictive testing for Huntington's disease. *Lancet* **2**: 603–605.

Croyle, R.T., Smith, K., Botkin, J., Baty, B. and Nash, J. (1997). Psychological responses to BRCA1 mutation testing. Preliminary findings. *Health Psychology* **16**: 63–72.

Huggins, M., Bloch, M., Kanani, S., Quarrell, O.W.J., Theilman, J., Hedrick, A. et al. (1990). Ethical and legal dilemmas arising during predictive testing for adult-onset disease: the experience of Huntington's disease. *American Journal of Human Genetics* **47**: 4–12.

Kash, K.M., Jacobsen, P.B., Holland, J.C., Miller, D.G. and Osborne, M.P. (1995). Development of an instrument to measure breast cancer anxiety (Meeting abstract). American Society of Preventive Oncology, 19th Annual Meeting, March 8–11, Houston, TX.

Leppert, M., Burt, R., Hughes, J.P., Smowitz, W., Nakamura, Y., Woodward, S., Gardner, E., Lalouel, J.M. and White, R. (1990). Genetic analysis of an inherited predisposition of colon cancer in a family with a variable number of adenomatous polyps. *New England Journal of Medicine* **322**: 904–908.

Lerman, C., Narod, S., Schulman, K., Hughes, C., Gomez-Caminero, A., Gold, K., Trock, B., Main, D., Bonney, G., Lynch, J., Fulmore, C., Snyder, C., Lemon, S.J. and Lynch, H. (1996). BRCA1 testing in hereditary breast-ovarian cancer families: a prospective study of patient decision-making and outcomes. *Journal of the American Medical Association* **275**: 1885–1892.

Miki, Y., Swensen, J., Shattuck-Eidens, D., Futreal, P.A., Harshman, K., Tavtigian, S., Liu, Q., Cochran, C., Bennett, L.M., Ding, W., Bell, R., Rosenthal, J., Hussey, C., Tran, T., McClure, M., Frye, C., Hattier, T., Phelps, R., Haugen-Strano, A., Katcher, H., Yakumo, K., Gholami, Z., Shaffer, D., Stone, S., Bayer, S., Wray, C., Bogden, R., Dayananth, P., Ward, J., Tonin, P., Narod, S., Bristow, P.K., Norris, F.H., Helvering, L., Morrison, P., Rosteck, P., Lai, M., Barrett, J.C., Lewis, C., Neuhausen, S., Cannon-Albright, L., Goldgar, D., Wiseman, R., Kamb, A. and Skolnick, M.H. (1994). A strong candidate for the breast and ovarian cancer susceptibility gene BRCA1. *Science* **266**: 66–71.

Nicolaides, N.C., Papadopoulos, N., Liu, B., Wei, YF., Carter, K.C., Ruben, S.M., Rosen, C.A., Haseltine, W.A., Fleischmann, R.D. and Fraser, C.M. (1994). Mutations of two PMS homologues in hereditary non-polyposis colon cancer. *Nature* **271**: 75–78.

Ostrer, H., Allen, W., Crandall, L.A. et al. (1993). Insurance and genetic testing: where are we now? *American Journal of Human Genetics* **52**: 565–577.

Peltomäki, P., Aaltonen, L.A., Sistonen, P., Pylkkänen, L., Mecklin, J.-P., Järvinen, H., Green, J.S., Jass, J.R., Weber, J.L., Leach, F.S., Petersen, G.M., Hamilton, S.R., de la Chapelle, A. and Vogelstein, B. (1993). Genetic mapping of a locus predisposing to human colorectal cancer. *Science* **260**: 810–812.

Prochaska, J.O., DiClemente, C.C. and Norcross, J.C. (1992). In search of how people change: applications to addictive behaviors. *American Psychologist* **47**: 1102–1114.

Redelmeier, D.A., Rozin, P. and Kahneman, D. (1993). Understanding patients' decisions: cognitive and emotional perspectives. *Journal of the American Medical Association* **270**: 72–76.

Rosenstock, I.M., Strecher, V.J. and Becker, M.H. (1988). Social learning theory and the health belief model. *Health Education Quarterly* **15**: 175–183.

Tibben, A., Duivenvoorden, H.J., Vegter-van der Vlis, M., Niermeijer, M.F., Frets, P.G., van de Kamp, J.J.P., Roos, R.A.C., Rooijmans, G.M. and Verhage, F. (1993). Presymptomatic DNA testing for Huntington's disease: identifying the need for psychological intervention. *American Journal of Medical Genetics* **48**: 137–144.

Wooster, R., Bignell, G., Lancaster, J., Swift, S., Seal, S., Mangion, J., Collins, N., Gregory, S., Gumbs, C., Micklem, G., Barfoot, R., Hamoudi, R., Patel, S., Rice, C., Biggs, P., Hashim, Y., Smith, A., Connor, F., Arason, A., Gudmundsson, J., Ficenec, D., Keisell, D., Ford, D., Tonin, P., Bishop, D.T., Spurr, N.K., Ponder, B.A.J., Eeles, R., Peto, J., Devilee, P., Cornelisse, C., Lynch, H., Narod, S., Lenoir, G., Egilsson, V., Barkadottir, R.B., Easton, D.F., Bentley, D.R., Futreal, P.A., Ashworth, A. and Strattoa, M.R. (1995). Identification of the breast cancer susceptibility gene BRCA2. *Nature* **378**: 789–792.

Wiggins, S., Whyte, P., Huggins, M., Adam, S., Theilman, J., Bloch, M. et al. (1992). The psychological consequences of predictive testing for Huntington's disease. Canadian Collaborative Study of Predictive Testing. *New England Journal of Medicine* **327**: 1401–1405.

23

Women at Increased Risk for Breast Cancer: Family Issues, Clinical Treatment, and Research Findings

DAVID K. WELLISCH and NANGEL LINDBERG

Department of Psychiatry and Biobehavioral Science, School of Medicine,
University of California at Los Angeles, CA, USA

Since the first chapter on this group of women at increased risk for breast cancer was written in the first edition of *Cancer and the Family* in 1996, both of these authors have continued in clinical and research work with this population (Wellisch et al., 1996). This chapter, then, is an update on the emergence and growth of our work in the UCLA–Revlon Breast Center High Risk Clinic. At this point in the history of the High Risk Clinic we have approximately 500 women enrolled and under clinical management and research evaluations of different types.

This chapter contains four basic sections which include: (a) an updated literature review since the last chapter, covering the years 1996–1998, dealt with by year (1996, 1997, and 1998)—it is not exhaustive, but covers some important issues in the area; (b) an updated outline of the High Risk Clinic structure; (c) some recent data focusing upon clinic demographics; having a mother with breast cancer (vs. not having a mother with breast cancer); having only family history, having breast disease only (not cancer), or both; comparing patients with multiple, one, two, or no biopsies; comparing having one or multiple sisters with breast cancer (i.e., mother, sisters, and other relatives); and comparing women with one vs. multiple relatives with breast cancer; and (d) case vignette descriptions.

LITERATURE REVIEW

1996

In this year, three key papers appeared in the literature. Two shared a focus on the issue of anxiety in this population (Drossaert et al., 1996; Thirlaway et al., 1996). In the Drossaert et al. (1996) paper, high-risk women were compared to women without a family history of breast cancer. Fully 46% of family history positives 'did not know

Cancer and the Family, 2nd Edn. Edited by L. Baider, C. L. Cooper and A. Kaplan De-Nour
© 2000 John Wiley & Sons, Ltd

their risk was increased by their family history', however, they had increased risk perception. Although family history positives had higher risk perceptions, no differences in early detection behavior(s) were found that could not be attributed to higher anxiety levels. The authors concluded that the higher risk perception was partly accounted for by having experience with the disease 'at close range.' Thirlaway et al. (1996) examined the issue of whether family history (high-risk) clinics exacerbate or alleviate anxiety in their patients. They compared women at risk in a tamoxifen prevention trial with at-risk women selected from the National Breast Screening Program (NBSP) who were not attending a high-risk clinic. Most anxiety was found in women with a family history in the NBSP program. Women in the high-risk clinic (on tamoxifen) had anxiety scores comparable to women without family histories in the NBSP program. The investigators concluded that high-risk clinics do not appear to cull or recruit a selected group of the most anxious high-risk women. A third paper from this year (Lerman et al., 1996) showed results from a randomized study where high-risk women received either individualized breast cancer risk counseling or general health education. Women who received the breast cancer risk counseling (BCRC) showed significantly less breast cancer-specific distress at 3 month follow-up, compared to the control group. In both groups, women with 'monitoring' (information-seeking) styles exhibited increases in general distress from baseline to follow-up.

1997

In this year, five key papers appeared in the literature. Three dealt with issues surrounding genetic testing and genetic counseling (Lerman et al., 1997; Croyle et al., 1997; Audrain et al., 1997). In the Lerman (1997) study, 149 high-risk women from hereditary cancer families were offered genetic counseling and testing. Of this group, 58% wanted to know their BRCA-1 status and 42% declined. After controlling for demographics and risk status, cancer-specific distress was related to BRCA-1 test use, while global distress was unrelated to test use. Croyle et al. (1997) evaluated very short-term distress (1–2 weeks post-test) of BRCA-1 gene mutation carriers vs. non-carriers. Positive carriers did not have significantly higher levels of (test-related) psychological distress. The highest level of distress was found in positive carriers with no history of cancer or cancer surgery. Audrain et al. (1997) performed a study on high-risk women volunteering for genetic counseling and BRCA-1 testing. The investigators sought: (a) to characterize the psychological status of these women; and (b) to identify specific demographic, personality, and appraisal factors (monitoring vs. blunting style of information seeking) that contribute to both cancer-specific and general distress in these women. Results revealed moderate (overall) distress in this population. Women with higher levels of general distress were less likely to: be married, have optimism, and have higher risk perceptions and lower perceptions of control over development of breast cancer. Women with higher levels of cancer-specific distress were: younger, non-Caucasian, and have lower perceptions of control over developing breast cancer. Two other papers in this year dealt with psychological symptoms of high-risk women (Gilbar, 1997; Zakowski et al., 1997). Gilbar (1997) psychologically tested 16 women with family histories of breast cancer vs. 37 while during a routine examination in a breast clinic. Results showed significantly more distress globally as well as on 6/10 subscales of a standardized instrument (Brief Symptom Inventory) in the family histories group. Most significantly different were: Depression, Somatization, and Hostility. Zakowski et al. (1997) attempted to predict intrusive thoughts and avoidance in women with family histories of breast cancer. The key aim of the study was to evaluate the contribution of death of a parent from (breast) cancer to distress at high risk. The high-risk group undergoing mammography was compared to a non-high-risk group not undergoing mammography on the day of mammography and 4–8 weeks after the notification of normal results. The high-risk group had higher levels of intrusive thoughts, avoidance, and perceived lifetime risk than the comparison group on both testing days. Among the high-risk group, those with parental death had the highest levels of intrusive thoughts, avoidance, and perceived risk, compared also with a subgroup of women with family histories of maternal breast cancer whose mothers had survived. Results suggested that perceived risk mediated the effects of mammography on intrusive thoughts and avoidance regarding breast cancer.

1998

In this year, three key papers appeared in the literature. One dealt with outcomes of genetic testing (Dudok de Wit et al., 1998), one with support needs of women at high-risk (Hopwood et al., 1998), and one with distress in women with benign breast problems (Cunningham et al., 1998). The Dudok de Wit et al. (1998) study followed three populations (Huntington's disease, HD; familial adenomatous polyposis, FAP; and hereditary breast and ovarian cancer, HBOC, at 1 week and 6 months post-genetic testing; psychological distress was measured by the Impact of Events Scale (IES). The results showed the Huntington's disease gene carriers to be significantly more distressed in terms of Intrusion (intrusively experienced ideas, images, feelings, or bad dreams) and Avoidance (consciously recognized avoidance of certain ideas, feelings, or situations) at both 1 week and 6 months post-genetic testing. The investigators felt that those gene carriers with FAP and HBOC are more inclined to be able to ward off the emotions involved than the HD carriers. The Hopwood et al. (1998) study followed 158 women who had received genetic counseling at a family history clinic. They were followed at baseline and at 3 months post-counseling. At baseline, only 10% of the population had accurate estimates of risk, while at 3 months 55.7% did ($p = 0.005$). Those women with accurate risk knowledge post-counseling had significantly lower distress ($p = 0.003$). Using standard assessment and diagnostic criteria (via interview), 13% of the population were diagnosed with an affective disorder at 3 months post-counseling. This is compared to 26% using a standardized psychological test. Another important conclusion was that psychiatric morbidity was apparently not caused by the genetic counseling. Themes of loss and unresolved grief were more central to mood disorder in these women, probably resulting from the impact of familial breast cancer. Also, past psychiatric disorder had a significant relationship with current distress/affective disorder. It was concluded that risk counseling does not adversely affect the general mental health of recipients, but a minority of women may need help and more intervention based on the impact(s) of breast cancer in the family and because of past psychiatric history. The Cunningham et al. (1998) study compared 66 women with a benign breast problem (BBP) (at least one breast biopsy) with 66 age-matched healthy comparison (HC) women. The BBP group reported significantly greater worry about cancer than did the HC women. Breast symptom incidence and breast cancer risk perceptions mediated group differences in breast cancer worry. Although both groups had the same median number of first-degree relatives with breast cancer histories, this study is of particular importance because a proportion of most high-risk breast clinic populations will include women with benign breast problems *with or without* a family history of breast cancer.

STRUCTURE OF THE REVLON–UCLA BREAST CENTER HIGH RISK CLINIC

The UCLA High Risk Clinic has now operated and cared for patients for 6 years. At present, the clinic continues to meet 1 half-day per week and will see three to four new patients and four to five follow-up patients each week. At present the clinic has more than 500 women enrolled and being followed in this matrix of care. Most patients are seen at 6 month intervals unless they are at ultra-high-risk, ultra-anxious, or being worked-up for a breast lump, where they will be seen every 3 months or more often. Such patients are in the distinct minority. The services offered and providers for those services are listed in Table 23.1. At the initial (baseline) visit, each patient will see and be counseled by each member of the team. Upon each follow-up visit selected members of the team will see the patient, according to the wishes of the patient and the evaluation and care plan of the team.

Since 1996, the staff structure and services provided have remained constant except for the addition of the Genetics Counselor. This is obviously a key position on the team. The Genetics Counselor sees every new patient and does an in-depth history of all cancers in several generations of the patient's family. This is structuralized in the form of a genogram, which is a multigenerational chart highlighting the presence of cancer(s) in family members in several generations of the family. This helps organize the family history and aids in beginning the process of educating the patient about risk and realistic risk estimation. The Genetics Counselor has several basic functions in her clinical role, including:

Table 23.1 Services and staff of the Revlon–UCLA Breast Center High Risk Clinic

Services offered	Provider
Medical counseling/risk counseling	Medical oncologist
Risk counseling	Genetics counselor
Psychological evaluation	Psychologist and psychology intern
Breast examination/evaluation, self-examination education	Nurse practitioner
Mammography/ultrasound	Radiologist specialist in breast-imaging
Exercise planning/instruction	Exercise specialist instructor
Nutritional counseling	Physician specialist in nutritional medicine

1. Collection of detailed family histories (both maternal and paternal) which serve to create the actual genogram.
2. Pedigree assessment and recognition of cancer susceptibility syndromes.
3. Cancer risk analysis, calculation, and presentation of these figures to the patient.
4. Discussion of basic principles of cancer biology and genetics as they relate to the patient.

The Genetics Counselor, in creating the family genogram, sets the basic pattern for the focus on the family for the rest of the team. The genogram experience sets the family history in an objective, multigenerational diagram that the patient can see and then begin to react to emotionally. In our clinic structure, we try to have the Psychologist meet with the patient after the genogram is created, so the patient can then, in further depth, react emotionally to this family history of illness (and often death) along the generations. This creates a distinct shift from intellectual considerations of risk calculations to the more emotional impacts that such risk calculations create in the individual.

Several of the other functions/services provided by the team members have a strong orientation toward a family component of the patient's past and present experiences. These might include:

1. Medical counseling by the Medical Oncologist. For example, in such counseling with a patient on hormone replacement medications, often the patient can be left with a choice of whether she will continue on these hormones. The choice is to reduce risk by stopping the hormones but incur added problems, such as possible diminution of sexual interest and vaginal dryness. This begins to have strong implications in the marital/relationship sector for the woman to consider and discuss.
2. Nutritional counseling by the physician specialist in nutritional medicine. We have come to learn that proposed changes in the patient's nutrition take place in a family context and not in isolation. If the patient is to eat differently, so in all likelihood will the family. Thus, consideration of the family and their motivations to make these changes is fundamental to the patient actually making the nutritional shifts toward the lower-fat and soy-based products that are often recommended. To ignore the family is to essentially defeat the patient's possible success in this area.
3. Exercise planning by the exercise specialist also involves a strong component of family motivation and willingness to reinforce and sometimes actually participate. We are asking the patient to adopt a lifestyle that incorporates exercise with the goal of reducing body fat percentage and elevating muscle mass percentage. The goal of this is to lower risk by lowering the basic level of circulating estrogen. Here again, we have learned that if the spouse or significant other supports and actually participates in such an undertaking, the likelihood of the patient being successful with this goes up dramatically. If the family sees the patient's participation in this as taking time or attention from them, the likelihood of the patient complying does down dramatically. Given all of this, family considerations in our counseling of the patient becomes central in this context.

4. Teaching breast self-examination (BSE) by the Nurse Practitioner. We have learned that consideration of family history is an essential component of patient receptiveness to learning BSE. If the patient evidences significant clinical anxiety in BSE, it is highly likely that she has one or two issues. Either she witnessed a relative who had significant anxiety in facing her own BSE and/or breast cancer, or she has unresolved grief and/or anxiety over a relative's breast cancer, or both. The ability of the Nurse Practitioner to understand and to begin to help the patient talk about such issues can make a significant difference in the patient's receptivity to learning BSE.

These are a few key examples of how family issues are relevant and considered by team providers in addition to the psychologists in the comprehensive clinical management of patients.

The role of the Psychologist, given the foregoing observations, is two-fold. The Psychologist must be a consultant to the other team providers on consideration and integration of these family issues into their clinical services and counseling of the patient. In direct counseling of the patient, the Psychologist must also closely keep to the family perspective in helping the patient deal with, integrate, and plan for the other providers' suggestions.

DATA RELEVANT TO FAMILY ISSUES
WITH HIGH-RISK PATIENTS

In this next section, data will be presented which relates to a family or personal experience of being at increased risk for breast cancer. This data comes from ongoing efforts to evaluate this population. This data represents a small subset of a larger ongoing project, and results from that project will be available elsewhere. This data comes from baseline interviews and psychological testing of these patients. The instruments used include: (a) a structured clinical interview developed by these authors specifically for this population (available from the first author by request); (b) the Spielberger State–Trait Anxiety Inventory (Spielberger et al., 1970); and (c) the Center for Epidemiologic Studies Depression Scale (CES-D) (Radloff, 1977).

DEMOGRAPHIC INFORMATION FROM THE HIGH RISK CLINIC

The data presented here comes from 430 patients seen at the UCLA High Risk Clinic. Demographic analyses of the data indicate that, at the time of their initial visit to the UCLA High Risk Clinic, participants are on average 42 years of age, range 15–78. Most patients are Caucasian (84.2%), with the remainder self-identifying as Asian–American (4.7%), African–American (1.6%), and Latino (1.6).

In terms of family composition, most participants are currently married (59.6%), although many are single and have never been married (25.7%). About half of patients have children (53%). Our patient population appears to be highly educated, with most patients having college or graduate degrees (33.7% and 40.1%, respectively), and only a few that did not complete High School (1.8%) or have only a High School diploma (5.7%). Most patients work full-time or part-time

(55.6% and 17.8%, respectively), with only 3.9% of the remainder actively seeking employment.

Comparing Patients with Mother with Breast Cancer vs. Mother without Breast Cancer

Women whose mothers had breast cancer were significantly younger ($M = 40.47$) than those whose mothers did not have breast cancer ($M = 50.53$), $t = 8.09$, $p < 0.001$. Women whose mothers had breast cancer were also significantly more likely to be single ($\chi^2 = 23.70$, DF $= 5$, $p < 0.001$) and to have fewer children than those whose mothers did not have breast cancer ($F = 26.17$, $p < 0.001$).

As shown in Table 23.2, examination of the symptoms of depression presented by Clinic patients showed no significant differences for women whose mothers had breast cancer, as compared to those whose mothers did not have the disease; however, a significant difference was observed for the STAI-state scores; the mean anxiety state scores for women whose mothers had breast cancer ($M = 39.08$) was significantly higher that that of women whose mothers did not have breast cancer ($M = 34.56$, $t = 2.67$, $p < 0.01$). Closer inspection of the data showed that, unlike women whose mothers were not afflicted by the illness, patients whose mothers had breast cancer have a mean state anxiety score above the 40th percentile, indicating clinically significant symptoms of anxiety ($t = 2.25$, $p < 0.05$). Along a related line, examination of the patients' perception of their personal risk for getting breast cancer revealed a non-significant trend, with patients whose mothers did not have breast cancer assessing their risk as lower ($M = 44.22$) than women whose mothers had breast cancer ($M = 51.03$, $t = 1.71$, $p = 0.8$).

Examination of the anxiety experienced by women regarding getting a Papanicolaou (PAP) smear, a mammogram, or performing BSE revealed no significant differences among the groups. Similarly, as shown in Table 23.3, in terms of patients' actual compliance with medical recommendations regarding diet, PAP smears, and BSE, no significant differences were found. However, in regard to compliance for mammogram screenings, patients whose mothers had breast cancer appeared to be significantly less likely to obtain mammograms than were individuals whose mothers did not have breast cancer ($t = 3.88$, $p < 0.001$).

Table 23.2 Comparison of daughters of mothers with breast cancer vs. mothers without breast cancer—anxiety, depression, and risk

| | Mean scores | | |
	STAI	CES-D	Risk-estimate*
Mothers with breast cancer	39.08 (SD 12.44)	11.87 (SD 11.57)	51.03 (SD 25.49)
Mothers without breast cancer	34.56 (SD 10.60) ($p = 0.015$)	9.97 (SD 10.02) ($p = 0.26$)	44.22 (SD 14.01) ($p = 0.087$)

*Scale: 0–100% likelihood of ever getting breast cancer.

Table 23.3 Comparison of daughters of mothers with breast cancer vs. mothers without breast cancer—compliance

	Mean scores		
	PAP Smear compliance[*]	Mammogram compliance[*]	Breast self-examination compliance[*]
Mothers with breast cancer	1.17 (SD 0.49)	1.59 (SD 0.99)	1.92 (SD 0.80)
Mothers without breast cancer	1.22 (SD 0.66) ($p = 0.532$)	1.16 (SD 0.60) ($p = 0.003$)	2.13 (SD 0.82) ($p = 0.092$)

[*]Scale: 1 = compliant; 2 = sometimes compliant; 3 = not compliant.

Comparing Patients Having Only Family History of Breast Cancer, Only Breast Disease, and Both

Women who presented to the High Risk Clinic with a family history of breast cancer as their primary risk factor tended to be significantly younger ($M = 41.68$) than those who presented with only breast changes ($M = 50.40$) and those with both a family history and breast changes ($M = 47.11$; $F = 10.02$, $p < 0.001$). Women from the three risk groups did not differ significantly in any other demographic variable.

Comparing Patients with Multiple, One or Two, or No Biopsies

Women who presented to the High Risk Clinic having never had a breast biopsy tended to be significantly younger ($M = 40.52$) than those with a history of only one or two biopsies ($M = 46.26$), or those who had had more than three biopsies ($M = 49$, $F = 15.99$, $p < 0.001$). Women with no biopsies also tended to have significantly fewer children ($M = 1.04$) than those with more than three biopsies ($M = 1.78$, $F = 5.27$, $p < 0.05$). No other significant differences emerged for these groups in the demographic variables assessed.

As shown in Table 23.5, no significant differences were observed in the depression and anxiety scores for women with few, multiple, or no biopsies. A non-significant trend suggested that women with a history of more than three breast biopsies assessed their risk for getting breast cancer as significantly higher ($M = 63.85$) than those with only one or two biopsies ($M = 48.74$) and those who had never had a biopsy ($M = 49.07$, $F = 2.14$, $p = 0.12$).

Examination of the anxiety experienced by women regarding obtaining a PAP smear revealed no group differences. Interestingly, however, a significant linear relationship emerged between the number of biopsies women had undergone, and the anxiety experienced by them regarding mammograms, with more biopsies associated with higher levels of anxiety ($R = 0.18$, $p < 0.005$). A similar, although non-significant, trend was found associating number of biopsies and anxiety regarding BSE, with women that had never had a biopsy experiencing less anxiety ($M = 1.95$) than those who had had one or two ($M = 2.19$) or multiple biopsies ($M = 2.43$, $F = 2.57$, $p = 0.08$). Tables 23.4 and 23.6 show the mean scores for anxiety and compliance regarding screening tests.

Table 23.4 Comparison of daughters of mothers with breast cancer vs. mothers without breast cancer—anxiety about screening tests

	Mean scores		
	Level of anxiety re: PAP smear[*]	Level of anxiety re: mammogram[*]	Level of anxiety re: breast self-examination[*]
Mothers with breast cancer	1.44 (SD 0.80)	2.25 (SD 1.16)	2.07 (SD 1.10)
Mothers without breast cancer	1.40 (SD 0.79) ($p=0.721$)	2.00 (SD 1.12) ($p=0.128$)	1.95 (SD 1.04) ($p=0.437$)

Scale: 1–4; 1 = minimal; 4 = maximal.

Table 23.5 Comparison of number of biopsies—anxiety, depression, and risk

	Mean scores		
	STAI	CES-D	Risk estimate[*]
No biopsy	37.44 (SD 11.91)	11.20 (SD 10.89)	49.07 (SD 25.26)
One or two biopsies	38.94 (SD 13.29)	11.03 (SD 12.11)	48.74 (SD 26.31)
Three or more biopsies	39.23 (SD 9.38) ($p=0.65$)	14.79 (SD 9.81) ($p=0.50$)	63.85 (SD 17.70) ($p=0.12$)

[*]Scale 0–100% likelihood of ever getting breast cancer.

Table 23.6 Comparison of number of biopsies—compliance

	Mean scores		
	PAP smear compliance[*]	Mammogram compliance[*]	Breast self-examination compliance[*]
No biopsy	1.19 (SD 0.55)	1.60 (SD 0.99)	2.00 (SD 0.79)
One or two biopsies	1.18 (SD 0.56)	1.31 (SD 0.76)	1.89 (SD 0.86)
Three or more biopsies	1.07 (SD 0.27) ($p=0.72$)	1.00 (SD 0.001) ($p=0.01$)	2.00 (SD 0.78) ($p=0.63$)

[*]Scale: 1 = compliant; 2 = sometimes compliant; 3 = not compliant.

Comparing Patients Having One or Multiple Sisters with Breast Cancer

Women who had only one sister afflicted with breast cancer were significantly younger ($M=45.97$) than those with several sisters affected with the disease ($M=52.95$; $F=8.31$, $p<0.005$). Compared to women with only one sister with breast cancer, women with multiple sisters afflicted with the illness were more likely to have only a high school diploma or to have not completed college ($\chi^2=17.8$, DF $=5$, $p<0.005$). A non-significant trend was observed, with women with only one sister with breast cancer having fewer children ($M=1.47$) than women with multiple sisters with breast cancer ($M = 2.05$, $F = 3.15$, $p < 0.08$). No other significant differences emerged in the demographic variables assessed.

No significant differences were found in the depression, anxiety, or personal risk perception scores of Clinic patients based on the number of sisters they had who were afflicted with breast cancer. As shown in Tables 23.7 and 23.8 no differences were found in terms of the anxiety they experienced, or their level of compliance, regarding BSE or mammograms. Specifically with regard to PAP smears, however, whereas the groups did not differ in terms of their experienced anxiety, the level of compliance was significantly better for women who had multiple sisters afflicted with breast cancer ($M = 1.00$) than for those with only one sister affected with the illness ($M = 1.14$, $t = 1.99$, $p < 0.05$).

Comparing Patients with One vs. Multiple Relatives with Breast Cancer

No significant differences were observed in the demographic variables between women with only one relative with breast cancer as compared to those with multiple relatives afflicted with the illness.

No significant differences emerged regarding the depression, anxiety, or personal risk perception scores of women, based on the number of relatives afflicted with breast cancer. Tables 23.9 and 23.10 show mean scores for compliance and anxiety with screening practices. As shown, no differences were found with regard to the

Table 23.7   Comparison of number of sisters with breast cancer—compliance

	Mean scores		
	PAP smear compliance*	Mammogram compliance*	Breast self-examination compliance*
One sister	1.14 (SD 0.49)	1.26 (SD 0.75)	1.92 (SD 0.75)
Two or three sisters	1.00 (SD 0.00)	1.07 (SD 0.26)	1.93 (SD 0.70)
	($p = 0.05$)	($p = 0.33$)	($p = 0.95$)

*Scale: 1 = compliant; 2 = sometimes compliant; 3 = not compliant.

Table 23.8   Comparison of number of sisters with breast cancer—anxiety about screening tests

	Mean scores		
	Level of anxiety re: PAP smear*	Level of anxiety re: mammogram*	Level of anxiety re: breast self-examination*
One sister	1.30 (SD 0.71)	2.01 (SD 1.20)	1.83 (SD 1.01)
Two or three sisters	1.40 (SD 0.83)	−2.31 (SD 1.25)	−2.25 (SD 1.13)
	($p = 0.65$)	($p = 0.37$)	($p = 0.14$)

*Scale 1–4; 1 = minimal; 4 = maximal.

Table 23.9 Comparison of number of relatives with breast cancer—compliance

	Mean scores		
	PAP smear compliance*	Mammogram compliance*	Breast self-examination compliance*
One relative	1.09 (SD 0.33)	1.48 (SD (0.92)	1.96 (SD 0.84)
Multiple relatives	1.22 (SD 0.61)	1.51 (SD 0.97)	1.96 (SD 0.80)
	($p = 0.04$)	($p = 0.80$)	($p = 0.96$)

*Scale: 1 = compliant; 2 = sometimes compliant; 3 = not compliant.

Table 23.10 Comparison of number of relatives with breast cancer—anxiety about screening tests

	Mean scores		
	Level of anxiety re: PAP smear*	Level of anxiety re: mammogram*	Level of anxiety re: breast self-examination*
One relative	1.34 (SD 0.68)	2.38 (SD (1.22)	2.14 (SD 1.15)
Multiple relatives	1.47 (SD 0.86)	2.06 (SD 1.14)	2.00 (SD 1.06)
	($p = 0.14$)	($p = 0.03$)	($p = 0.29$)

*Scale: 1–4, 1 = minimal; 4 = maximal.

actual compliance or anxiety experienced with BSE or mammograms. However, women with only one relative afflicted with breast cancer were found to be significantly more compliant with PAP smear recommendations ($M = 1.09$) than women that had multiple relatives affected with the illness ($M = 1.22$, $t = 2.03$, $p < 0.05$). Closer examination of the data revealed a linear relationship between the number of relatives affected with breast cancer, and the anxiety experienced by women regarding PAP smears, with more afflicted relatives associated with higher anxiety levels ($R = 0.13$, $p < 0.05$).

IMPLICATIONS OF DATA

Demographics

The present study involves a sample that tended to be overwhelmingly Caucasian, affluent, educated, and to have adequate networks of social support; as such, our findings may not be generalized to less affluent groups, or to women of other cultural backgrounds, and instead may be a function of this particular sample. It is clear that further efforts are needed to make multidisciplinary preventive services available to a wider and more heterogeneous population of women at risk for breast cancer.

Results

Comparing Patients with Mother with Breast Cancer vs. Mother without Breast Cancer The finding that women whose mothers have breast cancer tend to be younger at the time of presenting at the Clinic than those whose mothers do not have the disease may be explained by the fact that most patients whose mothers do not have breast cancer tend to be sisters of women of an older cohort that have developed the disease, and are older themselves.

Our study also found that women whose mothers have breast cancer were more likely to be single and to have fewer children than those whose mothers did not have breast cancer. Whereas this may be a cohort effect, it suggests the possibility that women whose mothers have breast cancer may have less available immediate family support, which may in turn impact the level of stress they experience. Given that many women whose mothers have had breast cancer at some point become the main providers of support and care for their mothers, which for many individuals constitutes a major stressor, it is possible that a lack of immediate family support may negatively impact on these women's health-related behaviors.

Whereas our study has found no differences in depressive symptomatology among women in terms of the breast cancer status of their mothers, our study found that having a mother with breast cancer constitutes a significant risk factor for developing high levels of anxiety. Attachment theory provides a useful framework from which to interpret this finding: the perception that the mother (who is usually considered the closest attachment object) may be in danger is likely to lead to a perception of threat to one's own safety. This perception of threat is likely to be greater among women who perceive their mothers to be particularly vulnerable to, or have died from, the disease, or among those who have seen the scars of radical mastectomies and for whom that constitutes a particularly stressful experience. It can be argued that the perception that their closest attachment object is under a potentially lethal threat leads daughters of women that have had breast cancer to see themselves at greater risk for developing the illness, thus increasing their anxiety levels. Supporting this explanation for the increased anxiety levels among patients whose mothers have had breast cancer is the finding of a trend showing that they see themselves as more likely to get breast cancer than do women whose mothers have not had the illness. It appears, then, that the relationship to the family member affected with breast cancer plays a key mediating role in the development of psychological symptoms among at-risk women; the perception of threat appears to increase in direct relationship with the degree to which one is emotionally attached to the ill relative.

An additional finding with significant implications for women's health-related behaviors is the finding that women whose mothers have had breast cancer are less likely to comply with medical recommendations regarding mammograms than do other women. It is possible that women whose mothers have had breast cancer use avoidance as a primary defense against anxiety, and thus prefer not to know what their breast cancer status is until it is unavoidable.

Comparing Patients

Having Only Family History of Breast Cancer, Only Breast Disease, and Both   Contrary to our expectations, we found no differences in psychological symptoms or level of compliance among women based on the type or number of their risk factors: in terms of the assessed group differences, our study only found age to be significant, with women with a family history of breast cancer being younger than those with breast changes. Whereas it is possible that a family history of breast cancer and pre-cancerous conditions do not, in fact, differ in terms of the psychological symptoms with which they are associated, further studies should be conducted to examine these populations more closely, to determine the extent to which age mediates the development of psychological symptoms among this at-risk population.

Comparing Patients with Multiple, One or Two, or No Biopsies   In line with previous findings of more likelihood of breast changes with increased age, our study found a linear relationship between age and number of biopsies, with older women having had more biopsies. It was perhaps more surprising that no significant associations were found between the number of biopsies experienced and levels of general anxiety or depression. While further analyses are needed, our study found a significant linear relationship between the number of biopsies and levels of anxiety regarding mammograms and BSE; women who have undergone more biopsies experience greater anxiety regarding screening tests, although their level of compliance does not differ from other women. It appears, then, that while experiencing high levels of anxiety when undergoing screening tests, women who have undergone invasive diagnostic tests are not likely to use avoidance to cope with their distress, and thus are able to maintain adequate levels of compliance. Their anxiety appears to manifest itself in their having a heightened perception of their own vulnerability to breast cancer, shown in this sample as a non-significant trend in which women who have never undergone biopsies provide lower estimates regarding their likelihood of developing breast cancer in their lifetime, as compared with women who have undergone biopsies.

Comparing Patients Having Only One or Multiple Sisters with Breast Cancer   Our study found no significant group differences in depressive or anxiety symptoms, or in the perception of vulnerability to breast cancer, based on the number of sisters afflicted with breast cancer. It appears, then, that having several siblings with breast cancer does not have an additive effect on one's feelings of anxiety and sense of personal vulnerability to the disease. In fact, the experience of anxiety, depression, and vulnerability to breast cancer appears to be similar for women who have ill sisters and for those who do not, but who do themselves present precancerous breast changes. We find that having to undergo increasing number of breast biopsies magnifies women's sense of vulnerability to breast cancer, but that having more sisters affected with the illness does not appear to exacerbate their feelings of threat. Stressing the powerful role that one's emotional closeness to an ill relative plays on psychological adjustment, our study found that women whose mothers had breast cancer experienced significantly more anxiety compared with those with an ill sister. It seems clear that the degree of emotional attachment to a family member with breast cancer is a key variable in the development of distress among women; furthermore, the emotional closeness one has to the afflicted relative appears to play a more powerful mediating role in the development of anxiety than simply the number of affected relatives.

Comparing Patients with One vs. Multiple Relatives with Breast Cancer   The importance of the nature of the relationship to the ill relative, as compared with the number of afflicted relatives, seems to explain the lack of significant differences in psychological symptoms between women with only one or with more relatives afflicted with breast cancer. Interestingly, only one difference emerged, involving the anxiety involved in, and the compliance with, PAP smear recommendations. Women with multiple relatives affected with breast cancer experience more anxiety regarding PAP smear tests, and are in fact less likely to comply with this screening tests than women that have only one ill relative. While the relationship between women having multiple relatives with breast cancer, and their own anxiety over a non-breast-related test seems unclear, it points out that anxiety over medical procedures is not necessarily specific to the domain for which individuals are at risk. In this regard, clinicians must be aware that while informing patients about risk and protective factors for their specific vulnerabilities may lessen some of their domain-specific anxieties, other health-related behaviors may continue to be a source of distress.

CASE VIGNETTES

Three case vignettes are given below of patients who have recently been seen in the High Risk Clinic, with an attempt to draw some clinical implications and interventional possibilities from them. These cases were not chosen because they generally reflect the clinic population, but rather because they raise provocative issues to be considered clinically.

VIGNETTE 1

A 29 year-old woman presented to the High Risk Clinic with her 34 year-old sister. This is not unusual, as we have had many experiences where two or even three sisters (see next vignette) present at the same time. The obvious implication of this is the family (vs. the individual) experience of breast cancer. Breast cancer in this family was traced back at least two generations. The patient's maternal grandmother had had breast cancer and had died at age 52. It was unknown whether her breast cancer was premenopausal, but the staff suspected that it had developed at this phase of life. The patient's mother was diagnosed with unilateral breast cancer at age 35, and died of breast cancer at age 40; thus, her breast cancer was absolutely premenopausal. The 29 year-old patient was 10 when her mother was diagnosed, and 15 when she died. Three things were highlighted in this patient's baseline interview. They included:

1. The fact that this woman had made many decisions not to establish or commit to an adult life out of fear that she will die at her mother's age of death. Her rationale, not uncommon for a subgroup of our clinic population, was, 'Why should I get involved and attached to people and things that I will surely come to lose?' Examples of this ranged from not seeking a relationship or even considering having children, to not buying a house or apartment, to not even being willing to buy carpeting for her apartment. We have come to term this 'life truncation syndrome,' reflective of the inability to allow life to progress around adult commitments. In this patient's psychological state, this was a majorly conscious series of decisions. We have also seen patients in whom this pattern has emerged, but at a far less conscious level than was evident in this patient.

2. The fact that her sister was 34 years old, 1 year from the age at which their mother was diagnosed with her breast cancer. Careful attention was paid to the developmental dynamics of this sibling relationship. It became evident that the older sister moved into the maternal role upon the diagnosis of their mother, and had remained in this role with her younger sister up to the present time. Thus, two fears were present for the younger sister; her fear of her becoming her mother's age and dying, *and* her fear of her sister becoming her mother's age and being diagnosed/dying.

3. The fact that this patient underwent puberty, the development of her own breasts, and the entire early phase of adolescence with her mother ill/dying of breast cancer. This appeared to lead this patient to become phobic about examining her own breasts and to renounce her breasts as an erotic area of sexuality. In short, her breasts became a 'forbidden area.' About 16% of our clinic population have experienced at least some changes in their feelings about their breasts sexually. This patient was referred for individual psychotherapy. The patient accepted this referral.

Clinical Issues

1. This patient can benefit from psychological intervention to resolve unresolved grief. From Freud's early writing on unresolved grief to the present, the theme that unresolved grief prevents an individual from re-attaching to people and things in later life is consistently described.

2. A sub-theme is the need to disentangle the patient's sense of identification/fusion with her mother. The interface of her early adolescent developmental phase with her mother's breast cancer seemed to have left her without the ability to separate/individuate/disentangle from her mother. Without this ability, she was unable to experience herself as separate from her mother and not 'be doomed' like her mother.

3. Wellisch et al. (1991) described the differences in developmental phases in daughters when their mothers were diagnosed and the impact of this on adjustment in adult life. In addition, an additional psychological risk factor described in this study is if the mother died from her disease. This patient was an adolescent (highest-risk developmental phase) when her mother was diagnosed and when her mother also died. These psychosocial risk factors correlate to predict that this woman will have a harder time adjusting to her high-risk status than many other women in our clinic population. This woman, therefore, can benefit from education about the 'normality' and predictability of her emotional state, given these factors in her life.

4. This patient can benefit from psychological intervention to separate/individuate from her sister. The replacement of the mother, psychologically, by the sister has added to the patient's inability to attach to another. Clinically, she presented as an adolescent still attached to her mother. This primarily calls for individual psychotherapy, with a particular focus on the sibling relationship. It would be all too easy to miss her issues about her sister and overfocus on the loss of her mother. Although critical, the loss of the mother is only part of this woman's psychological equation.

VIGNETTE 2

A 43 year-old woman presented at the High Risk Clinic with her 44 year-old sister. Cancer(s) in this family were traced back at least two generations. In the previous generation, their mother had never had cancer, but *all* four of their maternal aunts had died of ovarian cancer in their 50s. This is the exact same gene as the one for breast cancer. Among the sisters, the eldest (age 45) was diagnosed with breast cancer at age 35 and then with ovarian cancer at age 45. The eldest sister's medical oncologist decided to test her for the BRCA-1 gene. She was identified as a positive carrier. This led to consideration of testing the other two sisters for the BRCA-1 gene. This is where the trouble began for the 43 year-old sister. This woman and her 44 year-old sibling lived in different States than the oncologist and the eldest sister. They sent blood, but never actually saw the oncologist who did the evaluation. Both sisters were also identified as positive carriers of the BRCA-1 gene. Upon interview, the youngest sister reported an almost unbelievable story of how this information had been relayed back to her and her sister. The medical oncologist did not see or even speak on the telephone to the two sisters, but instead opted to relay this ultra-sensitive information via *his* patient, the eldest sister. Therefore neither sister had a chance to ask any questions or know what to do with this information. The middle (44 year-old) sister promptly underwent an oophorectomy. She presented at our clinic as relatively calm, however. The younger sister presented with a highly agitated depression, characterized by inability to sleep and ruminative, tormented thinking about her BRCA-1 carrier status. Her primary concern was about her 16 year-old daughter. She worried about how to tell her about her genetic testing results and worried that she had doomed her daughter to the same fate. A dual psychological intervention was suggested to this woman. First, we suggested that she immediately begin crisis intervention, combining psychopharmacology and supportive psycho-therapy. Second, we suggested that the family enter family therapy as soon as the patient was stabilized, especially in the area of sleep. We felt she was too acutely upset and distraught to deal directly and effectively with her daughter. We made an arrangement with both a psychopharmacologically experienced psychiatrist and a family therapist before the patient left the clinic. The patient also utilized the High Risk Clinic experience to ask the staff all the questions she never had the chance to ask the medical oncologist.

Clinical Issues

1. First and foremost is the lesson(s) learned about poor management of information about genetic testing results. The necessity of finding a program that will facilitate the preparation, delivery, and aftermath of genetic testing information for such a patient as this youngest sister is obvious in this clinical example.
2. The dilemma of *what* to tell the 16 year-old daughter was not the real dilemma in our combined staff perception. We counseled this woman to tell her daughter the truth about the situation, including the inability to know exactly what all of this might mean genetically for the daughter. The dilemma was to find the right

context and support to tell the daughter and work their feelings through to a point of functional adaptation as a family.

3. The necessity of psychopharmacological intervention for the patient that addresses the longer term depression element as well as the acute distress. It is likely that it will take a considerable amount of time for this patient to cope with her feelings about being a BRCA-1 positive gene carrier. This would call for antidepressant medication as well as anxiolytic medication. The other issue is that the adolescent daughter needs to see her mother calm down and model her ability to cope with her genetic status and to be able to talk about the situation effectively. A combined psychotherapeutic and pharmacologic intervention can be the shortest route to arrive at these outcomes.

VIGNETTE 3

An 18 year-old woman presented at the High Risk Clinic with her mother. The patient had finished the Freshman year at college and had returned to live with her parents for the summer. The family history revealed that only her mother had been diagnosed with breast cancer. Her mother was first diagnosed when the patient was 12 years old·and then suffered a recurrence when the patient was 17 years old. In the first episode, the mother had undergone a lumpectomy with radiation and chemotherapy. With the recurrence, the mother had undergone a bilateral mastectomy, more intensive chemotherapy, and then a tram-flap breast reconstruction. During the process of the interview, the patient was given the option of asking her mother to leave the room. Without hesitation, she chose to ask her mother to stay. The patient shifted her affect dramatically during the course of the interview. Initially she was 'calm, cool, and collected.' As she proceeded, she gradually became more upset and overtly emotional. It became relatively clear that the patient did not realize the extent of her unresolved grief. She also did not realize how impotent she had felt in relation to the wish to have helped her mother though her two breast cancer experiences. It was also evident that this daughter and her mother had never stepped back and jointly processed their feelings about the breast cancers. The daughter indicated in the interview that she had never seen her mother's breasts post-mastectomy or post-breast reconstruction. In our clinic, about 73% of women have viewed their relative's breasts post-surgery, and 27% have not had this experience. Thus, this daughter belongs to a smaller sub-group of our clinic matrix in this category. As the interview proceeded, it was clear that it was not the mother who did not want to show her breasts, but the daughter who was hesitant to look. This 18 year-old patient was referred to a therapist who had formerly trained in the High Risk Clinic. She was offered the option of individual therapy, with the ability to invite her mother in as she so desired. We felt the major focus, however, should be the identification and processing of her feelings about her experience of her mother's breast cancers.

After the initial interview, the Psychologist (DKW) consulted with the Nurse Practitioner, as is our usual custom and practice as a team. The Nurse Practitioner consulted with the Psychologist prior to her performing the breast examination on the 18 year-old patient. She decided to try a unique intervention during that examination. She wished to examine the patient in the presence of the mother, and then wished to have the patient view her mother's breasts during the same examination. She felt that the patient was 'stuck' emotionally, and that with her support in the examination, the patient could possibly become 'unstuck' in the process of viewing her mother. This Psychologist was dubious about the feasibility of this intervention. It was tried and the patient still declined to view her mother's breasts.

Clinical Issues

1. Daughters and mothers coming together to the High Risk Clinic is usually a statement that a powerful family experience will occur. This is usually the beginning of a joint process of looking at the family experience of breast cancer. It is, in short, the beginning of a form of family therapy. The daughter in this case gave at least one important clue that she was invested in such a process. She asked her mother to stay during her interview. She wished her mother to be involved as she explored her own feelings about her breast cancer(s). This was a statement, of 'I want us to do this together, at least for now.' Family therapy can begin in the High Risk Clinic, but cannot be ongoing. This requires an outside referral.
2. This daughter had the experience of her mother's breast cancer(s) at two critical points in her development. The first was at the outset of her adolescence and puberty. She was developing breasts just when her mother was threatened with the loss of hers. The second was at the time that the patient was preparing to leave the family home and go off to college. Both of these situations have a similar and predictable emotional outcome, that of guilt in the daughter. Thus, this should be expected as an important theme in this daughter's emotional development, current conflicts, and psychotherapy. Guilt was, in fact, an issue this daughter reported as important for her.
3. The daughter's inability to view her mother's breast surgery result is a complex, multi-thematic issue. Wrapped up in this may be elements of guilt, anxiety, fear of identification, and post-traumatic stress (a variant of anxiety). This Psychologist conceptualized the viewing as the *end* of a process of emotional resolution rather than the beginning of such a process. The Nurse Practitioner was well-intentioned, but premature in her wish to facilitate this 18 year-old to break out of her impasse. It was important, in retrospect, for the team to not view the patient's inability to view her mother during the examination as a failure on anyone's part. Rather, it was important to conceptualize it as an end goal in a process that may look far easier than it is in reality.

SUMMARY

This chapter reflects a mosaic of pieces, including recent literature, service delivery structure, original data, and case examples. All of these point to an underlying and consistent basic theme. That theme is the reverberation of a breast cancer diagnosis through generations of a family. If breast cancer becomes a multigenerational experience, then it can become a way of life for a family. The bottom line is that breast cancer is a biological event within an individual, but a family experience emotionally, sometimes for generations.

REFERENCES

Audrain, J., Schwartz, M.D., Lerman, C. et al. (1997).   Psychological distress in women seeking genetic counseling for breast-ovarian cancer risk: the contributions of personality and appraisal. *Annals of Behavioral Medicine* **19**(4): 370–377.

Croyle, R.T., Smith, K.R., Botkin, J.R. et al. (1997).   Psychological responses to BRCA-1 mutation testing: preliminary findings. *Health Psychology* **16**(1): 63–72.

Cunningham, L.C., Andrykowski, M.D., Wilson, J.F. et al. (1998).   Physical symptoms, distress, and breast cancer risk perceptions in women with benign breast problems. *Health Psychology* **17**(4): 371–375.

Drossaert, C.C.H., Baer, H. and Seydel, E.R. (1996).   Perceived risk, anxiety, mammogram uptake, and breast self-examination of women with a family history of breast cancer: the role of knowledge to be at risk. *Cancer Detection and Prevention* **20**(1): 76–85.

Dudok de Wit, A.C., Duivenvoorden, H.J., Passchier, J. et al. (1998).   Course of distress experienced by persons at risk for an autosomal dominant inheritable disorder participating in a predictive testing program: an explorative study. *Psychosomatic Medicine* **60**: 543–549.

Gilbar, O. (1997).   Women with high-risk for breast cancer: psychological symptoms. *Psychological Reports* **80**: 800–802.

Hopwood, P., Keeling, F., Long, A. et al. (1998).   Psychological support needs for women at genetic high-risk of breast cancer: some preliminary indicators. *Psycho-Oncology* **7**: 402–412.

Lerman, C., Schwartz, M.D., Lin, T.H. et al. (1997).   The influence of psychological distress on use of genetic testing for cancer risk. *Journal of Consulting and Clinical Psychology* **65**(3): 414–420.

Lerman, C., Schwartz, M.D., Miller, S,.M. et al. (1996).   A randomized trial of breast cancer counseling: interacting effects of counseling, educational level, and coping style. *Health Psychology* **15**(2): 75–83.

Radloff, L. (1977).   The CES-D Scale: a self-report depression scale for research in the general population. *Applied Psychological Measurement* **1**(3): 385–401.

Spielberger, C., Gorsuch, R. and Lushene, T. (1970).   State–Trait Anxiety Inventory Manual. Palo Alto, CA: Consulting Psychologists' Press.

Thirlaway, K., Fallowfield, L., Nunnerly, H. and Powles, T. (1996).   Anxiety in women 'at risk' of developing breast cancer. *British Journal of Cancer* **73**: 1422–1424.

Wellisch, D.K., Gritz, E. R., Schain, W. et al. (1991).   Psychological functioning of daughters of breast cancer patients. Part I. Daughters and comparison subjects. *Psychosomatics* **32**(2): 324–336.

Wellisch, D.K., Hoffman, A. and Gritz, E. (1996).   Psychological concerns and care of daughters of breast cancer patients. In L. Baider, C.L. Cooper and A. Kaplan De-Nour (Eds), *Cancer and the Family*. Chichester: Wiley.

Zakowski, S.G., Valdimarsdottir, H.B., Bovbjerg, D.H. et al. (1997).   Predictors of intrusive thought and avoidance in women with family histories of breast cancer. *Annals of Behavioral Medicine* **19**(4): 362–369.

Section VIII
TERMINAL ILLNESS AND SYSTEMS OF BELIEF

24

The Family in Terminal Illness

SIMON WEIN

Department of Oncology, Shaarei Zedek Medical Center, Jerusalem, Israel

> When I am dead my dearest
> Sing no sad songs for me;
> Plant thou no roses at my head,
> Nor shady cypress-tree:
> Be the green grass above me
> With showers and dewdrops wet;
> And if thou wilt, remember,
> And if thou wilt, forget.
> *Christina Georgina Rossetti*

People uncommonly die alone. They are accompanied on their final illness by family, friends, and health-care professionals. The past generation of clinicians and researchers has overseen an evolution in the concept of family and now defines the unit of treatment as the family, instead of the disease or the patient (Rait and Lederberg, 1989; Davies et al., 1994; Kristjanson, 1996). The concept of the family has developed from a rigid, objective, view, based on blood-ties, to a subjective, individually determined definition centered on relationships. This change in emphasis has a curious parallel with the doctor–patient relationship, which has also witnessed a transformation, from a paternalistic to an autonomic model. The Nuremberg trials following World War II emphasized the importance of patient consent, autonomy and rights, and arguably have had a significant impact in some of these broad cultural changes (Burt, 1996). The other dynamic force, especially in the Western world, has been the fragmentation into nuclei of the extended family due to the major socio-economic forces of the second half of the twentieth century. The nuclear family has wrought substantial changes to the family in terminal illness.

The family are not uninvolved mirrors, merely reflecting and acknowledging. The interdependence of family members and patient is a given, for better or worse. Family, both as individual members and as a symbolic concept, react and respond to the dying loved one. Their lives will be irrevocably altered after the death. They

Cancer and the Family, 2nd Edn. Edited by L. Baider, C. L. Cooper and A. Kaplan De-Nour
© 2000 John Wiley & Sons, Ltd

suffer, they nurture, and they will maintain the memory in grief, bereavement, and survival.

Much research has been done in recent years—both theoretical and practical—focusing on the interrelationships between the patient, family members, and health-care providers in terminal illness. The relationship between the family and the health-care professionals is often intense and under-reported, and carries by proxy and displacement a large emotional burden, which in turn impacts on the therapeutic alliance.

Fifty percent of cancer patients will die of their illness, whilst cancer accounts for 25% of adult deaths (Wingo et al., 1995). Some are diagnosed with potentially curable disease and then relapse, whilst others present for the first time with an advanced, incurable condition. Palliative care is defined by the World Health Organization as:

> the active total care of patients whose disease is not responsive to curative treatment. Control of pain, of other symptoms, and of psychological, social and spiritual problems is paramount...it affirms life and regards dying as a normal process...to neither hasten nor postpone death (WHO, 1990).

The different phases and transitions have characteristic psychosocial issues. In management of terminal illness in cancer, we will explore the key issues as they pertain to the family and its web of interrelations, whilst emphasizing the overall aim of facilitating communication between family members and patient in preparation and anticipation of separation, loss, and bereavement.

THE FAMILY AS THE TREATMENT UNIT

Viewing the family as the unit of treatment achieves two critical purposes. First, it acknowledges the patient as more and other than a disease process. This raises the question of why a patient might in the first place be perceived in an I–It relationship, to use Buber's (1973) evocative paradigm. The commonest cause for addressing the patient as an 'it' is to protect the medical and nursing staff from the embarrassing, emotionally revealing, and frightening task of addressing death. The second purpose achieved in treating the cancer as a family disease is to acknowledge that family members are emotionally affected and irrevocably changed by the individual's illness (Leis et al., 1997; Kaye and Gracely, 1991; Musci and Dodd, 1990). Research confirms the emotional and physical impact on family members and justifies describing family members as 'second-order patients' (Rait and Lederberg, 1989).

Care should be taken not to refer to cancer as a sentient being which 'disrupts all components of social integration' (Zabora and Loscalzo, 1998). It is not the cancer, but rather the individuals in the family, including the patient, their personal histories, and interrelationships, that cause and create disruptions.

Family is no longer appropriately defined along strictly biological lines (if ever it was). In the palliative care setting, the term 'family' develops three themes. First is the definition as a 'self-identified group of two or more individuals who may or may not be related by bloodlines or law, but who function in such a way that they consider themselves to be a family' (Whall, 1986). Second, the word 'family' (etymological origin is from the Latin for slave or servant) conjures a concept of protection against loneliness, insecurity, and death, particularly in sickness. Conceivably, the family concept can be compared with the idealized mother–child bond or the protective master–slave relationship, which goes part of the way to explaining the frequent unconscious need of healthy family members to protect and infantilize the patient by wanting to control food, activity, and information. Chochinov et al. (1995) found that social or family isolation was a significant co-morbid factor in depression and its relationship to desire for death in terminal illness. The third concept lies with the individuals that constitute the family. Each has his/her own psychological history, unique position, and pattern of relationship. Thus, in practical terms, when receiving a patient and family it is important to draw up a genogram, not just of medical history, but particularly to document the significant relationships and their natures.

The legal and ethical implications of family, particularly in palliative care, focus on confidentiality, transfer of information, decision-making, and end-of-life issues such as euthanasia, terminal sedation, and resuscitation. Underpinning this is the conflict between patient rights and family rights. Do families have rights *vis-à-vis* the patient? In the West, where patient autonomy is highly valued, the emphasis is heavily on the individual's rights. Yet we have just expended some effort in describing cancer as a family illness. Is the ethical corollary that family members therefore do have rights to information and decision-making? In cultures not of the Western sphere, the concept of family is often all-encompassing. There it might be more appropriate to view the *family* as the fundamental ethical unit of that society. However, by merging both views one can build an approach whereby individuals make decisions, albeit embedded in the collective interdependence of family and culture. Practically the need is to balance the conflicting and, at times, opposing needs and rights.

FAMILY: CLASSIFICATION, EVALUATION AND ASSESSMENT

Most families cope with and adapt to the changes and losses wrought by severe illness in a family member. The individual's coping style plays a key role. Nonetheless, evaluating and assessing the family is important, as it enables the health-carers to identify those families that might develop problems and to know best where to direct what resources. Or, as some authors put it, it is important to 'think family' (Rait and Lederberg, 1989). It is beyond the scope of this paper to analyze in depth the theory and research behind assessing families and identifying types, nevertheless it is important to have a conceptual framework in hand when interacting with families to enable an informed evaluation and timely referral.

Kissane and colleagues (1998) developed a classification of families (supportive, conflict-resolving, intermediate, sullen, and hostile) that enabled them to predict psychological outcome and devise suitable psychotherapeutic interventions. Their classification of family types, based on substantiated screening tools, used the characteristics of cohesiveness, level of conflict, and ability to express thoughts and feelings. Olson (1989) categorizes families using two dimensions: adaptability and cohesiveness. Adaptability is the ability to respond to the stress of cancer by reassigning roles, changing rules of day-to-day living, and adopting new problem-solving strategies. A rigid family will not adapt to stressors, as they are inflexible and unable to create fresh coping strategies. An adaptive or chaotic response, on the other hand, implies ability to innovate and try new strategies. Cohesion is the level of emotional bonding, and in this model reflects the amount of effective support the family can supply. Low cohesion means that family members are 'disengaged', whilst high cohesion implies 'enmeshment' where boundaries are blurred and support is ineffectual, even damaging. Weisman et al. (1980) emphasizes the power families have through their ability to encourage, coerce, reinforce, or shame. These word-concepts are helpful when evaluating a difficult family interaction.

Zabora and Loscalzo (1998) identified a number of problematic family behaviours: interference with delivery of medical care; non-compliance; coercion of the patient; excessive demands on staff; unrealistic expectations; formation of alliances with other families against the health-care team; and lack of cooperation with decision-making. Rait and Lederberg (1989) identified three common ways families attract the staff's attention: failure to care for the patient; overt psychiatric symptoms or signs (or reportage of) in family members; and conflict and non-compliance between staff, patient and family in any or all combinations. These are problems in their own rights and also indicators of underlying family distress.

The literature documents the impact of cancer on family members. Rait and Lederberg (1989) coined the expression 'second-order patients'. Although caring for a sick loved one is a powerful way to express feelings and duties, it can be frightening and stressful. Anxiety and depression are the commonest psychiatric problems in families. One study found that 39% of caregivers had psychiatric disorders prior to the death of a patient (Addington-Hall et al., 1992), whilst another, looking at depression amongst spouses, found that 50% had clinical depression (Siegel et al., 1996). Loss of job or significant reduction in income have also been documented as common, under-recognized problems (Murinen, 1986). The sequelae of cancer have been examined extensively amongst the children of cancer patients, and findings include psychological symptoms of depression and anxiety, acting-out, school problems, social isolation, disturbances of eating, sleeping, and self-care, and lowered self-esteem (Adams-Greenly, 1986).

INFORMATION AND COMMUNICATION

Communication in terminal care demands not only time and empathy, but also an ability to analyze the dynamics of emotional interactions between family members and towards staff, to think on one's feet, and to respond momentarily. The family meeting is an important tool to communicate information bidirectionally; identify practical and psychological problems; assess family dynamics; ventilate feelings; clarify misunderstandings; establish the ethical and emotional boundaries, and convey a sense of caring and availability. The family meeting may be with or without the patient, but it clearly requires the informed consent of the patient. Conversely, information communicated by a family member in confidentiality cannot be transmitted without consent. Ideally, a family meeting has only two or three staff representatives, in order not to appear overwhelming. As many members of the family as possible should be present and identification of a single spokesperson is preferable, so that needless calls are avoided and to ensure an unbroken message (Mount, 1998; Bascom and Tolle, 1995).

It is important to secure the confidence and trust of the family in order to provide medical care and emotional support. Availability around the clock is a first step. Giving access is a positive and generous show of trust that patients and families invariably value and rarely abuse. It adds a small strain to the doctor or nurse, but its importance in relieving anxiety cannot be overestimated. In the rare situation that abuse of privilege does occur, early and very firm limit setting, initially by telephone and then face-to-face, with agreed principles of engagement usually resolves the problem. If abuse repeatedly occurs, it may indicate psychiatric problems requiring more extensive intervention.

How does the staff communicate caring? Most information is communicated non-verbally, as is caring. Actively listening to the other person; trying to comprehend their experience and what it might feel like to have cancer; facial expression of empathic concern; holding a hand or putting an arm around a shoulder; getting up from behind the desk; making and holding eye contact at the critical moments; being silent when necessary and giving the family space when needed (Mount, 1998).

Information about the medical condition is paramount. Truth is preferable to uncertainty. No truth should be delivered without a tincture of hope, yet postponing the difficult discussion may encourage false hopes and contribute to inappropriate treatment choices (Rhymes, 1991). Information may not in general be passed to family members without obtaining the consent of the patient. However, it needs be acknowledged that it is important, and justly so, that families be involved with the dying person in making critical decisions. The staff serve well as facilitators of this communication. Since we do not always know what the dynamics of a family are, we must tread carefully. Many patients prefer not to confide in their loved ones in order to protect them (Davies et al., 1990). Conversely, many family members ask doctors not to tell the patient the bad news in order to protect him (Vess et al., 1985). This conspiracy of silence can reach absurd proportions and is an example of the importance of staff taking a proactive stance in directing communication. Concealment may be a sign of family pathology or previous adverse experiences. Tragically, this dance of silence can result in the patient dying without resolving outstanding issues or saying 'goodbye'.

Medical staff also find telling the truth difficult. No-one wants to hurt another person. Furthermore, by admitting that the disease is progressing implies, *ipso facto*, that we have failed to contain it. Experience and research has shown that lying is more problematic in the long run; it is unethical and illegal in many countries, and is simply disrespectful. Nevertheless, if the patient has stated clearly that he/she does not want to know the truth, or in specific cultural and psychiatric circumstances it is judged to be damaging and harmful, then truth is appropriately mitigated or withheld.

The staff should ensure that medical information comes from one source, which can be difficult to secure, especially if different teams are involved. If conflicting information is given, confusion and division can ensue within an already delicate situation. In a family with pathologic dynamics, this 'misinformation' might be used as ammunition for manipulation and acting-out. Thus, it is incumbent upon medical staff to ensure that the level of communication between themselves is also open! A precarious and common problem is the transition of care from the diagnostic unit, to the oncology unit, to the palliative care team. Each transfer carries great significance and marks changes in the goals of care. Clear directive communication relating to goals of care must be transmitted. More portentously to the family and patient is that, in a real and symbolic way, the transfer is experienced as a loss which anticipates the final loss. It is appropriate to reassure the family that care will continue and, at the same time, to explore fears and sadness of loss and abandonment.

Information should also be sought from the family. Have there been previous losses? How have members coped? Is this the first death that they have experienced? What is the nature of relationships within the family? What do the family understand of the illness? There are often significant lacunae of knowledge and remarkable myths about cancer. What are the thoughts about taking the patient home? In general the family should be actively encouraged to be the caregivers for the patient, unless after careful assessment it is apparent that they lack physical or emotional resources or the desire to do so, in which case the staff must supplant the family in this role.

The patient should also be consulted. What are the patient's wishes about caregivers? Does he want to go home? What does he see are the family's emotional, physical, and financial resources? What is the role of religious community support, including the pastor? Whom do you rely on most for support? Whom do you worry about most as being unable to cope?

PRACTICAL ISSUES AND INTERVENTIONS

The clinical practice of medicine is infinitely complex, subtle and varied. The following clinical observations based on broad experience should serve as an initial practical guide.

The psychological responses of families in distress depends on many factors. First, it is important to state that the family is not monolithic. It is composed of individuals with personal histories who fit uniquely into the web of inter-relations that constitutes family. Stress often unmasks prior problems that may be known or may surface for the first time. For example, the unfolding crisis might bring together mistresses and spouses; half-siblings; estranged siblings; and so forth. All potential oil for the fire, but if anticipated and managed appropriately this may be an opportunity for resolution and acceptance. The gamut of emotions expressed by family members include hostility, guilt, fear, anxiety, anger, ambivalence, powerlessness, dependency, and frustration. A recent study found, counterintuitively perhaps, that patients were less anxious than their spouses, although 'meaningfulness of life' was higher for the spouse, possibly reflecting the value and process of caring for the patient (Axelsson and Sjoden, 1998).

Patients often express concern about being a burden on the family and experience shame, guilt, embarrassment, and fear of abandonment, and seek ways to protect the family and expiate self. In response family members see the suffering and unconsciously wish it would be over, and their loved one would die. This ambivalence in turn generates guilt, shame, anxiety—and so the cycle continues. It is critical that the staff have their finger on the pulse and intervene bilaterally by opening the lines of communication. Often it is only a matter of breaking the ice in order to effect a catharsis. Anger, a common emotion, can be frightening to deal with. Maintaining poise and calm is critical. Clarifying the source of the anger, and then acknowledging that loss may be unjust, will often go a long way to dispersing the anger. Powerlessness and frustration in the family at the medical profession's inability to stem the progress of the disease can also lead to intense abreactions. The staff must identify these emotions early, provide careful explanations, and seek appropriate interventions, for example, involving the family in the physical caring of the patient such as administration of intravenous fluids, medications and analgesia. Empowerment can redirect the anger. In the absence of background psychiatric illness, it is uncommon for family members to require psychopharmacologic intervention. It is usually adequate to employ relaxation tapes or exercises, and brief psychotherapy.

A special situation of ruptured communication is between spouses. It is rather disturbing to hear silence with the storm gathering. Possible explanations include that they never spoke; that they are both unconsciously in denial to protect the other; or that it is a conscious plan to maintain a positive and fighting spirit. Direct questioning is needed to assess whether intervention is warranted.

Anticipatory grief is common in a prolonged illnesses such as cancer and can have beneficial and adverse consequences. On the one hand, by anticipating the death, the surviving family members prepare themselves for grief and bereavement. On the other hand, if the family behaves towards the dying patient as if he/she is already deceased, this can lead to premature emotional and physical withdrawl which in turn can lead to confusion, anger, and terror in the patient. Conversely, family members unconsciously feeling the emotional distance and, seeing the reaction in the patient, will experience guilt and shame. It is comforting to explain to family members that thoughts jumping ahead in anticipation are normal and not for undue concern.

A common source of family–patient friction with the medical staff concerns the ethical domain of confidentiality and information. Not infrequently, family members will ambush the medical staff in the corridor, demanding that their relative not be told the diagnosis of cancer. The ostensible reasons are that the patient does not know (although in truth, the majority of patients are at the least suspicious of the diagnosis) and that the bad news will destroy hope and kill him/her prematurely. This can generate anger in the staff for a number of reasons: their authority is undermined; the implied devaluation of the patient; and the presumptuousness of the family. The need for families to protect adult members in this way derives from a number of dynamics: first, the desire to nurture a sick loved one and unconsciously replay the parent–child role; second, it enables the family to deny the severity of the diagnosis—they can pretend there is no illness, using projective identification to protect themselves; third, there might be a genuine fear that the patient may be hurt by the bad news. It is always useful to invest time explaining to the family some of these issues, especially that living with uncertainty itself is anxiety provoking. Without some focus to battle, the fear of the unknown can grip the imagination and turn it feverish with anxiety. Nobody enjoys divulging a painful truth, even, or especially, doctors (Wein, 1999). The reality is that it is still a fundamental right of the patient to have charge of his/her body and fate. It is correct to ask the patient what he/she wants done with the information, whether or not to hear it and/or share it with loved ones. In our experience, it is often a relief for the family when patients are told the diagnosis by the doctor. Often their unstated fantasy is that the patient will die suddenly or even kill him/herself. The role of the staff is to educate and demonstrate that support and hope will continue.

Health-care is expensive and money can play a role as a metaphor for value, control, and power (Farkas and Loscalzo, 1987). At the outset, money is no object and no cost is too great. As the disease progresses, however, financial resources may be stretched, and with the realization that cure is not an appropriate goal, money will come to be seen as a metaphor for anger, loss of hope, and exhaustion. A metaphor is a signal to initiate open discussion, and in this situation to reconcile expectations and resources, both physical and emotional (Zabora and Loscalzo, 1998).

Accurate assessment of symptoms in terminal illness is critical in order to be able to deliver quality care. As more family members become involved in home care, it is important to assess the degree of congruence between patients' and family caregivers' assessment of distress. Kristjanson et al. (1998) looked at 78 couples and found a high correlation between family's symptom rating and patient's self-report, and that 71–91% of family caregivers were accurate in reporting individual symptoms. They conclude that health professionals can rely on family caregivers' assessments.

A special mention must be made of the attitude towards opioids (morphine, oxycodone, fentanyl, etc). Frequently, family members express reserve, even shock, at the use of opioids, and attempt to influence the medical staff and the patient against using them. Ignorance and prejudice against opioids are pervasive in society, but cannot justify withholding them if medically indicated. The reasons given for withholding morphine include that they are addictive, dangerous, and symbolically represent death. The fears are real, the reasons are not. Rarely (and never without an underlying psychiatric problem) do patients become addicted in the presence of cancer pain (American College of Physicians Health and Public Policy Committee, 1983). Fear of addiction is often based on the stereotype presented in the popular press. Physical dependence is not addiction. Addiction is a pattern of drug-seeking behavior, characterized by craving for an opioid drug to achieve a psychic effect (psychological dependence), and this behavior continues despite harm to self or others (Foley, 1989). Physical dependence is a pharmacologic property of opioids defined by the development of a withdrawal syndrome following abrupt or too rapid withdrawal of the medication. Opioids, when used with skill and knowledge, are not dangerous. 'Opioids as a harbinger of death' is only a partly correct concept. As the disease progresses, pain often becomes a problem requiring the introduction of opioids. Clear and informative explanations must be given to assuage fears by stating that the disease is progressing, but not because of the morphine, and that it is absolutely unacceptable for the patient to experience unnecessary pain. When the patient is relieved of pain and feels well, the family and patient usually accept the decision in retrospect.

Not infrequently, roles are exchanged and reversed within the family. This is significantly influenced by culture and stage in family life cycle. Vess et al. (1985) found that open communication between spouse and family members enables them to rationally and more effectively re-allocate roles and functioning. A common role reversal is an elder son stepping into the role as head of the family for a sick father. This can be stressful on the son, who is displacing the father whilst still alive, and might be subject to pressures from family members; conversely, the father will feel the symbolic significance of being replaced. Or a young daughter might step into the shoes of a sick mother, confusing previously established roles in the family.

Constant reassessment of the level of coping in the family is essential. If family caregivers are stressed and tired, then a respite admission for the patient is necessary. This is especially true in the elderly, in whom cancer is common and spouses have fewer resources, with children frequently out of the picture. The medical circumstances in advanced cancer can, within a day, suddenly change from palliative chemotherapy to terminal care, and the goals of care will flux dramatically. It is worth noting that 20–30% of patients with cancer die suddenly, which can have a devastating effect despite the known underlying illness (Tolle and Girard, 1982). It is difficult, if not impossible, to anticipate such events, but they demand a quick response from the staff by way of explanation, support, and guidance.

In recent years there has developed a strong trend to encourage patients to die at home. Surveys have suggested that 50–60% of advanced cancer patients would like to die at home, although in the final analysis less than 20% actually do so (Merrill and Mor, 1993). Dying at home is an idealized concept, recalling the security of a childhood home against the fear of the unknown and the emptiness of loneliness. It is also a symbol of what is meaningful to that person's life, especially family. Home provides privacy and supports intimacy. Other patients, despite exhortations from willing family members, prefer to die in an institution, as only there do they feel the security of around-the-clock medical and nursing staff. Dying at home is a complex procedure, demanding support and cooperation from family members, staff, and community resources. Often there is uncertainty about the ability to succeed. Symbolically, however, it is important to try, and if necessary fail, so that the family will feel they have done everything. The door should be left open for the patient to return at any time, either for respite or, as often happens, to die. Finally, it is important to emphasize that there is no moral premium on families looking after dying patients at home—some can, others cannot, and in the interests of all concerned the issues should not be forced. At times it is incumbent upon the medical staff to take a paternalistic and didactic stance and declare that the patient cannot go home if the staff assess that it would not be possible to manage. On the other hand, when a family is highly determined, remarkable achievements have been witnessed.

The management of advanced cancer is a complex sociomedical problem. In order to deal adequately with the patient and family, an interdisciplinary team of health-care professionals is required. This adds flexibility to respond to the different demands, personalities, and problems of families, especially during a difficult hospitalization. Sourkes (1997) points out the importance of the senior physician in staff–staff and staff–family meetings to serve as a role model. The involvement of a consultant-liason psychiatrist is important when conflict develops between family and staff. Teaching staff how to apply limits to intrusive family behaviour, explaining the psychological dynamics of an aggressive family, providing support as another hand on-board, and teaching problem solving are some useful interventions psychiatrists can initiate. Similarly, assessment of a difficult family is crucial: does the family understand the medical situation and prognosis? Do they have resources? Is any family member in acute psychiatric danger? What is the source and mechanism of conflict with the staff? How has the family functioning been imbalanced by the illness? Another important resource is the clergy, in order to address spiritual and community needs of families and patients. Emotional support and bonding between family and staff members is unpredictable and is not hierarchy-dependent, which emphasizes the importance of a team involvement. Finally, Steele (1990) and McCorkle (1998) have shown that effective psychosocial support of families during the terminal illness can result in a smoother and more integrated bereavement.

DYING AND DEATH

Death at the end of a period of prolonged suffering may be perceived as a relief. This sense of relief is experienced by patient, family and staff. It is incumbent upon the staff to attentively accompany the family during dying. The family may never have experienced a death, especially of a loved one, and staff should answer unasked questions, and fully mobilize resources. The ambiguity of wishing for relief of suffering and desperately not wanting to lose a family member can result in confusion, uncertainty, hostility, and guilt. It is important to share with the family that such feelings are common, but in no way diminish the love for, or value of, the patient.

Frequently, family will ask if members overseas should be contacted to return to the bed-side. The rule of thumb is that once it has been considered, and given the unpredictability of the final phases, it is prudent to advise the family to return forthwith. A more difficult request is to be asked to keep a patient alive long enough for a family member to arrive. This raises tricky ethical and practical questions; however, it serves to underly the symbolic and real importance of loved-ones being together at death (Lederberg et al., 1990).

As death approaches it is useful to arrange a family meeting to field questions, provide information, and agree upon the goal and plan of care. If the patient is competent, consent must be sought. It is not uncommon in advanced cancer for the patient to be incompetent due to coma or delirium. However, most families want to be involved in decision-making, and to the extent that they are partners, but without compromising the patient's autonomy, dignity, or rights, their requests should be accommodated.

Generally, the mode of death can be anticipated and measures to prevent suffering outlined. The main fears of family are pain, shortness of breath, the 'death-rattle,' massive bleeding, and delirium. Often at this stage, the family make it clear that they do not want the patient to suffer. This indicates two things to the doctor: first, that they have accepted the inevitability of death; and second, that discussion regarding resuscitation can be broached at this point. Cardiopulmonary resuscitation is never appropriate in terminally ill patients with advanced untreatable cancer. This is based on the medical judgment that resuscitation will not be effective—it is futile (Cherny et al., 1996). No religious or ethical system demands resuscitation in the face of imminent and irreversible death. In respecting religious sensitivities, it is important to discuss with and assist the family in reconciling their belief system with the facts. Staff should be available to consult with clergy as requested. Using the paradigm of the Do-Not-Resuscitate law in New York, Lederberg (1997) emphasized the importance of supporting families and patients in coming to terms with death rather than enforcing legal positions. Making decisions about resuscitation is 'emotionally taxing and ... traumatizing and can result in strong and sustained, even years later, feeling of guilt and responsibility' (Lederberg, 1997).

Uncontrolled pain and inability to breathe are universal fears. The gurgling of accumulated secretions causing the 'death rattle' in an unconscious patient is not distressing to the patient, but is to the family. Delirium, with hallucinations, confusion, and aggressive behavior, is particularly frightening as it touches on the indignity of 'losing the mind.' Explanations are not treatment enough. It is usually possible to control these symptoms with standard medications and procedures; however, occasionally in the imminently dying, when symptoms are refractory, sedation to unconsciousness is the only way to relieve suffering. This is a situation which requires careful explanation to the patient (if appropriate), staff and family, and equally careful documentation. The ethical dilemma that must be explained to the family is that some clinicians are concerned that sedation might shorten life, and itself be short-hand for euthanasia. In appropriately selected patients, with open family discussion, and skillful, ethically-minded doctors, sedation of the terminally ill 'is an indicator of impending death and not a cause of premature death' (Stone et al., 1997). The US Supreme Court in 1997 unanimously ruled 'that there is no constitutional right to physician-assisted suicide ... [that] terminal sedation intended for symptom relief is not assisted suicide ... [and the Court] licensed an aggressive practice of palliative care' (Burt, 1997). Occasionally, family will ask whether an injection can be given to 'put the patient to sleep.' Mostly it expresses the desire to see the suffering end, although sometimes it reflects a persistent request for euthanasia. A clear message acknowledging the suffering and reassurances that all efforts are being made to relieve it are usually adequate. It may be necessary to emphasize that euthanasia is not legal and is not practiced.

Another ethical question that is frequently asked is the role of hydration and nutrition. In the terminally ill, each case must be evaluated on its merits and this must be explained faithfully to the family members. For example, intravenous fluid is not always appropriate if a patient is not making urine due to renal failure. Giving fluid in this situation merely exacerbates uncomfortable fluid retention and edema. On the other hand, dehydration is known to exacerbate delirium and fluid should be repleted. Nutrition holds a very important symbolic place in any nurturing situation. Tending to a loved one at the end of life recalls and replays caring at the beginning of life. Unfortunately, there is no evidence that nutrition plays any role in the terminally ill, either to prolong life or to improve its quality. This should be carefully but firmly communicated, preferably at a family meeting.

Doctors are notoriously poor at predicting the time of death. This can be frustrating to the family. As death becomes imminent it is incumbent upon the doctor and staff to be with the family, explaining and supporting. The symptoms of dying can be controlled, and although dying has taken days or weeks, the moment of death is always significant. It is preferable that one of the staff be with the family at the time of death. To those inexperienced, death, even when expected, is frightening. Nothing happens. Everything just stops. It is incomprehensible. Relatives, family, and friends should be encouraged to be present. Participation begets healing. Children of all ages can attend and should be encouraged to do so (Mount, 1998). The key point is that a responsible, supportive adult, whom the child trusts, should accompany and monitor the child. It is important to tell the parents that no harm will come and it will not lead to nightmares. However, many cultures are strongly against bringing children, in which case, after a simple explanation the issue should be put aside.

Religious rituals must be encouraged, as there is good evidence that by 'plugging in' to rituals and customs the believer is helped in terms of grief and mourning (Koenig and Gates-Williams, 1995). There is a wide variation both, individually and culturally, in immediate grief customs. Some people wail, faint, or sob in waves. Others scream and yet others cry silently. If there is no self-harm, it is important to give time for the rituals and customs to take their course, as they invariably do. It is wise to give significant latitude and let the family members reach their closure, rather than enforce a hospital rule of half an hour! Rarely do grievers require emergency psychiatric aid. Only if inappropriate violence occurs should security guards be called, initially to show their presence, and only then act if necessary.

BEREAVEMENT

Part of the management of families during terminal illness is to keep in mind bereavement. Screening for psychosocial problems and interactive support should be done with the aim of preparing the family to live without. Studies have confirmed that there is increased morbidity and mortality for bereaved spouses (Helsing and Szklo, 1981). Researchers have identified a number of prognostic factors that predict for difficult bereavement: social isolation; previous psychiatric illness; previous adverse grief experiences; substance abuse; unexpected deaths; ambivalent relationships with the deceased; repression of emotional expression; concurrent life crises; excessive anger, blame or idealization of deceased; enmeshed, disengaged or rigid family dynamics; prolonged and overwhelming grief; and forbidden grief, as with a mistress or ex-spouse (Mount, 1998; Helsing and Szklo, 1981). The great majority of families grieve, resolve, and continue their lives appropriately.

All medical units treating palliative oncology should have a procedure whereby telephone or personal contact, not merely via a letter, is made with an identified family member a week or two after death. There are two main reasons to contact family. The first is to screen the family and to offer an opportunity to them to express doubts, gratitude, and love. The conversation should aim to convey commiseration and sorrow; to allow for questions; to review the death and its immediate aftermath; encourage reorganization; and for the health carers to express positive, personal and private observations about the deceased. In particular, the sudden breach of the family from the staff is also a sense of loss, if not abandonment. During the terminal illness, intense and rapidly intimate bonds are forged with the staff as the illness becomes an all-consuming—time, emotional, physical—experience. For the family it is unique. For some family members, the loss and grief opens conflicts that were previously buried within the family dynamics. Now is a window of opportunity for psychotherapy before the quotidian routine of daily life represses the issues and the chance for insight is lost. It is equally important not to 'over-diagnose' a pathological bereavement. The second reason to contact family is to enable staff to disengage emotionally; to grieve; to find answers to issues that maybe could not be broached in life; to accept thanks; to appreciate, despite the pain, how much was in fact achieved;

and to resolve the loss before the next bereavement, lest there be unhealthy accumulation without adequate ventilation.

CONCLUSION

Not all families need active therapeutic interventions; however, all families need guidance, support, and empathy. The family experiences the cancer in three ways: as a vicarious, emotional response to the patient; as second-order patients; and finally as survivors who perpetuate the memories.

A frequent frustration is that we meet our patients when their characters and personalities are laden and distorted with the trauma of cancer. Pain, anxiety, surgery, disfigurement all change the person superficially and more significantly. As newcomers we often come to know the patient in a curious and reverse way through the honour, respect, and care proffered by family and friends. In a sense, a life is summarized. The innermost threads of the web of human relations provides the fabric of life. Within this summary, the patient and family have the opportunity to establish mental health along the lines of Antonovosky—that life should be meaningful, manageable, and comprehensible.

The health-care team with skill, curiosity, and caring are there to provide support if required. It is critically important for mental health and emotional growth that the health-care practitioner provides space for the family to reach the conclusions and difficult decisions themselves. It is in making these decisions, informed, supported and guided by the doctor, that understanding, acceptance, maturation, and insight will occur. Most families benefit from this approach at some level. Some need more space and room, others less. Occasionally, a family is so poorly functioning, with little cohesiveness and limited adaptability, that the health team must adopt an overwhelmingly paternalistic approach and orchestrate and choreograph proceedings rigidly. Most families learn and evolve, with a guiding hand.

The family is the centrepiece of palliative care in cancer. The trauma of cancer depends very much on who the patient is, the stage of life-cycle events, and the care and guidance the family receives from the caregivers. The caregivers are often invited into the family circle and given temporary membership. This is not only because of the importance of the role of the doctor and nurse, or out of judicious self-interest, but is due to the nature of the relationship. The intimacy irresistibly draws the doctor or nurse into the most private of domains. Traditionally, caregivers have been taught not to become emotionally involved, but rather to maintain a professional distance, lest objective assessment be lost. This caveat is well heeded. Nevertheless, the importance of drawing close is critical to the family as it honors the intimacy being offered the caregivers. For the caregivers it is, in the end, a rewarding experience. It is the riches of life itself. The caregiver, through good health and colleagial support, will re-establish. The family will be forever altered by the death of a loved one. The health-care profession has an opportunity to shape that response in a favorable way. A rare privilege indeed.

REFERENCES

Adams-Greenly, M., Beldoch, N. and Moynihan, R. (1986). Helping adolescents whose parents have cancer. *Seminars in Oncology Nursing* **2**: 133–138.

Addington-Hall, J.M., MacDonald, L.D. and Anderson, H.R. (1992). Randomized controlled trial of effects of coordinating care for terminally ill cancer patients. *British Medical Journal* **305**: 1317–1322.

American College of Physicians Health and Public Policy Committee (1983). Drug therapy for severe chronic pain in terminal illness. *Annals of Internal Medicine* **99**: 870–880.

Axelsson, B. and Sjoden, R.-O. (1998). Quality of life of cancer patients and their spouses in palliative home care. *Palliative Medicine* **12**: 29–39.

Bascom, P.B. and Tolle, S.W. (1995). Care of the family when the patient is dying. *Western Journal of Medicine* **163**: 292–296.

Buber, M. (1973). *I and Thou*. Edinburgh: T. and T. Clark.

Burt, R.A. (1996). The suppressed legacy of Nuremberg. *Hastings Center Report* **5**: 30–33.

Burt, R.A. (1997). The supreme court speaks. *New England Journal of Medicine* **337**: 1234–1236.

Cherny, N.I., Coyle, N. and Foley, K.M. (1996). Guidelines in the care of the dying patient. In N. I. Cherny and K. H. Foley (Eds), *Pain and Palliative Care: Hematology/Oncology Clinics of North America* Vol. 10, (pp. 261–286). Philadelphia: Saunders.

Chochinov, H.M., Wilson, K.G. and Enns, M. (1995). Desire for death in the terminally ill. *American Journal of Psychiatry* **152**: 1185–1191.

Davies, B., Reimer, J.C. and Martens, N. (1990). Families in supportive care. Part I: The transition of fading away: the nature of the transition. *Journal of Palliative Care* **6**: 12–20.

Davies, B., Reimer, J.C. and Martens, N. (1994). Family functioning and its implications for palliative care. *Journal of Palliative Care* **10**: 29–36.

Farkas, C. and Loscalzo, M. (1987). Death without indignity. In A.H. Kutscher, A. Carr and L.G. Kutscher (Eds), *Principles of Thanatology*, New York: Columbia University Press.

Foley, K.M. (1989). The decriminalization of cancer pain. In C.S. Hill and H. Field (Eds), *Drug Treatment of Cancer Pain in a Drug-orientated Society. Advances in Pain Research and Therapy* Vol. 11 (pp. 5–18). New York: Raven.

Helsing, K.J. and Szklo, M. (1981). Mortality after bereavement. *Epidemiological Review* **114**: 41–52.

Kaye, J.M. and Gracely, E.J. (1991). Psychological distress in cancer patients and their spouses. *Journal of Cancer Education* **8**: 47–52.

Kissane, D.W., Bloch, S., McKenzie, M., McDowall, A.C. and Nitzan, R. (1998). Family grief therapy: a preliminary account of a new model to promote healthy family functioning during palliative care and bereavement. *Psycho-Oncology* **7**: 14–25.

Koenig, B.A. and Gates-Williams, J. (1995). Understanding cultural difference in caring for dying patients. *Western Journal of Medicine* **163**: 244–249.

Kristjanson, L.J. (1996). The family as a unit of treatment. In R. Portenoy and E. Bruera (Eds), *Supportive Care Medicine* (pp. 245–263). New York: Oxford University Press.

Kristjanson, L.J., Nikoletti, S., Porock, D., Smith, M., Lobchuk, M. and Pedler, P. (1998). Congruence between patients' and family caregivers' perception of symptom distress in patients with terminal illness. *Journal of Palliative Care* **14**: 24–32.

Lederberg, M.S., Massie, M.J. and Holland, J.C. (1990). Psychiatric consultation to oncology. In A. Tasman, S.M. Goldfinger and C.A. Kaufman (Eds), *Review of Psychiatry* Vol. 9 (pp. 491–514). Washington. DC: American Psychiatric Press.

Lederberg, M.S. (1997). Doctors in limbo: the United States 'DNR' debate. *Psycho-Oncology* **6**: 321–328.

Leis, A.M., Kristjanson, L., Koop, P.M. and Laizner, A., Lev, E. and Benoliel, J.Q. (1997). Family health and their palliative care trajectory: a cancer research agenda. *Cancer Prevention and Control* **1**: 352–360.

McCorkle, R., Robinson, L. and Nuamah, I. (1998). The effects of home nursing care for patients during terminal illness on the bereaved's psychological distress. *Nursing Research* **47**: 2–10.

Merrill, D. and Mor, V. (1993). Pathways to hospital death among the oldest old. *Journal of Aging and Health* **8**: 206–212.

Mount, B. (1998). Communications in terminal illness. In N. MacDonald (Ed.), *Palliative Medicine* (pp. 226–245). New York: Oxford University Press.

Murinen, J.M. (1986). The economics of informal care: labor market effects in the national hospice study. *Medical Care* **24**: 1007–1017.

Musci, E.C. and Dodd, M.J. (1990). Predicting self-care with patients and family members' affective states and family functioning. *Oncology Nursing Forum* **17**: 394–400.

Olson, D.H., McCubbin, H.I. and Barnes, H.L. (1989). Predicting conflict with staff among families of cancer patients during prolonged hospitalizations. *Journal of Psychosocial Oncology* **7**: 103–111.

Rait, D. and Lederberg, M.S. (1989). The family of the cancer patient. In J.C. Holland and J.H. Rowland (Eds), *Handbook of Psycho-oncology* (pp. 585–597). New York: Oxford University Press.

Rhymes, J.A. (1991). Clinical management of the terminally ill. *Geriatrics* **46**: 57–62.

Siegel, K., Karus, D.G. and Raveis, V.H. (1996). Depressive distress among the spouses of terminally ill cancer patients. *Cancer Practitioner* **4**: 25–30.

Sourkes, B. (1997). Facilitating family coping with childhood cancer. *Journal of Paediatric Cancer* **2**: 65–67.

Steele, L.L. (1990). The death surround: factors influencing the grief experience of survivors. *Oncology Nursing Forum* **17**: 235–241.

Stone, P., Phillips, C. and Spruyt, O. (1997). A comparison of the use of sedatives in a hospital support team and in a hospice. *Palliative Medicine* **11**: 140–144.

Tolle, S.W. and Girard, D.W. (1982). The physician's role in the events surrounding patient death. *Archives of Internal Medicine* **143**: 1447–1449.

Vess, J.D., Moreland, J.R. and Schwebel, A.L. (1985). An empirical assessment of the effects of cancer on the family role-functioning. *Journal of Psychosocial Oncology* **3**: 1–16.

Wein, S. (1999). Cancer. In R.G. Robinson and W.R. Yates (Eds), *Psychiatric Treatment of the Medically Ill*, (pp. 229–252). New York: Marcel Dekker.

Weisman, A.D., Worden, J.W. and Sobel, H.J. (1980). *Psychosocial Screening and Interventions with Cancer Patients: A Research Report.* Boston, MA: Harvard Medical School and Massachusetts General Hospital.

Whall, A.L. (1986). The family as the unit of care in nursing: a historical review. *Public Health Nursing* **3**: 240–249.

Wingo, P.A., Tong, T. and Bolden, S. (1995). Cancer statistics, 1995. *CA—A Cancer Journal for Clinicians* **45**: 8–30.

World Health Organization (1990). *Cancer Pain Relief and Palliative Care.* Geneva, World Health Organization.

Zabora, R.J. and Loscalzo, M.J. (1998). Psychosocial consequences of advanced cancer. In A.M. Berger, R.K. Portenoy and D.E. Weissman (Eds), *Principles and Practice of Supportive Oncology*, (pp. 531–548). Philadelphia, PA: Lippincott–Raven.

25

Religion, Cancer, and the Family

BERNARD SPILKA and SCOTT HARTMAN

Department of Psychology, University of Denver, Denver, CO, USA

It is not amiss to call cancer 'the scourge of the twentieth century'. To speak the word 'cancer' is to elicit images of death and disability (Curbow, 1986). Currently, however, 60% of patients survive at least 5 years, as opposed to 40 years ago when only 39% lived this long. Even at the millennium, with treatments proliferating, diagnosis is ahead of prevention and cure. This may, in part, account for the finding that cancer death rates are now higher than 30 years ago (American Cancer Society, 1998). Still, advances in treatment have often extended survival for many years, where previously the course of the disease may have been measured in months (American Cancer Society, 1998).

Statistics frequently convey a false impression. They imply that a patient is 'a statistic,' identifying cancer as primarily an individual tragedy. Today, it is increasingly seen as having familial roots and repercussions. The estimated 1.2 million new cases diagnosed in the USA in 1998 were rarely of isolated individuals. They are, as a rule, our nearest kin—somebody's son or daughter, sister or brother, mother or father. Simply put, cancer is a family illness.

Ever earlier detection and treatment of cancer have both positive and negative consequences. On the one hand, there is a greater likelihood of full recovery—on the other, increased therapeutic concerns and protracted periods of possible debilitation and handicap. These factors, along with the high heritability of many forms of the malady, emphasize that cancer will probably involve the entire family.

Just as the individual commonly resides within a family framework, the family is embedded in a cultural setting. It is thus affected by society's major cultural institutions. Central among these is religion, and it is known that the threat of cancer can be influenced by the way religion is employed within the family (Pargament, 1997). It must be understood at the beginning that religious adherence varies greatly. Even though, in the USA, most people assert a belief in God (95–97%), state that they pray (89%), and claim affiliation with religious institutions (63%), these and similar data do not actually reflect a comparably high level of devotion and personal involvement on the part of most Americans (Hood et al., 1996). The inclination, however, is present for increased ardor and piety when crisis strikes. This is the usual state of affairs families and patients confront when the diagnosis is cancer. Such a

Cancer and the Family, 2nd Edn. Edited by L. Baider, C. L. Cooper and A. Kaplan De-Nour
© 2000 John Wiley & Sons, Ltd

faith is largely extrinsic, functional, and utilitarian. In fact, it performs as desired, although not as effectively as an intrinsic dedication, in which there is a deep personal commitment to religious doctrines (Hood et al., 1996).

STRESS, CANCER AND THE IMMUNE SYSTEM

The core factor mediating familial responses to cancer is stress. Its effects are both physical and psychological, and are likely to influence both the patient and those close to the patient. In other words, stress pervades the family. We contend that the essential role of religion in these circumstances is to reduce such stress.

Among the more destructive effects of stress is its tendency to compromise the immune systems of all who must deal with this dilemma. Such immunosuppression increases the probability of more ill-health developing within the family. A circular pattern of worsening stress expectedly strains the coping resources of those connected to the patient (Bieliauskas, 1982).

The relatively new field of psychoneuroimmunology (PNI) studies the complex relationships between the various body systems—immune, nervous, and endocrine—involved in this 'collaborative informational network' (Pert, 1997). The detailed interaction of these systems with stress and emotion has been explicated elsewhere (Cohen and Herbert, 1996). Familial and individual strengths and weaknesses tie family members together in a matrix of mutual stressful influence that can greatly exacerbate both physical and psychological difficulties. Factors in this matrix that have been researched are genetic predispositions, poor health practices, depression, repression/denial, and pessimism, among others (Cohen and Herbert, 1996). There is also evidence that the equipping of individuals with resources to combat stress leads to significantly healthier outcomes for cancer patients (Leventhal et al., 1984). Research with metastatic breast cancer patients and others suffering from malignant melanoma reveal the considerable benefits of religious/spiritual supportive interventions on the operation of immune system defenses, quality of survival, longevity, and level of suffering (Fawzy et al., 1993).

Like the person diagnosed with cancer, the family has a prognosis regarding their well-being in response to the disease. Immunosuppression, sickness, and mental health correlates, such as anxiety and depression, are natural reactions to the stressful ordeal of cancer within the family setting.

RESPONDING TO CANCER AS POST-TRAUMATIC STRESS SYNDROME

Acute, chronic, and delayed stress responses to cancer in the family have recently been viewed as a form of Post-traumatic Stress Disorder (PTSD)(Kazak, 1998). This is especially true for long-term survivors. In terms of established PTSD stages and symptoms, the analogy is by no means far-fetched. It ties some reactions to cancer (nightmares, fears/phobias, anxiety) to a broader diagnostic framework, and permits insights from extensive experience with PTSD to be applied to work with cancer patients and their families.

A variety of treatment modes have been employed with PTSD, which appear relevant to cancer. Not the least of these involve spiritual and religious content and methods, particularly when depression and guilt are present (Green et al., 1998).

Because pastoral counseling is common in cancer, it has been suggested that clergy be trained to recognize PTSD and to utilize pastoral techniques that have shown promise with PTSD (Jimenez, 1993; Weaver et al., 1996). Although pastoral approaches usually stress the attainment of meaning and perspective, there are indications that the prime factor in PTSD may be empowerment; hence, treatment should also be directed at issues of mastery and control (Ell et al., 1989; Jimenez, 1993).

THE ROLE OF RELIGION

WHAT RELIGION DOES

There is a saying: 'When misery is the greatest, God is the closest' (Gross, 1982, p. 242). This is the time that 'God . . . is not understood; he is used' (James, 1902, p. 506). The need is for aid, and to the supplicant, the time may be past when human intervention is adequate. Something more is needed, and that more to religious people is the ultimate source of help—God.

The prime question concerns what religion and God-belief does for the patient and family when cancer strikes. We suggest that three basic needs, and possibly a fourth, are met. These are for meaningful information, for increased control and for the sustaining influence of others. A need to view oneself in positive terms, namely self-esteem, may be a result of meeting these more basic wants. In other words, religion offers to those who suffer: (a) meanings that convey hope and the potential of success; (b) increased power to counter the helplessness that accompanies despair, pain, and anguish; and (c) aid from others. Participating in religious activities such as prayer also encourages the belief that one is engaged in behavior that is effective. This framework has been extensively discussed elsewhere (Hood et al., 1996). It is specifically focused here on the family's efforts to cope with cancer.

RELIGION AS A COPING MECHANISM IN DEALING WITH CANCER

The Importance of Meaning

Fichter (1981) asserts that 'Religious reality is the only way to make sense out of pain and suffering' (p. 20). In part, this is confirmed by the research of Ersek and Ferrell (1994), who found that the meaning-making process involving one's faith is an important aspect of coping with pain from cancer. Establishing such meaning poses a quandary for cancer patients, as well as for family caregivers. The 'Why me?' question is generally left unsatisfied by naturalistic explanations, whereas religious answers are often more emotionally pleasing. A cancer patient in one of our studies illustrated this principle in a representative comment: 'I had no idea God could answer so many of my questions' (Johnson and Spilka, 1991, p. 30). Our observations confirm those of Ashbrook (1967), that 'No other sickness forces this dimension on us as cancer' (p. 69).

The search for meaning can also be distressing. One may see cancer as self-caused, the consequence of personal actions, for example smoking. When religious coping is employed, 'God's will' is one of the most frequently cited causes given by patients and family members (Taylor, 1995). In relatively rare instances, 'God's will' is punishment via cancer for sinful behavior (Burish et al., 1987). Among cancer patients, however, the dominant tendency is to invoke God as healer and not as the cause of cancer. Reluctance to blame God is transformed into 'God had a reason,' and whatever the reason is, it is regarded as right and proper. Although there has been some disagreement in the research, cancer is usually associated with increased religiosity (Moschella et al., 1997), which, in turn, engenders an enhanced sense of hope, and heightened well-being (Acklin et al., 1983; Galloway, 1995). Generally, religious ideas are paramount in the selection and creation of meanings that portend a positive resolution to the dilemma of cancer (Jenkins and Pargament, 1995).

The Role of Control

An oft-stated purpose of seeking meaning has been to control the outcomes of personal encounters with life's vicissitudes (Spilka et al., 1985). Jenkins and Pargament (1995) point out that religion may furnish meanings 'that control over cancer exists [and] may motivate efforts to seek control through interchange with God' (p. 62). This view is confirmed by Koenig (1994), who observed how faith counters depression in cancer via hopeful meanings that portend an increased sense of control.

The beneficial effects of personal autonomy and control in illness and cancer have been extensively documented (Lefcourt and Davidson-Katz, 1991; Taylor et al., 1984). Control, however, is a complex phenomenon. It may involve changing the conditions to which one is subject or turning inward to alter the way reality is perceived. Relative to cancer, patients and family members may take an active role in their own care and treatment plus volunteering to aid other families (Hill et al., 1986). Still, the feeling that one has lost all semblance of control often prevails in cancer (Burish et al., 1987). This may support the use of an external source of mastery, such as religion and, vicariously, God.

Changing one's self-image to perceive a sense of mastery counters depression and pessimism (Thompson et al., 1993). In a 17 year follow-up of cancer patients, a low sense of control along with depression correlated positively with mortality (Shekelle et al., 1981). The feeling of control religion sponsors is also associated with a greater sense of life's meaning, less despair, and less denial (Acklin et al., 1983).

A form of self-modification observed with breast cancer is termed 'positive reframing'—seeing the situation in the best light (Carver et al., 1993). This has been demonstrated in the making of 'downward' social comparisons. Women with breast cancer feel better when they can infer that others in similar straits are actually in worse condition than they (Wood et al., 1985). Overall, the more one uses religion to cope with cancer, the greater the likelihood of positive reframing (Carver et al., 1993). In addition, the role of prayer should not be overlooked as a means of increasing one's sense of control when under the stress of cancer (Hood et al., 1996; Johnson and Spilka, 1991).

The Role of Social Support

Like meaning and control, the need for others appears to be essential for survival and well-being. Evidence for the beneficial effects of social support for cancer patients and their families, in general, and specifically via religion, is overwhelming (Ell et al., 1989; Pargament, 1997). Spiritual support for family caregivers does reduce stress (Carson, 1997). The greater the religious commitment of the family, the more information is disseminated within the family and to close friends. There are, however, indications of a narrowing of the social field beyond these groups, with less information imparted to outside-others. Religion may thus serve a defensive-protective function that permits family members to cope more effectively with their predicament. Such restriction could minimize external sources of additional stress (Spilka et al., 1991).

The fact that social support, along with faith, also contributes to the attainment of meaning adds to its significance among cancer patients (O'Connor et al., 1990). Social support is also a solid predictor of spiritual well-being among those with cancer (Pace and Stables, 1997). One mechanism here may be that others act as sources of information that aid the creation of gratifying meanings.

A number of studies further reveal that immune system responses of both cancer patients and their spouses are positively related to social support (Baron et al., 1990). Insofar as formal religion and religious institutions provide support, one can expect favorable health effects (Hood et al., 1996).

The Role of Self-esteem

Well over a half century of research demonstrates that having information as opposed to ambiguity, a sense of control in contrast to feelings of helplessness, and being favorably regarded by others contribute to self-esteem (Wylie, 1979). Research findings also indicate that self-perceptions mediate psychological adjustment among cancer patients (Heidrich et al., 1994). Significant elements here are the achievement of meaning and a sense that one possesses control relative to one's cancer (Lewis, 1989).

RELIGION AS A STRESSOR AND A COUNTER TO STRESS

Some aspects of religion can be 'hazardous' to one's health. Much commentary and some research has indicted rigid fundamentalist outlooks and upbringing as sources of abnormal mental content (Hood et al., 1996). Pruyser (1977) claims that religious doctrines contain meanings that are at variance with reality, and cause what he termed a 'sacrifice of intellect.' Sometimes, simplistic polarizations (e.g., good vs. bad, etc.) may prevent proper understanding and treatment of ill-health. Invoking 'God's will' may then represent little more than pathological thinking (Hood et al., 1996).

In parallel, religion can be a source of abnormal motivation and cognition. Obsession with sin and guilt may stimulate bizarre thinking and behavior (Frank-Stromborg et al., 1984). This is representative of a wide variety of unrealistic attributions that ordinarily result from a combination of desperation with a pathological sense of sin.

Although religion has been overwhelmingly associated with effective coping with cancer, it may sometimes be distorted and employed inappropriately. In such circumstances, pastoral counseling might help the disturbed individual adapt in a more constructive manner (Mays, 1977).

INSTITUTIONAL RELIGION AND CANCER

Although the foregoing functions of religion seem to be the most significant, we are not suggesting that they are the only ones. Faith can buttress the immune system in other, more indirect, ways. Immune function may be enhanced through institutional religious backing for various health practices. The Church of Jesus Christ of Latter Day Saints (Mormons) has always strongly promoted good health and food practices, including proscriptions against the use of coffee, alcohol, and tobacco. The 'Mormon state,' Utah, has consistently demonstrated the lowest cancer death rates in the USA (American Cancer Society, 1998). In addition, religious beliefs and church involvement correlate positively with a reduced incidence of cancer (Jenkins, 1991).

CANCER, THE FAMILY, AND RELIGION

THE FAMILY AS A SOCIAL SYSTEM

Families are functional systems of relationships. The interplay between spouses, parents and children, and among the children themselves are part of an organized pattern of interdependencies. We will distinguish a few of these for the purposes of expedient illustration.

Regardless of who develops cancer, there are fairly general responses to its diagnosis (e.g., fear of death/pain/disfigurement, anxiety, depression, etc.). Still, each social position within the family—mother, father, husband, wife, adult, child, son, daughter—carries with it special burdens due to traditional familial roles. Parents as patients necessarily worry about the effects of heavy financial demands, inability to fulfill everyday responsibilities, separation in the hospital, creating severe emotional stresses on others, and becoming dependent on those who previously relied on them. Affectional relationships may be grievously strained as children witness the formerly powerful parent become weak and subordinate. Further, parents now have to relate differently to each other. Schedules are disrupted and new constraints on time interfere with old commitments. In sum, the family system goes through an extended period of reorganization as the afflicted individual experiences painful and taxing procedures—surgery, chemotherapy, radiation, and possible debility and decline. Ambivalence, where anger and bitterness alternate with fear and anxiety, continually intrudes and creates frustration and conflict, with depressing and unsettling consequences (Rosenbaum, 1975).

CANCER AND SPOUSAL RELATIONS

The family begins with the union of two individuals in which a secure attachment is normally based on love and affection. The diagnosis of cancer poses the direst of threats to this relationship; the image of death is ever-present. Studies of spouses with cancer, whether one or both are afflicted, reveal equally high levels of distress in the patient with the cancer and the healthy spouse (Baider et al., 1998). Spousal support *per se* apparently counters depressive responses that ordinarily develop in these trying circumstances (Blanchard et al., 1996).

Breast cancer in women is one of the most common cancers threatening the spousal relationship. Northouse (1989) found that survival concerns dominated the thoughts of both spouses following a mastectomy. Religion was a significant source of strength at this time, particularly in the hospital setting, where it seemed to mitigate anxiety. In other work, religion performed a similar function among early breast cancer patients, encouraging positive reframing as one form of active coping with their misfortunes (Carver et al., 1993). A spiritual outlook also correlates positively with a woman's willingness to be emotionally supportive of others in the same predicament (Kurtz et al., 1995).

In general, those favorably oriented towards their faith frequently benefit from religious involvement and connections—clergy visits, participation in public and private prayer and ritual, plus similar activities on their behalf by fellow parishioners (Johnson and Spilka, 1991; Spilka et al., 1983). Specifically, spiritual support countered feelings of hopelessness. A new sense of life's meaning was conveyed and reinforced via such religious 'growth' (Ferrell et al., 1998). Formal religion actually enters the picture in the diagnostic process, as church attendance correlates with better mammography status, even when income and education are controlled (Fox et al., 1998). It is possible that interactions among like-minded women within a church setting purvey meanings about cancer that stimulate preventive actions and early detection.

Most women outlive their husbands, hence loss of the latter from cancer generally occurs after many years of marriage. When cancer takes the husband, religious meanings, activities, and social support are especially noteworthy. They mitigate depression and subjective discomfort, and strengthen immune system function (Glick et al., 1974; Hood et al., 1996; Uchino et al., 1996). The chief mechanism here is social support from church-affiliated women's groups.

WHEN A PARENT HAS CANCER

The majority of the research on parents with cancer focuses on the mother, and breast cancer is the chief form studied. The illness invariably disrupts the maternal role in the home. Explaining this to young children is difficult. In multiple-child families, different understandings can lead to apprehension and confusion, especially among the youngest. Adolescent daughters are particularly anxious that they may carry a genetic propensity for breast cancer. In addition, during a period when teenage girls are gaining independence, they may be forced back into the home to take over various motherly duties (National Cancer Institute, 1980). Even younger children may become caregivers, reversing typical family roles. The church is regarded as an important source of reinforcement and support for the child's new duties (Gates and Lackey, 1998).

Children evidence a variety of fears—of death, separation, that cancer is contagious, that they may have caused the cancer, and that their lives will be changed for the worse. Associated with these concerns are a number of complicating responses, including anger at the sick parent. This may also be misplaced on the other parent and siblings. Seeing parental unhappiness and crying often elicits sadness and guilt. Feelings of isolation and separation are prevalent when the mother is hospitalized or goes for therapy. Finally, there is curiosity about not only the condition, but treatment, mastectomy, and their effects (Brzy and Ircink, 1998). God may perform as a surrogate in such conditions.

Despite early, often graphic, evidence of stress and anxiety affecting the children, the place of religion in this process is unclear, as empirical research is apparently lacking. Hart and Schneider (1997), however, propose a potentially useful guide for assessing and working with the spiritual needs of children. Placing behavioral signs of disturbed thinking and relationships in a religio-spiritual conceptual framework, they treat illness, pain, and death by emphasizing God, forgiveness, love, and afterlife ideas. The main issue is one of meaning and understanding. This is made appropriate for children of different ages via the developmental theories of Piaget, Erikson, and Fowler.

THE CHILD AS PATIENT

The thought of a child with cancer tears at the heart of our expectations about life. The core of the family, if not its primary purpose, is threatened. To comprehend in personal and human terms why a child may be stricken with cancer severely tests one's faith, yet religious answers often bring solace (Fichter, 1981).

Communication and Knowledge

When a diagnosis of cancer in a child is conveyed to parents, the initial problem concerns what knowledge is to be imparted to the child, his/her siblings, and others. Protecting the patient from the worst fears of the parents poses a serious dilemma. Considering the likelihood of hospitalization, a high probability of painful and invasive medical procedures, exposure to medical professionals, and other children in similar circumstances, it comes as no surprise that by age six, the child patient is well aware of the seriousness of the illness (Spinetta and Maloney, 1978). Most parents feel that they have communicated this information to the patient. To a lesser degree, patients and siblings agree that they have been told. Questions, of course, arise relative to how well those who are informed understand what they have been told (Zwartjes et al., 1979).

The Experiences and Feelings of Children with Cancer

That cancer is an extremely stressful experience for children goes without saying. It is a time of 'separation fears, loss of self-esteem, fear of mutilation . . . strange, painful procedures, frequent monitoring of bodily functions, tearful or tense facial expressions, secret conversations between parents and physicians, etc.' (Issner, 1972, p. 129). Anxiety about the sickness, its treatment, and potential death prevail. Although patient age is important, anxieties about these matters are expressed by children and adolescents of all ages. The dominant response to the diagnosis appears to be depression (Spilka et al., 1991).

The fundamental dilemma confronting these young people has been described as one of mastery and meaning (Hart and Schneider, 1997; Spinetta, 1977). Religious and spiritual resources have been recommended as means of meeting these needs (Hart and Schneider, 1997). Such seem to work, as religion counters fear, anger, and denial in these young patients (Spilka et al., 1991). The stronger the faith of the children, the more they feel they truly understand their condition. Coles (1990) describes the use of prayer, ritual, and Biblical readings with and by fairly young children, some terminally ill with cancer. This age group strongly believes that prayer is efficacious in enhancing control. For the very young who are troubled, the proposal has been made that pastoral counselors might utilize play therapy (Webb, 1991).

Denial has also been considered an adaptive coping mechanism for children with cancer (Derevensky et al., 1998). Apparently religion constructively aids this process (Pargament, 1997).

The Effects of Child Cancer on Parents

The diagnosis of cancer in a child is devastating to parents. Fearing the worst, virtually every undesirable reaction that can be conceived seems at one time or another to have been reported. This litany ranges from anxiety and depression to extreme marital distress (Enskar et al., 1997; Grootenhuis and Last, 1997; Hayout and Krulik, 1999; Leyn, 1976).

Social support and religion are repeatedly cited as resources for these disturbed families (Cook and Wimberly, 1983). Again, the issues are to make sense out of what has occurred, and somehow to gain a sense of control, not only of the child's ailment, but of parental relationships (Spilka et al., 1991).

The Effects of Child Cancer on Siblings

It seems anti-climactic to note the effects of childhood cancer on siblings, but considerable study has concentrated on what too often seems to be these almost forgotten family members when a child is struck by cancer.

In addition to the symptoms already listed for parents and patients in these pages, a few stand out among siblings. Not the least among these emphasize death. The hospital is likely to be viewed as a place of death. This sometimes relates to the development of an extreme fear of death. When a patient dies, pathological ideas may be expressed by the siblings. In one case, an identical twin was obsessed with joining his brother in death. This was associated with teeth grinding during sleep, sleep walking and talking. An older sibling vehemently blamed his parents for passing on a cancer gene to all of their children (Kaplan et al., 1972). Signs of shock, depression, guilt, denial, anger, and a variety of psychosomatic symptoms also put in an appearance. Ambivalence is likely to accompany the sense that parental attention has shifted toward the patient and away from the sibling (Zwartjes et al., 1979). These feelings may be realistic, as the presence of physical and psychological symptoms that would normally result in health care for the sibling are much less likely to do so when another child has cancer (Zeltzer et al., 1996). Familial religion performs a stabilizing function, bracing siblings against disruptive and stressful forces. Faith unifies the family and, as much as possible, maintains pre-illness behavior and performance on the part of the patient, siblings, and the parents themselves (Spilka et al., 1991).

CONCLUSIONS

Even though a considerable literature has been examined here, empirical research explicitly dealing with religious variables and cancer is rare. If one discusses social support or demographic factors, religion is frequently overlooked, or is not specified as possible content in the measures used. In one review of over 250 articles on psychosocial factors relating to cancer, a total of four studies treat religion, and in only two did religion receive more than a few words of explication (Cwikel et al., 1997). On the other hand, 'talk' papers averring the importance of religion abound. These, as a rule, speak less to cancer than to illness-in-general, and bereavement. Here is an area crying for research.

Studies examining issues of meaning are treated similarly. The significance of religion for endowing cancer, pain, death, etc. with meaning has been repeatedly demonstrated (Fichter, 1981; Hood et al., 1996; Taylor, 1995). Still, when efforts are made to assess meaning, the presence of religious content or the use of religious/spiritual items is rarely noted. Given these propensities, the role of faith is often more hypothetically suggestive than conclusive.

The evidence reviewed in these pages reinforces the view that religion and God-belief are active players in both individual and family trials with cancer. In most instances, the outcomes have been helpful and constructive; in relatively few cases, faith has been distorted and employed to create a pathology of meaning.

Customarily, when a family assimilates their misfortune into pre-existing religious notions, they essentially imbue the crisis with hope. Hope is an over-riding meaning that has been joined in research on cancer to religion, social support, and control (Bunston et al., 1995; Johnson and Spilka, 1991). Through these avenues, a broad spectrum of maladaptive and negative emotions and behavior are countered. Religion, *per se*, may well be the mobilizing force behind these coping efforts (Pargament, 1997). Given this likelihood, we believe that clergy might create an especially effective pastoral counseling methodology for those to whom faith is important. Finally, we recommend that a theoretically directed research program be undertaken to study the family as a unit using the guidelines suggested above.

REFERENCES

Acklin, M.W., Brown, E.C. and Mauger, P.A. (1983).   The role of religious values in coping with cancer. *Journal of Religion and Health* 22: 322–333.

American Cancer Society (1998).   *Cancer Facts and Figures—1998.* New York: American Cancer Society.

Ashbrook, J.B. (1967).   The impact of the hospital situation in our understanding of God and man. In D. Belgum (Ed.), *Religion and Medicine: Essays on Meanings, Values, and Health* (pp. 61–80). Ames, IA: Iowa State University Press.

Baider, L., Walach, N. Perry. S. and Kaplan De-Nour, A. (1998).   Cancer in married couples: higher or lower distress? *Journal of Psychosomatic Research* **45**(3): 239–248.

Baron, R.S., Cutrona, C.E., Hicklin, D., Russell, D.W. and Lubaroff, D.M. (1990). Social support and immune function among spouses of cancer patients. *Journal of Personality and Social Psychology* **59**: 344–352.

Bieliauskas, L.A. (1982). *Stress and Its Relationship to Health and Illness*. Boulder, CO: Westview.

Blanchard, C.G., Toseland, R.W. and McCallion, P. (1996). The effects of a problem-solving intervention with spouses of cancer patients. *Journal of Psychosocial Oncology* **14**(2): 1–22.

Brzy, J. and Ircink, M. (1998). Breast cancer: Common reactions of children and how to help. University of Wisconsin Internet site (http://www2.medsch.wisc.edu/childrenshosp/childrens.html).

Bunston, T., Mings, D., Mackie, A. and Jones, D. (1995). Facilitating hopefulness: the determinants of hope. *Journal of Psychosocial Oncology* **13**(4): 79–103.

Burish, T.G., Meyerowitz, B.E., Carey, M.P. and Morrow, G.R. (1987). The stressful effects of cancer in adults. In A. Baum and J.E. Singer (Eds), *Handbook of Psychology and Health. Vol. 5: Stress* (pp. 137–173). New York: Hillsdale.

Carson, V. B. (1997). Spiritual care: the needs of the caregiver. *Seminars in Oncology Nursing* **13**(4): 271–274.

Carver, C.S., Pozo, C., Harris, S.D., Noriega, V., Scheier, M.F., Robinson, D.S., Ketcham, A.S., Moffat, F.L. Jr and Clark, K.C. (1993). How coping mediates the effect of optimism on distress: a study of women with early stage breast cancer. *Journal of Personality and Social Psychology* **65**: 375–390.

Cohen, S. and Herbert, T.B. (1996). Health psychology: psychological factors and physical disease from the perspective of human psychoneuroimmunology. In J.T. Spence, J.M. Darley and D.J. Foss (Eds), *Annual Review of Psychology*, Vol. **47** (pp. 113–142). Palo Alto, CA: Annual Reviews.

Coles, R. (1990). *The Spiritual Life of Children*. Boston, MA: Houghton Mifflin.

Cook, T. and Wimberly, D. (1983). If I should die before I wake: religious commitment and adjustment to the death of a child. *Journal for the Scientific Study of Religion* **22**: 222–238.

Curbow, B., Andrews, R.M. and Burke, T.A. (1986). Perceptions of the cancer patient: causal explanations and personal attributions. *Journal of Psychosocial Oncology* **4**: 115–134.

Cwikel, J.G., Behar, L.C. and Zabora, J.R. (1997). Psychosocial factors that affect the survival of adult cancer patients: a review of research. *Journal of Psychosocial Oncology* **15**(3/4): 1–34.

Derevensky, J.L., Tsanos, A.P. and Handman, M. (1998). Children with cancer: an examination of their coping and adaptive behavior. *Journal of Psychosocial Oncology* **16**(1): 37–61.

Ell, K.O., Mantell, J.E., Haimovitch, M.B. and Nishimoto, R.H. (1989). Social support, sense of control, and coping among patients with breast, lung, or colorectal cancer. *Journal of Psychosocial Oncology* **7**: 63–89.

Enskar, K., Carlsson, M., Golsater, M., Hamrin, E. and Kreuger, A., (1997). Parental reports of changes and challenges that result from parenting a child with cancer. *Journal of Pediatric Oncology Nursing* **14**(3): 156–163.

Ersek, M. and Ferrell, B.R. (1994). Providing relief from cancer pain by assisting in the search for meaning. *Journal of Palliative Care* **10**(4): 15–22.

Fawzy, F.I., Fawzy, N.W., Hyun, C.S., Elashoff, R. and Guthrie, D. (1993). Malignant melanoma: effects of an early structured psychiatric intervention, coping, and affective state on recurrence and survival six years later. *Archives of General Psychiatry* **50**: 681–689.

Ferrell, B.R., Grant, N., Funk, B., Otis-Green, S. and Garcia, N. (1998). Quality of life in breast cancer. Part II: Psychological and spiritual well-being. *Cancer Nursing* **21**(1): 1–9.

Fichter, J.H. (1981). *Religion and Pain*. New York: Crossroads.

Fox, S.A., Pitkin, K., Paul, C. and Duan, N. (1998). Breast cancer screening adherence: does church attendance matter? *Health Education and Behavior* **25**: 742–758.

Frank-Stromborg, M., Wright, P.S., Segalla, M. and Diekman, J. (1984). Psychosocial impact of the cancer diagnosis. *Oncology Nursing Forum* **11**: 16–22.

Galloway, A.L. (1995, 9 June). Religiosity, quality of life and control in cancer patients. Unpublished Doctoral dissertation, Graduate School of Professional Psychology, University of Denver, CO.

Gates, M.F. and Lackey, N.R. (1998). Youngsters caring for adults with cancer. *Image: Journal of Nursing Scholarship* **30**(1): 11–15.

Glick, I.O., Weiss, R.A. and Parkes, C.M. (1974). *The First Year of Bereavement*. New York: John Wiley.

Green, B.L., Lindy, J.D. and Grace, M.C. (1998). Long-term coping with combat stress. *Journal of Traumatic Stress* **1**: 399–412.

Grootenhuis, M.A. and Last, B.F. (1997). Parents' emotional reactions related to different prospects for the survival of their children with cancer. *Journal of Psychosocial Oncology* **15**(1): 43–62.

Gross, L. (1982). *The Last Jews in Berlin*. New York: Simon and Schuster.

Hart, D. and Schneider, D. (1997). Spiritual care for children with cancer. *Seminars in Oncology Nursing* **13**(4): 263–270.

Hayout, I. and Krulik, T. (1999). A test of parenthood: dilemmas of parents of terminally ill adolescents. *Cancer Nursing* **22**(1): 71–79.

Heidrich, S.M., Forsthoff, C.A. and Ward, S.E. (1994). Psychological adjustment in cancer patients: The self as mediator. *Health Psychology* **13**: 346.

Hill, A.F., Hamilton, P.K., & Ringer, L. (1986). *I'm A Patient, Too*. New York: Nick Lyon Books.

Hood, R.W. Jr, Spilka, B., Hunsberger, B. and Gorsuch, R.L. (1996). *The Psychology of Religion: An Empirical Approach*. New York: Guilford.

Issner, N. (1972, June 22–24). Can the child be distracted from his disease? In *Proceedings of The American Cancer Society* (pp. 129–133). Atlanta, GA: American Cancer Society.

James, W. (1902). *Varieties of Religious Experience*. New York: Longmans, Green.

Jenkins, R.A. (1991). Toward a psychosocial conceptualization of religion as a resource in cancer care and prevention. *Prevention in Human Services* **10**: 91–105.

Jenkins, R.A. and Pargament, K.I. (1995). Religion and spirituality as resources for coping with cancer. *Journal of Psychosocial Oncology* **13**, 51–74.

Jimenez, M.J. (1993). The spiritual healing of post-traumatic stress disorder at the Menlo Park Veteran's Hospital. *Studies in Formative Spirituality* **14**(2): 175–187.

Johnson, S. and Spilka, B. (1991). Religion and the breast cancer patient: the roles of clergy and faith. *Journal of Religion and Health* **30**: 21–33.

Kaplan, D.M., Smith, A. and Grobstein, R. (1972, June 22–24). The problems of siblings. In *Proceedings of The American Cancer Society* (pp. 140–143). Atlanta, GA.

Kazak, A.E. (1998). Post-traumatic distress in childhood cancer survivors and their parents. *Medical and Pediatric Oncology* **1** (Suppl.): 60–68.

Koenig, H.G. (1994). *Aging and God: Spiritual Pathways to Mental Health in Midlife and Later Years*. New York: Haworth.

Kurtz, M.E., Wyatt, G. and Kurtz, J.C. (1995). Psychological and sexual well-being, philosophical/spiritual views, and health habits of long-term cancer survivors. *Nursing* **16**(3): 253–262.

Lefcourt, H.M. and Davidson-Katz, K. (1991). Locus of control and health. In C.R. Snyder and D.R. Forsyth (Eds.), *Handbook of Social and Clinical Psychology* (pp. 246–266). New York: Pergamon.

Leventhal, H., Nerenz, D.R. and Steele, D.J., 1984). Illness representations and coping with health threats. In A. Baum, S.E. Taylor and J.E. Singer (Eds), *Handbook of Psychology and Health*, Vol. IV (pp. 219–252). Hillsdale, NJ: Erlbaum.

Lewis, F.M. (1989). Attributions of control, experienced meaning, and psychosocial well-being in patients with advanced cancer. *Journal of Psychosocial Oncology* **7**(1/2): 105.

Leyn, R.M. (1976). Terminally ill children and their families: a study of the variety of responses to fatal illness. *Maternal–Child Nursing Journal* **5**: 179–188.

Mays, L.H. (1977, September 7–9). Cancer management: the role of the clergy. In *Proceedings of the American Cancer Society Second National Conference on Human Values and Cancer* (pp. 122–127). New York: American Cancer Society.

Moschella, V.D., Pressman, K.R., Pressman, P. and Weissman, D.E. (1997). The problem of theodicy and religious response to cancer. *Journal of Religion and Health* **36**: 17–20.

National Cancer Institute (1980). *The Breast Cancer Digest.* NIH Publication No. 81-1691. Bethesda, MD: National Cancer Institute.

Northouse, L.L. (1989). The impact of breast cancer on patients and husbands. *Cancer Nursing* **12**(5): 276–284.

O'Connor, A.P., Wicker, C.A. and Germino, B.R. (1990). Understanding the cancer patient's search for meaning. *Cancer Nursing* **13**(3): 167–175.

Pace, J.C. and Stables, J.L. (1997). Correlates of spiritual well-being in terminally ill persons with AIDS and terminally ill persons with cancer. *Journal of the Association of Nurses in AIDS Care* **8**(6): 31–42.

Pargament, K.I. (1997). *The Psychology of Religion and Coping.* New York: Guilford.

Pert, C. (1997). *Molecules of Emotion: Why You Feel the Way You Feel.* New York: Scribner.

Pruyser, P.W. (1977). The seamy side of current religious beliefs. *Bulletin of the Menninger Clinic,* **41**: 329–348.

Rosenbaum, E.H. (1975). *Living with Cancer.* New York: Praeger.

Shekelle, R.B. Raynor, W.J., Ostfeld, A.M., Garron, D.C., Bieliauskas, L.A., Liu, S.C., Maliza, C. and Oglesby, P (1981). Psychological depression and 17-year risk of death from cancer. *Psychosomatic Medicine* **43**: 117–125.

Spilka, B., Shaver, P. and Kirkpatrick, L.A. (1985). A general attribution theory for the psychology of religion. *Journal for the Scientific Study of Religion* **24**: 1–20.

Spilka, B., Spangler, J.D. and Nelson, C.B. (1983). Spiritual support in life-threatening illness. *Journal of Religion and Health* **22**: 98–104.

Spilka, B., Zwartjes, W.J. and Zwartjes, G.M. (1991). The role of religion in coping with childhood cancer. *Pastoral Psychology* **39**: 285–304.

Spinetta, J.J. (1977). Adjustment in children with cancer. *Journal of Pediatric Psychology* **2**(2): 49–51.

Spinetta, J.J. and Maloney, L.J. (1978). The child with cancer: patterns of communication and denial. *Journal of Consulting and Clinical Psychology* **46**: 1540–1541.

Taylor, E.J. (1995). Whys and wherefores: adult patient perspectives of the meaning of cancer. *Seminars in Oncology Nursing* **11**(1): 32–40.

Taylor, S.E., Lichtman, R.R. and Wood, J.V. (1984). Attributions, beliefs about control, and adjustment to breast cancer. *Journal of Personality and Social Psychology* **46**: 489–502.

Thompson, S.C., Sobolew-Shubin, A., Galbraith, M.E., Schwankovsksy, L. and Cruzen, I.D.. (1993). Maintaining perceptions of control in low-control situations. *Journal of Personality and Social Psychology* **64**: 293–304.

Uchino, B.N., Cacioppo, J.T. and Kiecolt-Glaser, J.K. (1996). The relationship between social support and physiological processes: a review with emphasis on underlying mechanisms and implications for health. *Psychological Bulletin* **119**: 488–531.

Weaver, A.J., Koenig, H.G. and Ochberg, F.M. (1996). Post-traumatic stress, mental health professionals and the clergy. *Journal of Traumatic Stress* **9**: 847–855.

Webb, N.-B. (1991). *Play Therapy with Children in Crisis: A Case Book for Practitioners.* New York: Guilford.

Wood, J.V., Taylor, S.E. and Lichtman, R.R. (1985). Social comparison in relation to breast cancer. *Journal of Personality and Social Psychology* **49**: 1169–1183.

Wylie, R.C. (1979). *The Self Concept,* Vol. 2, 2nd Edn. Lincoln, NE: University of Nebraska Press.

Zeltzer, L.K., Dolgin, M.J., Sahler, O.J., Roghmann, K., Barbarin, O.A., Carpenter, P.J., Copeland, D.R., Mulhern, R.K. and Sargent, J.R. (1996). Sibling adaptation to childhood cancer collaborative study: Health outcomes of siblings of children with cancer. *Medical and Pediatric Oncology* **27**(2): 98–107.

Zwartjes, W.J., Spilka, B., Zwartjes, G.M., Heidemann, D.R. and Cilli, K.A. (1979). *School Problems of Children with Malignant Neoplasms.* Report of National Cancer Institute Project No. 212-46-1061. Denver, CO: The Children's Hospital.

Coping with Cancer:
Religion as A Resource for Families

S. BRYANT KENDRICK
Wake Forest University School of Medicine, Winston-Salem, NC, USA
HAROLD G. KOENIG
Duke University Medical Center, GRECC, VA Medical Center, Durham, NC, USA

The purpose of this chapter is to examine the role that religion plays in the coping process of family members of cancer patients. To date, a significant amount of research has focused primarily on the relationship of religion and cancer in two areas: the variation of cancer rates by different religious groups (Koenig et al., in press) and the role that religion plays in assisting the cancer patient him/herself in coping with the disease (Larson et al., 1997). By contrast, research studies specifically examining family coping in relation to religion are few. The plan of this chapter, then, is three-fold:

1. To present a brief review of the research examining the relationship between religion and the cancer patient's ability to cope with cancer.
2. To introduce the available research that has examined the relationship of religion and family coping in response to cancer.
3. To supplement and illustrate the research findings on family coping and religion with cases from the authors' clinical experience in working with cancer patients and their families.

It is our hope that this information will help the reader develop a deeper appreciation of the complex role that religion plays as a family copes with cancer in one of its members.

RELIGION AND COPING WITH CANCER:
THE EXPERIENCE OF PATIENTS

When a person is diagnosed with a life-threatening disease, it is a time of significant crisis. The individual's life course is likely to be dramatically altered by the impact of the disease on the sense of self and relationships, by the effects of the treatment

Cancer and the Family, 2nd Edn. Edited by L. Baider, C. L. Cooper and A. Kaplan De-Nour
© 2000 John Wiley & Sons, Ltd

process, and by the long-term impact on the physical and mental capabilities of the patient. Coping with these changes becomes the major agenda of these persons as they seek to come to terms with perceptions of suffering, changes in lifestyle, and the possibility of death.

While the path that an individual takes in coping with the crisis will be molded by personality factors, past experiences, and family norms, religious preferences may also be influential. In a study of coping activities in response to a crisis, Charismatic Catholics were more likely to use their church group for emotional support, while Bahais focused on sacred writings and Christian Scientists on positive thinking (Ebaugh et al., 1984). Further, within any given religious tradition, there may be more than one legitimate way to interpret its major theological doctrines as individuals make meaning of their disease experiences; e.g., in a study of one group of Protestants, three distinct coping styles were found, based on different assumptions about God (Pargament et al., 1988).

While cognizant of the potential diversity of responses, some order within this arena is to be expected. For example, it is probable that each patient's account will be a more-or-less individualized rendering of the major themes developed within his/her faith tradition. All of the world's great religions concern themselves with the polarities of health/sickness and well-being/suffering within their teachings about human 'being' and ultimate reality. While religions differ in important ways, each provides a set of largely parallel resources. These include: interpretive schemata, which enable individuals to discern spiritual meaning in experience; a supportive community, in which adherents have access to contextualized relationships; and rituals, which assist them to respond to the predictable crises of life, including the disease of cancer (Numbers and Amundsen, 1986).

Another factor which provides some order to the variability in faith-based coping is the fact that patients facing serious disease tend to focus religious responses around three existential axes: power/powerlessness, connection/disconnection, and meaning/meaninglessness (Burton, 1998). In the power axis, the patient is concerned about who or what is in charge of his/her life and how much control remains with the patient. In the connection/disconnection axis, patients express concerns about changes in the relationships with family, friends, and the Divine. In the meaning/meaningless axis, patients examine themes related to the significance of the disease for the patient's overall understanding of his/her life. These three axes form the primary spiritual coping agenda for patients.

Each religious tradition addresses these axes with questions and teachings that are characteristic of that tradition. While healthcare providers may not share the same set of beliefs as a patient, they may access these three axes by asking questions that enable patients to discuss their experience in spiritually meaningful ways. A list of questions that focus on spiritual issues and provide a structure for assessing the three existential axes has been developed by Burkhardt and Nagi-Jacobson (1997). Many of their questions are denominationally 'neutral', yet encourage genuine spiritual responses.

While it is obvious that many patients will use religious resources in coping with cancer, what researchers have determined about the efficacy of this approach is limited. From an empirically-oriented research perspective, the relationship between religion and coping is difficult to assess for at least three reasons: the complex nature of religion itself; the effect of the coping process on a person's religious beliefs and practices; and the use of a wide variety of measures of religiosity.

Religion is a multifaceted and dynamic reality that defies simplistic operational definitions. Providing guidance in coping with the crisis of a disease such as cancer is only one of its myriad functions. Primarily, religion provides an effective framework for meaning rooted in a relationship to the ultimate or Divine One that addresses the full range of human experiences. This framework is a rich tapestry, composed of worship experiences, interpretive symbols, and community experiences. While not primarily 'coping methods' *per se*, they form the experiential, relational, and cognitive matrix within which individuals, families, and communities create religious coping responses.

The process individuals use to develop religious coping responses is not well understood. A model being tested by Pargament and colleagues (1992) suggests that the coping response must involve a movement from the symbolic and general to the concrete and personal dimensions of faith. As these researchers point out:

> People do not face stressful events without resources. They bring with them a system of generalized beliefs, practices, aspirations, and relationships which affect how they deal with difficult moments. Religion is, to a greater or lesser extent, part of this general orienting system. In the coping process, both the religious and non-religious elements of this orienting system are translated into concrete, situationally-based appraisals, activities, and goals (Pargament et al., 1992).

As aids to coping, religious beliefs and practices interact with the unique group of life-changing events brought on by the presence of a serious disease and its concomitant therapy, a dynamic process in which the beliefs themselves may undergo change. For example, some persons may become more or less religious during the coping experience. Other people may experience a shift in the meaningfulness of certain aspects of their religious experiences as the significance of a disease unfolds, for example, a person may find that corporate worship experiences have become less (or more) important than before, and intense periods of personal meditation have become more (or less) meaningful (Pargament et al., 1995).

To make matters even more difficult, there is little agreement among researchers on how to measure 'religion,' leading to a lack of consistency in measures across research designs. Typical measures of religion include religious denomination, rates of church attendance, and single-item scales indicating the importance of religion in the life of the patient. Taking all of this into consideration, it is not surprising to find that the research presents a distinctly mixed view, with many studies finding positive correlation, others none, and some even finding negative effects of religion on patient coping. What the research may indicate is that religion plays a positive role in the adaptation of some patients, will have no effect in others, and be associated with a negative effect in a very few others (Jenkins and Pargament, 1995).

A number of studies of cancer patients find a positive correlation between religious beliefs and practices and important aspects of successful coping. Indicators of effective coping associated with patients' religious behavior include: less hostility, reduced social isolation, and greater levels of transcendent meaning (Acklin et al., 1983); higher levels of self-esteem (Jenkins and Pargament, 1988); greater sense of psychological well-being (Eil et al., 1989); less anxiety (Kaczorowski, 1989); and higher levels of hope (Mickley and Soeken, 1993).

In studies involving breast cancer patients, religion has not only been found to be helpful in coping (Johnson and Spilka, 1991), but also to be one of the most prevalent coping strategies used (Carver et al., 1993). In a study of patients with gynecologic cancer, Roberts et al. (1997) found that 49% of subjects became more religious since having the cancer, while no subjects became less religious. In studies of cancer patients in Switzerland, faith in God and prayer were important for 36% of the subjects (Kesselring et al., 1986). In a study of lung cancer patients in Ontario, Canada, Ginsburg et al. (1995) found that 79% of subjects identified family and 44% identified religion as major sources of support. Spilka et al. (1983) found the use of prayer to be a supportive practice in patients facing life-threatening illness.

As part of a larger review of the relationship between religion and coping in chronic disease, Dein and Stygall report on a variety of studies that have examined the relationship between cancer and religion (Dein and Stygall, 1997). Several studies found that many cancer patients have unmet spiritual and existential needs and that over one-third of patients use religion as a source of support. One study found that one-third of 190 metastatic cancer patients became more religious following diagnosis. However, other studies find no dramatic shifts in religious beliefs in the face of life-threatening illness.

A positive correlation between religion and effective coping by cancer patients was further identified in many of the studies reviewed by Dein and Stygall (1997). In these, religion was correlated with lower levels of pain, anxiety, and hostility and with higher levels of life satisfaction, increased ability to cope with survival concerns among women post-mastectomy, and with enhanced adjustment in the face of death among children and adolescents. On the other hand, three studies reviewed found no relationship between religion and coping, and two studies found religion associated with a negative effect on coping.

Agreeing with Jenkins and Pargament (1995; see above), Dein and Stygall (1997) point out that conflicting data are not surprising when one realizes that the measures of religion used in the studies reviewed vary considerably from indexes of belief to frequency of worship attendance. As an overall conclusion, they find that the research which does exist indicates the importance of spiritual concerns to patients, families, and the healthcare professionals caring for them.

RELIGION AND COPING WITH CANCER:
THE EXPERIENCE OF THE FAMILY AS REVEALED IN RESEARCH

Many and difficult are the burdens associated with care-giving for patients with severe illness. For cancer patients, the disease often entails dependency on family members (Siegal 1991), who are themselves impacted as their focus on care-providing activities increases. In one study of 2661 seriously ill patients, 34% of the patients required major commitment of family members' time to provide needed daily assistance; and in 20% of cases, a family member had to quit work or make other major life changes in order to assume new care-giving roles. Loss of family savings was reported by 31% of the study subjects; 29% reported loss of a major source of income (Covinsky et al., 1994). In addition to changing family roles, important emotional issues emerged: anxiety, fear, and anticipatory grief impacted relationships and communication patterns (Aldredge-Clanton, 1998).

What people believe about experiences directly impacts how they cope with them. Family members are often influenced by a legacy of religious beliefs about health and disease. These beliefs, comprising rules, rituals, and relevant myths, are handed down within the family from one generation to the next and provide a way to interpret traumatic events. Major ideas about the Divine, what is right and wrong, and the degree of human freedom and responsibility, are core parts of these legacies (Burton, 1992).

No matter how revered these beliefs may be, it is apparent that some facilitate coping by individuals and family members better than others. In their work on family beliefs and illness, Wright et al. (1996) divided beliefs about illness into two types: constraining beliefs, which restrict consideration of options, and facilitative beliefs, which increase options for consideration. Religious beliefs can certainly function in either manner. For example, Prong (1995) looked at the cultural factors associated with healthy grieving among Cambodian children, and found that religious beliefs related to discussion about death and dying were associated with open communication and environmental stability. By contrast, some beliefs that constrain options have been found to be associated with diminished levels of active coping. In a study of breast cancer in 33 Jewish women living in Israel, subjects who identified with an Oriental (non-rational, magical) perspective, as opposed to a Western (rational, scientific) perspective, were more likely to attribute the cause of their cancer to God or to fate and were more likely to feel helpless, resigned and submissive (Baider and Sarell, 1983).

Do families whose beliefs constitute a 'facilitative spiritual core' do better over the long haul in coping with illness? Wright et al. (1996) answer in the affirmative. The central issue that has emerged from their studies involves the notion of spiritual distress. Families who are able to invest the events associated with the disease and their coping with a meaning that is personally significant have lower levels of spiritual distress over the long term (Wright et al., 1996).

Religious resources are also called on in responding to crisis periods within the long-term adaptational sequence. In coping with the immediate crisis of hospitalization, Koller found that the five most effective mechanisms used by family members of patients in an adult intensive care unit were communication with other family members, prayer, positive thinking, thinking about good things in their life, and hope (Koller, 1991).

The emotional impact of long-term care responsibilities was studied by Rabins et al. (1990b) in two groups of caregivers: 32 Alzheimer's care-givers and 30 caregivers of cancer patients. The researchers administered a neuroticism–extraversion–openness questionnaire, a family adaptability and cohesiveness scale, and other measures of health, mood states, and grief. They found that a positive emotional state was associated with the number of social contacts and feeling supported by one's religious faith. These two factors, social contacts and support from one's religious faith, were also found to be significantly correlated with positive emotional adaptation to the caregiving role after 2 years (Rabins et al., 1990a).

The stress on a family involved in caring for a patient with cancer is perhaps no more acute than when that patient is a child. Spilka et al. (1991) examined the role of religion in the coping process of children with cancer and their family members through interviews with 66 pediatric patients and 112 mothers and 81 fathers of these patients. At the time of the interviews, 5.2 years (on average) had elapsed since the diagnosis; the patients' average age was 15.1 years and the average ages of the parents were 42.1 years (mothers) and 45.3 years (fathers). The results of this research, although only a pilot study, reveal fascinating glimpses into familial coping responses to pediatric cancers and their relationship to family and patient religion. Included in their study are the effects of religious belief on several significant aspects of family life: (a) parental perceptions of the child diagnosed with cancer; (b) family behaviors and behavioral norms; (c) the quality of relationships within the family; and (d) the number and quality of relationships outside the family.

The parents who scored higher on the religion measure were more likely to state that their child had less understanding of his/her diagnosis than the children of less religious parents. Parents who scored lower on the religion measure reported that their child expressed emotions of anger, fear, and denial in reacting to the disease, while parents who scored high on the religious variable reported that their child responded with more depression that was verbally communicated. Perceptions of activity levels also varied by parental religiosity, with 'high-religious' parents seeing a greater reduction in overall activity level of the child than parents with 'low' religiosity. As one example, these children were more likely to be restricted in what they could do after school. Assessment of overall personality change in the child also varied with parental religiosity, i.e., more religious parents reported less change in the child's personality.

In commenting on these findings, the authors point out that, while the parents may have underestimated the child's comprehension of the diagnosis as a defense mechanism, the children themselves reported understanding the nature and implications of their illness as their faith became more important:

> 'It is possible that strengthening the significance of religion counters potential depression and the tendency to verbalize about the illness permits more solid knowledge to be gained about it than is true of the less religious children (Spilka et al., 1991, p. 299).

The authors note that resistance to change, both perceived and real, is often associated with religiosity, and infer that religious parents may work to maintain the status quo of their family life as a way to provide a reassuring sense of continuity. This is seen as a coping strength if it does not degenerate into unrealistic denial.

Parental perceptions of good quality relationships within the family (mother–patient, father–patient, sibling–patient) are positively correlated with religion, both in pre- and post-diagnosis time periods:

> 'Not only do the more religious families appear closer under normal and crisis conditions, but with the growing importance of religion following diagnosis, these connections increase in strength for the patient with both parents and siblings. In other words, a strong faith implies a close-knit family, the bonds of which are reinforced when the stress of life-threatening illness enters the picture (Spilka et al., 1991, p. 299).

For the more religious patients and families, the actual number of social contacts goes down in the period following the diagnosis, and fewer people are initially informed about the diagnosis. However, those who are involved in the life of the patient and family are usually closer friends, with many of these individuals being part of the family's religious community. While the use of introvertive fantasies in coping might account for this 'turning inward,' it is also possible that the more religious family is strengthening bonds with those within their intimate family, social, and religious network who are perceived to be helpful in the tasks of coping with their child's cancer. The findings in this study suggest that religion plays a role in successful adaptation to the needs of families who are caring for a child with cancer by serving as a '... protective–defensive system that motivates efforts to cope actively and constructively ...' (Spilka et al., 1991, p. 303).

Another study (using oral history techniques) focused on the sibling relationship of a pair of sisters, one of whom developed childhood leukemia (Lehna, 1998). Data were gathered from a 22-year-old sibling of a leukemia survivor through taped interviews that were transcribed and analysed for thematic content. Six themes emerged: closeness, activity, fearfulness, anger, worry, and spirituality. The information about spirituality revealed its role in helping to deal with death anxiety and in facilitating an acceptance of death as a natural part of life. Also, the family participated in a church-wide celebration thanking God for the patient's subsequent survival, an event that involved many in the community and served as a joyful reaffirmation of bonds and belongings.

In contrast to these positive findings, Barbarin and Cheslar (1986) found no significant correlation between religion and the coping strategies of parents of children with cancer. However, they did find a high correlation between coping and the quality of the relationships with medical staff.

WHAT IMPACT DOES BELONGING TO A RELIGIOUS COMMUNITY HAVE ON THE FAMILY MEMBERS OF A PERSON DIAGNOSED WITH CANCER?

Religious communities may be conceived of as organized around two orienting dimensions: the vertical and the horizontal. The vertical dimension comprises the group's relation to the Divine, as communicated in tradition and experienced in ongoing worship. The horizontal dimension comprises the group's orientation to the secular, in terms of distinctive lifestyles modeled on the basic beliefs and values transmitted in the vertical dimension. All religious groups provide ritual structure, cultic relationships, sources of meaning, and avenues of personal praxis for their members to use in coping with the fundamental issues associated with transiting the human journey. As socializing forces, religious communities teach their members what to expect from the community and how to relate to community members in a time of crisis. Through participation in the rites of passage of others, individuals and families learn in an experiential way how they, in their turn, will be related to when similar crisis events occur which involve them directly. Thus, religious communities function as 'hands-on teachers' of faith-based coping styles.

The family unit is of basic concern to all religious groups, and support of both the individual and family during times of disease is a natural expression of any religious group's ethos. Understanding how this natural form of support actually influences family coping is complicated by the fact that religious communities usually link to all members of the family through a variety of sub-group memberships. In a modern urban setting, these would include participating in educational classes, mission groups, choirs, committees, athletic teams, and administrative bodies, in addition to participating in worship experiences intended for all the members. A variety of relationships, then, may exist between any given family and its religious community, with family members themselves active in different subgroups, with different levels of attachment, and attributing different levels of significance across these multiple contact points. Assessing the importance of religion in the coping process of any particular family will require a robust theoretical model that can account for fluctuations in these multiple contact points.

As the research reviewed thus far indicates, support from the religious community seems to have a generally positive impact on the ability of the cancer patient and family to cope with the illness. While these results are not surprising, new research findings are providing quite unexpected results indicating that religion may have a direct impact on the *survival* of the patient. Spiegel and colleagues (Spiegel et al., 1989; Spiegel, 1992) at Stanford University and Fawzy et al. (1990a, 1993) at the University of California at Los Angeles have discovered that *group support* may directly influence survival. Physiological mechanisms are now being uncovered by means of which social support may be significantly altering immune system functioning, i.e. the ability of the body to contain the spread of cancer (Rabin, 1999).

The religious community may literally be a life-giving source of supportive friendships for the cancer patient and his/her family. Because the patient's family is often the most important source of support for the patient, it is essential that family members caring for the patient receive support from their religious leaders and religious community. This will help prevent burnout and increase the family members' emotional reserves so that they can be emotionally available to the patient. Thus, the religious community plays an important role in supporting both the patient and his/her family—support that may have both psychological as well as physical health benefits.

One of the main contacts between the family experiencing a crisis brought on by the illness of one of its members and its religious community is the relationship provided by the family's clergyperson. It is at the heart of the pastoral role to participate in the various passages of the life cycle through which the family moves. Birth and coming-of-age ceremonies, weddings and funerals are some of the times when the clergyperson's presence intersects the family's life course. Having 'been with' families through the normal transformations associated with human experience, it is not surprising that clergy are able to provide an important supportive ministry to patients and families responding to the crisis of cancer. In a study comparing hospital chaplains and 'home pastors' of parents of children with cancer and cancer patients, it was found that subjects actually prayed more with home pastors than with hospital chaplains, and the prayer experiences with home pastors were more highly valued than those with hospital chaplains (Spilka et al., 1983). This difference may be based in the often long-standing connection of the religious leader with the family, one which enables the familiar minister to play a more facilitative role as the family begins to cope with the meaning of the illness of one of its members.

The role of the clergy as 'mediators' can assist families in adjusting to the uncertainties of a new diagnosis of serious illness. In many situations families need help in determining what issues can be discussed together and which may be too burdensome to share openly. A desire to protect each other may limit important discussions, since at the initial diagnosis some patients '... tend to become secretively protective and work towards sparing their families and loved ones the devastation they feel' (Burton, 1992). Clergy, especially those who know the family from past involvement, can serve as 'ears to hear' what others may not be ready to process.

As the full range of issues unleashed by the diagnosis become clearer to family members, the first stage of adapting to the disease may become a time of potential conflict if ways to balance and address competing needs are not found. Learning how to strike this balance may require new information on how to manage emotions. A practical guide for families has the following advice:

> Each has to deal with individual feelings, while trying to be sensitive to those of the person who has cancer. Being part of the family doesn't mean you can make people talk about their feelings before they are ready, but you need outlets, too. There are ways to encourage openness. Be ready to listen when others are ready to talk and let your continued presence show your support. But remember, the person with cancer gets to set the timetable (National Cancer Institute, 1999).

One of the major roles of the clergy is to provide guidance at times like these, guidance that may require 'normalizing' new communication experiences that will be helpful to the patient and family. One way to 'bridge' the world of the familiar and known to experiences that are unique, complex, and threatening involves the creative use of religious rituals and other symbolic forms. One Hospice chaplain described this way of providing spiritual support to families in the following manner:

> It can be a religious ceremony like communion but constructed in a way that enables family members to share among themselves as part of the liturgy. The patient is included too. Sometimes this is the first time they all come to grips with the issues they need to focus on. Similar things can happen even if you do not use religious liturgies. You can encourage the telling of family stories by using a family photograph album. Everyone starts laughing, crying, expressing anger, but they are making closure. The ritual aspect helps give them the structure to do this (Kendrick, 1999b).

Through these experiences, clergy may help patients and family members discover new patterns of communication that they can then use to enhance their own problem solving and to interact around issues that were initially perceived as too painful to share. In addition, information developed in these exchanges may alert clergy to the need for referrals to the various types of support groups provided by both the religious and secular community (Cunningham and Edmonds, 1996).

The relationship of the religious community to the family of a person with cancer goes far beyond that provided by the clergy. With variations dependent on the size of the religious community, the complexity of its administrative structure, and organizational norms, support to a family may include:

1. A constant stream of cards and letters sharing supportive thoughts and prayers.
2. Focused prayers during corporate worship.
3. Provision of food during stressful times.
4. Assistance with transportation to and from treatment.
5. Respite opportunities for fatigued caregivers.
6. Assistance with house and yard work.
7. Visitation in the home.
8. A communication service which keeps people informed about needs and progress.
9. Hosting fund-raising events to provide financial assistance to families who face mounting medical bills.

Another resource which membership in a religious community provides for family members of cancer patients involves individuals who can help overcome problems posed by the family's communication pattern. Families develop distinctive ways of talking, which includes limits on expressing strong emotions, deep-felt needs, and ideas that diverge from those generally viewed as 'acceptable' by the family. When a family member develops cancer, the communication needs of the patient and the family members may exceed what is allowable within the long-established family communication norms. This creates a communication crisis superimposed on the original problems posed by the diagnosis. The relationships provided by the religious community provide opportunities to share feelings openly with others and meet some of the needs family members have without forcing discussion of topics that, while important, may be too volatile to manage within the family's existing communication norms.

In many cultures under the influence of modern medical care, families have lost the skills associated with caring for a chronically ill family member. These skills must be re-learned 'on the job'. Within the religious community there are usually several individuals and families who have acquired these skills by caring for a person with cancer. They have 'been this way before' and can provide valuable guidance, an informed listening, and a helping hand to those recently initiated into their journey as caregivers to a family member with cancer. Thus, the religious community represents a repository of wisdom that can nurture the modern urban family by providing access to people who can, through personal experience, identify closely with the needs, fears, problems, and distress of family members and provide an introduction to the skills needed to care for a loved one who suffers from cancer.

As repositories of wisdom, most religious communities have libraries well-stocked with books and other educational media to assist families deal with the predictable crises of life. For example, a bibliotherapy bibliography for children from preschool to sixth grade, provided by the Church and Synagogue Library Association, contains a section entitled 'Illness, Health, and Medical Care' which addresses cancer, dentists, doctors, and hospitals. The section entitled 'Death' contains titles that discuss the death of children, an older person, parent, grandparent, and pets (Pearl, 1990). Additional information on a broad base of supportive resources (including spirituality) for cancer patients and their families can be found at the OncoLink website of the University of Pennsylvania (http://www.oncolink.upen.edu); select 'Psychosocial Support and Personal Experiences'.

The existence of an ongoing relationship with a religious community in which one is known and supported by an ethic of caring during times of personal and familial crisis is a 'built-in' advantage for family members. In these communities, permission to connect with others around significant personal and family events is the norm; and, through participation over the years, the family members have observed how this information is generated, communicated, and responded to. The expectation of a supportive and caring response beyond the merely casual and socially accepted becomes one of the facilitative coping beliefs which families who participate meaningfully in religious communities bring to the task of adapting to the diagnosis of cancer in one of their members.

While membership of a religious community all but guarantees the development of supportive relationships for cancer patients and their families, some religious groups look outside their membership and provide ministries to meet the needs of cancer patients and their families who may not be attached to any religious group. In one project, volunteers were recruited from churches and trained to deal with health issues and cancers prevalent among African–Americans, questions of spirituality and death and dying, and communication skills. Among the services provided were transportation to and from medical appointments, grocery shopping, banking, medication pick-up, and respite time for caregivers (Brown-Hunter and Price, 1998). In addition, many religious groups offer their meeting rooms for support groups of patients and/or patient family members and provide special 'retreat' experiences through regional and national organizations.

A new form of congregation-based health care ministry called the Parish Nurse Program has been evolving among religious groups in the USA since 1984. This program was envisioned by the Reverend Granger Westberg to meet religious and health needs that were often unaddressed in standard health care systems. The parish nurse supports patients and families by providing health counseling and education, coordinating support groups within the community and participating congregations, and facilitating referrals to community-based resources. In addition to providing nursing care during home visits, the parish nurse provides spiritual care in the form of prayer, reading of scripture, and worship services for home-bound individuals and family members. The parish nurse serves as a mediator between the questions that patients and family members have about complex treatments and the often difficult to comprehend medically-based explanations (Djube and Westberg, 1995). As regular visitors in the home, parish nurses offer a known and trusted resource when patients and family members face difficult treatment decisions.

From the original group of six churches located near Chicago (three Lutheran, one Methodist, and two Roman Catholic), the movement has expanded across the USA and now serves as a model for similar initiatives sponsored by other religious groups. The American Nurses Association has established professional standards for parish nurse programs that cover the areas of Spirituality, Health Educator, Health Counselor, Liaison to Community Resources, Coordinator of Volunteers, and Professional Development (Spikes, no date available). More information is available from the National Parish Nurse Resource Center, 1-800-556-5368.

RELIGION AND FAMILY COPING:
PRACTICAL EXAMPLES FROM CLINICAL PRACTICE

When discussing the process of coping with cancer in a family member, the religious dimension of the family's experience emerges quite freely if the family actively participates in a faith tradition. The authors have had numerous discussions with patients and families related to coping with cancer in which the religious dimension was more or less clearly in focus. The examples used to highlight this relationship presented in this section are all drawn from the authors' own clinical experience. Some serve to illustrate themes identified in the research literature, while others indicate areas of potential future investigations.

In our experience of working with cancer patients and families in North Carolina, one of the most positive coping resources mentioned by adults was the importance of the Sunday School Class. This is usually a small group in which the individual caregiver feels known and valued. It is a group in which it is easy to share what really happens in the caregiver role. It is a place where family caregivers confidently expect their feelings to be understood and accepted, since they know from their own participation in the group over the years that others sitting in the same room within them have faced similar situations. In addition to receiving expressions of support, they are able to tap into a repository of personal wisdom and expertise that allows them to test out strategies and reactions. Most importantly, the frustration and exhaustion which sometimes arise in caregiving for a family member with cancer can be vented in the forgiving and understanding acceptance provided by the group.

Another important religious resource identified in our experience by family caregivers involves the availability of clergy to provide specific counseling related to questions of meaning, to help with the stress of coping, and to provide worship experiences in the home. In many situations, attendance at worship becomes impossible for both the patient and the family caregiver. Specific worship practices, such as praying together, holding a brief service, reading and discussing scripture, or participating in other religious rituals, provide times of meaningful encounter for the patient and family. Family members value the experience because it enables the reaffirmation of a sense of connectedness to the Divine and the affirmation of a 'purpose' at work, even in the midst of pain and suffering. While many family members are motivated to provide care out of the love they feel for their family member, it is also true that these feelings are often linked to religious values. Home worship experiences assist family members in reaffirming this vital level of meaning.

Home visitation by the clergy provides opportunities for several kinds of interventions. Assessments of family stress and coping can be made, and needed resources can be identified and communicated to the larger membership. Conversations with the patient and family allow for the exploration of spiritual issues and resources, as these become more relevant during the progression of the disease.

The following account illustrates the value of a minister as a 'family member mediator.' In discussing the last week of a patient's life in an interview, one spouse described how a minister had been helpful when the spouse had noticed a change in her husband's attitude. He had become restless and upset, but was not able to communicate the basis of his distress to his wife. In a conversation with a hospice chaplain, the patient revealed a need to bring closure to the relationship with his daughter, and he and the chaplain agreed that a letter from him expressing his love for her and pride in her accomplishments would be the best approach. The wife agreed to write the letter for him as he dictated it. 'Though he was very weak and it was hard for me to hear him, I know that each word came from his heart, and I know that our daughter will cherish this letter. With a weak and trembling hand, he signed it, "Love, Dad"' (Kendrick, personal interview with M.F., 1999).

Family members adjust as they can to the many changes in their lives brought on by becoming caregivers. Perhaps the most important role that religion plays is providing new attitudes to support significant changes in behavior required by new caring responsibilities. One spouse of a cancer patient had to leave a job she had performed for 27 years and had no sense of what the future would really be like for her. She described herself as a 'power person' who wanted to be in control, and the uncertainty of a future without a job—and with a husband suffering from an incurable cancer—placed her close to the end of her coping abilities. However, her sense of dread was replaced by a profound peace during a worship service in which her minister (during the sermon) recounted the tradition of God's daily provision for the Israelites during their desert wanderings. A startling awareness of the providence of God filled her mind and overcame her anxiety. From that point on she was able to trust that God would care for her and her husband. 'I didn't know where we were going with this cancer, but God did. And that was enough for me' (Kendrick, personal interview with M.F., 1999).

This is a clear example of one of the most powerful ways in which religious beliefs support effective adaptation among family members of persons with cancer. Religious belief systems provide believers with traditional concepts, metaphors, and stories that allow them to reframe current experiences in ways that foster enhanced coping. Leaving the known and relatively secure for the unknown and threatening calls on faith resources that enable caregivers to look beyond the present and trust in a Higher Power to journey with them and provide guidance.

Another indication of the many kinds of supportive roles that religious communities may play in family coping was related by the spouse of a couple whose long-range plan had been to travel upon the husband's retirement. Since an earlier than expected retirement was required by his disease, the couple spent as much time as they could traveling while the patient was yet able, participating often in trips sponsored by their religious community. As their trips increased, so did the number and richness of relationships within their religious community, which served to balance the loss of important relationships that had been developed with people at work and in other community activities. The unexpected alteration in the life course resulted in the enhancement of the network of relationships that provided important sources for support for the family and patient as the impact of the disease grew over time.

Some family members reported the frustrations they felt when their desire to be involved in caring for the patient was blocked by forces beyond their control. For example, the adult son of one middle-aged couple was planning to be involved in the daily home-based care of his father to provide back-up and support for his mother, who had left her job in order to take the major burden of care for her terminally ill husband. Unfortunately, after several weeks of providing care and 'fine tuning' their process, the son was informed at his job that he was being transferred to another part of the country. Since he was married and had two children, he did not think he could refuse the transfer. This meant a major revamping of the support-system for his mother. Since the beginning of their experience with the cancer, the family had practiced openness in communication about matters related to the disease and their feelings about it. This attitude of openness was one practical result of their belief that nothing in the experience of the disease was shameful or removed them from their understanding of the nature of God. This belief contributed to the family's ability to thoroughly discuss this problem and to develop an alternative plan to provide assistance to the mother.

Coping with the numerous weighty decisions associated with cancer therapy is yet another component of family stress. Family members will necessarily be involved in the deliberations related to treatment-level decisions (e.g., what kind of chemotherapy to take) and management-level decisions (e.g., who will be up with the cancer patient during the evening). The number, significance, and unfamiliarity of decisions that need to be made add the stress of anxiety to the family system. Ready access to concerned clergy and friends within the religious community provide the cognitive and emotional support which keep the family from being overwhelmed by demands that are often perceived to outstrip abilities or understanding.

The decision to end curative and accept palliative treatment only stands as a watershed moment in the experience of most caregivers. In cultures where this decision is primarily a personal one based on the beliefs, desires, and experience of the patient, the relationship to others and the need to have them understand and validate this decision remains important. This may be especially true for family caregivers, who otherwise may fear being judged as having 'quit caring' or as having succumbed to compassion fatigue. Participation within a religious community, allows others to see the faith of the family and patient as well as the struggle with the disease. When this experience has been shared, close friends and members of the religious community, far from being 'shocked,' often offer validation for this most difficult decision.

The role of the religious community and its meaning for patients and family members may additionally contribute to terminal phase issues by helping some patients 'let go' of some important concerns for the family after death. It is clear that one of the needs of the patient in the terminal phase of the disease involves assurances that his/her family members will be able to cope after his/her death. This is especially true when the biological family is geographically dispersed. In this situation, the religious community often becomes a substitute family. One spouse reported: 'The presence of the church family in our home and providing assistance in transportation and in other ways, helped him know that I would not be alone and without assistance' (Kendrick, personal interview with S.R., 1999).

Some family members reported times when they saw 'guidance from above' and 'little miracles' in which unexpected positive events occurred. In addition, patients would describe experiences in which they 'saw ancestors,' 'felt drawn to a beautiful garden,' or experienced other mystical events that fell outside the norm of their usual experience. Other family caregivers reported deep moments of connection to the Divine associated with participation in care-giving activities. These experiences tended to confirm their beliefs that God was intimately linked to the illness experience of patients and the care-giving roles of the family, a perception that is generally agreed to be the most supportive of all awareness. The existence of a religious perspective enabled these experiences to be identified and interpreted in a way that provided patients and families with a sense of a Divine connection that brought profound peace, even as the reality of the disease pressed toward inevitable death.

The examples from the authors' clinical experience presented thus far highlight the more obvious ways in which religion assists families in coping creatively with cancer in one of its members. However, there are many subtle aspects of this relationship that may go unnoticed when only the usual measures of religion are inquired about. One example from our database of discussions with family members will conclude this section.

In an account of the ways in which religion aided her family to cope with the anticipated loss of her husband, an informant shared the following story. One day her grandson expressed his concern about how he would make gingerbread cookies for a religious holiday, since he had always done that with his grandfather who, at this point, was close to death. She told the child that when the holiday arrived next year, she and he would make the cookies in exactly the same way that he and his grandfather had always done it. Furthermore, she wanted him to help her remember the steps involved. This plan for the next celebration of the holiday eased her grandson's mind (Kendrick, personal interview with A.B.W., 1999).

Through this response, this wise grandmother both helped her grandson to value the unique meaning of this activity with his grandfather and also provided for continuity for that experience in an altered future. She preserved—and yet expanded—the meaning of the experience, so that at the next celebration of the holiday, there would be grief and remembrance, but also gingerbread! In this account we see how faithful observance of the religious calendar can be a strong support for families, as religious holidays provide heightened symbolic moments whose meaning is deepened through the care and remembrance of the family with cancer.

CONCLUSIONS

It is clear that the religions of the world provide adherents with comprehensive systems of meaning, networks of supportive relationships, and familiar rites and rituals. The family active in a faith group has a multi-faceted, if hard-to-measure, resource which can play a vital role in helping family members cope in ways that enhance family function and resolve the crises imposed on it by the sickness of one of its members. While the available empirical research and the authors' clinical experience are generally positive, not enough is known concerning the specific ways in which religion—in all of its complexity—interacts with and influences family coping. Additional research, primarily of a qualitative nature, is needed to help us understand this dynamic process more accurately. As a prelude to future research, however, much work on foundational theoretical models is needed to truly capture the full range of dynamic interactions between religion and family coping processes.

ACKNOWLEDGMENT

Support for this work was provided in part by the John Templeton Foundation, Radnor, PA, USA.

REFERENCES

Acklin, M.W., Brown, E.C. and Mauger, P.A. (1983).   The role of religious values and coping with cancer. *Journal of Religion and Health* **22**: 323–333.

Aldredge-Clanton, J. (1998).   *Counseling People with Cancer*. Louisville, KY: Westminster John Knox Press.

Baider, L. and Sarell, M. (1983).   Perceptions and causal attributions of Israeli women with breast cancer concerning their illness: the effects of ethnicity and religiosity. *Psychotherapy and Psychosomatics* **39**: 136–143.

Barbarin, O.A. and Cheslar, M. (1986).   The medical context of parental coping with childhood cancer. *American Journal of Community Psychiatry* **14**: 221–235.

Brown-Hunter, M. and Price, L.K. (1998).   The good neighbor project; volunteerism and the elderly African–American patient with cancer. *Geriatric Nursing* **19**(3): 139–141.

Burkhardt, M.A. and Nagai-Jacobson, M.G. (1997).   Spirituality and Healing. In B.M. Dossey (Ed.), *Core Curriculum for Holistic Nursing*. Gaithersburg, MD: Aspen.

Burton, L.A. (1992).   Families with cancer: insights from family therapy. In L.A. Burton and G. Handzo (Eds), *Health Care Chaplaincy in Oncology* (pp. 57–72). Binghamton, NY: Haworth Pastoral Press.

Burton, L.A. (1998).   The spiritual dimension of palliative care. *Seminars in Oncology Nursing* **14**(2): 121–128.

Carver, C.S., Pozo, C., Harris, S.D., Noriega, V., Scheier, M.F., Robinson, D.S., Ketcham, A.S., Moffat, F.L. and Clark, K.C. (1993).   How coping mediates the effect of optimism on distress: a study of women with early stage breast cancer. *Journal of Personality and Social Psychology* **65**: 375–390.

Covinsky, K.E., Goldman, L., Cook, E.F., Oye, R., Desbiens, N., Reding, D., Fulkerson, W., Connors, A.F., Lynne, J. and Phillips, R.S. (1994).   The impact of serious illness on patients' families. *Journal of the American Medical Association* **272**(23): 1839–1844.

Cunningham, A.J. and Edmonds, C.V. (1996).   Group psychological therapy for cancer patients: a point of view and discussion of the hierarchy of options. *International Journal of Psychiatry in Medicine* **26**(1): 51–82.

Dein, S. and Stygall, J. (1997). Does being religious help or hinder coping with chronic illness? A critical literature review. *Palliative Medicine* **11**: 291–298.

Djube, A.M. and Westberg, G. (1995). Congregation-based health programs. In M.A. Kimble, S.H. McFadden, J.W. Ellor and J.J. Seeber (Eds), *Aging, Spirituality, and Religion* (pp. 325–334). Minneapolis, MN: Fortress.

Ebaugh, H., Richman, K. and Chafetz, J. (1984).   Life crises among the religiously committed: do sectarian differences matter? *Journal for the Scientific Study of Religion* **23**: 19–31.

Ell, K.O., Mantell, J.E., Hamovitch, M.B. and Nishimoto, R.H. (1989).   Social support, sense of control, and coping among patients with breast, lung, or colorectal cancer. *Journal of Psychosocial Oncology* **7**: 63–89.

Fawzy, F.I., Cousins,. N., Fawzy, N.W., Kemeny, M.E., Elashoff, R. and Morton, D. (1990a).   A structured psychiatric intervention for cancer patients: I. Changes over time and methods of coping and affective disturbance. *Archives of General Psychiatry* **47**: 720–725.

Fawzy, F.I., Fawzy, N.W., Hyun, C.S., Elashoff, R., Guthrie, D., Fahey, J.L. and Morton, D.L. (1993).   Malignant melanoma: effects on an early structured psychiatric intervention, coping, and affective state on recurrence and survival 6 years later. *Archives of General Psychiatry* **50**: 681–689.

Fawzy, F.I., Kemeney, M.E., Fawzy, N.W., Elashoff, R., Morton, D., Cousins, N. and Fahey, J.L. (1990b). A structured psychiatric intervention for cancer patients: II Changes over time in immunological measures. *Archives of General Psychiatry* **47**: 729–735.

Ginsburg, M.L., Quirt, C., Ginsburg, A.D. and MacKillop, W.J. (1995). Psychiatric illness and psychosocial concerns of patients with newly diagnosed lung cancer. *Canadian Medical Journal* **152**: 701–708.

Jenkins, R.A. and Pargament, K.I. (1988). Cognitive appraisals in cancer patients. *Social Science and Medicine* **26**: 625–633.

Jenkins, R.A. and Pargament, K.I. (1995). Religion and spirituality as resources for coping with cancer. *Journal of Psychosocial Oncology* **13**(1/2): 51–74.

Johnson, S.C. and Spilka, B. (1991). Coping with breast cancer: the roles of clergy and faith. *Journal of Religion and Health* **30**: 21–33.

Kaczorowski, J.M. (1989). Spiritual well-being and anxiety in adults diagnosed with cancer. *The Hospice Journal* **5**: 105–116.

Kendrick, S.B. (1999b). Personal interview with F.M.

Kesselring, A., Dodd, M.J., Lindsey, A.M. and Strauss, A.L. (1986). Attitudes of patients living in Switzerland about cancer and its treatment. *Cancer Nursing* **9**: 77–85.

Koenig, H.G. (2000). Cancer—Part 1: importance, causes, and prevalence in different religious groups. In: Koenig, H.G., McCullough, M. and Larson, D.B. (Eds), *Religion and Health*. New York, NY: Oxford University Press. Forthcoming.

Koller, P.A. (1991). Family needs and coping strategies during illness crisis. *AACN Clinical Issues in Critical Care Nursing* **2**: 338–344.

Larson, D.B., Swyers, J.P. and McCullough, M.E. (Eds) (1997). *Scientific Research on Spirituality and Health: A Consensus Report*. Washington, DC: National Institute for Healthcare Research.

Lehna, C.R. (1998). A childhood cancer sibling's oral history. *Journal of Pediatric Oncology Nursing* **15**(3): 163–171.

Mickley, J.R. and Soeken, K. (1993). Religiousness and hope in Hispanic- and Anglo-American women with breast cancer. *Oncology Nursing Forum* **20**: 1171–1177.

National Cancer Institute (1999). Taking time: support for people with cancer and the people who care about them. National Institutes of Health. Available at: http://rex.nci.gov/PATIENTS/INFOR_PEOPL_DOC.html.

Numbers, R.L. and Amundsen, D.W. (Eds) (1986). *Caring and Curing: Health and Medicine in the Western Religious Traditions*. New York: Macmillan.

Pargament, K., Crevengoed, N., Hathaway, W., Kennell, J., Newman, J. and Jones, W. (1988). Religion and problem solving: three styles of coping. *Journal for the Scientific Study of Religion* **27**: 90–104.

Pargament, K.I., Olsen, H., Reilly, B., Falgout, K., Ensing, D. and Van Haitsma, K. (1992). God help me (II): the relationship of religious orientations to religious coping with negative life events. *Journal for the Scientific Study of Religion* **31**(4): 504–513.

Pargament, K.I., Van Haitsma, K.S. and Ensing, D. (1995). Religion and Coping. In M.A. Kimble, S.H. McFadden, J.W. Ellor and J.J. Seeber (Eds), *Aging, Spirituality, and Religion* (pp. 47–67). Minneapolis, MN: Fortress.

Pearl, P. (1990). *Helping Children Through Books: A Selected Booklist* (3rd Edn). Portland, OR: Church and Synagogue Library Association.

Prong, L.L. (1995). Childhood bereavement among Cambodians: cultural considerations. *Hospice Journal* **10**(2): 51–64.

Rabin, B.S. (1999). *Stress, Immune Function, and Health: The Connection*. New York: Wiley-Liss.

Rabins, P.V., Fitting, M.D., Eastham, J. and Zabora, J. (1990a). Emotional adaptation over time in care-givers for chronically ill elderly people. *Age and Aging* **19**, 185–190.

Rabins, P.V., Fitting, M.D., Eastham, J. and Zabora, J. (1990b). The emotional impact of caring for the chronically ill. *Psychosomatics* **31**: 331–336.

Roberts, J.A., Brown, D., Elkins, T. and Larson, D.B. (1997). Factors influencing views of patients with gynecological cancer about end-of-life decisions. *American Journal of Obstetrics and Gynecology* **176**: 166–172.

Siegal, K., Raveis, V.H.P.H. and Mor, V. (1991). Caregiver burden and unmet patient needs. *Cancer* **68**: 1131–1140.

Spiegel, D. (1992). Effects of psychosocial support on patients with metastatic breast cancer. *Journal of Psychosocial Oncology* **10**: 113–120.

Spiegel, D., Bloom, J.R., Kraemer, H.C. and Gottheil, E. (1989). Effect of psychosocial treatment on survival of patients with metastatic breast cancer. *Lancet* **2**(8668): 888–891.

Spikes, J.M. (undated). Standards of Parish Nurse Practice: A Presentation at the 5th Annual National Parish Nurse Conference, St. Louis, Available at: http://hymancare.Icms.org/hm/spikes.htm.

Spilka, B., Spangler, J.D. and Nelson, C.B. (1983). Spiritual support in life-threatening illness. *Journal of Religion and Health* **22**: 98–104.

Spilka, B., Zwartjes, W.J. and Zwartjes, G.M. (1991). The role of religion in coping with childhood cancer. *Pastoral Psychology* **39**(5): 295–304.

Wright, L.M., Watson, W.,L. and Bell, J.M. (1996). *Beliefs: The Heart of Healing in Families and Illness* (1st Edn). New York, NY: Basic Books.

Section IX
MEDICAL ETHICS AND COMMUNICATION

Patient–Family Communication with Physicians

CHRISTINA G. BLANCHARD,* TERRANCE L. ALBRECHT**
and JOHN C. RUCKDESCHEL**†

Medical Interaction Research Group,
H. Lee Moffitt Cancer Center and Research Institute, Tampa, FL, USA

For a patient with a potentially life-threatening illness, such as cancer, the relationship with the physician assumes particular significance. From pre-diagnosis concerns and tests through diagnosis, treatment, and survivorship or terminal illness, the patient turns to the physician for ongoing information and support. The physician frames the information and support based on an assessment of the disease and prognosis and ideally places these in the context of the patient's style, abilities, and needs. The interaction dynamics between the patient and physician also impact on the delivery and reception of the messages exchanged (Ruckdeschel et al., 1994).

Additionally, the patient presents to the physician bringing not only a set of physical problems but also a social context which includes his/her family, job, and community relationships (Waitzkin and Britt, 1989). The family must deal with the emotional impact of the disease and its impact on familial roles. At the same time, the family is involved directly in obtaining information regarding the disease and treatment, in decision making regarding treatment, and in care of the patient, especially if the disease progresses (see Lederberg, 1998). Thus, Doherty (1985) noted that 'every individual patient intervention in health care is simultaneously a family intervention' (p. 131). This is particularly true in the case of serious illness. Hence, the provider–patient relationship is inherently a triad (not a dyad), consisting of the health care professional, the patient, and the family. Each party supports or

* Also at The Cancer Center of Albany Med, Albany Medical Center, Albany, NY, USA
**Also at Department of Community and Family Health, College of Public Health, University of South Florida, Tampa, FL, USA
† Also at Department of Internal Medicine, College of Medicine, University of South Florida, Tampa, FL, USA

Cancer and the Family, 2nd Edn. Edited by L. Baider, C. L. Cooper and A. Kaplan De-Nour

undermines the relationship between the other two. Each party thus is affected by what else happens in the triad.

The physician, of course, also brings aspects of his/her social, cultural, familial, and professional context to the interaction. Our focus is primarily on the *principles* (see also Charles et al., 1997) and resulting *skills* that the *physician* must exhibit to foster the most effective and successful physician–patient–family relationship as defined by the patient and family.

Clearly, the US Census Bureau's traditional definition of the family as 'two or more persons living together who are related by blood, marriage, or adoption,' no longer applies to many who define themselves as a family. A family can now be defined more broadly as 'the nexus of people living together or in close contact, who take care of one another' (see Patterson and Garwick, 1994). Further, the family is subjectively defined (i.e., the family itself defines who is and who is not part of the 'family'). Components of family functioning including flexibility, cohesion, problem solving, and affective expression are likely to determine the ways in which the family copes with the cancer (see Patterson and Garwick, 1994, for a more complete discussion of a family system perspective of chronic illness in the family).

The boundaries of a family define who is 'in' and who is 'out'. An important implication is that key family members may be psychologically present but physically absent. Thus, the family member accompanying the patient to the physician visit may or may not be the one to whom the patient turns to for assistance in decision making or even physical care. Indeed, the physician may be contacted by several family members for information, questions, or complaints. Care must be taken to assess this entire family constellation. Familial boundaries also differ in terms of openness to input from outside systems. For example, members of a family system may refuse referral to a home care agency, citing a need for privacy, or conversely, incorporate the agency personnel into the family as additional family members.

We will examine patient–family communication with the physician by first discussing the patient–physician relationship, as the research to date has primarily focused on this dyad, with relatively little attention given directly to the impact of the family on this relationship and the resulting transformation of the dyad into a triad. Next, we briefly address studies of family concerns/needs. Finally, studies of the patient–family–physician relationship are summarized, and directions for research suggested.

TOWARD A PARTNERSHIP MODEL OF THE PHYSICIAN–PATIENT RELATIONSHIP

While technologies continue to be developed with ever-increasing sophistication, face-to-face communication remains the primary mode of information exchange between physician and patient (Ong et al., 1995). Until the past 25 or so years, this interaction was characterized by physician power and control, with the physician possessing the expertise telling the patient what action should be taken. This paternalistic model did have several benefits (Quill and Brody, 1996). Physicians made the best decisions they could for patients, and their families were spared from agonizing about decisions regarding the use of interventions that might have limited effectiveness. Physicians also had more control over the ways medical technology was used, with its increasing ability to help as well as harm. However, the obvious problem with the model was that patients were often deprived of the opportunity to make decisions that reflected their circumstances and reality (determined in part by their gender, race, socio-economic status, family dynamics, and personality style).

The pendulum first swung from paternalism to patient autonomy, in which patients and families were asked to make critical medical decisions on the basis of neutrally presented data, as free as possible from physician bias. Causes of this trend include the consumer movement, which taught patients to be more assertive, to question physicians, and often to take some responsibility for obtaining their own information to discuss with their physician (a trend hastened by the availability of National Cancer Institute and American Cancer Society 800 toll-free telephone numbers and the Internet). The difficulty is that the physician's recommendations, based on expertise and experience, may not be presented to the patient, possibly short-changing the patient this input and appropriate medical guidance.

A new model has been developed which encourages patient participation but provides the patient and family with opinions and recommendations to assist with the decisions. Originally termed a 'mutual participation' model by Szasz and Hollender (1956), this has more recently been called an 'enhanced autonomy model' by Quill and Brody (1996). Others have called it a 'shared decision-making model' (Charles et al., 1997). This is a relationship-centered model, with the patient and physician (and often the family) participating in the information exchange and in decision-making. The model is based on the premise that open dialogue, in which the physician expresses his/her view, is the best 'protector' of patient autonomy. It explicitly acknowledges the values and views of the physician. Additionally, dialogues that enhance autonomy include explorations of the assumptions, values, and perspectives of both the patient and physician, improving the extent to which communication behavior is sensitive to the patient's culture (Deber, 1994). 'Patients want physicians who are not afraid to use their power, but they also want to trust them to use that power to assist them through a crisis and not to control or coerce them' (Quill and Brody, 1996, pp. 764–765).

We prefer the term 'partnership' to describe the emerging relationship. This suggests that each party has rights and responsibilities and that to exercise them requires them to interact. Partnership is a broader term than 'shared decision-making', which implies that the decisions *must* be shared. We suggest that the key is the *negotiation* between the physician and the patient as the physician obtains information and asks questions, sensitive to the patient's social context, so that patient preferences for degree of information and participation in decision-making can be ascertained.

A successful patient–physician encounter would include the following components. The physician must establish an environment in which the patient's views about decision making, and thus treatment options, are valued and discussed in the context of a patient's life. Information on the diagnosis and treatment options, with discussion of the risks and benefits of each, needs to be presented clearly, with the patient encouraged to ask questions and the physician attuned to the degree to which the patient desires and can process information. The physician should share his/her recommendations with the patient. For an effective partnership, the patient must be willing to disclose preferences for information and involvement in decision making by asking questions and stating opinions. Ideally, patient and physician reach a consensus, with the patient encouraged to have the degree of input into the decision that he/she desires (see Charles et al., 1997, who discuss these components as they apply to the shared decision-making model).

Empirical studies have shown that enhanced patient autonomy or participation has been associated with a variety of improved outcomes in emotional health, substance abuse treatment, weight reduction, pain control, and adherence to treatment regimens (see Quill and Brody, 1996; Stewart, 1995). A recent review of research, both for an against patient participation in decision-making, by Guadagnoli and Ward (1998) concluded that patients want to be informed of treatment alternatives and, in general, want to be involved in treatment decisions when there is more than one treatment alternative. A variety of physician factors (e.g., lack of knowledge of communication skills) and patient variables (e.g., past experience with the health care system reinforcing physician paternalism, age, or cultural variables supporting a more dominant role of the physician) operate to influence the degree of a partnership between the patient and physician. Guadagnoli and Ward (1998) support the enhanced autonomy model of decision-making and suggest that Prochaska and colleagues' theory of receptivity to change in behaviors be applied to an analysis of patients' 'readiness' to participate in decision-making with interventions to foster patient participation appropriate to his/her level of readiness.

DOES THE PARTNERSHIP MODEL
FIT THE CANCER PATIENT–PHYSICIAN RELATIONSHIP?

Does the partnership model fit when the patient has a chronic, life-threatening disease such as cancer? The communication process between the cancer patient and physician is particularly challenging due to the fear and stigma associated with cancer, the complexity of the medical information, and the uncertainty regarding the course of the disease (see Siminoff, 1992). Perhaps the partnership model is most critical in the setting of cancer as the patient is facing the possible loss of life. The responsibilities of each party that foster a partnership for decision making have been outlined by Schain (1990) (Table 27.1). Although she was describing the interaction of a physician and a breast cancer patient, the same elements would be present regardless of disease site. It is particularly important to assist the cancer patient to be as comfortable as possible with the decisions made regarding treatment. Wendy S. Harpham, M.D., writing as a physician and cancer survivor, said: '... health care professionals must help all people to understand that the 'best treatment choice' is one based on foresight, not retrospect. Assuming that medically sound decisions are being made, when a person's cancer progresses unexpectedly during a first course of treatment, only to respond dramatically to a change in treatment, the person must perceive the first course of treatment, not as a poor choice or, worse, as a mistake, but as the best choice with the information available' (1995, pp. 96–97). We suggest that this is a prototype for interaction, regardless of the treatment outcome. This will help to avoid guilt or second guessing and should thus assist in psychological adjustment.

Table 27.1 Responsibilities of the parties in decision making about breast cancer treatment

Physician	Patient
Encourage questions about alternatives	Ask for information about options and side effects
Provide 'congruent' information	Tell doctor if she feels rushed or confused
Provide supplemental aids, e.g., audio tapes	Ask doctor about training, experience, fees, and payments
Integrate information about psychosocial, functional, and cosmetic needs	Explain wishes and needs for functional and cosmetic results
Provide risk and benefit information alternatives	Question informed consent
Inquire and integrate information about sexual and reproductive needs	Explain specific sexual and reproductive concerns
Recommend baseline and follow-up tests	Inquire about follow-up tests and schedule
Know community resources (self-help, professional)	Tell doctor whether or not she feels satisfied or needs additional services
Ask patient about needs for participation	Explain needs for disclosure and participation at various stages
Know clues to a dysfunctional relationship	Know clues, i.e., loss of faith, trust, or respect

Reprinted from Schain, W.S. Physician–patient communication about breast cancer. *Surgical Clinics of North America*, 70: 917–936 (1990). With permission from W.B. Saunders Company, Philadelphia, PA.

How much of a partnership now exists? There is near-universal agreement by physicians today that cancer patients should be told their diagnosis (Novak et al., 1979).* Patients also believe they should be told all information, good or bad, about their illness (Blanchard et al., 1988; Cassileth et al., 1980). Not surprisingly, the physician is the primary person patients turn to for information, while empathic support is required from the physician and family and friends (Neuling and Winefield, 1988). It should be noted that the provision of information itself can be seen as a supportive behavior (see Albrecht and Adelman, 1987; Wortman, 1984).

Unfortunately, information also may not be heard accurately (even if transmitted). This may be particularly true when 'bad news' is conveyed. One study found that only half the patients whose physicians thought they were incurable realized this prognosis. The other half thought they had a chance of cure. Only 37% of the patients' expectations of cure agreed with those of the physicians (Mackillop et al., 1988). Siminoff and colleagues (1989) found that 60% of breast cancer patients overestimated their chance of cure by 20% or more, compared with physician estimates. It is not clear whether this information gap reflects a failure of communication or represents a coping mechanism employed by the patient.

Recognizing the negative impact of 'bad' news on the patient, Creagan (1994) provided guidelines to assist the physician in this communication. He stressed the importance of: (a) providing a quiet, confidential setting; (b) assessing the patient's

---

*Although it is beyond the scope of this chapter to examine the doctor–patient relationship in other cultures, one recent study showed that 80% of a sample of hospitalized patients in Japan wanted candid information about their diagnosis and prognosis. This is a culture in which direct communication between patient and physician rarely occurs, especially if there is a poor prognosis (see Kai et al., 1993).

level of understanding and assumptions; and (c) attending to the patient's reactions to guide the interaction. Bennett and Alison (1996) stress the importance of breaking the news at a pace appropriate to the cancer patient's verbal and non-verbal behavior and provide helpful suggestions for the physician to be an effective communicator.

Certainly a major function of the provision of information is that it serves to reduce uncertainty at a time of great stress and crisis. While information is critical for the making of clinical decisions, several studies have suggested that not all patients want to participate in clinical decision-making. Although over 90% of cancer patients wanted information about their illness (good or bad), a smaller percentage (older, sicker males) wanted the physician to make treatment decisions (Blanchard et al., 1988; see also Beisecker and Beisecker, 1990; Fallowfield et al., 1995). Several possible reasons for these findings have been suggested. First, the preference to have the physician make the decision may reflect an underlying personality construct. Second, patients may feel they do not possess the skills necessary to process the information. Third, the patient may have learned passive role-taking during previous interactions with health care professionals. Fourth, there may be a generational cohort effect, with older persons deferring more to the physician for decision-making (Charles et al., 1997).

Of course, patients do not always participate in decision-making to the extent they prefer. Degner and colleagues (1997) reported that 22% of breast cancer patients wanted to select their own treatment, 47% wanted the treatment decisions to be made collaboratively with the physicians, and 34% wanted the physicians to decide. However, 42% achieved their desired goal in decision-making. Interestingly, the two most highly ranked types of information desired were knowing the chances of cure and spread of the disease. These ranked above discussions of treatment alternatives, again showing that preference for information does not always mean preference for shared decision-making. The possible relationship between ratings of information and psychological adjustment was examined by Butow et al. (1996) in a study of Australian breast and melanoma patients. They found that psychological adjustment was related to patient ratings of the quality of physician discussions about treatment options, not about the diagnosis of cancer and its implications.

Ford et al. (1996) audiotaped consultations between five oncologists and 117 outpatients in a large London teaching hospital. Patients were given a large volume of biomedical information ('bad news') and treatment options were offered. They received counseling concerning their medical condition. However, there were few open-ended questions and few psychosocial questions from physicians, despite the potential toxicity of treatments that were being recommended. Patients were rarely given space to express their feelings, and the level of patient-centeredness was low. There were suggestions in the data that three of the physicians varied their behaviors depending on the patient's age and prognosis, but the number of patients per oncologist was too small for further analysis.

The relationship between preference for decisional control and illness information among 35 women with breast cancer was studied by Hack et al. (1994). A card-sort measure was used to determine patient decisional preference and information needs. Patients who desired an active role in treatment decision making also desired detailed information. There was not a clear relationship for passive patients. The authors suggest that the advantages of active and passive roles may differ at different stages of the illness process. Furthermore, it cannot be assumed that those with an active role preference are better adjusted or that passive patients' desire for minimal information should be targeted for an intervention.

THE CANCER PATIENT–PHYSICIAN RELATIONSHIP AND THE DECISION TO ACCRUE TO CLINICAL TRIALS

One specific patient–physician communication that has been recognized as particularly significant is that in which the physician presents to the patient the possibility of entering a clinical trial. Clearly, the effectiveness and efficacy of new treatments depend on patients participating in clinical trials, yet fewer than 3% of all cancer patients are enrolled on a protocol (Gotay, 1991). While several reasons exist why patients accrue or do not accrue, communication behaviors between patient and physician are a major determining factor.

We have videotaped 48 patient–physician interactions, involving 12 oncologists, in which a clinical trial option was presented to the patient (Albrecht et al., 1999). A coding system, the Moffitt Accrual Analysis System (MAAS) was developed to code behaviors representing both the *legal–informational* and *social influence/support* models of communication behavior. The first model is a study-centered framework represented by the informed consent form, a legal document which contains required information about the study, including the title, investigators and institutions participating, purpose and description of the study, risks and benefits, randomization (if a Phase III trial), alternative treatments, confidentiality of results, payment expectations of costs involved, voluntary nature of participation, liabilities related to possible injury, persons to contact if there are questions, and the need for patient (and witness if appropriate) signatures.

The second model is a person-centered strategy. The physician's goal is to connect with the patient's needs. Thus, from a social exchange standpoint, the patient's perceived benefits of study enrollment are maximized while perceived barriers are directly addressed, with the desired result being that benefits outweigh the barriers.

Results showed that physicians who were observed to use both models of influence were found to enroll more patients. Thus, patients were more likely to accrue to a trial when the physician verbally presented items included in the informed consent document and when they also behaved in a reflexive, patient-centered supportive, and responsive manner. As expected, discussion of benefits, side effects, patient concerns, and resources (tangible as well as emotional support) were each associated with accrual. Additional studies will examine the impact of patient and protocol characteristics on the accrual decisions. The impact of a third party (i.e., a family member) on the decision is also being investigated.

THE RELATIONSHIP BETWEEN PHYSICIAN BEHAVIOR AND CANCER PATIENT SATISFACTION

Patient satisfaction is perhaps the most common outcome measure used to evaluate the physician–patient relationship (see Ong et al, 1995 for a review of the consequences of doctor–patient communication on patient satisfaction, adherence to treatment, recall and understanding of information, and health status/ psychiatric morbidity). Several studies that have focused on cancer patient satisfaction are reviewed here.

To examine the possible relationship between physicians' actual behaviors, patient perceptions of these behaviors, and patient satisfaction, Blanchard et al. (1990) measured physician behaviors in 366 encounters with hospitalized adult cancer patients on morning rounds. There was no 'standard' set of behaviors across physicians. Patient satisfaction was high ($X = 87.8$ mm on a 100 mm scale). Path analysis showed that four variables predicted 62% of the variance in patient satisfaction: (a) perception of needs met that day; (b) perception of emotional support; (c) patient age (older) and (d) one physician behavior, discusses treatment. Perception of needs met or emotional support provided were predicted by patient perceptions of the occurrence of physician behaviors involving the transmission of information, such as the diagnosis, and explaining future tests and treatment. Physician behaviors, particularly 'identifying tests and treatments' and 'inquiring about signs and symptoms' were predictive of patient perceptions of these behaviors. Patient satisfaction was interpreted to represent the patient's affective evaluation ('needs met') of the cognitive aspects of the physician–patient interaction, i.e., the provision of information.

Wiggers et al. (1990) assessed the perceptions of 232 ambulatory patients, in four oncology clinics in Australia, about the importance of and satisfaction with several aspects of care. They found that greatest importance was given to the technical quality of medical care, the interpersonal and communication skills of physicians, and the accessibility of care. Most patients were satisfied with the opportunities to discuss their needs with doctors, the interpersonal support of doctors, and the technical competence of doctors. They were less satisfied with the provision of information concerning their disease, treatment, and symptom control, with the provision of home care, and with the support for family and friends.

Bertakis et al. (1991) reported on a study in 11 institutions examining the association between patient medical interview style (measured by the Roter Interaction Analysis System) and patient satisfaction in a chronic disease clinic visit. Task-directed satisfaction was the most important subscale affecting overall satisfaction with the visit. Further analysis showed that patients were most satisfied by interviews encouraging them to talk about psychosocial issues in an atmosphere that was characterized by less physician dominance.

These studies are consistent with research on patient satisfaction by Inui and Carter (1985), who concluded that patient satisfaction is maximized when the physician responds to the patient's expectations and concerns; communicates with warmth, interest, and concern; and provides information to the patient. Similar findings were reported by Hall et al (1988), who summarized 41 studies containing objectively measured physician behavior and patient outcome variables. Meta-analysis showed that patient satisfaction was related to the amount of information given by providers, greater technical and interpersonal competence, more partnership building, more social conversation, more positive and less negative talk, and more communication overall.

IMPACT OF PATIENT AND PHYSICIAN STYLES ON THE RELATIONSHIP

Several studies have broadened the exploration of physician–cancer interaction by assessing the relationship between the patients' coping style and mood and their impact on the evaluation of the interaction. Dermatis and Lesko (1991) studied 39 adult bone marrow transplant patients. Results showed a positive relationship between perceived quality of the physician–patient relationship and two factors: problem-focused coping style and perceived autonomy in decision-making. Although patients exhibited significantly higher psychological distress (measured by the Brief Symptom Inventory) than the normal population, it was striking that this variable was unrelated to either the coping style or perceived quality of the physician–patient interaction. The authors suggested that patients received sufficient emotional support from their family and friends and did not turn to physicians for this support.

A few studies have used the Miller Behavioral Style Scale (MBSS) to assess coping style. Coping style was assessed as either monitoring (information-seeking) or blunting (distraction/avoidance of information). Steptoe et al. (1991) found that hospitalized cancer patients reported high satisfaction levels. However, patients who were less than completely satisfied with communications had higher 'monitoring' scores.

In contrast, Lerman et al. (1993) reported that 84% of the 97 breast cancer patients studied reported communication difficulties with the medical team. The 11-item Medical Interaction component of the CARES (Cancer Rehabilitation Evaluation System) was used to measure specific areas of difficulty. The most commonly reported problems were difficulty in understanding physicians (49.5%), difficulty in expressing feelings (46.3%), desiring more control over doctors (45.3%), and difficulty in asking physicians questions (42.6%). Fewer communication problems were reported by patients with a blunting/avoidant style. They also found that those reporting communication problems were more distressed, less optimistic, and felt more helpless about their disease. The association between communication problems and mood disturbance remained significant, although small, at 3 month follow-up, after adjusting for baseline mood disturbance, coping style, and sociodemographic variables.

The Steptoe et al. (1991) and Lerman et al. (1993) studies reporting high satisfaction/fewer communication difficulties related to an avoidant/blunting style may mean that the information expectations of these patients are met. These patients may be more likely to be buffered from the acute stress of the disease and thus may experience lower distress levels. Conversely, high levels of monitoring may be self-defeating and produce anxiety when individuals believe the situation is unchangeable, hopeless, or when it is uncontrollable. Thus, more information may exacerbate feelings of powerlessness and helplessness (see also Glanz and Lerman, 1992).

Miller (1995) concluded that, in general, patients with a monitoring style do better with more information; those with a blunting style with less. However, patients with a monitoring style who are pessimistic about their future or who face long-term uncontrollable medical situations may not only require additional information but more emotional support from their physicians to assist in coping with the disease.

Turning briefly to the physician's style and its possible impact on the relationship, it is clear that some physicians have a 'patient-centered' approach that solicits patient questions, provides information and addresses patient needs. Others have a more 'physician-centered' approach, characterized by more closed questions and directives (see Street, 1992). Taylor (1988) also reported that physician style was an important variable influencing whether a clinical trial was presented to a cancer patient. Those physicians with an experimental style were more likely to discuss the options of a clinical trial than were those with a therapeutic style.

SUMMARY AND IMPLICATIONS

Certainly, the model of the physician–patient relationship in the USA has moved from one that is paternalistic, to one providing the patient with virtual autonomy, to the current model suggesting a partnership between patient and physician. The vast majority of patients want information about their illness, good or bad, but it does not necessarily follow that they want all the details of the information, or that they want to use the information to assist them in a shared decision-making relationship with the physician. More research is necessary to clarify the impact of patient styles regarding the desire for information (monitor or blunter) and the relationship between that style, sociodemographic variables—particularly age, gender, and socio-economic status—preference for participation in treatment decision-making, stage of disease, and outcome measures including psychological morbidity, satisfaction, accrual to clinical trial, and adherence (see also Ong et al., 1995). Research is also needed to further examine the physician's communication behaviors and the ways in which patient and physician styles are congruent or conflict. It is hypothesized that when the patient and physician styles are congruent, both are likely to find the interaction of benefit and satisfying. On the other hand, when styles are incongruent, e.g., the physician has an experimental style (i.e., one that promotes clinical trials) while the patient has an informational avoidant style, difficulties result, with both becoming frustrated (Humphrey et al, 1992; see also Ruckdeschel et al., 1994).

Interventions can increase congruence, not only by teaching patients to modify their style by asking questions (as was reported by Greenfield and colleagues, 1985), but also by teaching physicians to adapt their styles to that characteristically used by the patients. Many medical schools now offer courses assisting students to develop effective communication skills with patients. Furthermore, several books and videos are available, leading one writer to entitle his article, 'Talking to patients about cancer: no excuse now for not doing it' (Buckman, 1996; see Roter and Fallowfield, 1998, for a review of physician training programs in communication skills).

CANCER AS A FAMILY ILLNESS

...One of the ways that all of us avoid thinking about death is by concentrating on the details of our daily lives...A year after I had my lung removed, my doctor asked me what I cared about most...I told him that what was most important to me was garden peas. What was extraordinary to me after that year was that I could again think that peas were important, that I could concentrate on the details of when to plant them and how much mulch they would need...The strength of my love for my children, my husband, my life, even my garden peas, has probably been more important than anything else in keeping me alive. The intensity of this love is also what makes me so terrified of dying . . . We will never kill the dragon. But each morning we confront him. Then we give our children breakfast, perhaps put a bit more mulch on the peas, and hope that we can convince the dragon to stay away for a while longer (Trillin, 1981).

The importance of the family to the patient is seen in this quote. Cancer is not a disease of one individual but impacts the entire family system. The family must confront and attempt to understand the meaning of cancer for the patient, for each family member individually, and for the family system as a whole. As the medical course of the disease moves through phases from pre-diagnosis, to diagnosis, to treatment, to remission, cure, relapse, or death, psychosocial transitions are also apparent. These transitions hopefully occur in ways that facilitate the performance of role functioning and functional communication patterns that enhance family flexibility for meeting the changing demands that result from the illness. Lewis (1993) described how families break down (destructure) operational and communication patterns that no longer respond to their new role responsibilities and functions, and rebuild (restructure) to meet the new responsibilities, always attempting to balance the needs of the individual with those of the family. There are times of reflection, searching, conflict, disappointment, and fear as the restructuring is occurring. Expectations or role transitions characterizing other major family changes, such as weddings or graduations, are not available to guide families as the disease status changes. Perhaps this is a major reason for the popularity of support groups where shared experiences facilitate the development of meaning and discussions of appropriate behavioral and emotional responses provide reassurance and comfort.

Of course, attempts by the family to manage the demands caused by cancer occur in the presence of other family maintenance tasks—family members must all eat, sleep, engage in employment and education roles, and maintain their other relationships. These are structured by the developmental stage of the family, socio-economic status, belief systems, past coping styles, and familial role of the patient. All these variables contribute to the specific concerns of the family and to the meanings ascribed to the cancer (see also Sales *et al.*, 1992).

In addition to family context variables, the stage of the illness is another major factor determining patient and family concerns (Sales, 1991). In the initial diagnostic phase, families and patients are confronted with a range of emotional reactions to the disease (i.e., anger, fear, sadness, helplessness) as the continuity of the family and future hopes are disrupted. Contacts with the health care delivery system are frightening and confusing, but also generally supportive. Families may attempt to conceal their own fears in an effort to focus on those of the patient (see Gotay, 1984), who may hesitate to share his/her concerns so as not to burden the family. The family may also try to protect the patient by requesting (sometimes ordering) the physician not to give 'bad news' to the patient. During treatment, the family may feel ignored by the medical staff while also needing to be patient advocates. Role overload and exhaustion are common. Dealing with side effects may require not only support but also family caretaking. After treatment is concluded, the family must adapt to new role configurations, depending on the degree of disability or disfigurement.

Cancer patients also live with the uncertainty of recurrence; the distress accompanying recurrence may equal or surpass that of the initial diagnosis (see Sales, 1991) as patients and families become aware that the initial treatment did not control the disease. It should be noted, however, that clinically we have often heard patients and families discuss the positive changes in priorities and emphasis on living in the present that have developed as the family copes with the cancer.

The physical and emotional demands on the family reach a peak if the illness progresses to the terminal stage. Family members must assume new caregiving tasks and not feel they lack the skills, information, or assistance to perform them. Their own needs may be neglected, leading to emotional isolation, exhaustion, and alienation. The assistance provided by the health care team and/or hospice may help to address these problems and may further facilitate completing any 'unfinished business' prior to the death, while finally assisting family members in their bereavement.

THE PATIENT–FAMILY–PHYSICIAN/TEAM RELATIONSHIP

The importance of the treatment team, particularly the physician, for the family cannot be overestimated. Particularly during times of acute crises, the family revolves around 'illness issues' and turns to the medical team for information, support, and guidance. The family interprets both overt and covert messages from the team to better comprehend the patient's condition and its meaning. If clear communication and shared values are present and the family is functional, the interface between family and staff is likely to operate well, with greater satisfaction. If there is not a 'good fit,' frustration increases on both sides, with the team expressing annoyance and perhaps being slower to answer phone calls or questions. Family dissatisfaction is expressed in increased demands, phone calls, or even a decision to switch to another health care provider.

In a large medical system, it is difficult to control the flow of information and impossible to insure that different physicians give similar messages. Mixed messages create confusion, anxiety, and anger among patients and family members. The team may overestimate the family's desire for information and overwhelm them or underestimate this desire, making the family more passive than they would prefer. Similarly, complications may occur when family patterns are dysfunctional, sometimes reflecting long-standing conflicts, which may result in several family members communicating conflicting messages to the staff regarding the patient. Additionally, families from other cultures bring differing values and traditions regarding disease, treatment, and death that may further complicate interactions with the staff.

The family, like the patient, turns to the physician primarily for information. Information needed is directly related to stage of the disease, with information regarding diagnosis, treatment, side effects, support groups and other community resources changing as the stage of the disease changes, and with it, goals of treatment move from diagnosing, to curing, to palliative care (Northouse and Peters-Golden, 1993). It is essential that hope be maintained throughout the disease process, but it should be realistic, based on anticipated disease outcomes (Northouse and Northouse, 1987). It is likely that the transitions between the stages (pre-diagnosis,

diagnosis, treatment, survivorship, recurrence, death) represent the most difficult points for the physician as the patient/family must be prepared for the change, reflecting the change in treatment goals.

Little is known about the experience of the patient, family, and health care professional when the patient has advanced cancer and is involved in experimental therapy. Stetz (1993) interviewed 24 patients with advanced liver cancer and 16 of their spouses before, during, and after receiving chemotherapy at a major cancer center. Three phases were evident. The first was termed 'engaging', i.e., persistent behavior engaged in by the patient and spouse to find treatment after the prognosis was given by the physician. The patient and spouse sought information and decided to be treated. Physicians encouraged patients to consent to the treatment and administered the treatment. The second stage was 'monitoring'. This was the stage of guarded optimism during treatment. The spouse was supportive; the physician the messenger of good or bad news. In the third stage, 'carrying on', the patients primarily dealt with living as normally as they could in their remaining time, and spouses assumed increasing responsibilities while physicians disengaged and referred patients back to their community oncologists.

As was noted earlier, families often want to help and protect the patient, sometimes resulting in attempts to protect the patient (and themselves) from 'bad news' or particularly difficult decision making, such as 'Do Not Resuscitate' decisions. The principles of doing good to the patient and not harming the patient (beneficence and non-maleficence), respecting the patient (autonomy), and being fair and not discriminating (justice) are to be followed to determine a course of action to a patient (see Surbone, 1996). This generally means that patients should be told the truth about their disease. However, how should the beneficent views of a family, who have generally known the patient longer than the physician, be considered? In a study of 30 cancer patients in the UK, Benson and Britten (1996) found that all patients wished doctors to respect their views rather than those of their family, should they differ. With their consent, subjects favored close family receiving information about their illness. Most rejected unconditional disclosure of information without their consent, and rejected the notion of having their family influence what information they would be given. The authors concluded that the patients valued respect for their autonomy more highly than beneficence. In short, they felt that their own needs took priority over the needs of their family.

Information and support can be provided to the family directly by the physician, as would be done during office or hospital visits or at family meetings. These should occur with the patient present whenever possible to reduce the chances of misinformation being transmitted to family members, to encourage open discussion among the family, and, most importantly, because the primary relationship is between the patient (not the family) and the physician. When there is conflict between family and patient regarding treatment options, clinical trials, resuscitation status, or hospice care, the physician may reduce the conflict by speaking to the entire family together, often with the assistance of a social worker to facilitate discussion (see also Faulkner and Maguire, 1994). Of course, information and support are also provided by other health care team members, particularly nurses and social workers, and by information from the National Cancer Institute and the American Cancer Society.

THE IMPACT OF FAMILY PRESENCE ON THE PATIENT–PHYSICIAN RELATIONSHIP

Patients are generally encouraged to bring a family member with them to an office visit. The presence of a third person, however, makes possible a coalition of 'two against one' (Wolff, 1950). Coe and Pendergast (1985) compared encounters of the same elderly patient with, and without, companions present, finding that more than one coalition emerged within a single visit when a companion was present. Companions can be advocates, passive participants, or antagonists (Adelman et al., 1987), medical managers or supervisors, interpreters, negotiators, or caretakers (Coe & Pendergast, 1985), watchdogs, significant others, or surrogate patients (Beisecker, 1989).

Beiscker and Moore (1994) interviewed 12 oncologists regarding their perceptions of the effects of cancer patients' companions on physician–patient interactions. The physicians estimated that three-quarters of patients brought companions, most often spouses, to the visit. They overwhelmingly favored the presence of a companion during the visit but noted that the companion was occasionally a problem and generally made the visit more complex. The behaviors of a companion varied from domination to note-taking. Physicians judged companions who were young, professional men or older women to be the most assertive and as asking the majority of questions. Physicians noted that the following alliances might develop during the visit: patient and physician (to control or persuade a companion); companion and physician (to persuade the patient); patient and companion (often asking the physician's blessing to obtain a second opinion), and family coalition (particularly evident when several family members visiting from out of town attempt to direct family members who are in immediate contact with the patient).

Despite the view that cancer impacts the entire family and the studies showing needs of patient and family for information and support, our study (Labrecque et al., 1991) is the only one of which we are aware that examined the cancer patient–physician interaction when the family is present. We compared patient–physician interactions in the outpatient setting with a family member present ($n = 99$) with those without a family member present ($n = 374$).

Patients with a family member present for the visit were significantly more likely to have a poorer performance status ($\chi^2 = 45.6$, $p < 0.001$) and to be undergoing active treatment. Neither sex nor age predicted whether the patient would be accompanied by a family member. Factor analysis of physician behaviors (measured by the Physician Behavior Check List; Blanchard et al., 1983) produced six Factors: (1) discussing future treatment; (2) discussing current treatment; (3) discussing current medical status; (4) greeting the patient; (5) providing emotional support; and (6) providing reassurance. The physician provided significantly more information when the family member was present (Factors 1,3) and also was more likely to greet the patient (Factor 4). However, there was no main effect of family presence on reassurance provided (Factor 6), and the physician provided less emotional support (Factor 5) when the family member was present.

Main effects for performance status were also found. For Factors 1–3, which pertain to the provision of information, the physician provided significantly more information to the sicker patients. However, the physician was significantly less likely to greet the sicker patient (Factor 4) or to provide emotional support (Factor 5). There was no difference in Factor 6 (reassurance).

Significant univariate interactions were found between family presence and performance status on Factors 1,3,4, and 5. Table 27.2 shows the means and *post hoc* comparisons for factor scores with significant multivariate interactions of family presence by performance status. Table 27.2 shows that the physician provided the most information on future treatment when the family was present and the patient was symptomatic. Current medical treatment was discussed more frequently when the family was present, regardless of symptoms. If the family was not present and the patient was sicker, the physician greeted the patient less often. When a family member was not present, the physician provided more emotional support to the patient who was asymptomatic.

Thus, physicians provided more information under conditions of potential uncertainty. These included when the patient was symptomatic or when the family was present, bringing them up to date and responding to their concerns about the future. It is likely that a sense of support was offered through the transmission of information. The physician offered emotional support significantly more often when the medical issues seemed less critical (i.e., the patient is asymptomatic), no family present. Not surprisingly, the physician spent more time when the family member was present. Patient satisfaction and quality of life were rated lower for sicker patients and were unrelated to physician behaviors.

THE SPECIAL CASE OF CHILDREN/ADOLESCENTS

Foley (1993) recently addressed the issue of child–family health care team communication. Using an historical perspective, she noted that the belief in the pre-1960s that the child should be protected from knowing his/her disease or prognosis was gradually replaced in the 1970s by the realization that children coped more effectively when told their diagnosis. Currently, the challenge is to promote effective communication between the child, the parents, and the team. This facilitates the child/adolescent's participation and may enhance self-esteem and development and increase cooperation. It also assists patient and family coping at all stages of the disease process.

Table 27.2 Means and *post hoc* comparisons for factor scores with significant multivariate interactions of family presence by performance status

	Patient only		Family present	
Factor	No symptoms	Symptoms	No symptoms	Symptoms
1 Future treatment	1.743[a]	1.772[a]	1.696[a]	1.882[b]
3 Current medical	2.195[a]	2.248[b]	2.381[c]	2.381[c]
4 Greeting	0.470[a]	0.436[b]	0.496[a]	0.478[a]
5 Emotional support	0.500[a]	0.432[b]	0.390[b]	0.412[b]

Means within a row which have different superscripts are significantly different at $p < 0.05$.
Reprinted from Labrecque M.S., Blanchard, C.G., Ruckdeschel, J.C. and Blanchard, E.B. The impact of family presence on the physician-cancer patient interaction. *Social Science and Medicine*, **33**: 1253–1261 (1991). With permission from Elsevier Science Ltd.

FUTURE DIRECTIONS

As we have discussed, the prevailing model of a partnership between physician and patient does characterize the physician–cancer patient relationship. This is particularly true of information, as both patient and physician believe that information (good or bad) should be shared with the patient. It is less true of decision-making, with a smaller percentage of patients preferring less autonomy and more physician guidance than a partnership would suggest.

Given that cancer has a major impact on the family and the assertion that every interaction with the physician involves the family, it is surprising that so few studies exist examining the changes in the interactions that occur when the family is actually present and the impact of these on patient decision-making and satisfaction. Much work remains regarding our understanding of communication processes and structures that shape the cognitions, emotions, and behaviors of each party to the triad: patients, families, and physicians. For example, longitudinal studies of the initiation, maintenance, and dissolution of these complex relational ties among the patient, physician, close and perhaps distal kin/friends (including the shifting structural coalitions that may occur; see Coe and Pendergast, 1985) are needed to better predict and understand requirements for consistency vs. flexibility in decision-making processes. Further investigation of the impact of stage of the disease, along with sociodemographic variables including gender, age, and socio-economic status, are also needed to understand communication behaviors and messages.

In addition, more developed measures of characteristic patient, family, and physician communication styles/patterns/expectations will assist in evaluating the extent of congruence/compatibility of styles. Areas of congruence and beneficial outcomes include: (a) cognitive congruence, related to meaning, recall, and interpretation of information; (b) affective congruence, related to perceptions of social support, reassurance, acceptance, and hopefulness, and (c) behavioral congruence, most generally related to patient adherence.

Research efforts of this nature carry the potential to develop theoretical frameworks, given the dearth of models to date. At the clinical level, such model building can guide the development of interventions to improve patient, family, and physician relationships. At the educational level, it may lead to improved training of physicians and other health care professionals.

REFERENCES

Adelman, R.D., Greene, M.G. and Charon, R. (1987). The physician–elderly patient–companion triad in the medical encounter: the development of a conceptual framework and research agenda. *Gerontologist* **27**: 729–734.

Albrecht, T.L. and Adelman, M.B. (1987). *Communicating Social Support*. Newbury Park, CA: Sage.

Albrecht, T.L., Blanchard, C.G., Ruckdeschel, J.C., Coovert, M. and Strongbow, R.M. (1999). Strategic physician communication and oncology clinical trials. *Journal of Clinical Oncology* **17**: 3324–3332.

Beisecker, A.E. (1989). The influence of a companion on the doctor–elderly patient interaction. *Health Communication* **1**: 55–70.

Beisecker, A.E. and Beisecker, T.D. (1990). Patient information-seeking behaviors when communicating with physicians. *Medical Care* **28**: 19–28.

Beisecker, A.E. and Moore, W.P. (1994).   Oncologists' perceptions of the effects of cancer patients' companions on physician–patient interactions. *Journal of Psychosocial Oncology* **12**: 23–39.

Bennett, M. and Alison, D. (1996).   Discussing the diagnosis and prognosis with cancer patients. *Postgraduate Medical Journal* **72**: 25–29.

Benson, J. and Britten, N. (1996).   Respecting the autonomy of cancer patients when talking with their families: qualitative analysis of semi-structured interviews with patients. *British Medical Journal* **313**: 729–731.

Bertakis, K.D., Roter, D. and Putnam, S.M. (1991).   The relationship of physician medical interview style to patient satisfaction. *Journal of Family Practice* **32**: 175–181.

Blanchard, C.G., Ruckdeschel, J.C., Blanchard, E.B., Arena, J.C., Saunders, N.L. and Malloy E.D. (1983).   Interactions between oncologists and patients during rounds. *Annals of Internal Medicine* **99**: 694–699.

Blanchard, C.G., Labrecque, M.S., Ruckdeschel, J.C. and Blanchard, E.B. (1988).   Information and decision-making preferences of hospitalized adult cancer patients. *Social Science and Medicine* **27**: 1139-1145.

Blanchard, C.G., Labrecque, M.S., Ruckdeschel, J.C. and Blanchard, E.B. (1990).   Physician behaviors, patient perceptions, and patient characteristics as predictors of satisfaction of hospitalized adult cancer patients. *Cancer* **65**: 186–192.

Buckman, R. (1996).   Talking to patients about cancer. *British Medical Journal* **313**: 699–700.

Butow, P.N., Kazemi, J.N., Beeney, L.J., Griffin, A.M., Dunn, S.M. and Tattersall, M.H.N. (1996).   When the diagnosis is cancer. *Cancer* **77**: 2630–2637.

Cassileth, B.R., Zupkis, R.V., Sutton-Smith, K. and March, V. (1980).   Information and participation preferences among cancer patients. *Annals of Internal Medicine* **29**: 832–836.

Charles, C., Gafni, A. and Whelan, T. (1997).   Shared decision-making in the medical encounter: what does it mean? (or, it takes at least two to tango). *Social Science and Medicine* **44**: 681–692.

Coe, R.M. and Pendergast, C.G. (1985).   The formation of coalitions: interaction strategies in triads. *Sociology of Health and Illness* **64**: 236–247.

Creagan, E.T. (1994).   How to break bad news and not devastate the patient. *Mayo Clinic Proceedings* **69**: 1015–1018.

Deber, R.B. (1994).   Physicians in health care management: 7. The patient–physician partnership: changing roles and the desire for information. *Canadian Medical Association Journal* **151**: 171–176.

Degner, L.F., Kristjanson, L.J., Bowman, D., Sloan, J.A., Carriere, K.C., O'Neil, J., Bilodeau, B., Watson, P. and Mueller, B. (1997).   Information needs and decisional preferences in women with breast cancer. *Journal of the American Medical Association* **277**: 1485–1492.

Dermatis, H. and Lesko, L.M. (1991).   Psychosocial correlates of physician–patient communication at time of informed consent for bone marrow transplantation. *Cancer Investigation* **9**: 621–628.

Doherty, W.J. (1985).   Family intervention in health care. *Family Relations* **34**: 129–137.

Fallowfield, L., Ford., S. and Lewis, S. (1995).   No news is not good news. Information preferences of patients with cancer. *Psycho-oncology* **4**: 197–202.

Faulkner, A. and Maguire, P. (1994).   *Talking to Cancer Patients and Their Relatives.* Oxford: Oxford University Press.

Foley, G.V. (1993).   Enhancing child–family health team communication. *Cancer* **71** (Suppl.): 3281–3289.

Ford, S. Fallowfield, L. and Lewis, S. (1996).   Doctor–patient interactions in oncology. *Social Science and Medicine* **42**: 1511–1519.

Glanz, K. and Lerman, C. (1992).   Psychosocial impact of breast cancer: a critical review. *Annals of Behavioral Medicine* **14**: 204–212.

Gotay, C. (1984). The experience of cancer during early and advanced stages: the view of patients and their mates. *Social Science and Medicine* **18**: 605–613.

Gotay, C.C. (1991). Accrual to cancer clinical trials: directions from the research literature. *Social Science and Medicine* **5**: 569–577.

Greenfield, S., Kaplan, S. and Ware, J.E. Jr (1985). Expanding patient involvement in care: effects on patient outcomes. *Annals of Internal Medicine* **102**: 520–528.

Guadagnoli, E. and Ward, P. (1998). Patient participation in decision-making. *Social Science and Medicine* **3**: 329–339.

Hack, T.F., Degner, L.F. and Dyck, D. G. (1994). Relationship between preferences for decisional control and illness information among women with breast cancer: a quantitative and qualitative analysis. *Social Science and Medicine* **39**: 279–289.

Hall, J.A., Roter, D.L. and Katz, N.R. (1988). Meta-analysis of correlates of provider behavior in medical encounters. *Medical Care* **26**: 657–675.

Harpham, W.S. (1995). Psychosocial oncology: a view from the other side of the stethoscope. *Journal of Psychosocial Oncology* **13**: 89–105.

Humphrey, G.B., Littlewood, J.L. and Kamps, W.A. (1992). Physician–patient communication: a model considering the interaction of physicians' therapeutic strategy and patients' coping style. *Journal of Cancer Education* **7**: 147–152.

Inui, T.S. and Carter, W.B. (1985). Problems and prospects for health services research on provider–patient communication. *Medical Care* **23**: 521–538.

Kai, I., Ohi, G., Yano, E., Kobayashi, Y., M., Yama, T., Nhno, N. and Naka, K. (1993). Communication between patients and physicians about terminal care. A survey in Japan. *Social Science and Medicine* **36**: 1151–1159.

Labrecque, M.S., Blanchard, C.G., Ruckdeschel, J.C. and Blanchard, E.B. (1991). The impact of family presence on the physician–cancer patient interaction. *Social Science and Medicine* **11**: 1253–1261.

Lederberg, M.S. (1998). The family of the cancer patient. In J. Holland (Ed.), *Psycho-oncology* (pp. 981–993). New York: Oxford University Press.

Lerman, C., Daly, M., Walsh, W.P., Resch, N., Seay, J., Barsevick, A., Berenbaum, L., Heggan, T. and Martin, G. (1993). Communication between patients with breast cancer and health care providers. *Cancer* **72**: 2612–2620.

Lewis, F.M. (1993). Psychosocial transitions and the family's work in adjusting to cancer. *Seminars in Oncology Nursing* **9**: 127–129.

Mackillop, W.J., Stewart, W.E., Ginsberg, A.D. and Stewart, S.S. (1988). Cancer patients' perceptions of disease and its treatment. *British Journal of Cancer* **58**: 355–358.

Miller, S. (1995). Monitoring versus blunting styles of coping with cancer influence the information patients want and need about their disease. *Cancer* **76**: 167–177.

Neuling, S.J. and Winefield, H.R. (1988). Social support and recovery after surgery for breast cancer: frequency and correlates of supportive behaviors by family, friends, and surgeon. *Social Science and Medicine* **27**: 385–392.

Northouse, P.G. and Northouse, L.L. (1987). Communication and cancer: issues confronting patients, health care professionals, and family members. *Journal of Psychosocial Oncology* **5**: 17–46.

Northouse, L.L. and Peters-Golden, H. (1993). Cancer and the family: strategies to assist spouses. *Seminars in Oncology Nursing* **9**: 74–82.

Novak, D.H., Plummer, R., Smith, R.L., Ochitill, H., Morrow, G.R. and Bennett, J.M. (1979). Change in physicians' attitudes toward telling the cancer patient. *Journal of the American Medical Association* **241**: 897–900.

Ong, L.M.L., DeHaes, J.C.J.M., Hoos, A.M. and Lammes, F. B. (1995). Doctor–patient communication: a review of the literature. *Social Science and Medicine* **40**: 903–918.

Patterson, J.M. and Garwick, A.W. (1994). The impact of chronic illness on families: a family systems perspective. *Annals of Behavioral Medicine* **16**: 131–142.

Quill, T.E. and Brody, H. (1996). Physician recommendations and patient autonomy: finding a balance between physician power and patient choice. *Annals of Internal Medicine* **125**: 763–769.

Roter, D. and Fallowfield, L. (1998). Principles of training medical staff in psychosocial and communication skills. In J.C. Holland (Ed.), *Psycho-oncology* (pp. 1074–1082). New York: Oxford University Press.

Ruckdeschel, J.C., Blanchard, C.G. and Albrecht, T. (1994). Psychosocial oncology research: where we have have been, where we are going, and why we won't get there. *Cancer* **74**: 1458–1463.

Sales, E. (1991). Psychosocial impact of the phase of cancer on the family: an updated review. *Journal of Psychosocial Oncology* **9**: 1–18.

Sales, E., Schulz, R. and Biegel, D. (1992). Predictors of strain in families of cancer patients: a review of the literature. *Journal of Psychosocial Oncology* **10**: 1–26

Schain, W.S. (1990). Physician–patient communication about breast cancer. *Surgical Clinics of North America* **70**: 917–936.

Siminoff, L.A. (1992). Improving communication with cancer patients. *Oncology* **6**: 83–87.

Siminoff, L.A., Fetting, J.H. and Abeloff, M.D. (1989). Doctor–patient communication about breast cancer adjuvant therapy. *Journal of Clinical Oncology* **7**: 1192–1200.

Steptoe, A., Sutcliffe, I., Allen, B. and Coomes, C. (1991). Satisfaction with communication, medical knowledge, and coping style in patients with metastatic cancer. *Social Science and Medicine* **32**: 627–632.

Stetz, K.M. (1993). Survival work: the experience of the patient and the spouse involved in experimental treatment for cancer. *Seminars in Oncology Nursing* **9**: 121–126.

Stewart, M.A. (1995). Effective physician–patient communication and health outcomes: a review. *Canadian Medical Association Journal* **152**: 1423–1433.

Street, R.L. (1992). Communicative styles and adaptations in physician–parent consultations. *Social Science and Medicine* **34**: 1155–1163.

Surbone, A. (1996). The patient–doctor–family relationship: at the core of medical ethics. In L. Baider, C. L. Cooper and A. K. De-Nour (Eds), *Cancer and the Family* (pp. 389–405). Chichester: Wiley.

Szasz, T. and Hollender, M. (1956). A contribution to the philosophy of medicine: the basic models of the doctor–patient relationship. *Archives of Internal Medicine* **97**: 585–592.

Taylor, K.M., (1988). Telling bad news: physicians and the disclosure of undesirable information. *Sociology of Health and Illness* **10**: 109–132.

Trillin, A. S. (1981). Of dragons and garden peas: a cancer patient talks to doctors. *New England Journal of Medicine* **304**: 699–701.

Waitzkin, H. and Britt, A. (1989). A critical theory of medical discourse: how patients and health professionals deal with social problems. *International Journal of Health Services* **19**: 577–597.

Wiggers, J.H., Donovan, K.O., Redman, S. and Sanson-Fisher, R.W. (1990). Cancer patient satisfaction with care. *Cancer* **66**: 610–616.

Wolff, K.H. (1950). *The Sociology of George Simmel*. Glencoe, IL: Free Press.

Wortman, C. (1984). Social support and the cancer patient. *Cancer* **53**: 2339–2360.

28

Cancer, Medical Ethics, and the Family

CARL CHRISTOPHER HOOK
Mayo Clinic, Rochester, MN, USA

Medicine is above all else a relationship. It is a covenant between one person who is afflicted with some malady or concern, the patient, and one who offers to help the other, the physician or caregiver. This relationship provides the framework in which all the other aspects of medicine—the science, the diagnostic tests, and the therapeutic interventions—take place and are given context. Even when we have no more medications or procedures that can be employed, the relationship itself remains, providing comfort and healing. The caregiver–patient relationship is, in fact, one of the most powerful tools medicine has to offer, and this is especially true in the case of our patients with malignant diseases.

This relationship does not exist alone, but occurs in the context of other important relationships in the life of each individual. The most important of these relationships are the ones we often call 'family.' Unfortunately, the bioethics literature has not focused much on the role of family in the healing relationship, except perhaps as surrogate decision makers, or as sources of conflict over requests for 'futile' therapy. This has been a serious error and is the consequence of the Western focus on the principle of autonomy. As we shall see, the exclusion of the family as an integral part of the patient's concerns, decision making, support and source of identity and meaning, has actually diminished the fundamental concern of the principle of autonomy—that is, respect for the individual patient as a person.

While 'family' has traditionally been understood as our spouses, parents, siblings, children and other extended 'blood' relatives, cultures around the world are experiencing significant changes in the understanding of who constitutes 'family.' Divorce and remarriage, assisted reproductive technologies and non-traditional arrangements (couples living together but remaining unmarried, homosexual couples, etc.) all have brought significant challenges to the concept of family. For the purposes of this discussion, 'family' will be understood as:

> ... any social configuration that incorporates at least most of the morally significant features of, say, marital and parent–child relationships .... These features include

Cancer and the Family, 2nd Edn. Edited by L. Baider, C. L. Cooper and A. Kaplan De-Nour
© 2000 John Wiley & Sons, Ltd

long-standing, committed relationships; blood ties; emotional intimacy; shared histories; shared projects that produce solidarity among family members (Nelson and Nelson, 1995).

THE NATURE AND GOALS OF MEDICINE AND CANCER

Illness of any kind is an existential crisis. Distracting or disabling symptoms, and the concrete realization of our mortality, alters our concept of self. The enjoyment of life, our future plans, and our visions of who we are, where we are going, or what we are becoming, may be lost or significantly compromised.

Cancer particularly is such a life-altering illness. Not only may we face the cause of our demise, but invariably this destroyer from within, this part of self turned killer, alters the integrity of our being. Surgery, radiation, and/or chemotherapy each impact our comfort, function, energy level, and body image. Even if we are lucky enough to survive the assault of malignant disease, the fear of relapse, or a second malignancy, remains.

Healers may help patients struggle with cancer in a number of ways, all vital goals of medicine. These include cure, when possible, palliation of symptoms, prevention or limitation of harm, and restoration—not only restoration of bodily function, but also restoration of self. As healers are so often limited in the ability to cure, helping a patient confront the existential crisis of cancer, helping the patient live with his/her disease and minimizing the erosion of self, becomes the greatest service given to the patient. Families are often crucial components of a patient's self-identity and therefore must be considered as partners in the restorative mission of medicine.

THE PRINCIPLES OF MEDICAL ETHICS AND THE IMPORTANCE OF FAMILY

'Declare the past, diagnose the present, foretell the future: practice these acts. As to diseases, make a habit of two things—to help, or at least do no harm' (Hippocrates, trans. Jones, 1964). This phrase from the Hippocratic writings is one of the fundamental expressions of the medical ethic and provides a succinct statement of the principles of beneficence and non-maleficence. The fundamental goal of medicine is to help, to contribute to the good of the patient, and, in so doing, to avoid harming the patient as much as possible.

Despite much literature to the contrary, *beneficence* is still the first principle of medicine. Much of contemporary bioethics focuses instead on the principle of *autonomy*. This ascendance of autonomy as *the* ethical principle, however, is primarily an American and European phenomenon, rooted in Western concepts of the supreme value of the individual and the importance of self-rule. But in medical ethics autonomy can be seen as contained in, or coupled with, the principle of beneficence. The art of respecting patient autonomy is recognizing the unique meaning of beneficence for each patient. The healer must recognize the intrinsic and inestimable value of each person. This requires that the patient be seen and respected as a person, an individual, a unique and wonderful miracle of life. For each individual patient the idea of good or benefit is dependent upon several different levels of concern: (a) biomedical good, (b) personal or social good, and (c) ultimate or spiritual good. Biomedical good is the physical benefit, the pathophysiologic alteration to remove the harmful agent or to repair compromised activity. Typically in medicine the focus is only on this concept of the good. However, patients are frequently just as concerned about the psychological/social/spiritual context of their illnesses. If a treatment may leave them with a disability unacceptable to them, or cause them to violate their spiritual or religious convictions, their personal good and/ or their ultimate or spiritual good may not only be hindered, but in fact the result may be seen as harmful. Understanding and respecting these personal definitions of benefit are what the concept of autonomy should be concerned with. Because families help shape, provide meaning for, and enable fulfillment of, these personal definitions of the good, caregivers must include the family in considerations meant to respect the autonomy of, and achieve benefit for, the patient.

Indeed, the family is often viewed as critical to personal and spiritual fulfillment in the world's great religious traditions. From the Jewish and Christian scriptures: 'For this reason a man will leave his father and mother and be united to his wife, and they become one flesh' (Genesis, 2:24); and the Fifth Commandment, 'Honor your father and your mother, so that you may live long in the land that the Lord your God is giving you' (Exodus, 20:12—New International Version). In the Hindu scriptures, it is written with regard to family members: 'Be not parted—growing old, taking thought, thriving together, moving under a common yoke, come speaking sweetly to one another; I'll make you have one aim and be of one mind' (Atharva Veda, 3:30). Confucian writings state: 'There are five relations of utmost importance under Heaven . . . between prince and minister; between father and son; between husband and wife; between elder and younger brothers; and between friends' (Doctrine of the Mean, 20:8). Even if these are viewed as ideals, and recognizing that few families truly achieve this degree of closeness, respect and harmony, it is clear that families are critical to the nature and nurture of the individual person.

In the USA and other Western countries, family may not seem to be as important an issue for some patients. Extended family relationships are less common and pursuit of individual happiness is a prominent cultural icon. Nevertheless, family members are often involved in the care of a patient when that individual becomes critically ill and disabled. Family members are increasingly and intimately involved in terminal care, especially as hospice care becomes more common. In other cultures, such as sub-Saharan cultures, the person is identified primarily as a 'familial self.' Illness is not an individual matter, but a family matter (Olweny, 1998). By compromising the health and longevity of the individual patient, familial roles and relationships are effected. Therefore, regardless of culture, it is clear that severe illness, like cancer, necessarily becomes a family concern, from the perspective of both the patient and the family.

Hampe has identified eight needs of family members of dying (and, one would infer, critically ill) patients (Hampe, 1975):

1. To be with the dying person.
2. To be helpful to the dying person.
3. To receive assurance of the dying person's comfort.
4. To be informed of the dying person's condition.

5. To be informed of impending death.
6. To ventilate emotions.
7. To receive comfort and support from family members.
8. To receive acceptance, support and comfort from health-care professionals.

Items 3, 4, 5, 6, and 8 are communication issues involving physicians, nurses, and other care-providers and illustrate the importance of the fundamental ethical virtues in medicine.

THE FUNDAMENTAL VIRTUES OF MEDICINE

With restoration/preservation of self as a major goal of medicine, and the principles of beneficence and autonomy as guides to achieve that goal, it can be seen that there are some basic virtuous behaviors that all caregivers should exhibit. These behaviors have significant ethical importance because they support and empower the healing relationship, and without the relationship the beneficial goal may not be achieved. These virtues include Presence, Attention, Respect, Gentleness and Patience (Adson, 1995).

When we are with a patient we should be *fully* present for the patient. That is, the patient should know that we are there for him/her. So often we are distracted by the need to write a note, to move on to the next patient, the pager going off, etc. Rather than flying through, dropping off a package of 'care', barely deviating from our flight path, we must be willing to land and be with the patient, thus acknowledging his/her importance to us. In this way we mirror patients' intrinsic dignity back to them. In this manner, Attention is a part of Presence. The patient needs to know that we hear him/her, see him/her and that he/she is the center of our focus. The cancer patient may feel his/her life already ended and we can inadvertently confirm this mistaken notion with our actions and demeanor. Demonstrating respect is also critical because it underscores the point that the patient is important and a life of value.

Cancer and the available treatments are often harsh, battering the body and robbing it of strength. Consequently, the physician/caregiver must always treat the patient with gentleness. We must avoid further assaults upon the emotions and spirit of the patient.

So much is at stake with the diagnosis of cancer. The diseases and their treatments are often complex and the concepts foreign. Assimilating all the information necessary is difficult and may require repetition over several sessions. Because the implications are so far-reaching, physicians must be patient, willing to take the time for patients and family members to process the information. Thus, patience becomes another virtue that supports and helps restore the patient. If we are not patient we demean the afflicted, generating fear and anger as they struggle with their uncertainties and apprehensions.

So too, all these virtues are equally important for our interactions with family members and for the family's comfort with the care of their loved one. Families often feel extremely protective of the ill family member. The patient is very important to them and therefore should be important to us. If we do not demonstrate this by our actions and demeanor, the family may become angry and mistrustful of our care. All too often, family are seen as impediments to our mission, taking time, distracting us from 'more important things.' They are people as well, equally possessing infinite, intrinsic value and worthy or our respect. Because they are important to our patient and may be instrumental in battling with a disease, they should be important to us. Family members are also traumatized by the diagnosis of cancer in a loved one and require a gentle touch. And they also require our patience in assimilating the information and experience. Well-educated loved-ones can be tremendously helpful assistants in helping a patient to come to grips with an illness. In the final analysis, family members should be accorded the benefit of the same virtuous behaviors as the patient.

The remainder of this chapter will focus on specific areas of ethical concern for patients and their family members as all face the challenge of cancer.

COMMUNICATING BAD NEWS AND TRUTH TELLING

The first major hurdle in the relationship between physician and patient in the struggle against cancer (aside for what difficulties may have occurred in the process of establishing the diagnosis) is communicating the existence of the malignant process. Generally in modern times, especially in the West, it is believed that full, accurate disclosure must occur in order to respect the patient's rights of autonomy and informed consent. Indeed, lying to patients can damage the patient–care-giver relationship that is so crucial to healing. As difficult as the truth may sometimes be, patients need to know various facts about the disease, prognosis and treatment options in order to make appropriate care decisions, plan for the future, and resolve personal and interpersonal affairs.

However, there are often significant concerns about such disclosure expressed by family members. These concerns include emotional harm to the patient, loss of hope by the patient and the power of words to create reality and lock in destiny. This latter is especially true of many Native American and South-east Asian patients and families. Often in Islamic, Asian (Kashiwagi, 1998; Chau et al., 1998) and many Mediterranean (Trill and Holland, 1993; Surbone, 1992) cultures it is the family's duty to hear the diagnosis and bad news, make decisions regarding care and shield the patient from such devastating information. In a 1992 survey performed by the Japanese Ministry of Health and Welfare, it was found that only 18.2% of patients who died of cancer had been told of their diagnosis. However, 98.1% of families had been told of the patient's diagnosis (Ishikawa et al., 1992). Some prefer to use the term 'tumor' instead of 'cancer' because of the significant negative connotations of the 'C' word. While these attitudes toward disclosure may be more fully expressed and expected by some cultures, it would be an error to assume that such sentiments are restricted to these groups. Similar requests may just as readily come from families of English or Northern European decent as from patients from these other cultures.

With this variability in cultural and familial practice, how should caregivers proceed? The patient must be respected and given the information he/she desires, but one does not want to do violence to family and cultural expectations that may be valuable to the patient. Buckman (1998) has proposed a method of disclosure that addresses and respects these potentially conflicting concerns.

First, before the conversation begins in earnest, it is important to get the physical context correct. As much as possible, all distractions should be removed to promote attention and ease of listening and speaking. Only those individuals whom the patient desires be present should be in the room. The physician should introduce him/herself to all present and try to establish the relationship of each person to the patient. The virtues of presence, attention and respect should then be demonstrated by sitting down, fully facing the patient and with eyes meeting on a level plane. Any physical objects between the physician and the patient should be removed to the extent possible.

Then, as the conversation begins, the physician should elicit from the patient what is already known about the situation. This is critical in setting the content and flow of the remainder of the discussion. This is also a time in which a family member who is to serve as the major decision-maker and spokesperson may be identified.

The next step is perhaps the most important. Find out what the patient wants to know. This will allow the patient to guide the discussion, yet allows respect for cultural and familial expectations if the patient wishes to follow those norms and expectations. Similarly, it is important to find out how much the patient wants to know concerning a given issue. Families may insist before the meeting that no disclosure occur. However, if the patient wants to know certain information, he/she does, indeed, have the right to the truth. Consequently, it is important to instruct the family that: (a) you will not lie to the patient at any time, but that (b) you will not blurt out a lot of information without first allowing the patient to control the type and extent of information he/she receives. If another family member is to serve as the major decision maker, a subsequent discussion can be arranged with that individual so that fuller disclosure necessary for informed decision-making can occur.

During this communication the physician should acknowledge and respond supportively to expressed emotions from the patient and/or family members. There should also be plans made for future communications and follow-up discussions. It should be clear that access to the care provider is possible, and the patient and the family members should be made aware of the avenue(s) of access.

SURROGATE DECISION MAKING

When a patient lacks decision-making capacity, or, according to family or cultural tradition, this role falls to another family member, a surrogate decision maker must be utilized. In some countries this surrogate decision-maker may be identified by an advance directive, such as a durable power of attorney for health care. In this case, the patient specifically chooses who will serve as his/her spokesperson in the event he/she cannot speak for him/herself.

The role of the surrogate or proxy is to stand in for the incapable patient, making decisions and authorizing or refusing interventions as the patient would if he/she could speak for him/herself at that time. To perform this function, the surrogate must know deeply the ideals, goals, fears, and values of the patient, if not have explicit knowledge of the patient's choices concerning certain types of treatment, such as cardiopulmonary resuscitation (CPR). This type of surrogacy is referred to as 'substituted judgement', that is, 'standing in the shoes of the patient' and voicing what would otherwise be the words of the patient. Family members are usually assumed to have this type of intimate knowledge and understanding, and should, therefore, have more insight than acquaintances or friends. It is also commonly held that the family should be more concerned about the patient's welfare than others 'less connected.' This may not always be the case, and is why advance directives allowing the patient specifically to identify the individual he/she believes most able to represent his/her concerns have been created and recognized by law. However, when no such individual has been appointed, the usual order of authority for surrogate decision making is: (a) the (current) spouse; (b) an adult child, or the majority of adult children; (c) a parent; (d) an adult sibling or the majority of adult siblings; (e) a close family (blood) member, if no other closer family exists or is available; and finally, a friend with a close relationship with the patient.

In some, if not many, cases, the surrogate may not know the specific choices the patient would make for the situation or question at hand. Despite the close relationships within many families, often these issues are not discussed. When family members are separated by many miles and/or years, lack of such insight may be common. In this situation, the standard of the patient's best interests should be followed. Here the surrogate works with the caregivers to decide what seems to be in the best interest of the patient. The value of this process is improved when the surrogate can at least identify some basic values and goals of the patient with which to help judge the options available.

Uhlmann et al. (1988) and other investigators (Zweibel and Cassel, 1989; Gerety et al., 1993) have demonstrated the unfortunate fact that families do not always accurately choose what the patient would choose regarding life-sustaining care in a variety of clinical scenarios. Depending upon the specific scenario, ranging from present health, to coma or vegetative state, agreement between patients and their chosen surrogates ranges from 90% for current health to only 33–56% for situations of severe disability. In other words, the flip of a coin may prove as accurate. For this reason, involvement of the family in important discussions about goals of treatment and life and health care values is extremely important. Patients should be encouraged to discuss these concerns with their family members, if possible, in the company of the physician, to lay out these issues so that all hear what is said together, and understanding can be confirmed. This discussion is crucial in laying the groundwork of information that may be referenced when a surrogate family member later instructs the care providers to embark on a course contrary to the expressed wishes of the patient, or when there is disagreement among family members about what the patient would want.

The importance of discussing concepts and critical definitions with patients and family members cannot be emphasized enough, especially as advance directives are being created or given to a physician. A case is illustrative. A 68 year-old male was transferred interinstitutionally for treatment of advanced-stage, aggressive, malignant lymphoma, non-Hodgkin's type. Upon arrival, the patient was obtunded and no meaningful conversation was possible. An advance directive had been prepared at the transferring institution while the patient was still decisionally capable, in the presence of and with the assistance of his family. This directive was given to the physicians at the receiving hospital and stated that: 'Until I am declared brain-dead by two independent physicians, I want all life-sustaining care provided.' When the care team at the receiving hospital approached the accompanying family about the contents of the directive, it became quite clear that the family members, and by their report the patient, did not know what 'brain death' was, neither did they understand that 'life-sustaining care' potentially included cardiopulmonary resuscitation, mechanical ventilation, and dialysis, all of which looked likely to become necessary in the patient's near future. Of even more concern was the finding that, when the treatments and terms were more accurately understood by the family members, the directive was dictating care what all agreed was really not in keeping with what the patient and family had in mind at all. This case is not mentioned to challenge the usefulness or validity of advance directives in general, but to demonstrate how important education of patients and families is, and how essential a discussion of values, goals, and patient preferences with physicians, while the patient possesses decision-making capacity, may be.

RESOLVING ETHICAL DISPUTES

Good communication is the best preventive measure for avoiding disputes with family members. However, despite the best of intentions, disagreements and misunderstandings do occur. Ethics consultation can be a useful tool for helping to diffuse and/or resolve these disagreements. Sometimes a neutral, third party is necessary to conduct the discussion. This does not imply that the primary physician and/or the care team are not doing an excellent job of communicating. Strong emotions within the family, or within individual family members, particularly anger about the loved one's illness, may interfere with communication despite the best of efforts.

The primary care providers are ideally suited to facilitate a family care conference. Getting the whole family, or as many members as possible, together along with multiple members of the care team, including nursing and social service colleagues, can create an open forum so that all are hearing the same thing and have a chance to air concerns. All should be introduced and, when possible, the major spokesperson and decision-maker for the family should be identified, be it the spouse, someone appointed by an advance directive, etc. Of course, demonstrating the fundamental virtues of medicine, discussed above, is of great benefit in conducting a family conference.

The discussion plan for the meeting should follow an organized approach, at least in the early fact-summarization portion. The method of Jonsen et al. (1998) is an excellent tool for conducting a care-planning or dispute-resolution conference. These authors recommend organizing the information concerning a specific patient into four categories: medical indications, patient preferences, quality of life and contextual features.

'*Medical indications*' are the basic pathophysiologic elements of the situation, the diagnoses and/or clinical problems, the current treatments, and any proposed interventions. This is objective information. Clarification of these issues is essential to frame the remainder of the discussion and it is important that all understand this information.

'*Patient preferences*' reviews what the patient's values, goals and choices are concerning health and health care in general, and/or choices regarding the specific situation if they are known. In this section, the advance directive, if one exists, will be reviewed. Family members will have the opportunity to report pertinent discussions that have occurred with the patient that illustrate the patient's values, preferences for treatment, etc. There may be disagreement among family members in this portion and the care providers should work to elicit as much pertinent information and support for any claims as possible. The goal is to try to achieve consensus among the family. When consensus is not possible, and this is not unusual, it needs to be reiterated who in the family possesses final decision-making authority.

The '*quality of life*' section could more clearly be named 'probable outcomes.' In this portion the probable outcomes of the various treatment options are discussed. In addition to likelihood of success, each option is evaluated for the likely quality of life the patient will experience in the course of treatment and in its aftermath. This is the section where various proposed courses can be evaluated with the yardstick of the patient's values, fears, and goals. Often, although not always, the best choice becomes obvious or at least rises to the surface for all to see. This portion of the discussion affords an excellent opportunity for educating the family members of realistic probabilities of outcomes. Several studies have shown that patients, and presumably family members, dramatically overestimate the likelihood of surviving a cardiopulmonary arrest with cardiopulmonary resuscitation and advanced cardiac life support techniques (see, e.g., Miller et al., 1992). Murphy et al. (1994) have shown that simply making patients aware of the real probability of surviving an arrest often reduces by 50% the patients' desire to undergo a resuscitation attempt. Ideally, many of these questions should be addressed with the patient while he/she is still capable, but this is not always possible, particularly in modern health care settings, where many different teams of physicians may become involved over a given patient's course.

'*Contextual features*' ensures that other important issues and facts are recognized and considered. These include: the patient's social situation, financial concerns, religious issues, legal considerations, institutional policy, and so on. The items considered in this section are often essential to the potential realization of the projected courses and outcomes reviewed in the '*quality of life* section'.

MEDICAL FUTILITY

Some conflicts between family members and physicians come down to conflicts of world view, the basic belief systems of the participants. In these cases, no amount of education and sharing of information may resolve the disagreement. Many such cases often revolve around the concept of 'medical futility.' In these cases, families are often requesting interventions that the physicians believe offer the patient no, or a remote, chance of benefit. The family wants 'everything' to be done to try to keep a patient alive, or to treat the underlying malignancy. If there is any chance at all of the treatment working, then it must be given. The family is awaiting the 'miracle' or has a religious belief that life must be preserved as long as possible. The physician, on the other hand, is trying to follow the basic principle of non-maleficence. Often the requested intervention has a significantly greater likelihood of harming the patient, diminishing the patient's quality of life, or even potentially shortening the patient's remaining life. The physician(s) may not share the family's belief that quantity of life is more important than quality of life. The request, therefore, seems wrong to the caregiver. It is beyond the scope of this chapter to present a complete analysis of the 'futility' question (for a more detailed discussion, see Hook, 1996), but a few points are germane to this discussion.

Some have proposed that physicians be empowered to unilaterally decline or withhold interventions deemed 'futile' (Schneiderman et al., 1990). This presupposes that we have a clear understanding or definition of what constitutes futile therapy. If we are willing to utilize the true definition of the term 'futility'—'leaky, hence untrustworthy, vain, failing of the desired end through intrinsic defect' (*Oxford English Dictionary*)—then we can rightly declare a proposed medical intervention 'futile' if it will not succeed no matter how many times it is tried. For instance, if there is no pathophysiologic rationale for the intervention, it will fail, being 'vain . . . failing of the desired end through intrinsic defect'. Unfortunately, many use the term when the more correct description would be 'unlikely to succeed' or 'small chance of success'. It is rare that we can declare treatments truly futile, for most may have at least some small possibility of achieving the desired result. However, 'futile' is a more potent and judgmental term and that is why it is so often used, albeit incorrectly. To use the term 'futile' for anything less than a truly futile situation is dishonest and leads to potentially inappropriate clinical decisions (Curtis et al., 1995).

The conflict over futility threatens the very foundation of the healing relationship. Medicine is not a game where one side attempts to triumph over the other, pitting patient autonomy against physician authority. The power of medicine is in the relationship, and as caregivers we must do what we can to preserve and strengthen the relationship.

It is also important that the ethical and personal integrity of all parties in the relationship be recognized and respected. Physicians, nurses, and other caregivers do not cease being independent moral agents when serving in their various healing capacities. On the contrary, to neuter the consciences of healthcare professionals would be gravely dangerous to the individual practitioners, to the professions, and to our patients. Our approach to futility and other serious ethical disputes must work to bring the involved parties to a mutually acceptable resolution, or, if this is not possible, to transfer care to another physician, hospital, etc., where the treatment in question can be provided. This 'due process' approach does not depend on flawed and arbitrary definitions of 'futility' (Christian Medical and Dental Society, 1994).

In essence, multiple steps should be followed to attempt to defuse the disagreement. First, the primary physician should hold a discussion with the family, as outlined above, taking care to focus on the best interests of the patient, including the multiple levels of benefit that are important to the patient. A second-opinion consultation should be offered. If this discussion does not lead to an agreed-upon course of action, then third party mediation may be helpful. This includes assistance from nursing, chaplaincy, patient liaisons, and/or ethics consultation. At all times it should be clear that the patient and/or family is free to transfer care to another physician. If resolution still cannot be reached, transfer of care should be attempted. If this is not possible, Halevy and Brody (1996) recommend convening an independent committee to hear the case and render an opinion regarding the appropriateness of the treatment in dispute. If the committee finds that the requested intervention is appropriate, it will be provided, whereas if not, then the treatment will not be undertaken. This approach goes to the greatest extent possible to preserve the integrity of all parties involved and is less subject to unilateral abuse that is inherent in the Schneiderman et al. (1990) approach.

CONFLICT BETWEEN THE PATIENT AND THE FAMILY

Not all disagreements about the goals and choices of care occur between the caregivers and the patient or the patient's surrogates. There are often disputes between the patient him/herself and the family. Patients may come to terms with their cancers and be willing to accept their ultimate demise long before the family achieves such acceptance. Patients may choose to forego more chemotherapy or life-sustaining treatments, wishing instead to enjoy their remaining days as much as possible, unencumbered by the side effects of anti-cancer treatments. Their goals are to spend as little time as necessary in physicians' offices or the hospital. Families, however, may not be willing to face the prospect of life without the loved-one with cancer. They, therefore, may push the patient to receive undesired treatment. In some situations the family may try to coerce the patient to receive aggressive treatment by using guilt or emphasizing the patient's 'duty' to the family to do everything possible. The case of *Lane v. Candura* (1978) from Massachusetts illustrates the extent to which a family member may try to override a patient's refusal of therapy. The patient was a 77 year-old female with a gangrenous leg, who refused amputation. The patient was fully competent. Her daughter sued to have the patient declared incompetent, so that the patient could then be forced by a court-appointed guardian to have the amputation.

In these circumstances, the physician should serve as the patient's advocate. If a family member directs the physician to override a competent patient's refusal of treatment, the family member should be reminded that the physician's obligation is to the patient and that the patient's instructions, consents, and refusals will be respected. Should the patient then become incompetent, the physician should still abide by the patient's last instructions on the matter, even if the family member requesting the change in plan is a formally, patient-designated, surrogate. In this instance, the surrogate is violating the substituted judgment standard when it is clear what the patient would choose if he/she could still competently speak, and is thus invalidating his/her moral authority as a surrogate decision-maker.

In the case mentioned earlier about the man with advanced non-Hodgkin's lymphoma, there was a clear dispute between the patient's advanced directive and what the family unanimously stated were the choices that the patient really desired. In that case, however, the directive was not 'competent' ethically, because it was clear that the patient did not fully understand what it was he was requesting. It was, in essence, an invalid directive because the patient did not provide true *informed* consent to the procedures and treatments requested. In cases when the patient possesses decision-making capacity and has sufficient information to make informed medical choices, the physicians should respect the patient's wishes over the direction of the family. While recognizing the importance of the family, our primary obligation is to the patient.

Some very troubling situations arise in which it is clear that a patient does not want further chemotherapy, a surgical procedure, or life-sustaining treatments, but consents to these interventions as a consequence of coercion from the family. It is tempting to refuse to provide these treatments, knowing the patient's true feelings and wishes. However, the patient has competently chosen to disregard his/her own choices for the 'good' of the family. This is an expression of value, acknowledging that his/her role as a member of that family is one of the most important aspects of his/her identity. Because we should respect the patient as a person, in all of the various facets that may define personhood for a given individual, we should respect the choice.

CONFIDENTIALITY

Alhough it has been stated above that family members consider accurate information regarding the status of the patient's disease, the nature of treatments utilized and particularly prognosis, especially if death is imminent, one of their fundamental needs, patients themselves may request that this information be kept confidential. They do not want their health status shared with anyone, and sometimes particularly not with family members, or at least specific family members. Here again is a situation when we must remember that our primary commitment is to the patient, and these requests for confidentiality should in general be respected. It is within the purview of the caregiver to encourage the patient to share critical information with individuals who have just reason to know the information. It may be helpful to the patient to experience reconciliation over past disagreements or harms, etc. However, the patient's final word should be the rule for subsequent disclosures or lack thereof.

Typically, the family member has great concern about the health and prognosis of the patient, but the issues to be disclosed do not personally affect the physical health of the family member. As genetic testing for a familial predisposition to cancer becomes more common, family members may have a very direct personal stake in a patient's history and medical information. Consider the situation of a middle-aged female with end-stage breast cancer who consented to be part of a research protocol and was found to be positive for BRCA1, one of the so-called 'breast cancer genes'. She consented to participate because she wanted to help other women. However, she and her daughter have been estranged for years. When approached to allow the physicians to contact the daughter to make the daughter aware of the potential for inheriting the gene, the patient refuses. In this circumstance, a known, specific individual is potentially at significantly increased risk for developing breast cancer and may benefit from enhanced surveillance or prophylactic mastectomy. How should the physicians respond? Is the obligation to maintain strict confidentiality, or is the caregiver obligated to warn others of potential harm?

George Annas and his colleagues have stated in their proposed Genetic Privacy Act that no such duty to warn or protect exists legally (in the USA) and they would strictly prohibit any disclosure of genetic information to relatives over a patient's refusal (Annas et al., 1995a). Annas (1995b) writes:

> This 'no exception rule' also maximizes the privacy between individuals who receive services that result in private genetic information and their health care providers. It also places the responsibility for informing relatives of their potential genetic risks on the family member who has such knowledge, which is where we believe it morally belongs.

Further, we think it is reasonable to assume that with proper counseling and guidance from supportive and informed practitioners, family members will act in a protective manner toward other family members.

Andrews (1991) believes that trying to protect other family members will have serious downstream effects. It will transform a right to disclose into a duty to disclose and it will be hard to know where to establish legal limits to that duty. Consequently, any relative who had not been contacted could potentially sue the caregiver. Therefore, it is best to maintain a strict wall of confidentiality and not allow any disclosure to occur without the patient's consent.

While these arguments are strong and the approach taken may in the final analysis prove to be the most practical, there are still deeply troubling ethical concerns here. It is difficult to conceive of a compelling or convincing ethical argument justifying the concealment of information that might prevent a family member from an early death or severe disability from cancer, unless physical abuse or emotional instability were the underlying issues. Often the underlying motivation is spite, anger, selfishness, and/or some interpersonal conflict with the family. While counseling may bring about a more appropriate response in some, no amount of counseling or encouragement may induce all patients to do the right thing, despite Mr Annas' optimism. True, the primary responsibility does lie with the patient, but as physicians, we are also obligated to prevent harm when possible. Acknowledging that there may be difficulty in establishing legal limits to a potential duty to inform or protect is insufficient ethical justification to preclude all attempts to share critical information to protect *known* individuals at risk. Physicians have a higher ethical calling than legal risk management.

It is also unclear how the courts may respond to this type of question. Two US cases have wrestled with the issue of a physician's duty to warn and protect on the basis of a familial predisposition to cancer. The results have been contradictory. In the Florida case of *Pate v. Threlkel* (1995) the daughter of a woman who had been treated 3 years earlier for medullary cancer of the thyroid sued her mother's physician when she herself was diagnosed with thyroid cancer, claiming that her mother's physician had had a duty to warn her mother and her mother's children that there was a familial tendency to this type of cancer. The Florida Supreme Court ruled that the physician should at least have warned the mother (his patient) that there was a familial tendency to this type of malignancy, but that the physician did not have a duty to directly contact other family members. In the case of *Safer v. Pack* (1996), however, the New Jersey Superior Court ruled that the physician had a duty to warn not only the patient, but also family members at risk of inheriting a tendency to colorectal cancer. What is particularly interesting about this case is that the patient had specifically requested that the physician not reveal his diagnosis to family members when he was treated for colorectal cancer some 40 years earlier. The physician had respected the request. Suit was brought by one of the patient's children when she developed colorectal cancer, claiming that in spite of the patient's request for confidentiality, the physician had a duty to warn the children of their risk for developing cancer. The Court found for the daughter plaintiff.

Neither of these cases is satisfying, reflecting the ethical tension involved. Perhaps the best solution would be guidelines to allow physicians, under strict criteria, to contact at-risk, known family members over a patient's objection, but specifically not creating a mandate that this must be done. Two groups have suggested such criteria: the President's Commission for the Study of Ethical Problems in Medicine and Biomedical and Behavioral Research (1983), and the Committee on Genetic Risks of the United States Institute of Medicine in 1994 (Andrews et al., 1994). These groups have stated that relatives could be informed if: (a) all attempts to elicit voluntary disclosure from the patient have failed; (b) there is a high probability of irreversible or fatal harm to the relative without disclosure; (c) the disclosure of the information will prevent the harm; and (d) the disclosure is limited to the information necessary for the diagnosis and/or treatment of the relative.

We have examined a number of ethical concerns in the relationships between caregivers, patients, and family members. This has been a brief survey of some rather complex issues and space limitations have prevented more exhaustive analysis. However, there are several key points that the reader should take away from this discussion:

1. Restoration and preservation of the self is a major goal of treating cancer patients.
2. Family relationships are critical to the identity and healing of many, if not the vast majority of, cancer patients.
3. It is important to recognize and respect all the facets of 'benefit' from the patient's perspective, not just focus on biomedical benefit.
4. Demonstration of the basic virtues of medicine (attention, presence, respect, gentleness, and patience) is critical to our relationships with patients and their families.
5. While respecting cultural and familial traditions in communication, decision-making, etc., it is of great importance that the patient and his/her desires should guide our interaction with the patient and the family.
6. Education and open communication are key tools to preventing and resolving ethical disputes.
7. Our primary obligation is to the patient and his/her needs, unless the fundamental health and safety of family members may be put at risk.

Let us always remember to follow the Hippocratic admonition, 'to help, or at least do no harm'.

REFERENCES

Adson, M. (1995). An endangered ethic—the capacity for caring. *Mayo Clinic Proceedings* **70**: 495–500.

Andrews, L.B. (1991). Legal aspects of genetic information. *Yale Journal of Biology and Medicine* **64**: 29–40.

Andrews, L.B., Fullerton, J.E., Holtzman, N.A. and Motulski, A.G. (eds) (1994). Committee on Assessing Genetic Risks: Division of Health Sciences Policy, Institute of Medicine. *Assessing Genetic Risks: Implications for Health and Social Policy* (pp. 278–279). Washington, DC: National Academy Press.

Annas, G.J., Glantz, L.H. and Roche, P.A. (1995a). *The Genetic Privacy Act and Commentary*. Health Law Department, Boston University School of Public Health.

Annas, G.J., Glantz, L.H. and Roche, P.A. (1995b). Drafting the Genetic Privacy Act: science, policy and practical considerations. *Journal of Law, Medicine and Ethics* **23**: 360–366.

Buckman, R. (1998). Communication in palliative care: a practical guide. In In D. Doyle, G.W.C. Hanks, and N. MacDonald (Eds), *Oxford Textbook of Palliative Medicine*, 2nd Edn (pp 141–156). New York: Oxford University Press.

Chan, K.S. et al. (1998). Chinese patients with terminal cancer. In D. Doyle, G.W.C. Hanks and N. MacDonald (Eds), *Oxford Textbook of Palliative Medicine*, 2nd Edn (pp. 793–795). New York: Oxford University Press.

Christian Medical and Dental Society. (1994). Statement on Medical Futility.

Council on Ethical and Judicial Affairs, American Medical Association (1999). Medical futility in end-of-life care. *Journal of the American Medical Association* **281**: 937–941.

Curtis, J.R. et al. (1995). Use of the Medical Futility rationale in Do-Not-Resuscitate Orders. *Journal of the American Medical Association* **273**: 1214–128.

Gerety, M.B., Chiodo, L.K., Kanten, D.N. et al. (1993). Medical treatment preferences of nursing home residents: relationship to function and concordance with surrogate decision-makers. *Journal of the American Geriatric Society* **41**: 953–960.

Hampe, S.O. (1975). Needs of the grieving spouse in a hospital setting. *Nursing Research* **24**:113–119.

Havely, A. and Brody, B.A. (1996). A multi-institution collaborative policy on medical futility. *Journal of the American Medical Association* **276**: 571–574.

Hippocrates (trans. Jones, W.H.S., 1964). *Epidemics* 1, XI. Cambridge, MA: Harvard University Press.

Hook, C.C. (1996). Medical futility. In J.F. Kilner, A.B. Miller, and E.D. Pellegrino (Eds), *Dignity and Dying* (pp. 84–95). Grand Rapids: William B. Eerdmans.

Ishikawa, Y. et al. (1992). Cancer death in middle age. Report of the Statistics Bureau, Ministry of Health and Welfare, Japan.

Jonsen, A.R., Siegler, M. and Winslade, W.J. (1998). *Clinical Ethics: A Practical Approach to Ethical Decisions in Clinical Medicine*, 4th Edn. NewYork: McGraw-Hill.

Kashiwagi, T. (1998). Palliative care in Japan. In D. Doyle, G.W.C. Hanks, and N. MacDonald (Eds), *Oxford Textbook of Palliative Medicine*, 2nd Edn (pp. 797–798). New York: Oxford University Press.

Lane v Candura (1978). 6 Mass App Ct 377.

Miller, D.L. et al. (1992). Cardiopulmonary resuscitation: how useful? Attitudes and knowledge of an elderly population. *Archives of Internal Medicine* **152**: 578–582.

Murphy, D.J. et al. (1994). The influence of the probability of survival on patients' preferences regarding cardiopulmonary resuscitation. *New England Journal of Medicine* **330**: 545–549.

Nelson, H.L. and Nelson, J.L. (1995). Family. In W.T. Reich (Ed.), *Encyclopedia of Bioethics*, Revised Edn, Vol. 6 (p. 802).

Olweny, C.L.M. (1998). Cultural issues in sub-Saharan Africa. In D. Doyle, G.W.C. Hanks, and N. MacDonald (Eds), *Oxford Textbook of Palliative Medicine*, 2nd Edn (pp. 787–791). New York: Oxford University Press.

Pate v. Threlkel (1995). 661 So 2d 278 (Fla).

President's Commission for the Study of Ethical Problems in Medicine and Biomedical and Behavioral Research (1983). *Screening and Counseling for Genetic Conditions: A Report on the Ethical, Social and Legal Implications for Genetic Screening, Counseling and Education Program*. Washington, DC: US Government Printing Office.

Safer v. Pack (1996). 667 A 2d 1188 (NJ).

Schneiderman, L.J., Jecker, N.S. and Jonsen, A.R. (1990). Medical futility: it's meaning and ethical implications. *Annals of Internal Medicine* **112**: 949–954.

Surbone, A. (1992). Truth telling to the patient. *Journal of the American Medical Association* **268**: 1661–1662.

Trill, M.D., and Holland, J. (1993). Cross-cultural differences in the care of patients with cancer: a review. *General Hospital Psychiatry* **15**: 21–30.

Uhlmann, R.F., Pearlman, R.A., Cain, K.C. (1988). Physicians' and spouses' predictions of elderly patients' resuscitation preferences. *Journal of Gerontology* **43**(Suppl): M115–121.

Zweibel, N.R. and Cassel, C.K. (1989). Treatment choices at the end of life: a comparison of decisions by older patients and their physician-selected proxies. *Gerontologist* **29**: 615–621

The Role of the Family in the Ethical Dilemmas of Oncology*

ANTONELLA SURBONE

Memorial Sloan-Kettering Cancer Center and
Cornell University Medical College, New York, USA

The patient–doctor–family relationship is at the core of medical ethics. Such complex and delicate relationship never occurs in the void: rather, it occurs in a context—familiar, cultural, social, historical—where certain values have been previously acquired and established. Therefore, like any other relationship in life, the patient–doctor–family relationship is never morally neutral. Medical ethics reflects the contextual character of the patient–doctor–family relationship, while at the same time it expresses and articulates certain theoretical principles. In this chapter, I first briefly outline some essential steps in the history of bioethics, including the fundamental principles involved in Western bioethics. I later explore the character-istics of the patient–doctor–society relationship, of which the patient–doctor–family relationship is the primary component. In the final section, I present and analyze cases with respect to their ethical implications.

A BRIEF HISTORY OF WESTERN MEDICAL ETHICS AND ITS PRINCIPLES

The Hippocratic Oath is usually referred to as the first document on medical ethics in Western cultures (Hippocrates, 420 BC), and has retained its validity throughout the centuries. In the past few decades, however, the interest in medical ethics has greatly increased. In fact, with the development of modern technology, a concomitant expansion has occurred in the realm of possibilities in medicine.

We can now prolong life in its late stages, and mimic nature in the early phases. We are facing an unexpected amplification of what appears to be at our will through medicine (Thomas, 1990). Thus, medicine finds itself facing new horizons and, with

---

*This chapter is dedicated to my patients, from whom I learned about courage in facing suffering and dying, and to my son Francesco Akira, from whom I learned about courage in facing life itself.

Cancer and the Family, 2nd Edn. Edited by L. Baider, C. L. Cooper and A. Kaplan De-Nour
© 2000 John Wiley & Sons, Ltd

them, their consequences—not only medical, but also moral–ethical. The results of this expansion of medical possibilities impact upon all of us as individuals and upon our societies. The recent developments of genetics represent a striking example, which will be discussed in Case A (see below).

Due to the apparent novelty of the questions and answers proposed and imposed by modern technology, the field of medical ethics is rapidly growing, under the common academic name of 'bioethics' (*bios*=life, *ethos*=ethics). This term, first used by an American oncologist (Potter, 1971) in a descriptive naturalistic way, encompasses all ethical issues related to medicine and biotechnology. The role of ethics in medicine is not purely academic, however (Brewin, 1993); ethics first involves the fundamentals of medicine, being at the root of the patient–doctor–society relationship.

Ancient Greeks approached ethics from their complex philosophical standpoint, whereby there was no distinction between the sphere of ethics (from *ethos*=custom, character) and the sphere of aesthetics (from *aisthetikos*=of sense perception). Courage and beauty were equivalent to Aristotle (384–322 BC). Modern philosophy looks upon ethics either from a more deontic viewpoint, whereby ethics is governed by the universal moral law and its consequent obligations—duties (Kant, 1785); or from a teleological viewpoint, aiming at the greatest happiness for the greatest number, as in utilitarianism (Mill, 1806). Contemporary philosophy, particularly through the contribution offered by feminist moral theorists, moves from a more Humean approach (Hume, 1751), and stresses the role of trust and care in moral deliberation (Baier, 1994) as well as the importance of a shared moral understanding which takes into account the 'situation' of each moral agent (Walker, 1998).

Bioethics also adds a more pragmatic dimension to the theoretical moral preoccupation. Thus, we find that it makes use of certain fundamental principles, which have a two-level purpose of universality and practicality. Such principles often conflict, and the moral deliberation in medical ethics requires open debate as well as honest mediation in a communicative spirit (Habermas, 1990). In medical ethics, three principles appear fundamental: doing good to the patient and avoid harming (beneficence and non-maleficence), respecting the patient's right to self-determination (autonomy), and being fair and not discriminating among patients (justice). While the Hippocratic tradition was entirely focused on the first principle, modern medicine is strongly influenced by contemporary emphasis on individual freedom and autonomy, and by predominant utilitarian views of social justice.

The principles of beneficence and non-maleficence need not be inevitably seen as paternalism, such as in the Hippocratic Oath and in the still dominant climate of medicine in many countries. Rather, they have been elaborated in light of the therapeutic alliance and the concept of trust in the patient–doctor relationship (Pellegrino and Thomasma, 1988). This relationship stems from a fiduciary act, whereby a person in need asks for the help of an expert. Be it perceived in a more old-fashioned paternalistic way or in a more contractual way, this relationship is based on implicit trust. In this fiduciary essence lie both the motivation and the aim of the patient–doctor relationship, and within the frame of trust it is possible to set a common goal for both patient and doctor: the restoration of a lost good, i.e., health. Beneficence does include respect for autonomy, but autonomy is not seen as absolute. Rather, there may be limitations on autonomy as a beneficent act, namely when there is harm to others which is definable, clear, probable, and grave. In this perspective, 'good' precedes 'right' (Pellegrino, 1985). As a consequence of the nature of disease, which in itself limits the autonomy, of the subject, a hierarchy of principles is set. Priority is given to the patient's good, whenever conflicts arise between patient's good and patient's autonomy, or between the patient and the doctor (Pellegrino, 1985).

The growing perception of and request for autonomy as the guiding principle of social coexistence is of tremendous relevance to modern medical ethics, and in the patient–doctor relationship the moral obligation of the doctor to respect, to restore, and to foster the patient's autonomy becomes the leading principle (Cassel, 1977). The contractual nature of the patient–doctor relationship, based on autonomy, has been emphasized in bioethics by authors who make use of a procedural approach. Its basis is a practical—rather than theoretical—consensus, and the ethical justification rests upon the consensus reached by persons with the status of moral agents (Engelhardt, 1986). (It should be noticed how the term 'contractual' is also commonly used to refer to the post-paternalistic patient–doctor relationship in a broad and generic sense.) The priority of autonomy is an affirmation of the precedence of rights over goods.

Different schools of bioethics have, on the other hand, ranked the value of goods as hierarchically superior to rights in an ontological sense. The affirmation of life as the necessary condition for all values (including freedom) to be expressed derives from the catholic moral tradition (Sgreccia, 1991). This view—often referred to as 'personalism'—is ontologically founded, and emphasizes the person as first a living, rather than a moral, agent. The distinction is of paramount importance, as, for instance, the embryo, or the handicapped, or the comatose patients are considered to be full persons. The principles by which personalistic ethics is articulated in its normative function include: the principle of freedom–responsibility, the therapeutic–global principle and the principle of social help.

The utilitarian perspective emphasizes social justice; here the determining consideration of right conduct is the usefulness of its consequences. In bioethics, it demands that the doctor acts in the best interest of the patient and of society, and this may somehow take precedence over the patient's self-determination. In a teleologic perspective, the justification of such ethics is based on considerations of justice and injustice with regard to the maximization of happiness/pleasure and the minimization of unhappiness/pain. Thus, the ability of the conscious human being to feel is a criterion used to determine the just equalitarian conduct in medicine (Singer, 1979).

Finally, the principles of beneficence, non-maleficence, autonomy and justice have been assumed to be 'prima-facie principles' in the attempt to create a solid framework for the resolution of ethical issues and dilemmas within the existing pluralism (Beauchamp and Childress, 1994). The distinction between actual and prima-facie ethical obligations can be understood by seeing the first as absolute and the second as conditional ethical duties. Prima-facie duties are conditional upon stronger counter-considerations that may arise and make them inoperative, and moral conflicts are seen as the inevitable consequence of our imperfect understanding of the duties involved in each case (McConnell, 1972). The distinction between actual and prima-facie duties, however, appears to invalidate the concept of moral obligations, as exemplified in bioethics, where both autonomy and beneficence can be used to justify opposing medical and moral choices. Therefore, while a certain weakness is intrinsically bound to the definition of prima-facie principles, they are meant to have a relative and instrumental value. Prima-facie principles are useful tools for a preliminary reading of the moral experience, somehow at the interface between a systematic deductive moral theory and the truths emerging from an inductive–narrative method (Cattorini, 1993).

A purely descriptive approach to bioethics is not sufficient when we move from the level of the abstract debate to that of real circumstances in life and medicine. Bedside practice shows ethical dilemmas to be at least as innumerable as patients and their individual circumstances. A code of ethics should provide guidelines, rather than procedural instructions or algorithms, for determining what to do in difficult real-life cases. It delimits the range of acceptable actions (provides for constraints), but it does not necessarily determine particular acts (Rescher, 1987).

Moral dilemmas are a quandary of life, and they appear magnified in medicine. While in the ideal Kantian world duties and ethical rules cannot generate conflicts, in the imperfect and largely yet unexplored world of medicine moral dilemmas based on conflictual obligations are often encountered, although they may not always be recognized or openly faced. Moral dilemmas are a consequence of what 'good' is, not always and simply a choice between mutually exclusive alternatives, but often—in Plato's words—the result of blending and proportion, of combining and harmonizing.

THE PATIENT–DOCTOR–FAMILY RELATIONSHIP: AT THE CORE OF MEDICAL ETHICS

Exploring the patient–doctor–society, and especially the patient–doctor–family relationship, brings us to the core of medical ethics and illuminates its principles and their interactions. The philosophical foundation of medical ethics rests, in fact, upon the nature of the patient–doctor relationship (Pellegrino and Thomasma, 1981). This always includes a third party: society. There is no patient–doctor relationship outside the family and the social context. Family can be seen as the micro-environment, while society in its entirety is the macro-environment. But, family is more than a simple reflection of society: it is the first reality that surrounds the patient during disease, and it is generally also the only lasting reality, when disease has progressed to a stage where the patient can no longer work or engage in social activities.

A disease such as cancer, chronic and often life-threatening in nature, is charged with many psychological implications, and invariably affects the life of relatives and friends, as well as that of the patient. Cancer alters normal family dynamics, as this book describes in detail (Baider et al., 1996). The presence of cancer can create a profound re-evaluation of priorities and improve the quality of significant relations, but it can also negatively impact on pre-existing relationships, especially in the family.

Family is thus a key element in the patient–doctor–society relationship, and it plays a particularly important role in oncology, where the doctor must often interact with both the patient and the family simultaneously to achieve the therapeutic goals of care and cure. Most often, however, there is a tendency towards treating the disease in a purely medical sense, while negating its more complex nature. Disease becomes reified and the patient's life becomes 'over-medicalized'. The patient is seen only as the subject/object of pathological changes first, and of therapeutic and research efforts next. The patient becomes progressively isolated, and his/her disease is confined to its technical dimension. Disease, however, always has two dimensions, the objective and the subjective. In the latter, the patient is primarily interacting with his/her own environment—hence with his family—while in the former it is the medical world that predominates, with its rules, its rhythms, and its struggle to obtain control over the disease process.

Respect for patients' autonomy in view of a chronic disease is only reached by considering them in their environment, surrounded by the ones who love them. As cancer is seldom a surgical problem, which can be solved in an operating session, beneficence includes providing long-term support, which comes also and primarily from the family.

FIVE CASES FOR ETHICAL DISCUSSION

In this section, I have selected five cases which emphasize the importance of family in the patient–doctor–society relationship. To protect patients' confidentiality, their personal data have been slightly modified to prevent any possible identification. I have chosen to lead the reader through these clinical cases, in which the fundamental issues of bioethics can be recognized in a real situation, and can be better appreciated even without a formal academic background in ethics. Various methodologies for analysing individual cases, with respect to their ethical implications, have been standardized and published, and the most widely adopted in North America are known under the names of the centers where they have been developed: the Kennedy methods (by Pellegrino and Sass), the Hastings method (by Wolf), the San Francisco–Chicago methods (by Jonsen, Siegler and Winslade) (reviewed by Guillen, 1991). I have chosen to examine these cases from the perspective of the ethical principles involved, as well as in light of the role and the responsibilities of each partner in the patient–doctor–family relationship, by pointing out their possible breakdowns and distortions.

CASE A

The patient was a young, educated woman with a strong family history of breast and ovarian cancer. She was married, with two daughters in their 20s and a very close family. She was seen once in consultation for widely metastatic ovarian cancer. The consultation focused only on the pressing medical issues of the patient, and the patient returned to the primary care of her treating physician. The patient's course of disease was, unfortunately, rapidly progressing, and she soon developed brain metastases. She died a few months after the initial consultation. Her treatment and her death occurred at a different hospital; however, the consulting specialist continued to be involved by telephone. A few days prior to dying, the patient called the specialist, asking to be tested for a BRCA mutation (mutations of BRCA1 and -2 genes are present in high-risk families with a strong history of breast and/or ovarian cancers in young members of the same family; the presence of such mutations confers a particularly high risk of developing breast and/or ovarian cancer; the mutations can be inherited by the offspring, who may also be at similar high risk). The patient sounded very clear on the telephone, although she stated that she was in pain. She specifically said 'Doctor, please help me to do something for my daughters. I trust you and I know that you will take care of them, if needed, after I die.' The specialist arranged for a blood sample to be collected from the patient and brought to the consulting institution by her husband. An informed consent was obtained, signed by the patient and by her husband, where the husband was designated to receive the results of the genetic testing. The patient died within 48 hours of obtaining the blood sample. Several months later, the specialist received a standard call from the genetic laboratory, informing him that the results were available, and conveyed the information to the patient's husband. In order to protect the patient's confidentiality, the specialist was not told whether the results were positive or negative, but the husband decided to let the specialist know that his wife had been BRCA1-positive, and that he was undergoing active genetic counseling by an expert. In the following weeks, both of the patient's daughters called the specialist with general concerns about possible life-style contraindications in view of their mother's death from cancer and the possibility of her having been BRCA1-positive. Neither of them directly asked for the test results and it was obvious that they had not yet been informed by their father. The ethical dilemma for the specialist was whether or not he should personally disclose to the daughters the genetic information about their mother's BRCA status or whether he should let their father decide if and when to disclose it. The specialist chose to answer the questions appropriately on the basis of the available knowledge, taking into account the extremely high family risk, but without specifically informing the two daughters of the BRCA1-positive status of the mother.

The following is an attempt to dissect the case and analyze its ethical implications in order to understand the moral justification for the specialist's choice, as well as to explore alternative choices.

> The field of genetic screening in oncology has extensive social and ethical ramifications, and this case will illustrate three points: (a) the possible ways of solving medical dilemmas in medicine; (b) the depth of ethical dilemmas in medicine; (c) the impact of genetic testing on the entire family.

Solving Ethical Dilemmas in Medicine

Traditionally, two approaches to the resolution of an ethical dilemma have been described: one is legal, the other ethical. Under the ethical approach, there are three subdivisions. First, the moral foundations for the decision, i.e. the sources of moral justification, involving the choice of a theory (principles, utility, virtue, casuistry, etc.). Second is the use of the theory in the clinical situation (clinical ethics). Third, the underlying problem, is how to move from moral theory and justification to the particular case. In analysing case A, I wish to adopt an alternative classification, whereby the resolution of an ethical dilemma in medicine is possible from three different standpoints: the legal, the theoretical, and the clinical.

The Legal Standpoint   Many equate ethics with deontology and legality. From the medical–legal standpoint the case can be solved relatively easily. In fact, the issues involved from a legal point of view are: (a) privacy and confidentiality; (b) informed consent; (c) rights. If one looks at the details of the case, it is clear that privacy and confidentiality were respected, and an informed consent had been properly obtained. Such consent designated the husband to receive the results; therefore, there was no particular obligation for the specialist to discuss the results of the genetic testing with the daughters.

With respect to the issues of rights, many of the ethical dilemmas in medicine are phrased in the language of rights and this reflects a tendency in democratic societies to stress individual rights. In genetic testing there are issues of rights in access to genetic information—including rights of the person tested, rights to know the results of someone else's test, rights to have a fetus or a child tested, and rights of the research community to use archived material from deceased patients or to process samples for anonymous research. If we look at the issue of rights from a legal point of view, the daughters did not have any legal right to know their mother's BRCA status, since they were not involved or mentioned in the informed consent. Moreover, the daughters did not specifically ask for the results. This might have reflected their awareness of the fact that they did not bear any particular right.

There are many other ethical issues in genetic testing for cancer predisposition, such as the risk of discrimination in health insurance, in the workplace, in adoption, and possibly in gaining access to an education; the ethical implications of prenatal susceptibility testing including counseling, abortion, embryo selection, and eugenics; and finally, major considerations of justice in the allocation of resources, both in the Western context and in a worldwide perspective that includes less affluent areas (see Table 29.1). For case A, however, only the issues of privacy, confidentiality, informed consent, and rights were involved.

The Theoretical Standpoint   A theoretical approach to case A would focus on privacy, confidentiality, and rights. Ample debate in the ethical literature in the USA and worldwide centers on whether or not genetic information might be so important as to call for a reappraisal of the concept of privacy. Most Western societies, and particularly the USA, place tremendous importance on privacy and confidentiality as part of a liberal tradition, but the developments of computerized information, particularly in the health care field, inevitably weaken the ability to assure privacy and confidentiality of medical information. Moreover, the relevance that genetic testing might have with respect to the possibility of predicting a person's future and acting on such information may justify giving up some privacy in view of a higher

Table 29.1   Ethical issues in genetic testing for cancer predisposition

Information and informed consent
Confidentiality and privacy
Rights in access to genetic information
Risk of discrimination
Consequences of prenatal diagnosis
Issues of justice and economy

personal and societal good (Gostin, 1995). On one hand, the more information is available about our health care and the more insurance companies have access to it, the more we lose in terms of privacy. On the other hand, enhancing the exchange of information might prove to be beneficial in terms of the rapid collection of scientific data and furthering medical progress. The balance between privacy and private and public gain is therefore at stake.

A theoretical approach might also look at whether or not the language of right is the only appropriate one to frame an ethical issue and an ethical dilemma. Respect for human rights founded on personal liberty is the foundation of our democratic societies, and medicine accordingly must place particular emphasis on autonomy to protect patients' dignity and their right to self-determination. Emphasis on personal rights does not, however, change the relational essence of our being human. By increasingly revealing the links that unite mankind, genetics itself comes as a reminder of our connectedness (Lenoir, 1997), and being part of a community does not mean abdicating one's autonomy, but merely redefining it. It is therefore possible to approach the issue of rights from different theoretical perspectives.

The fundamental theoretical philosophical issue in genetic testing is whether genetic knowledge expands or restricts the control that we have on our lives. We are not our genome, and genetics helps us predict our future only in part, if at all. Genetic risks should therefore not be different from all other risks that we encounter in the course of our lives. However, we tend to see genetic data as more fundamental and more unalterable than any other variable in the equation of life, and the meaning and value attributed to genetic predisposition is greatly exaggerated. In the case of BRCA testing, the knowledge of a very high risk of developing breast or ovarian cancer has a profound and limiting effect on the personal choices of some women, who see in the haunting specter of cancer the final negation of freedom, so that their life is determined by the expectation of a dire future. On the contrary, some women who have already been cancer patients feel that the quality of their lives, in terms of intensity and depth, has improved after they have confronted the disease, and they consider genetic risk as any other risk in life—something to be dealt with and possibly to be overcome. Finally, other women hold the more abstract belief that knowledge, in itself, always contributes to control and freedom.

Philosophers have long debated the meaning of freedom, and have either stressed the importance of free will or followed more deterministic views of causation of life events. The case of genetic testing does not differ philosophically from any other type of predestination. However, traditional philosophical thinking has been centered around principles that tend to underestimate relational aspects, especially in regard to what is perceived as controllable, not only by 'me', but also by 'us'. The repercussions of testing positive for genetic testing do not depend only on individual reactions but also on the societal attitudes towards disease and on the collective perception of what constitutes a genetic abnormality. Indeed, if it is through the research community that we know our genome and that we face genetic diversity, it is through society that we attribute values. Society attributes meaning to normalcy and to diversity (Reilly, 1995). Society—which means all of us—determines the acceptability of sickness and disability, and attaches or does not attach a negative connotation to diversity. Moreover, disease is not only a pathological entity but also a social construct, which is often accompanied by a change in the ontological status of the ill person (Rollin, 1978). This is a particularly worrisome consequence of the medicalization of our modern lives as well as of the reification of disease. Indeed, any illness should be inscribed into our ontology, rather than determining it. How genetic risk is perceived and how much it will empower people with more control of their lives depends both on how society faces diversity and on whether the scientific community will privilege genotypical or phenotypic information.

The Clinical Standpoint   The ethical implications of Case A can be analyzed from a more clinical standpoint. Here we deal with the rich particularity of a clinical case and the interpersonal and sociological desiderata appear in all their uniqueness. The specialist chose to solve this case from a clinical standpoint, by attempting to establish a proper balance between his patient's good, her autonomy, and the good of her daughters. To do so a physician must assess: (a) the real meaning of the questions asked by patients and relatives; (b) the clinical situation; (c) the risk and benefits of disclosure of genetic information; (d) his/her obligation.

He first had to understand the questions that were posed to him. Were the two daughters trying to ask about the BRCA status of their mother, or were they only concerned with their general high risk? In order to give an answer to such question, one needs to evaluate the personal and family background of the patients. Physicians, however, work under extreme pressure in terms of time and economical constraints, and they can rarely reach a sufficient knowledge of their patients' lives and of their family dynamics. Moreover, physicians seldom meet their patients' relatives, and they know very little about their grieving processes. It would be particularly difficult for a physician who has only met a patient once or twice to understand the possible hidden meaning of questions posed over the telephone.

The main task of the physician is to assess the clinical situation—never an easy task. In Case A, the patient not only suffered from extensive metastatic ovarian cancer but she also had brain metastases. This raises questions with regard to the mental status of the patient at the time of the request for the genetic testing. Although the consent was a valid one, the patient might not have been completely clear in expressing her desire to inform the two daughters about a possible BRCA positivity, and indeed, she had not given any specific instruction to the specialist or to her husband. The case occurred in early 1995 (Miki et al., 1994) and at the time there was limited knowledge of the impact of BRCA1 and BRCA2 allele-specific penetrance (Struewing et al., 1997). Therefore, the possibility of making predictions based on being a carrier of a particular BRCA mutation was even more limited than it is now. Moreover, in 1995 there were major limitations with respect to available preventive and therapeutic options for BRCA mutation carriers. Even now, BRCA1 and BRCA2 sensitivity, specificity, and reproducibility are sufficiently high to provide accurate information regarding what the test purports to measure (i.e. the presence or absence of certain mutations), but the ability to predict future development of breast and ovarian cancer is still uncertain. Moreover, available preventive measures and treatment options—lifestyle changes, close follow-up, chemoprevention, and even prophylactic surgery—do not yield complete protection against breast and ovarian cancer. In 1995, and still nowadays, counseling on the sole basis of the known family history was therefore medically and ethically appropriate.

The specialist had to estimate the risk–benefit ratio of the disclosure of the genetic information regarding the mother to the two daughters. The specialist had knowledge of the BRCA positivity of the mother, which, as discussed above, had limited impact on the immediate treatment and counseling needed for the two daughters. The specialist also had to estimate the possible family disruption that might ensue from disclosing the BRCA positivity to the two daughters at a time when the father had not yet informed them. Such interference in the father–daughter relationship might have had a major negative impact, particularly since the events occurred shortly after the mother's death. (It must be noticed that the specialist might have chosen to disclose the genetic data of the mother, had the information prevented harm or provided benefit to the daughters.)

Finally, a doctor always has to account for his/her obligations. Is the obligation of the doctor exclusively toward the patient, or are there broader obligations? In particular, does the doctor have an obligation towards the family, toward the scientific community, toward society? Finally, in the case of a deceased patient, does the doctor's obligation somehow cease or does it extend to the relatives?

The Depth of the Ethical Dilemma   Case A shows the intricacy of the ethical ramifications of genetic testing, as well as the many layers involved in the solution of an ethical dilemma in medicine. A merely legal and deontological approach is not satisfactory in yielding answers to complex ethical dilemmas. In case A, the patient had designated two different persons in 'providing help to her daughters via the BRCA information', i.e. her husband and the specialist. On one hand, the patient had signed the informed consent, where she designated her husband as the one to be informed of the results. On the other hand, the patient had spoken directly to the specialist and expressly stated that she wanted to be tested for her daughters. She had also entrusted the specialist with providing care for her daughters, if ever necessary, after her death. In view of this ambiguity, a pure legalist view would betray the complexity of the case. A mere theoretical approach, no matter how philosophically provocative and challenging, is also rarely helpful when an immediate clinical decision needs to be made. The solution to an ethical dilemma in medicine, therefore, mostly relies on the clinical standpoint, where the ethical choice stems from an ethical theory as well as from the estimate of the individual and sociological aspects.

The patient–doctor relationship is a covenant where the primary obligation of the doctor is toward the patient (Pellegrino, 1988). In this case the patient had spoken to the specialist and had specified that she wanted to be tested for her daughters. The specialist, therefore, might have felt entitled to inform the daughters of the BRCA status of their mother independently of their father, because of his direct obligation to his patient under the covenant. On the other hand, the specialist had somehow inherited a broader obligation towards the entire family and he chose to counsel the daughters on the basis of their high-risk family history. Moreover, he contacted the husband and discussed with him the need to inform the daughters as a way to respect their mother's wishes and to enable them to take advantage from any future development of medical research.

The ethical dilemma is very deep, as both alternatives appear valid and ethically tenable. Different doctors choose differently on the basis of equally justified moral considerations. Rarely is there a unique correct answer to an ethical dilemma in medicine, and in most cases the solution admits of the same existential ambiguity which is characteristic of our human condition (Merleau-Ponty, 1962). In his *Letters to a Young Poet* of July 16, 1903, Rainer Maria Rilke wrote: 'Try to care for the questions themselves, as if they were locked rooms or books written in a very foreign language' (Rilke, 1929). Medical ethics is also somehow more about posing the moral questions than about finding uncontroversial answers.

CASE B

The patient, a 50 year-old woman, had been hospitalized on an emergency basis in a state of cachexia due to gastric ulcer (found to be benign at subsequent biopsy) and erosive esophagitis with resulting malnutrition, unresponsive to standard treatment with ranitidine, sucralphate and antacids. The patient had been an invalid for many years, under the care of her treating physician, due to previous mastectomy followed by massive lymphedema. Her son–physician was very close to her and had been at her side in the weeks immediately preceding hospitalization. The patient had been in excruciating unrelenting epigastric and retrostemal pain for several days. This had been unresponsive to analgesia. Upon the patient's request, no narcotic had been administered. After 5 days of hospitalization, a major conflict had arisen between the patient, the son–physician, the family, and the medical team around the issue of an aggressive diagnostic procedure, which the patient asked to postpone, after discussing it with her son–physician. They had evaluated the risks and benefits of this aggressive procedure, and concluded that it was unnecessarily painful and invasive at that particular time in the patient's course (the procedure was not an emergency and no proper analgesia could be offered). During a quiet week-end the patient had a remarkable night. She was a very caring and loving person, and had been informed on that particular day of the sudden death of a young friend. She had broken into tears, and had fallen asleep with an intense headache, for which she was not given any analgesia due to the still unclear diagnosis. The patient fell asleep while the TV was on in her room. In the morning she described her falling asleep as fainting. Here is a transcript of what she recalled:

> My fainting was such that my personality—not in its emotional part, but in what concerns my thoughts—had become a shining line, almost as a lightning. From my eyes this line was as high as the TV screen. It was not shaped as an arrow, nor was it dazzling as a lightning, nor was it blinking. On the contrary, instead of having acute angles, it resembled the domes of street signs for up and down hills. Two hours later I felt as if coming back to life. I felt crazy for anguish and I was terrified at the idea of having become a line. Therefore, I made major efforts to go back to who I am. Thus, I repeated to myself that I am the person—not the line—living in that particular home, with those particular paintings, and so on. Then I told myself that I was the person who previously had lived in a different place, and before in another city. Then I decided to start thinking of all my pets. I wanted to see my cat, and I succeeded in seeing it. I saw the cat when going outdoors, facing the lawn filled with intensely perfumed flowers and colorful butterflies. Then I decided to go back with my memory to my second home, which was as beautiful as a castle, with space for everybody. Then I looked at the cats living in that home, because I wanted to. Two were on the balcony. Then I felt desperate again, because I could not see my third cat. Finally, with major effort, I was able to see it. It

was 6.30 a.m. and I felt back to myself again, ready for the daily pain, but—more than anything—quite ready for a difficult meeting with the doctors. I still had dull headache.

Case B raises many issues: (a) the possible conflicts of the patient–doctor–family relationship; (b) the ethics of caring for a close relative; (c) the depersonalization of the patient in the hospital environment (and in disease itself); and (d) the conscious effort that needs to be made to 'remain oneself.'

Possible Conflicts in the Patient–Doctor–Family Relationship

While this case is influenced to some extent by the fact that the son was a physician, it is possible to separate the two issues, and to analyze them in detail. The principles involved are that of autonomy, beneficence, and justice. We should be extremely careful to respect the individual patient's perception of beneficence and autonomy, aiming at a harmonious relationship with patients and their families or significant others. There are instances, though, where conflicts do arise, as on occasion when the patient's autonomy and beneficence are not the same, or are perceived differently by the partners in the relationship. This becomes more and more true when we consider the family also as an essential third partner in the relationship. Most conflicts arise from lack of proper communication, and they can be solved by clarifying issues and by discussing roles and responsibilities.

However, we cannot deny the presence of objective obstacles to communication, such as major differences in cultural background, language problems and religious beliefs. Also, the physician is exposed to pressure from the outside, such as 'economic pressure' and 'scientific pressure.'

The case described above first shows a mismanagement on the part of the health care team, since no invasive procedure should be performed at substantial patient cost, unless it is a real emergency. However, we can examine the above case also as a clear example of the different objectives and view-points of the patient–family and the medical team. For the patient and the family, the priority was to obtain the maximum patient comfort first, along with the diagnosis and correct etiological treatment. For the doctor, the priority was efficiency (i.e. obtaining a diagnosis as quickly as possible, both for economic reasons—justification for the insurance company—and for prestige/image reasons—the center was well known for being extremely efficient). An invasive test had been scheduled for day X, and to postpone it for 3 days was seen as a loss of time, hence a loss of prestige.

The principle that needs to be considered in this and similar situations is that of *justice*. While justice primarily involves being fair toward the single patient and not discriminating among patients, this principle is also applied to a broader context. At an institutional level, social and distributive justice must be faced and, on occasion, the physician is also confronted with this aspect of justice in his daily practice. In the expensive field of oncology, the growing economic pressure is likely to increase greatly the need for the oncologist to be aware of possible conflicts, and to learn ethical ways to face them. Excellent ways of cost-control measures that are also ethical have been proposed, such as education, peer-review, and contained bureaucracy (Sulmasy, 1992). To these, especially in oncology, we should certainly add international cooperation: the duplication of experiments and data, for instance, is such that there is major economic waste due to the lack of open and timely international sharing of scientific knowledge.

It is essential to notice that ethics is never, and never should be, distinct from economy, science, medicine, or culture: only when ethics is an integral part of our thinking and decision-making process, can we see problems in their complexity and globally as well, and never get trapped into misleading *non-existent dichotomies*. The dichotomy between ethics and the rest of the world should simply not exist. Thus, the conflict which results from an outside imposition on the health care workers, needs to be resolved in favor of a better patient–doctor–family relationship. Whoever is not convinced by the ethical imperative of a good relationship as a priority, might consider how much time (i.e., cost) is involved in working in a confrontational milieu!

The Ethics of Caring for a Close Relative

The presence of a physician in the family modifies the *dynamics* of the patient–doctor–family relationship. A physician–relative, even when not directly involved in the care, represents a destabilizing element. The fundamental principles involved are again autonomy and beneficence.

In the above case, there was an active involvement, mostly due to a justified need *to protect* the patient–mother from aggressive maneuvers which were medically not necessary, and the physician–son acted with the informed consent of the patient–mother. In other cases, the physician–relative is the one who assumes the entire burden of communication, as it is delegated to him/her by the patient: again, the main objective is to protect the patient. Also in these cases there is generally the patient's consent, although often not verbalized.

The protective role of the family with respect to disease, as well as to all traumatic events of life, is a well-known fact of family dynamics. It is an essential and valid function of family also in those cultures where the emphasis is placed on individual autonomy and on personal rights. While close family ties are more prominent in some cultures, nurturing, mutual help, and protection are what family is about the world around (Surbone and Zwitter, 1997).

When a relative is a physician, this protection extends beyond normal limits and the result is always an imbalanced relationship with the doctor. In fact, responsibilities are not as clearly defined as they should be, and all partners find it hard to identify the proper interlocutor. At times, it is necessary for the doctor to confront the physician–relative and clarify the intrinsic dangers of a dual role. The illness of a relative is a painful event, and the additional stressor of 'direct medical responsibilities' is unlikely to make it easier for the physician–relative. However, after a kind and truthful confrontation, the doctor should be prepared to accept this new figure in the play. Some physician–relatives might in fact very well understand the difficulty of their role, but still wish to undertake certain medical responsibilities. However, the doctor needs to make it very clear from the beginning that he is there, fully in charge of the case, open to the input of the physician–relative, but also available to alleviate the relative's responsibilities whenever requested by the family or the patient, by assuming them entirely upon himself. The role of the doctor includes fostering *the patient's autonomy*, and the doctor should be extremely sensitive to those instances where 'protection' is a signal of unresolved conflicts within the family, and a substitute for true confrontation of the real issues. While it is not the physician's responsibility to judge or to decide the best way to deal with family problems, he/she must assure high quality of care involving counseling for the entire family, in order to be *beneficent*. Disease is not necessarily to be looked upon as a state from which the patient has to go back to normal, but rather as an event of life which might well be the beginning of something new. It is then worthwhile to foster interfamily confrontation of unresolved issues, providing the appropriate support and counseling.

When the patient is a cancer patient, there are responsibilities that a doctor should simply not allow a relative to take—these include the administration of chemotherapy and of narcotics for pain control. The doctor will easily convince a physician–relative not to assume these responsibilities, provided he/she fully meets the appropriate standards of care for the patient. A doctor who delegates responsibility for narcotic administration to a physician–relative is unfair and unethical, and this should never happen. We have a *responsibility* toward the hopelessly ill patient (Wanzer et al., 1989), and we cannot escape from it.

Which brings us to the issue of 'responsibility'. Responsibilities in the patient–doctor–family relationship are different, well-defined, and mutual. Upon the doctor always rests the responsibility for the medical intervention, and this is by no means alleviated by the presence of an 'informed consent' (World Medical Association, 1964). Informed consent, when true and no matter how technically expressed (verbal vs. written depends on many cultural variables), assures that the best effort has been made by the doctor to act as both an expert and an educator; but it should never imply that the burden of medical choices is put upon the patient. The patient, no matter how educated and understanding, is in a 'uniquely dependent state' due to disease itself (Pellegrino, 1987). He/she should not be urged to make a medical decision, but rather be counseled and kindly given as much explanation as possible about the disease and its course. After doing so, the doctor will face a vast array of patient responses: from denial to non-compliance to desire to 'be in control'. In none of these instances is the doctor's professional responsibility diminished. Accepted or refused, and in the best of cases shared, the medical responsibility rests with the expert.

Once again, *communication* appears to be the password for most ethical dilemmas in the patient–doctor–family relationship (Surbone and Zwitter, 1997). It is, in fact, by means of communication that *mutual trust* can be achieved. And it is only within the frame of trust that the mutual responsibilities of the patient, the doctor, and the family can be clearly defined (Pellegrino and Thomasma, 1988).

Depersonalization

The case presented is paradigmatic of how depersonalization can be experienced by the hospitalized patient, and to a larger extent in disease itself. Such depersonalization is likely to affect the family dynamics too, and should be examined also from that perspective.

It is said that, when sick, animals tend to isolate themselves; we as human beings do not. However, a component of *isolation* is always present in disease and serves to protect all partners of the patient–doctor–family relationship from overexposure to pain and suffering. Ethics should be questioned, with respect to the principle of autonomy, when isolation leads to lack of control by the patient on his health and life.

At times, and depending on cultural variables too, a ritual starts between the patient and the family, leading to everyone pretending that disease is not so severe (or does not exist at all) and that normal life can still go on. Occasionally, the doctor can become the only person from whom the patient does not hide his/her true feelings and fears. However, the time constraints of the patient–doctor encounter are such that the doctor, even when able to share the patient's concerns (what we call empathy or inclusion; Buber, 1967; Bellet and Malony, 1991; Spiro, 1992), can only temporarily alleviate the patient's tension.

Disease is not a response in itself, and is seldom a solution for previous problems. Disease itself is a major problem, which adds to the existing ones in a family. No easy answers are ever provided by disease. On the contrary, many questions arise which are likely to remain unsolved and to create additional stress. Within this frame, it is easier to understand the actual and metaphorical role of hospitalization in the course of a chronic disease such as cancer. When the patient is hospitalized, the isolation of disease from the context of normal life is accomplished. Hospital life and rhythms and rituals take over daily habits, and drastically change them. Hospital hours subvert the normal routine; the patient lies in bed wearing a hospital gown or pyjamas, surrounded by physicians and nurses properly dressed and further protected by their white coats; therapeutic and diagnostic procedures are the dominant events in the day. The patient feels more and more isolated, as the hospital raises its barriers against the patient. He/she can grow in his/her anxiety as isolation fosters the development of *metaphorical interpretation* of events which are so unusual. How many of my patients describe with tremendous fear the 'infusion pump' as a machine which 'forces chemicals inside the bloodstream'—a true invasion from the outside!

The health care team, on the other hand, and the family too, need to protect themselves against a tremendous emotional overflow. They achieve this by way of limiting and ritualizing the exposure to the patient and his/her disease. Thus, the same isolation which is likely to be perceived by the patient as a depersonalization can be positive for the health care team and for the family. This issue is of great importance when considering the role of *supportive care in cancer* in a broad sense. Some figures, by becoming more active in the hospital setting, can represent a liaison with the outside world—a way to restore the patient's *autonomy* while allowing doctors, nurses and family to detach themselves from the patient. Such figures can be psychologists, spiritual advisors, social workers, volunteers; they all have the capacity to positively affect the course of the disease (Surbone, 1993) and especially the patient's stay in hospital. For the patient too, in fact, the isolation created by the hospital need not be necessarily synonymous with depersonalization, and could instead turn into a positive moment of pause and reflection, far from the daily routine. At times, this can result in major positive steps forward in understanding the disease and its implications, and in facing disease, life, and death.

The Conscious Effort to Remain Oneself

Isolation can, however, progress towards a feeling of depersonalization, and lead to the need for a conscious effort to remain oneself. The principle involved is again that of autonomy.

The case described illustrates this aspect most powerfully. The Roman Emperor Hadrianus once said, 'It is difficult to remain the Emperor in front of a physician' (Yourcenar, 1974). In our case, the patient was afraid of her personality having become a line, and she described in detail that her fear concerned her thoughts rather than her emotions. While the patient was unaware of the words of St Augustine in his *Confessions*, her description is reminiscent of them. In the *Confessions*, St Augustine dedicates several chapters to memory and how he thought he could access it. One passage reads as follows:

> *I* will go through the webs of my memory, where I find the treasures of the endless images which have been stored through all perceptions. Whenever I enter that realm, I ask it to produce whatever it is that I wish to remember. Some impressions it produces immediately; some need to be searched for longer...others come spilling from the memory, thrusting themselves upon us when what we want is something quite different.... With a voluntary act I push them away from the vision of memory, up until what I wish to see stands out dearly and emerges from the background.... All this is inside of me, in the vast cloisters of my memory. In it are the sky, the earth, the sea, and all perceptions, ready at my summons.... In it I meet myself as well' (St Augustine, 398 AD). It is worth remembering that the *Confessions*, in their acute existential and phenomenological analysis based on ferocious self-honesty, have always been valued for their profound psychological insight (Mohrmann, 1958).

It is essential for any human being to *maintain control* over his/her life, thoughts, and self. One of the major faults of modern medicine is, indeed, the growing tendency to take away control from the subject. If we want to foster our patients' autonomy, we as health care workers must understand this need to remain oneself, and try to help our patients in achieving such a goal. This is certainly part of our ethical obligations.

CASE C

A 34 year-old Mediterranean man, PhD in mathematics, presented with re-lapsed non-Hodgkin's lymphoma, for which high-dose chemotherapy with bone marrow transplantation was indicated. The patient was informed of his disease and of his prognosis. Bone marrow transplantation was the indicated therapy. However, when he and his family were presented with this therapeutic option, an irrational drastic reaction manifested from the family members. His mother acted violently against the physician, who had very properly conveyed detailed information about the therapy. His fiancée felt that bone marrow transplantation would diminish him ('my future husband should not have it!'). As a result, the patient did not undergo the recommended procedure, and became depressed. The family accused the doctor of having been the cause of the patient's suicidal ideation (something that was never apparent to the doctor himself. A psychiatric consultation was offered and refused by the family). The doctor withdrew from the care, but subsequently took charge, when the patient—almost in a terminal condition—asked him to 'be his doctor again.'

CASE D

A 47 year-old woman, an unmarried physician in the USA, refused adjuvant chemotherapy because of her dread of sterility. The patient's doctor, herself without children, while accurately providing information on the risks and benefits of chemotherapy, was unable to openly confront the patient about her unrealistic expectations from life. The patient did not undergo adjuvant chemotherapy and relapsed 2 years later. She had always seen the doctor alone, never bringing any family member.

In cases C and D, the issue of information is raised. Both cases emphasize (a) cultural influences on the expression of the principles of medical ethics; they also illustrate the difficulty encountered in (b) defining the respective roles of ethics, deontology, and law.

Cultural Influences on the Expression of the Principles of Medical Ethics

In societies where *autonomy* is synonymous with freedom, such as in most of the USA, truth-telling is possible and beneficial to the patient and gives rise to a very direct patient–doctor relationship. In societies where autonomy is synonymous with *isolation*, such as in most Mediterranean countries, direct truth-telling in an 'American way' is neither always possible nor always beneficial (Surbone, 1992; Pellegrino, 1992). In our multi-ethnic societies we should learn how to recognize different patterns of communication and how to modulate our language (global language, including the non-verbal one) according to the patients' cultural background (Stiefel and Senn, 1992).

Cross-cultural analysis is very important, as it allows us to face the dilemma apparently created by *pluralism*. The existence of pluralism challenges the idea that ethical principles are absolute. Cultural relativism and the consequent ethical relativism have often been seen as intrinsically pessimistic, insofar as they appear to negate universal values. In contrast, pluralism can enrich ethics by adding an historical perspective, through a more concrete vision of values, which have a contextual dimension (Bellino, 1993). Some ethical principles appear universal (Thompson, 1987)—for example, the basis for the Universal Declaration of Human Rights (General Assembly of the United Nations, 1948). The effect of culture is a modulation of the expression of these principles. The universality of ethical principles can, however, only be appreciated when these principles are perceived as being equally valid and intercorrelated—rather than antagonistic—principles. Autonomy cannot be true without beneficence, and beneficence is never such without autonomy.

Defining the Respective Roles of Ethics, Deontology and Law

Ethics finds itself at the crossroads of many different disciplines, and its relationship with law and deontology are not always clearly defined. While apparently an unnecessary subtlety, the clarification of this issue is relevant to the patient–doctor–family relationship, since some discordances arise simply due to the physician's lack of familiarity with the different sphere of influence of law (related to liability issues), deontology (the ethical obligations of a certain professional category), and ethics (confronting moral issues and involving the individual conscience first) (Documento di Erice, 1991; Canale, 1992). Truth-telling is a powerful example, since the physician, in deciding what to convey to the patient, should take into consideration many different elements, from the cultural background to the psychological state of the individual patient and the medico-legal milieu.

In case C, by sharing accurate information with the patient, the doctor bypassed the strong cultural belief favoring 'protection of the patient from painful truths', rather than truth-telling. The reaction of the family, while inappropriately predominating over the patient's autonomy, found the support of the deontology in that particular country (Surbone, 1992). In case D, the US physician's response to her patient, while inappropriate from an ethical point of view, was clearly supported by the strong request for patient autonomy in the US culture and deontology. The doctor had not recognized that her judgment had been somehow distorted by her own background, and she had confused 'respect for the patient's autonomy' with a more complex situation where counseling for the patient would have been indeed appropriate and truly ethical.

It should be stressed that bioethics is not only the systematic study of medical behavior in light of moral principles (Reich, 1978), but also a means of influencing the prevailing cultures. Although bioethics focuses on medical issues, the discussion and deliberation involved can contribute to a better understanding of moral issues, which goes far beyond medicine. Thus, the debate on truth-telling in medicine can foster a broader discussion on individual autonomy in all cultures.

CASE E

An unmarried North American couple lived very closely and intensely the experience of breast cancer. While she underwent difficult surgery and chemotherapy, he succeeded in protecting her from the disclosure of complete truth, repeatedly telling the doctor that she could not bear the truth. The doctor referred the couple for psychological evaluation and counseling. When learning of the particular dynamics of unresolved guilt in the couple, he agreed not to provide details in his explanations to the patient. The patient, who had felt guilt toward a family member in need whom she had abandoned to become involved in her present relationship, eventually recovered from her cancer. In the following years, the patient remained cancer-free and her long suffering enabled her to overcome her guilt and resume a healthy relationship with the person she had abandoned. The partner, who had assumed upon himself the heavy burden of being the only one totally informed and aware of all risks, became seriously depressed and was repeatedly diagnosed as experiencing anticipatory grief. Even many years later, the partner continued to be severely psychologically distressed. They remained close and never ceased to live together.

In case D, cancer is the metaphor for an unresolved issue, and suffering has a symbolic value.

Cancer as a Metaphor

The oncologist should learn about metaphors and symbols too (Sontag, 1978, 1989), in order to achieve beneficence and to respect autonomy. At times, disease represents the solution, or the apparent solution, to pre-existing issues or problems. In this case, the patient saw in her being sick a 'redemption' from her perceived guilt. Also she attributed an additional symbolic value to her suffering, which helped her to get over a long-lasting guilt. The partner had also attributed to her disease and suffering a redeeming value which he did not experience. On the contrary, he insisted on experiencing an anticipatory grief, in which he possibly saw a similar redeeming value.

It is most important for the health care team to make efforts at understanding the *value* that the patient and the family attribute to *disease and suffering*, for this can dramatically change the attitude required of the physician. We have learned from Freud that human suffering is nourished by a fountain which never drains. Therefore, suffering cannot be assumed as the ultimate criterion to apply when judging life, its quality or its value. Suffering is so deeply rooted in our being human that we should always consider it also within the personal perspective of the patient. In oncology, for instance, acknowledging the positive value which some religions attribute to suffering and understanding the patient's own metaphor can lead to more appropriate and more efficacious pain control (Kryspin and Heather, 1987).

Finally, the way disease itself is perceived vastly influences the therapeutic interventions. For some patients, disease is a *traumatic event*, from which one has to be cured in order to go *back to* normal life. This can, indeed, be a very useful way to look upon disease, and needs to be encouraged. Such patients, even when affected by cancer, should maintain a high level of planning for the future, if only the near future. For them, identifying and meeting short-term goals is a determinant for a positive attitude. Other patients, however, see in disease not only a traumatic and undesirable event, but also as a potential for change—a milestone in their development and an 'occasion' to reset priorities. For these patients, going back to previous situations in life is not at all desirable; and their aim is at finding a better level rather than returning to normal. The physician has to be always aware of different attitudes, and should avoid generalizations which undermine the true meaning of both autonomy and beneficence. Beneficence, *the patient's good*, always includes an active effort to modulate all interventions on the basis of the individual patient and of his/her personal and family values (Thomasma, 1992).

CONCLUDING REMARKS

The five cases illustrate the importance of the patient's cultural, social, and historical context and of the family in our efforts to solve the many ethical dilemmas of modern medicine. Ethical issues and conflicts appear magnified in oncology, where life-and-death decisions are common, and the patient's suffering is often prolonged and intense. Moreover, the recent developments of cancer genetics add a new and broader dimension to ethical deliberation in oncology. A key word to access the realm of ethics is 'communication', and the health care worker should regard communication as a priority in his/her relationship with patients and their families.

Many of the quandaries of bioethics, however, go beyond the interpersonal dimension of communication and are rather related to social, economical, and political considerations. While in the present chapter on cancer and the family I have focused more on the interpersonal aspects of the ethical dilemmas of medicine, it would be extremely misleading to stop at these only. The role of justice and fairness in our ethical debate is paramount and a comprehensive approach to bioethics should always take the social dimension into proper consideration. If family is isolated from society at large, we operate in a reductive perspective. On the contrary, we are members of a family, but also of a society, and finally of mankind.

ACKNOWLEDGEMENTS

I am deeply indebted to Mrs Kristine Salerno for her valuable assistance in preparing this manuscript. I am also very thankful to Dr Vicki Currie for our constructive ongoing discussions of the patient–doctor–family relationship and for her support throughout my writing of this chapter. Lastly, I would like to thank Dr Edmund E. Pellegrino for his critical comments of Case A.

REFERENCES

Aristotle (384–322 BC). *Etica Nichomachea*. Milan: Laterza (1973).
Baider L., Cooper C.L., and De-Nour A.K. (Eds). (1996). *Cancer and the Family*, 1st Edn. Chichester: Wiley.
Baier, A.C. (1994). *Moral Prejudices: Essays on Ethics*. Cambridge: Harvard University Press.
Beauchamp, T.L. and Childress, J.F. (1994). *Principles of Biomedical Ethics*, 4th Edn. New York: Oxford University Press.
Bellet, P.S. and Maloney, M.J. (1991). The importance of empathy as an interviewing skill in medicine. *Journal of the American Medical Association* **266**: 1831–1832.
Bellino, F. (1993). *I Fondamenti Della Bioetica*. Rome: Citta' Nuova.
Brewin, T.B. (1993). How much ethics is needed to make a good doctor? *Lancet* **341**: 161–163.
Buber, M. (1967). *Between Man and Man*. New York: Macmillan.
Canale, M. (1992). Scienza e Coscienza: due consiglieri insidiosi. *Federazione Medica* **7**: 391–393.
Cassel, E.J. (1977). The function of medicine. *Hastings Center Report* **7**: 16–19.
Cattorini, P. (1993). *Sotto Scacco: Bioetica di Fine Vita*. Naples: Liviana Medicina.
Documento di Erice sui rapporti della Bioetica e della deontologia medica con la medicina legale (1991). Erice: Convegno di Bioetica.
Engelhardt, T.H. Jr (1986). *The Foundations of Bioethics*. New York: Oxford University Press.
General Assembly of the United Nations (1948). *Universal Declaration of Human Rights*. Geneva: United Nations.
Gostin, L.O. (1995). Genetic Privacy. *Journal of Medicine and Ethics* **23**: 320–330.
Guillen, D.G. (1991). Clinical bioethics. In S. Spinsanti (Ed.), *Bioetica e Antropologia Medica* (p. 429). Rome: La Nuova Italia Scienfifica.
Habermas, J. (1990). Discourse ethics: notes on a program of philosophical justification. In *Moral Consciousness and Communicative Action*. Cambridge: Polity.
Hippocrates (420 BC). Oath of Hippocrates. In W.H.S. Jones, *Hippocrates* (p. 289). Cambridge: Cambridge University Press (1972).
Hume, D. (1751). In J.B. Scherwind (Ed.), *An Enquiry Concerning the Principles of Morals*. Indianapolis, IN: Hackett (1983).

Kant, I. (1785). *Groundwork of the Metaphysics of Morals* (translated by H.J. Pekou). New York: Harper and Row.

Kryspin, J. and Heather, P. (1987). Beyond beneficence, an ethical perspective in terminal care. *Humane Medicine* **1**: 82–91.

Lenoir, N. (1997). UNESCO, genetics and human rights. *Kennedy Institute of Ethics Journal* **7**: 31–42.

McConnell, T.C. (1972). Moral dilemmas and consistency in ethics. *Canadian Journal of Philosophy* **8**: 269–287.

Merleau-Ponty, M. (1962). *Phenomenologie de la Perception*. London: Routledge and Kegan Paul.

Miki, Y., Swenson, J., Shattuck-Eidens, D., Futreal, P.A., Harshman, K. and Tavtigian, S. (1994). A strong candidate for the breast and ovarian cancer susceptibility gene BRCA1. *Science* **266**: 66–71.

Mill, J.S. (1806). *Utilitarianism, On Liberty, Essay on Bentham: Together with Selected Writings by Jeremy Bentham and John Austin*. Meridian: New American Library (1974).

Mohrmann, C. (1958). *Introduction to the Confessions*. Milan: Rizzoli.

Pellegrino, E.D. (1985). *Moral choice, the good of the patient and the patient's good*. In J. Moskop and L. Kopelman (Eds), *Ethics and Critical Care Medicine* (pp. 117–136). Dordrecht: Reidel.

Pellegrino, E.D. (1987). Altruism, self-interest, and medical ethics. *Journal of the American Medical Association* **258**: 1939–1940.

Pellegrino, E.D. (1992). Is truth-telling to patients a cultural artifact? *Journal of the American Medical Association* **268**: 1734–1735.

Pellegrino, E.D. and Thomasma, D.C. (1981). *A Philosophical Basis of Medical Practice*. New York: Oxford University Press.

Pellegrino, E.D. and Thomasma, D.C. (1988). *For the Patient's Good: The Restoration of Beneficence in Health Care*. New York: Oxford University Press.

Potter, V.R. (1971). *Bioethics: Bridge to the Future*. Englewood Cliffs, NJ: Prentice Hall.

Reich, W.T. (1978). *Encyclopedia of Bioethics*. New York: Macmillan–Free Press.

Reilly, P.R. (1995). Panel comment: The impact of the genetic privacy act on medicine. *Journal of Law, Medicine and Ethics* **23**: 378–81.

Rescher N. (1987). *Ethical Idealism. An Inquiry into the Nature and Function of Ideals*. Berkeley, CA: University California Press.

Rilke, R.M. (1929). *Briefe an einen jungen Dichter* (translated by L. Traverso). Milano: Adelphi.

Rollin, B. (1978). On the nature of illness. *Man and Medicine* **4**: 157–172.

Saint Augustine (398 AD). *Confessions: Book X*. Milan: Rizzoli.

Sgreccia, E. (1991). *Manuale di Bioetica*. Roma: Vita e Pensiero.

Singer, P. (1979). *Practical Ethics*. Cambridge: Cambridge University Press.

Sontag, S. (1978). *Illness as Metaphor*. New York: Farrar, Straus and Giroux.

Sontag, S. (1989). *AIDS and its Metaphors*. New York: Farrar, Straus, and Giroux.

Spiro, H. (1992). What is empathy and can it be taught? *Annals of Internal Medicine* **116**: 843–846.

Stiefel, F. and Senn, J.H. (1992). Cancer diagnosis disclosure in a Spanish hospital: how do they discuss treatment options? *Annals of Oncology* **3**: 422.

Struewing, J.P., Hartage, P., Wacholder, S. et al. (1997). The risk of cancer associated with specific mutations of BRCA1 and BRCA2 among Ashkenazi Jews. *New England Journal of Medicine* **336**: 1401–1408.

Sulmasy, D.P. (1992). Physicians, cost control and ethics. *Annals of Internal Medicine* **116**: 920–926.

Surbone, A. (1993). The information to the cancer patient: psychosocial and spiritual implications. *Supportive Care in Cancer* **1**: 89–91.

Surbone, A. (1992). Truth telling to the patient. *Journal of the American Medical Association* **268**: 1661–1662.

Surbone A. (1997). Information, truth and communication: for an interpretation of truth-telling practices throughout the world. In A. Surbone and M. Zwitter. *Communication with the Cancer Patient. Information and Truth.* New York: Annals of the New York Academy of Sciences, Vol. 809.

Surbone, A. (in press). The ethical challenge of genetic testing for breast cancer. *Medicina e Morale.*

Thomas, J.P. (1990). *Misere de la Bioethique.* Paris: Albin Michel.

Thomasma, D.C. (1992). The ethics of caring for the older patient with cancer: defining the issues. *Oncology* **6**(Suppl.): 124–130.

Thompson, I.E. (1987). Fundamental ethical principles in health care. *British Medical Journal* **295**: 1461–1465.

Yourcenar, M. (1974). *Memories d'Hadrien suivi de Carnets de Notes de Memoires d'Hadrien.* Paris: Gallimard.

Walker M.V.(1998) *Moral Understandings. A Feminist Study in Ethics.* New York: Routledge.

Wanzer, S.H., Federman, D.D., Adelstein, S.J. et al. (1989). The physician's responsibility toward hopelessly ill patients. A second look. *New England Journal of Medicine* **320**: 844–849.

World Medical Association (1964). *Declaration of Helsinki. Recommendations Guiding Physicians in Biomedical Research Involving Human Subjects.* Adopted by the 18th World Assembly, Helsinki, Finland, June 1964; amended by the 29th World Medical Assembly, Tokyo, Japan, October 1975, and the 35th World Medical Assembly, Venice, Italy, October 1983.

Index

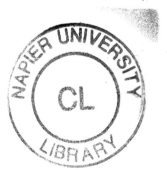